MOSBY'S

GUIDE TO

NURSING DIAGNOSIS

MOSBY'S GUIDE TO NURSING DIAGNOSIS

Second Edition

Gail B. Ladwig, MSN, RN, CHTP
Betty J. Ackley, MSN, EdS, RN

MOSBY

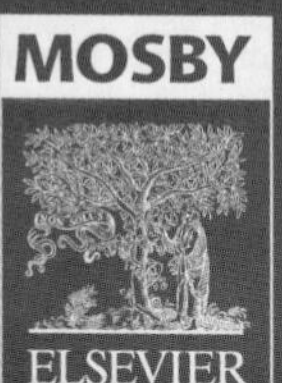

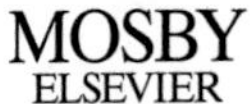

11830 Westline Industrial Drive
St. Louis, Missouri 63146

MOSBY'S GUIDE TO NURSING DIAGNOSIS, SECOND EDITION
ISBN: 978-0-323-05192-7

Notice

Knowledge and best practice in this field are constantly changing. As new research and experience broaden our knowledge, changes in practice, treatment and drug therapy may become necessary or appropriate. Readers are advised to check the most current information provided (i) on procedures featured or (ii) by the manufacturer of each product to be administered, to verify the recommended dose or formula, the method and duration of administration, and contraindications. It is the responsibility of the practitioner, relying on their own experience and knowledge of the patient, to make diagnoses, to determine dosages and the best treatment for each individual patient, and to take all appropriate safety precautions. To the fullest extent of the law, neither the Publisher nor the Authors assume any liability for any injury and/or damage to persons or property arising out or related to any use of the material contained in this book.

The Publisher

Previous edition copyrighted 2006

Library of Congress Control Number 2007929361

Senior Acquisitions Editor: Sandra Clark Brown
Senior Developmental Editor: Cindi Anderson
Publishing Services Manager: Deborah L. Vogel
Senior Project Manager: Steve Ramay
Design Direction: Julia Dummitt

Printed in the United States of America

Last digit is the print number:
9 8 7 6 5 4 3 2

To:

Dale Ackley, the greatest guy in the world, without whose support this book would have never happened, and my daughter, Dr. Dawn and her husband Cameron Goulding. And the absolute joy of my life, granddaughter Althea Rose Goulding.

Jerry Ladwig, my wonderful husband, who after 43 years is still supportive and helpful—he is "my right hand man" in revising this book every two years. Also to my very special children, their spouses and all of my grandchildren; Jerry, Kathy, Alexandra, Elizabeth, and Benjamin Ladwig; Christine, John, Sean, Ciara and Bridget McMahon; Jennifer, Jim, Abby, Katelyn, Blake and Connor Martin; Amy, Scott, Ford and Vaughn Bertram—the greatest family anyone could ever hope for.

A special thank you to Cindi Anderson, Senior Developmental Editor for Elsevier. She has worked tirelessly on this project for many editions. She is not only a colleague but has become a treasured and very special friend.

Acknowledgments

The authors would like to thank the following individuals for their contributions to *Nursing Diagnosis Handbook: An Evidence-Based Guide to Planning Care,* Eighth Edition, by Betty Ackley and Gail Ladwig, from which this book has been developed:

Nadine M. Aktan, MS, RN, APN-C
Donna L. Algase, PhD, RN, FAAN, FGSA
Keith A. Anderson, PhD
Sharon Baranoski, MSN, RN, CWOCN, APN, FAAN
Nancy Albright Beyer, RN, MSN, CEN
Kathaleen C. Bloom, PhD, CNM
Lisa Burkhart, PhD, RN
Stacey M. Carroll, PhD, APRN, BC
Susan Mee Coleman, RN PhDc, CPNP
June M. Como, RN, MSA, MS, CCRN, CCNS
Elizabeth Crago, RN, MSN, CEN, CCRN
Maryanne Crowther, MSN, RN, APNC, CCRN
Ruth Davidhizar, RN, CNS, ARNP, BC, FAAN
Rebecca L. Davis, RN, PhD
Mary DeWys, RN, BS
Brenda Emick-Herring, RN, MSN, CRRN
Dawn Fairlie, MS, ANP, FNP, GNP
Arlene T. Farren, RN, PhD, AOCN
Terri A. Foster, RN, BSN, CNOR
Judith A. Floyd, PhD, RN, FAAN
Joseph E. Gaugler, PhD
Judith R. Gentz, APRN-BC
Marie Giordano, RN, MS
Joyce Newman Giger, PhD
Barbara Given, RN, PhD, FAAN
Mikel Gray, PhD, FNP, PNP, CUNP, CCCN, FAANP, FAAN
Pauline M. Green, PhD, RN
Sherry A. Greenberg, MSN, APRN, BC, GNP
Elizabeth A. Henneman, RN, PhD, CCNS
T. Heather Herdman, RN, PhD
Paula D. Hopper, MSN, RN
Teresa Howell, MSN, RN

Jean D. Humphries, MSN, RN
Mike Jacobs, RN, DNS
Rebecca A. Johnson, PhD, RN
Beverly Kopala, PhD, RN
Barbara Kraynyak Luise, RN, EdD
Margaret Lunney, RN, PhD
Margo McCaffery, MS, RN-BC, FAAN
Ruth McCaffrey, DNP, ARNP-BC
Graham J McDougall Jr., PhD, APRN, BC, FAAN
Laura H. Mcilvoy, PhD, RN, CCRN, CNRN
Dale A. Nasby, MA, MS, RN, CNS
DeLancey Nicoll, SN
Leslie H. Nicoll, PhD, MBA, RN, BC
Katherina A. Nikzad, MSW
Lisa Oldham, PhD, MSN, RN, BC, CAN, FABC, GCM
Barbara J. Olinzock, MSN, EdD, RN
Peg Padnos, AB, BSN, RN
Chris Pasero, MS, RN-BC, FAAN
Kathleen L. Patusky, PhD, APRN-BC
Lori M. Rhudy, RN, PhDc
Susan Rosenberg, RN, MSN, CNRN, CHI
Julie T. Sanford, DNS, RN
Marilee Schmelzer, PhD, RN
Paula R. Sherwood, RN, PhD, CNRN
Mary T. Shoemaker, RN, MSN, SANE
Sheryl K. Sommer, PhD, RN
Mary Stahl, RN, CEN, MSN-NEdu
Elaine E. Steinke, PhD, RN
Michele Walters, MSN, ARNP
Linda S. Williams, MSN, RNBC
Diane Wind Wardell, PhD, RNC

How to Use Mosby's Guide to Nursing Diagnosis

ASSESS

Assess the client using the format provided by the clinical setting. Collect data including client's symptoms, clinical state, and known medical or psychiatric diagnoses.

DIAGNOSIS

Using Section I, Guide to Nursing Diagnoses, locate the client's symptoms, clinical state, medical or psychiatric diagnoses, and anticipated or prescribed diagnostic studies or surgical interventions (listed in alphabetical order). Note suggestions for appropriate nursing diagnoses.

Use Section II, Guide to Planning Care, to evaluate each suggested nursing diagnosis and "related to" etiology statement. Section II is a listing of care plans according to NANDA-I, arranged alphabetically by diagnostic concept, for each nursing diagnosis referred to in Section I. Determine the appropriateness of each nursing diagnosis by comparing the Defining Characteristics and Risk Factors to the client data collected.

DETERMINE OUTCOMES

Use Section II, Guide to Planning Care, to find appropriate Client Outcomes for the client.

PLAN INTERVENTIONS

Use Section II, Guide to Planning Care, to find appropriate Nursing Interventions for the client.

GIVE NURSING CARE

Administer nursing care following the plan of care based on the interventions.

EVALUATE NURSING CARE

Evaluate nursing care administered using the Client Outcomes. If the outcomes were not met, and the nursing interventions were not effective, it may be appropriate to reassess the client and determine if the appropriate nursing diagnoses were made.

DOCUMENT

Document all of the previous steps using the format provided in the clinical setting.

Contents

Section I **Guide to Nursing Diagnosis, 1**

An alphabetized list of medical-surgical and psychosocial diagnoses, diagnostic procedures, clinical states, symptoms, and problems, with suggested nursing diagnoses

Section II **Guide to Planning Care, 167**

The definition, defining characteristics, risk factors, related factors, client outcomes, interventions, pediatric and geriatric interventions (when appropriate), home care interventions, culturally competent nursing interventions (when appropriate), and client/family teaching for each alphabetized nursing diagnosis

MOSBY'S

GUIDE TO

NURSING DIAGNOSIS

SECTION

I

Guide to Nursing Diagnoses

Section I is an alphabetical listing of client symptoms, client problems, medical diagnoses, psychiatric diagnoses, and clinical states. Use this section to find suggestions for nursing diagnoses for your client.

First assess the client using the format provided by the clinical setting. Then use this section to locate the client's symptoms, problems, clinical state, diagnoses, surgeries, and diagnostic testing. Note suggestions given for appropriate nursing diagnoses.

Using information found in Section II, evaluate each suggested nursing diagnosis to determine if it is appropriate for the client.

A

Abdominal Distention

Acute **Pain** r/t retention of air, gastrointestinal secretions

Constipation r/t decreased activity, decreased fluid intake, decreased fiber intake, pathological process

Delayed **Surgical** recovery r/t retention of gas, secretions

Imbalanced **Nutrition**: less than body requirements r/t nausea, vomiting

Nausea r/t irritation of gastrointestinal tract

Abdominal Hysterectomy

See Hysterectomy

Abdominal Pain

Acute **Pain** r/t injury, pathological process

Imbalanced **Nutrition**: less than body requirements r/t unresolved pain

See cause of Abdominal Pain

Abdominal Surgery

Acute **Pain** r/t surgical procedure

Constipation r/t decreased activity, decreased fluid intake, anesthesia, narcotics

Imbalanced **Nutrition**: less than body requirements r/t high metabolic needs, decreased ability to ingest or digest food

Ineffective **Health** maintenance r/t knowledge deficit regarding self-care after surgery

Ineffective **Tissue** perfusion: peripheral r/t immobility, abdominal surgery

Risk for **Infection**: Risk factor: invasive procedure

See Surgery, Perioperative Care; Surgery, Postoperative Care; Surgery, Preoperative Care

Abdominal Trauma

Acute **Pain** r/t abdominal trauma

Deficient **Fluid** volume r/t hemorrhage

Disturbed **Body** image r/t scarring, change in body function, need for temporary colostomy

Ineffective **Breathing** pattern r/t abdominal distention, pain

Risk for **Infection**: Risk factor: possible perforation of abdominal structures

Abortion, Induced

Acute **Pain** r/t surgical intervention

Chronic low **Self-esteem** disturbance r/t feelings of guilt

Chronic **Sorrow** r/t loss of potential child

Compromised family **Coping** r/t unresolved feelings about decision

Ineffective **Health** maintenance r/t deficient knowledge regarding self-care after abortion

Risk for delayed **Development**: Risk factors: unplanned or unwanted pregnancy

Risk for imbalanced **Fluid** volume: Risk factor: possible hemorrhage

Risk for **Infection**: Risk factors: open uterine blood vessels, dilated cervix

Risk for **Post-trauma** syndrome: Risk factor: psychological trauma of abortion

Risk for **Spiritual** distress: Risk factor: perceived moral implications of decision

Abortion, Spontaneous

Acute **Pain** r/t uterine contractions, surgical intervention

Chronic **Sorrow** r/t loss of potential child

Disabled family **Coping** r/t unresolved feelings about loss

Disturbed **Body** image r/t perceived inability to carry pregnancy, produce child

Fear r/t implications for future pregnancies

Grieving r/t loss of fetus

Ineffective **Coping** r/t personal vulnerability

Ineffective **Health** maintenance r/t deficient knowledge regarding self-care after abortion

Interrupted **Family** processes r/t unmet expectations for pregnancy and childbirth

Risk for deficient **Fluid** volume: Risk factors: hemorrhage

Risk for **Infection**: Risk factors: septic or incomplete abortion of products of conception, open uterine blood vessels, dilated cervix

Risk for **Post-trauma** syndrome: Risk factor: psychological trauma of abortion

Risk for **Spiritual** distress: Risk factor: loss of fetus

Self-esteem disturbance r/t feelings of fetus

Abruptio Placentae <36 Weeks

Acute **Pain** r/t irritable uterus, hypertonic uterus

Anxiety r/t unknown outcome, change in birth plans

Death **Anxiety** r/t unknown outcome, hemorrhage, or pain

Fear r/t threat to well-being of self and fetus

Impaired **Gas** exchange: placental r/t decreased uteroplacental area

Impaired **Tissue** integrity: maternal r/t possible uterine rupture

Interrupted **Family** process r/t unmet expectations for pregnancy and childbirth

Ineffective **Health** maintenance r/t deficient knowledge regarding self-care with disorder

Risk for deficient **Fluid** volume: Risk factor: hemorrhage

Risk for disproportionate **Growth**: Risk factor: uteroplacental insufficiency

Risk for ineffective **Tissue** perfusion: fetal: Risk factor: uteroplacental insufficiency

Risk for **Infection**: Risk factor: partial separation of placenta

Abscess Formation

Impaired **Tissue** integrity r/t altered circulation, nutritional deficit or excess

Ineffective **Health** maintenance r/t deficient knowledge regarding self-care with abscess

Ineffective **Protection** r/t inadequate nutrition, abnormal blood profile, drug therapy, depressed immune function

Abuse, Child

See Child Abuse

Abuse, Spouse, Parent, or Significant Other

Anxiety r/t threat to self-concept, situational crisis of abuse

Caregiver role strain r/t chronic illness, self-care deficits, lack of respite care, extent of caregiving required

Compromised family **Coping** r/t abusive patterns

Defensive **Coping** r/t low self-esteem

Impaired verbal **Communication** r/t psychological barriers of fear

Insomnia r/t psychological stress

Interrupted **Family** process: alcoholism r/t inadequate coping skills

Post-trauma syndrome r/t history of abuse

Powerlessness r/t lifestyle of helplessness

Risk for self-directed **Violence**: Risk factor: history of abuse

Self-esteem disturbance r/t negative family interactions

A

A

Accessory Muscle Use (to Breathe)

Ineffective **Breathing** pattern (See **Breathing** pattern, ineffective, Section II)

See Asthma; Bronchitis; COPD (Chronic Obstructive Pulmonary Disease); Respiratory Infections, Acute Childhood

Accident Prone

Acute **Confusion** r/t altered level of consciousness

Adult **Failure** to thrive r/t fatigue

Ineffective **Coping** r/t personal vulnerability, situational crises

Risk for **Injury**: Risk factor: history of accidents

Achalasia

Acute **Pain** r/t stasis of food in esophagus

Impaired **Swallowing** r/t neuromuscular impairment

Ineffective **Coping** r/t chronic disease

Risk for **Aspiration**: Risk factor: nocturnal regurgitation

Acidosis, Metabolic

Acute **Pain**: headache r/t neuromuscular irritability

Decreased **Cardiac** output r/t dysrhythmias from hyperkalemia

Disturbed **Thought** processes r/t central nervous system depression

Imbalanced **Nutrition**: less than body requirements r/t inability to ingest, absorb nutrients

Impaired **Memory** r/t electrolyte imbalance

Ineffective **Tissue** perfusion: cardiopulmonary r/t progressive shock

Risk for **Injury**: Risk factors: disorientation, weakness, stupor

Acidosis, Respiratory

Activity intolerance r/t imbalance between oxygen supply and demand

Decreased **Cardiac** output r/t dysrhythmias associated with respiratory acidosis

Disturbed **Thought** processes r/t central nervous system depression

Impaired **Gas** exchange r/t ventilation perfusion imbalance

Impaired **Memory** r/t hypoxia

ACS (Acute Coronary Syndrome)

See Myocardial Infarction

Acne

Disturbed **Body** image r/t biophysical changes associated with skin disorder

Impaired **Skin** integrity r/t hormonal changes (adolescence, menstrual cycle)

Ineffective management of **Therapeutic** regimen r/t deficient knowledge (medications, personal care, cause)

Acquired Immunodeficiency Syndrome

See AIDS (Acquired Immunodeficiency Syndrome)

Acromegaly

Disturbed **Body** image r/t changes in body function and appearance

Impaired physical **Mobility** r/t joint pain

Ineffective **Airway** clearance r/t airway obstruction by enlarged tongue

Sexual dysfunction r/t changes in hormonal secretions

Activity Intolerance

Activity intolerance (See **Activity** intolerance, Section II)

Activity Intolerance, Potential to Develop

Risk for **Activity** intolerance (See **Activity** intolerance, risk for, Section II)

Acute Abdomen

Acute **Pain** r/t pathological process

Deficient **Fluid** volume r/t air and fluids trapped in bowel, inability to drink

See cause of Acute Abdomen

Acute Alcohol Intoxication

Disturbed **Thought** processes r/t central nervous system depression

Dysfunctional **Family** processes: alcoholism r/t abuse of alcohol

Ineffective **Breathing** pattern r/t depression of the respiratory center

Risk for **Aspiration**: Risk factor: depressed reflexes with acute vomiting

Risk for **Infection**: Risk factor: impaired immune system from altered nutrition

Acute Back

Acute **Pain** r/t back injury

Anxiety r/t situational crisis, back injury

Constipation r/t decreased activity, effect of pain medication

Impaired physical **Mobility** r/t pain

Ineffective **Coping** r/t situational crisis, back injury

Ineffective **Health** maintenance r/t deficient knowledge regarding self-care with painful back

Acute Confusion

See Confusion, Acute

Acute Respiratory Distress Syndrome

See ARDS (Acute Respiratory Distress Syndrome)

Adams-Stokes Syndrome

See Dysrhythmia

Addiction

See Alcoholism; Drug Abuse

Addison's Disease

Activity intolerance r/t weakness, fatigue

Deficient **Fluid** volume r/t failure of regulatory mechanisms

Disturbed **Body** image r/t increased skin pigmentation

Imbalanced **Nutrition**: less than body requirements r/t chronic illness

Ineffective **Health** maintenance r/t deficient knowledge

Risk for **Injury**: Risk factors: weakness

Adenoidectomy

Acute **Pain** r/t surgical incision

Ineffective **Airway** clearance r/t hesitation or reluctance to cough as a result of pain, fear

Ineffective **Health** maintenance r/t deficient knowledge of postoperative care

Nausea r/t anesthesia effects, drainage from surgery

Risk for **Aspiration**: Risk factors: postoperative drainage, impaired swallowing

Risk for deficient **Fluid** volume: Risk factors: decreased intake as a result of painful swallowing, effects of anesthesia

Risk for imbalanced **Nutrition**: less than body requirements: Risk factors: hesitation or reluctance to swallow

Adhesions, Lysis of

See Abdominal Surgery

Adjustment Disorder

Anxiety r/t inability to cope with psychosocial stressor

Disturbed personal **Identity** r/t psychosocial stressor (specific to individual)

Risk-prone health **Behavior** r/t assault to self-esteem

Impaired **Social** interaction r/t absence of significant others or peers

Situational low **Self-esteem** r/t change in role function

Adjustment Impairment

Risk-prone health **Behavior** (See health **Behavior,** risk-prone, Section II)

Adolescent, Pregnant

Anxiety r/t situational and maturational crisis, pregnancy

Decisional **Conflict**: keeping child versus giving up child versus abortion r/t lack of experience with decision making, interference with decision making, multiple or divergent sources of information, lack of support system

Deficient **Knowledge** r/t pregnancy, infant growth and development, parenting

Delayed **Growth** and development r/t pregnancy

Disabled family **Coping** r/t highly ambivalent family relationships, chronically unresolved feelings of guilt, anger, despair

Disturbed **Body** image r/t pregnancy superimposed on developing body

Fear r/t labor and delivery

Health-seeking behaviors r/t desire for optimal maternal and fetal outcome

Imbalanced **Nutrition**: less than body requirements r/t lack of knowledge of nutritional needs during pregnancy and as growing adolescent

Impaired **Social** interaction r/t self-concept disturbance

Ineffective **Coping** r/t situational and maturational crisis, personal vulnerability

Ineffective **Denial** r/t fear of consequences of pregnancy becoming known

Ineffective **Health** maintenance r/t deficient knowledge with denial of pregnancy, desire to keep pregnancy secret, fear

Ineffective **Role** performance r/t pregnancy

Interrupted **Family** processes r/t unmet expectations for adolescent, situational crisis

Noncompliance r/t denial of pregnancy

Risk for **Constipation**: Risk factors: hormonal effects, inadequate fiber in diet, inadequate fluid in diet

Risk for delayed **Development**: Risk factor: unplanned or unwanted pregnancy

Risk for impaired parent/child **Attachment**: Risk factors: anxiety associated with the parent role

Risk for impaired **Parenting**: Risk factors: adolescent parent, unplanned or unwanted pregnancy, single parent

Risk for urge urinary **Incontinence**: Risk factor: pressure on bladder by growing uterus

Situational low **Self-esteem** r/t feelings of shame and guilt about becoming or being pregnant

Social isolation r/t absence of supportive significant others

Adoption, Giving Child Up for

Chronic **Sorrow** r/t loss of relationship with child

Decisional **Conflict** r/t unclear personal values or beliefs, perceived threat to value system, support system deficit

Ineffective **Coping** r/t final decision

Insomnia r/t depression or trauma of relinquishment of child

Interrupted **Family** processes r/t conflict within family regarding relinquishment of child

Grieving r/t loss of child, loss of role of parent

Readiness for enhanced **Spiritual** well-being: harmony with self regarding final decision

Risk for **Post-trauma** syndrome: Risk factor: psychological trauma of relinquishment of child

Risk for **Spiritual** distress: Risk factor: perceived moral implications of decision

Social isolation r/t making choice that goes against values of significant others

Adrenal Crisis

Deficient **Fluid** volume r/t insufficient ability to reabsorb water

Delayed **Surgical** recovery r/t inability to respond to stress

Ineffective **Protection** r/t inability to tolerate stress

See Addison's Disease; Shock

Advance Directives

Death **Anxiety** r/t planning for end-of-life health decisions

Decisional **Conflict** r/t unclear personal values or beliefs, perceived threat to value system, support system deficit

Grieving r/t possible loss of self, significant other

Readiness for enhanced **Spiritual** well-being: harmonious interconnectedness with self, others, higher power, God

Affective Disorders

Adult **Failure** to thrive r/t altered mood state

Chronic low **Self-esteem** r/t repeated unmet expectations

Chronic **Sorrow** r/t chronic mental illness

Constipation r/t inactivity, decreased fluid intake

Insomnia r/t inactivity

Fatigue r/t psychological demands

Hopelessness r/t feeling of abandonment, long-term stress

Ineffective **Coping** r/t complicated grieving

Ineffective **Health** maintenance r/t lack of ability to make good judgments regarding ways to obtain help

Risk for complicated **Grief**: Risk factors: lack of previous resolution of former grieving response

Risk for **Loneliness**: Risk factors: pattern of social isolation, feelings of low self-esteem

Risk for **Suicide**: Risk factor: panic state

Self-care deficit: specify r/t depression, cognitive impairment

Sexual dysfunction r/t loss of sexual desire

Social isolation r/t ineffective coping

See specific disorder: Depression; Dysthymic Disorder; Manic Disorder, Bipolar I

Age-Related Macular Degeneration

See Macular Degeneration

Aggressive Behavior

Fear r/t real or imagined threat to own well-being

Risk for other-directed **Violence** (See **Violence,** other-directed, risk for, Section II)

Risk for self-directed **Violence**

*See **Violence,** self-directed, risk for, Section II*

Aging

Adult **Failure** to thrive r/t depression, apathy, fatigue

Chronic **Sorrow** r/t multiple losses

Death **Anxiety** r/t fear of unknown, loss of self, impact on significant others

Disturbed **Sensory** perception: visual or auditory r/t aging process

Functional urinary **Incontinence** r/t impaired vision, impaired cognition, neuromuscular limitations, altered environmental factors

Grieving r/t multiple losses, impending death

A

Health-seeking behaviors r/t knowledge about medication, nutrition, exercise, coping strategies

Impaired **Dentition** r/t ineffective oral hygiene

Ineffective management of **Therapeutic** regimen r/t deficient knowledge: medication, nutrition, exercise, coping strategies

Ineffective **Thermoregulation** r/t aging

Readiness for enhanced community **Coping** r/t providing social support and other resources identified as needed for elderly client

Readiness for enhanced family **Coping** r/t ability to gratify needs, address adaptive tasks

Readiness for enhanced **Knowledge**: specify: need to improve health

Readiness for enhanced **Nutrition**: need to improve health

Readiness for enhanced **Sleep**: need to improve sleep

Readiness for enhanced **Spiritual** well-being: one's experience of life's meaning, harmony with self, others, higher power, God, environment

Readiness for enhanced **Urinary** elimination: need to improve health

Risk for **Caregiver** role strain: Risk factor: inability to handle increasing needs of significant other

Risk for **Injury**: Risk factor: disturbed sensory perception

Risk for **Loneliness**: Risk factors: inadequate support system, role transition, health alterations, depression, fatigue

Sleep deprivation r/t aging-related sleep stage shifts

Agitation

Acute **Confusion** r/t side effects of medication, hypoxia, decreased cerebral perfusion, alcohol abuse or withdrawal, substance abuse or withdrawal, sensory deprivation or overload

Sleep deprivation r/t sundown syndrome

Agoraphobia

Anxiety r/t real or perceived threat to physical integrity

Fear r/t leaving home, going out in public places

Impaired **Social** interaction r/t disturbance in self-concept

Ineffective **Coping** r/t inadequate support systems

Social isolation r/t altered thought process

Agranulocytosis

Delayed **Surgical** recovery r/t abnormal blood profile

Ineffective **Health** maintenance r/t deficient knowledge of protective measures to prevent infection

Ineffective **Protection** r/t abnormal blood profile

AIDS (Acquired Immunodeficiency Syndrome)

Disturbed **Body** image r/t chronic contagious illness, cachexia

Caregiver role strain r/t unpredictable illness course, presence of situation stressors

Chronic **Pain** r/t tissue inflammation and destruction

Chronic **Sorrow** r/t living with long-term chronic illness

Death **Anxiety** r/t fear of premature death

Diarrhea r/t inflammatory bowel changes

Disturbed **Energy** field r/t chronic illness

Fatigue r/t disease process, stress, poor nutritional intake

Fear r/t powerlessness, threat to well-being

Grieving: family/parental r/t potential or impending death of loved one

Grieving: individual r/t loss of physio-psychosocial well-being

Hopelessness r/t deteriorating physical condition

Imbalanced **Nutrition**: less than body requirements r/t decreased ability to eat and absorb nutrients as a result of anorexia, nausea, diarrhea; oral candidiasis pathology in gastrointestinal tract

Ineffective **Health** maintenance r/t deficient knowledge regarding transmission of infection, lack of exposure to information, misinterpretation of information

Ineffective **Protection** r/t risk for infection secondary to inadequate immune system

Ineffective **Sexuality** pattern r/t possible transmission of disease

Interrupted **Family** processes r/t distress about diagnosis of human immunodeficiency virus (HIV) infection

Risk for deficient **Fluid** volume: Risk factors: diarrhea, vomiting, fever, bleeding

Risk for impaired **Oral** mucous membranes: Risk factor: immunological deficit

Risk for impaired **Skin** integrity: Risk factors: immunological deficit, diarrhea

Risk for **Infection**: Risk factor: inadequate immune system

Risk for **Loneliness**: Risk factor: social isolation

Risk for **Spiritual** distress: Risk factor: physical illness

Situational low **Self-esteem** r/t crisis of chronic contagious illness

Social isolation r/t self-concept disturbance, therapeutic isolation

Spiritual distress r/t challenged beliefs or moral system

See AIDS, Child; Cancer; Pneumonia

AIDS Dementia

Chronic **Confusion** r/t viral invasion of nervous system

Disturbed **Thought** processes r/t viral infection in the brain

See Dementia

AIDS, Child

Impaired **Parenting** r/t congenital acquisition of infection secondary to intravenous (IV) drug use, multiple sexual partners, history of contaminated blood transfusion

Parental role conflict r/t intimidation with invasive or restrictive modalities

See AIDS (Acquired Immunodeficiency Syndrome); Child with Chronic Condition; Hospitalized Child; Terminally Ill Child, Adolescent; Terminally Ill Child, Infant/Toddler; Terminally Ill Child, Preschool Child; Terminally Ill Child, School-Age Child/Preadolescent; Terminally Ill Child/Death of Child, Parent

Airway Obstruction/Secretions

Ineffective **Airway** clearance (See **Airway** clearance, ineffective, Section II)

Alcohol Withdrawal

Acute **Confusion** r/t effects of alcohol withdrawal

Anxiety r/t situational crisis, withdrawal

Chronic low **Self-esteem** r/t repeated unmet expectations

Disturbed **Sensory** perception: visual, auditory, kinesthetic, tactile, olfactory r/t neurochemical imbalance in brain

Disturbed **Thought** processes r/t potential delirium tremors

Dysfunctional **Family** processes: alcoholism r/t abuse of alcohol

Imbalanced **Nutrition**: less than body requirements r/t poor dietary habits

Ineffective **Coping** r/t personal vulnerability

Ineffective **Health** maintenance r/t deficient knowledge regarding chronic illness or effects of alcohol consumption

Insomnia r/t effect of depressants, alcohol withdrawal, anxiety

A

Risk for deficient **Fluid** volume: Risk factors: excessive diaphoresis, agitation, decreased fluid intake

Risk for other-directed **Violence**: Risk factor: substance withdrawal

Risk for self-directed **Violence**: Risk factor: substance withdrawal

Alcoholism

Acute **Confusion** r/t alcohol abuse

Anxiety r/t loss of control

Chronic **Confusion** r/t neurological effects of chronic alcohol intake

Defensive **Coping** r/t alcoholism

Ineffective **Denial** r/t refusal to acknowledge alcoholism

Insomnia r/t irritability, nightmares, tremors

Disabled family **Coping**: alcoholism r/t codependency issues

Imbalanced **Nutrition**: less than body requirements r/t anorexia

Impaired **Home** maintenance r/t memory deficits, fatigue

Impaired **Memory** r/t alcohol abuse

Ineffective **Coping** r/t use of alcohol to cope with life events

Ineffective **Protection** r/t malnutrition, sleep deprivation

Interrupted **Family** process: alcoholism r/t alcohol abuse

Powerlessness r/t alcohol addiction

Risk for **Injury**: Risk factor: alteration in sensory or perceptual function

Risk for **Loneliness**: Risk factor: unacceptable social behavior

Risk for other-directed **Violence**: Risk factors: reactions to substances used, impulsive behavior, disorientation, impaired judgment

Risk for self-directed **Violence**: Risk factors: reactions to substances used, impulsive behavior, disorientation, impaired judgment

Risk-prone health **Behavior** r/t lack of motivation to change behaviors

Self-esteem disturbance r/t failure at life events

Social isolation r/t unacceptable social behavior, values

Alcoholism, Dysfunctional Family Processes

Dysfunctional **Family** processes: alcoholism (See **Family** processes, dysfunctional: alcoholism, Section II)

Alkalosis

See Metabolic Alkalosis

Allergies

Ineffective **Health** maintenance r/t deficient knowledge regarding allergies

Latex **Allergy** response r/t hypersensitivity to natural rubber latex

Risk for latex **Allergy** response: Risk factor: repeated exposure to products containing latex

Alopecia

Deficient **Knowledge** r/t self-care needed to promote hair growth

Disturbed **Body** image r/t loss of hair, change in appearance

Altered Mental Status

See Confusion, Acute; Confusion, Chronic; Memory Deficit

ALS (Amyotrophic Lateral Sclerosis)

See Amyotrophic Lateral Sclerosis (ALS)

Alzheimer's Type Dementia

Adult **Failure** to thrive r/t difficulty in reasoning, judgment, memory, concentration

Disturbed **Thought** processes r/t chronic organic disorder

Caregiver role strain r/t duration and extent of caregiving required

Chronic **Confusion** r/t Alzheimer's disease

Compromised family **Coping** r/t interrupted family processes

Fear r/t loss of self

Hopelessness r/t deteriorating condition

Impaired **Environmental** interpretation syndrome r/t Alzheimer's disease

Impaired **Home** maintenance r/t impaired cognitive function, inadequate support systems

Impaired **Memory** r/t neurological disturbance

Impaired physical **Mobility** r/t severe neurological dysfunction

Ineffective **Health** maintenance r/t deficient knowledge of caregiver regarding appropriate care

Insomnia r/t neurological impairment, daytime naps

Powerlessness r/t deteriorating condition

Risk for **Injury**: Risk factor: confusion

Risk for **Loneliness**: Risk factor: potential social isolation

Risk for other-directed **Violence**: Risk factors: frustration, fear, anger

Risk for **Relocation** stress syndrome: Risk factors: impaired psychosocial health, decreased health status

Self-care deficit: specify r/t psychological or physiological impairment

Social isolation r/t fear of disclosure of memory loss

Wandering r/t cognitive impairment, frustration, physiological state

See Dementia

AMD (Age-Related Macular Degeneration)

See Macular Degeneration

Amenorrhea

Imbalanced **Nutrition**: less than body requirements r/t inadequate food intake

Risk for **Sexual** dysfunction: Risk factor: altered body function

See Sexuality, Adolescent

AMI (Acute Myocardial Infarction)

See MI (Myocardial Infarction)

Amnesia

Acute **Confusion** r/t alcohol abuse, delirium, dementia, drug abuse

Dysfunctional **Family** processes: alcoholism r/t alcohol abuse, inadequate coping skills

Impaired **Memory** r/t excessive environmental disturbance, neurological disturbance

Post-trauma syndrome r/t history of abuse, catastrophic illness, disaster, accident

Amniocentesis

Anxiety r/t threat to self and fetus, unknown future

Decisional **Conflict** r/t choice of treatment pending results of test

Risk for **Infection**: Risk factor: invasive procedure

Amnionitis

See Chorioamnionitis

Amniotic Membrane Rupture

See Premature Rupture of Membranes

Amputation

Acute **Pain** r/t surgery, phantom limb sensation

Chronic **Pain** r/t surgery, phantom limb sensation

Chronic **Sorrow** r/t grief associated with loss of body part

Disturbed **Body** image r/t negative effects of amputation, response from others

Grieving r/t loss of body part, future lifestyle changes

A

Impaired physical **Mobility** r/t musculoskeletal impairment, limited movement

Impaired **Skin** integrity r/t poor healing, prosthesis rubbing

Ineffective **Health** maintenance r/t deficient knowledge of care of stump, rehabilitation

Ineffective **Tissue** perfusion: peripheral r/t impaired arterial circulation

Risk for deficient **Fluid** volume: Risk factors: hemorrhage, vulnerable surgical site

Amyotrophic Lateral Sclerosis (ALS)

Chronic **Sorrow** r/t chronic illness

Death **Anxiety** r/t impending progressive loss of function leading to death

Decisional **Conflict**: ventilator therapy r/t unclear personal values or beliefs, lack of relevant information

Impaired spontaneous **Ventilation** r/t weakness of muscles of respiration

Impaired **Swallowing** r/t weakness of muscles involved in swallowing

Impaired verbal **Communication** r/t weakness of muscles of speech, deficient knowledge of ways to compensate and alternative communication devices

Ineffective **Breathing** pattern r/t compromised muscles of respiration

Risk for **Aspiration**: Risk factor: impaired swallowing

Risk for **Spiritual** distress: Risk factor: chronic debilitating condition

See Neurological Disorders

Anal Fistula

See Hemorrhoidectomy

Anaphylactic Shock

Impaired spontaneous **Ventilation** r/t acute airway obstruction

Ineffective **Airway** clearance r/t laryngeal edema, bronchospasm

Latex **Allergy** response r/t abnormal immune mechanism response

See Shock

Anasarca

Excess **Fluid** volume r/t excessive fluid intake, cardiac/renal dysfunction, loss of plasma proteins

Risk for impaired **Skin** integrity: Risk factor: impaired circulation to skin

See cause of Anasarca

Anemia

Anxiety r/t cause of disease

Delayed **Surgical** recovery r/t decreased oxygen supply to body, increased cardiac workload

Fatigue r/t decreased oxygen supply to the body, increased cardiac workload

Impaired **Memory** r/t anemia

Ineffective **Health** maintenance r/t deficient knowledge regarding nutritional and medical treatment of anemia

Ineffective **Protection** r/t bleeding disorder

Risk for **Injury** r/t alteration in peripheral sensory perception

Anemia, in Pregnancy

Anxiety r/t concerns about health of self and fetus

Fatigue r/t decreased oxygen supply to the body, increased cardiac workload

Ineffective **Health** maintenance r/t deficient knowledge regarding nutrition in pregnancy

Risk for delayed **Development**: Risk factor: reduction in the oxygen-carrying capacity of blood

Risk for **Infection**: Risk factor: reduction in oxygen-carrying capacity of blood

Anemia, Sickle Cell

See Anemia; Sickle Cell Anemia/Crisis

Anencephaly

See Neural Tube Defects

Aneurysm, Abdominal Surgery

Risk for deficient **Fluid** volume: Risk factor: hemorrhage r/t potential abnormal blood loss

Risk for ineffective **Tissue** perfusion: peripheral or renal Risk factor: impaired arterial circulation

Risk for **Infection**: Risk factor: invasive procedure

See Abdominal Surgery

Aneurysm, Cerebral

See Craniectomy/Craniotomy; Subarachnoid Hemorrhage (if aneurysm has ruptured)

Anger

Anxiety r/t situational crisis

Defensive **Coping** r/t inability to acknowledge responsibility for actions and results of actions

Fear r/t environmental stressor, hospitalization

Grieving r/t significant loss

Powerlessness r/t health care environment

Risk for compromised human **Dignity**: Risk factors: inadequate participation in decision making, perceived dehumanizing treatment, perceived humiliation, exposure of the body, cultural incongruity

Risk for other-directed **Violence**: Risk factors: history of violence, rage reaction

Risk for **Post-trauma** syndrome: Risk factor: inadequate social support

Risk for self-directed **Violence**: Risk factors: history of violence, history of abuse, rage reaction

Risk-prone health **Behavior** r/t assault to self-esteem, disability requiring change in lifestyle, inadequate support system

Angina Pectoris

Activity intolerance r/t acute pain, dysrhythmias

Acute **Pain** r/t myocardial ischemia

Anxiety r/t situational crisis

Decreased **Cardiac** output r/t myocardial ischemia, medication effect, dysrhythmia

Grieving r/t pain, lifestyle changes

Ineffective **Coping** r/t personal vulnerability to situational crisis of new diagnosis, deteriorating health

Ineffective **Denial** r/t deficient knowledge of need to seek help with symptoms

Ineffective **Health** maintenance r/t deficient knowledge of care of angina condition

Ineffective **Sexuality** pattern r/t disease process, medications, loss of libido

Angiocardiography (Cardiac Catheterization)

See Cardiac Catheterization

Angioplasty, Coronary

Decreased **Cardiac** output r/t ventricular ischemia, dysrhythmias

Fear r/t possible outcome of interventional procedure

Ineffective **Health** maintenance r/t deficient knowledge regarding care after procedures, measures to limit coronary artery disease

Risk for deficient **Fluid** volume: Risk factors: possible damage to coronary artery, hematoma formation, hemorrhage

Risk for ineffective **Tissue** perfusion: peripheral/cardiopulmonary: Risk factors: vasospasm, hematoma formation

Anomaly, Fetal/Newborn (Parent Dealing with)

Anxiety r/t threat to role functioning, situational crisis

A

Chronic **Sorrow** r/t loss of ideal child, inadequate bereavement support

Decisional **Conflict**: interventions for fetus or newborn r/t lack of relevant information, spiritual distress, threat to value system

Deficient **Knowledge** r/t limited exposure to situation

Effective **Therapeutic** regimen management r/t verbalized intent to reduce risk factors for progression of illness and sequelae associated with anomaly

Fear r/t real or imagined threat to baby, implications for future pregnancies, powerlessness

Hopelessness r/t long-term stress, deteriorating physical condition of child, lost spiritual belief

Disabled family **Coping** r/t chronically unresolved feelings about loss of perfect baby

Impaired **Parenting** r/t interruption of bonding process

Ineffective **Coping** r/t personal vulnerability in situational crisis

Interrupted **Family** processes r/t unmet expectations for perfect baby, lack of adequate support systems

Parental role **Conflict** r/t separation from newborn, intimidation with invasive or restrictive modalities, specialized care center policies

Powerlessness r/t complication threatening fetus or newborn

Risk for disorganized **Infant** behavior: Risk factor: congenital disorder

Risk for complicated **Grief**: Risk factor: loss of perfect child

Risk for impaired parent/child **Attachment**: Risk factor: ill infant unable to effectively initiate parental contact as result of altered behavioral organization

Risk for impaired **Parenting**: Risk factors: interruption of bonding process; unrealistic expectations for self, infant, or partner; perceived threat to own emotional survival; severe stress; lack of knowledge

Risk for **Spiritual** distress: Risk factor: lack of normal child to raise and carry on family name

Situational low **Self-esteem** r/t perceived inability to produce a perfect child

Social isolation r/t alterations in child's physical appearance, altered state of wellness

Spiritual distress r/t test of spiritual beliefs

Anorectal Abscess

Acute **Pain** r/t inflammation of perirectal area

Disturbed **Body** image r/t odor and drainage from rectal area

Risk for **Constipation**: Risk factor: fear of painful elimination

Anorexia

Deficient **Fluid** volume r/t inability to drink

Delayed **Surgical** recovery r/t inadequate nutritional intake

Imbalanced **Nutrition**: less than body requirements r/t loss of appetite, nausea, vomiting

Anorexia Nervosa

Activity intolerance r/t fatigue, weakness

Chronic low **Self-esteem** r/t repeated unmet expectations

Constipation r/t lack of adequate food, fiber, and fluid intake

Defensive **Coping** r/t psychological impairment, eating disorder

Diarrhea r/t laxative abuse

Disabled family **Coping** r/t highly ambivalent family relationships

Disturbed **Body** image r/t misconception of actual body appearance

Disturbed **Thought** processes r/t anorexia, impaired nutrition

Imbalanced **Nutrition**: less than body requirements r/t inadequate food intake, excessive exercise

Ineffective **Denial** r/t fear of consequences of therapy, possible weight gain

Ineffective family **Therapeutic** regimen management r/t family conflict, excessive demands on family associated with complexity of condition and treatment

Ineffective **Sexuality** pattern r/t loss of libido from malnutrition

Interrupted **Family** processes r/t situational crisis

Risk for **Infection**: Risk factor: malnutrition resulting in depressed immune system

Risk for **Spiritual** distress: Risk factor: low self-esteem

See Maturational Issues, Adolescent

Anosmia (Smell, Loss of Ability to)

Disturbed **Sensory** perception: olfactory r/t altered sensory reception, transmission, integration

Imbalanced **Nutrition**: less than body requirements r/t loss of appetite associated with loss of smell

Antepartum Period

See Pregnancy, Normal; Prenatal Care, Normal

Anterior Repair, Anterior Colporrhaphy

Risk for urge urinary **Incontinence**: Risk factor: trauma to bladder

Urinary retention r/t edema of urinary structures

See Vaginal Hysterectomy

Anticoagulant Therapy

Ineffective **Health** maintenance r/t deficient knowledge regarding precautions to take with anticoagulant therapy

Ineffective **Protection** r/t altered clotting function from anticoagulant

Risk for deficient **Fluid** volume: hemorrhage: Risk factor: altered clotting mechanism

Antisocial Personality Disorder

Defensive **Coping** r/t excessive use of projection

Disturbed **Thought** processes r/t internal turmoil and conflict (intrusive thinking)

Hopelessness r/t abandonment

Impaired **Social** interaction r/t sociocultural conflict, chemical dependence, inability to form relationships

Ineffective **Coping** r/t frequently violating the norms and rules of society

Ineffective family **Therapeutic** regimen management r/t excessive demands on family

Risk for impaired **Parenting**: Risk factors: inability to function as parent or guardian, emotional instability

Risk for **Loneliness**: Risk factor: inability to interact appropriately with others

Risk for other-directed **Violence**: Risk factor: history of violence

Risk for **Self-mutilation**: Risk factors: self-hatred, depersonalization

Spiritual distress r/t separation from religious or cultural ties

Anuria

See Renal Failure

Anxiety

Anxiety (See **Anxiety**, Section II)

Anxiety Disorder

Anxiety r/t unmet security and safety needs

Death **Anxiety** r/t fears of unknown, powerlessness

Decisional **Conflict** r/t low self-esteem, fear of making a mistake

Defensive **Coping** r/t overwhelming feelings of dread

Disabled family **Coping** r/t ritualistic behavior, actions

Disturbed **Energy** field r/t hopelessness, helplessness

Disturbed **Thought** processes r/t anxiety

Ineffective **Coping** r/t inability to express feelings appropriately

Ineffective **Denial** r/t overwhelming feelings of hopelessness, fear, threat to self

Insomnia r/t psychological impairment, emotional instability

Powerlessness r/t lifestyle of helplessness

Risk for **Spiritual** distress: Risk factor: psychological distress

Self-care deficit r/t ritualistic behavior, activities

Sleep deprivation r/t prolonged psychological discomfort

Aortic Aneurysm Repair (Abdominal Surgery)

See Abdominal Surgery; Aneurysm, Abdominal Surgery

Aortic Valvular Stenosis

See Congenital Heart Disease/Cardiac Anomalies

Aphasia

Anxiety r/t situational crisis of aphasia

Impaired verbal **Communication** r/t decrease in circulation to brain

Ineffective **Coping** r/t loss of speech

Ineffective **Health** maintenance r/t deficient knowledge regarding information on aphasia and alternative communication techniques

Aplastic Anemia

Activity intolerance r/t imbalance between oxygen supply and demand

Anxiety r/t deficient knowledge of disease process and treatment

Delayed **Surgical** recovery r/t risk for infection

Impaired **Protection** r/t inadequate immune function

Risk for **Infection**: Risk factor: inadequate immune function

Apnea in Infancy

See Premature Infant (Child); Premature Infant (Parent); SIDS (Sudden Infant Death Syndrome)

Apneustic Respirations

Impaired **Breathing** pattern r/t perception or cognitive impairment, neurological impairment

See cause of Apneustic Respirations

Appendectomy

Acute **Pain** r/t surgical incision

Deficient **Fluid** volume r/t fluid restriction, hypermetabolic state, nausea, vomiting

Ineffective **Health** maintenance r/t deficient knowledge regarding self-care after appendectomy

Risk for **Infection**: Risk factors: perforation or rupture of appendix, surgical incision, peritonitis

See Hospitalized Child; Surgery, Postoperative

Appendicitis

Acute **Pain** r/t inflammation

Deficient **Fluid** volume r/t anorexia, nausea, vomiting

Delayed **Surgical** recovery r/t risk for infection

Risk for **Infection**: Risk factor: possible perforation of appendix

Apprehension

Anxiety r/t threat to self-concept, threat to health status, situational crisis

Death **Anxiety** r/t apprehension over

loss of self, consequences to significant others

AMD (Age-Related Macular Degeneration)

See Macular Degeneration

ARDS (Acute Respiratory Distress Syndrome)

Death **Anxiety** r/t seriousness of physical disease

Delayed **Surgical** recovery r/t complications associated with respiratory pathology

Impaired **Gas** exchange r/t damage to alveolar-capillary membrane, change in lung compliance

Impaired spontaneous **Ventilation** r/t damage to alveolar capillary membrane

Ineffective **Airway** clearance r/t excessive tracheobronchial secretions

See Child with Chronic Condition; Ventilator Client

Arrhythmia

See Dysrhythmia

Arterial Insufficiency

Delayed **Surgical** recovery r/t ineffective tissue perfusion

Ineffective **Tissue** perfusion: peripheral r/t interruption of arterial flow

Arthritis

Activity intolerance r/t chronic pain, fatigue, weakness

Chronic **Pain** r/t progression of joint deterioration

Disturbed **Body** image r/t ineffective coping with joint abnormalities

Impaired physical **Mobility** r/t musculoskeletal impairment

Ineffective **Health** maintenance r/t deficient knowledge regarding care of arthritis

Self-care deficit: specify r/t pain, musculoskeletal impairment

See JRA (Juvenile Rheumatoid Arthritis)

Arthrocentesis

Acute **Pain** r/t invasive procedure

Arthroplasty (Total Hip Replacement)

Acute **Pain** r/t tissue trauma associated with surgery

Constipation r/t immobility

Impaired physical **Mobility** r/t decreased muscle strength, surgery

Impaired **Walking** r/t decreased muscle strength, surgery

Risk for **Infection**: Risk factors: invasive surgery, foreign object in body, anesthesia, immobility with stasis of respiratory secretions

Risk for **Injury**: Risk factors: interruption of arterial blood flow, dislocation of prosthesis

Risk for perioperative positioning **Injury**: Risk factors: immobilization, muscle weakness

Risk for **Peripheral** neurovascular dysfunction: Risk factor: orthopedic surgery

See Surgery, Perioperative; Surgery, Postoperative; Surgery, Preoperative

Arthroscopy

Ineffective **Health** maintenance r/t deficient knowledge regarding procedure, postoperative restrictions

Ascites

Chronic **Pain** r/t altered body function

Imbalanced **Nutrition**: less than body requirements r/t loss of appetite

Ineffective **Breathing** pattern r/t increased abdominal girth

Ineffective **Health** maintenance r/t deficient knowledge of care with condition of ascites

See cause of Ascites; Cancer; Cirrhosis

A

Asphyxia, Birth

Fear (parental) r/t concern over safety of infant

Grieving r/t loss of "perfect" child, concern of loss of future abilities

Impaired **Gas** exchange r/t poor placental perfusion, lack of initiation of breathing by newborn

Impaired spontaneous **Ventilation** r/t brain injury

Ineffective **Breathing** pattern r/t depression of breathing reflex secondary to anoxia

Ineffective **Coping** r/t uncertainty of child outcome

Ineffective **Tissue** perfusion: cerebral r/t poor placental perfusion or cord compression resulting in lack of oxygen to brain

Risk for delayed **Development**: Risk factor: lack of oxygen to brain

Risk for disorganized **Infant** behavior: Risk factor: lack of oxygen to brain

Risk for disproportionate **Growth**: Risk factor: lack of oxygen to brain

Risk for impaired parent/child **Attachment**: Risk factors: ill infant who is unable to initiate parental contact, hospitalization in critical care environment

Risk for **Injury**: Risk factor: lack of oxygen to brain

Risk for **Post-trauma** syndrome: parental: Risk factor: psychological trauma of sudden potential for loss of newborn

Aspiration, Danger of

Risk for **Aspiration** (See **Aspiration, risk for,** Section II)

Assault Victim

Post-trauma syndrome r/t assault

Rape-trauma syndrome r/t rape

Risk for **Post-trauma** syndrome: Risk factors: perception of event, inadequate social support, unsupportive environment, diminished ego strength, duration of event

Risk for **Spiritual** distress: Risk factors: physical, psychological stress

Assaultive Client

Disturbed **Thought** process r/t use of hallucinogenic substance, psychological disorder

Ineffective **Coping** r/t lack of control of impulsive actions

Risk for **Injury**: Risk factors: confused thought process, impaired judgment

Risk for other-directed **Violence**: Risk factors: paranoid ideation, anger

Asthma

Activity intolerance r/t fatigue, energy shift to meet muscle needs for breathing to overcome airway obstruction

Anxiety r/t inability to breathe effectively, fear of suffocation

Disturbed **Body** image r/t decreased participation in physical activities

Impaired **Home** maintenance r/t deficient knowledge regarding control of environmental triggers

Ineffective **Airway** clearance r/t tracheobronchial narrowing, excessive secretions

Ineffective **Breathing** pattern r/t anxiety

Ineffective **Coping** r/t personal vulnerability to situational crisis

Ineffective **Health** maintenance r/t deficient knowledge regarding physical triggers, medications, treatment of early warning signs

Sleep deprivation r/t ineffective breathing pattern, cough

See Child with Chronic Condition; Hospitalized Child

Ataxia

Anxiety r/t change in health status

Disturbed **Body** image r/t staggering gait

Impaired physical **Mobility** r/t neuromuscular impairment

Risk for **Falls**: Risk factors: gait alteration, instability

Atelectasis

Impaired **Gas** exchange r/t decreased alveolar-capillary surface

Ineffective **Breathing** pattern r/t loss of functional lung tissue, depression of respiratory function or hypoventilation because of pain

Atherosclerosis

See MI (Myocardial Infarction), CVA (Cerebrovascular Accident), Peripheral Vascular Disease

Athlete's Foot

Impaired **Skin** integrity r/t effects of fungal agent

Ineffective **Health** maintenance r/t deficient knowledge regarding treatment and prevention of athlete's foot

See Itching; Pruritus

ATN (Acute Tubular Necrosis)

See Renal Failure

Atrial Fibrillation

See Dysrhythmia

Atrial Septal Defect

See Congenital Heart Disease/Cardiac Anomalies

Attention Deficit Disorder

Disabled family **Coping** r/t significant person with chronically unexpressed feelings of guilt, anxiety, hostility, and despair

Risk for delayed **Development**: Risk factor: behavior disorders

Risk for impaired **Parenting**: Risk factor: lack of knowledge of factors contributing to child's behavior

Risk for **Loneliness**: Risk factor: social isolation

Risk for **Spiritual** distress: Risk factor: poor relationships

Risk-prone health **Behavior** r/t intense emotional state

Self-esteem disturbance r/t difficulty in participating in expected activities, poor school performance

Social isolation r/t unacceptable social behavior

Autism

Compromised family **Coping** r/t parental guilt over etiology of disease, inability to accept or adapt to child's condition, inability to help child and other family members seek treatment

Delayed **Growth** and development r/t inability to develop relations with other human beings, inability to identify own body as separate from those of other people, inability to integrate concept of self

Disturbed personal **Identity** r/t inability to distinguish between self and environment, inability to identify own body as separate from those of other people, inability to integrate concept of self

Disturbed **Thought** processes r/t inability to perceive self or others, cognitive dissonance, perceptual dysfunction

Impaired **Social** interaction r/t communication barriers, inability to relate to others, failure to develop peer relationships

Impaired verbal **Communication** r/t speech and language delays

Risk for delayed **Development**: Risk factor: autism

Risk for **Loneliness**: Risk factors: health alterations, change in cognition

Risk for other-directed **Violence**: Risk factors: frequent destructive rages toward others secondary to extreme response to changes in routine, fear of harmless things

Risk for self-directed **Violence**: Risk factors: frequent destructive rages toward self, secondary to extreme response to changes in routine, fear of harmless things

Risk for **Self-mutilation**: Risk factor: autistic state

See Child with Chronic Condition; Mental Retardation

Autonomic Dysreflexia

Autonomic dysreflexia r/t bladder distention, bowel distention, noxious stimuli

Risk for **Autonomic** dysreflexia: Risk factors: bladder distention, bowel distention, noxious stimuli

Autonomic Hyperreflexia

See Autonomic Dysreflexia

B

Back Pain

Acute **Pain** r/t back injury

Anxiety r/t situational crisis, back injury

Chronic **Pain** r/t back injury

Disturbed **Energy** field r/t chronic pain

Impaired physical **Mobility** r/t pain

Ineffective **Coping** r/t situational crisis, back injury

Ineffective **Health** maintenance r/t deficient knowledge regarding prevention of further injury, proper body mechanics

Risk for **Constipation**: Risk factors: decreased activity, side effect of pain medication

Risk for **Disuse** syndrome: Risk factor: severe pain

Bacteremia

Ineffective **Protection** r/t compromised immune system

See Infection; Infection, Potential for

Barrel Chest

See Aging (if appropriate); COPD (Chronic Obstructive Pulmonary Disease)

Bathing/Hygiene Problems

Bathing/hygiene **Self-care** deficit (See **Self-care** deficit, bathing/hygiene, Section II)

Impaired bed **Mobility** r/t chronic physically limiting condition

Battered Child Syndrome

Chronic **Sorrow** r/t situational crises

Dysfunctional **Family** processes: alcoholism r/t inadequate coping skills

Risk for **Aspiration**: Risk factor: propped bottle

Risk for **Post-trauma** syndrome: Risk factors: physical abuse, incest, rape, molestation

Risk for **Self-mutilation**: Risk factors: feelings of rejection, dysfunctional family

Sleep deprivation r/t prolonged psychological discomfort

See Child Abuse

Battered Person

See Abuse, Spouse, Parent, or Significant Other

Bed Mobility, Impaired

Impaired bed **Mobility** (See **Mobility**, impaired bed, Section II)

Bedbugs, Infestation

Impaired **Home** maintenance r/t deficient knowledge regarding prevention of bedbug infestation

Impaired **Skin** integrity r/t bites of bedbugs
See Itching; Pruritus

Bedrest, Prolonged

Deficient **Diversional** activity r/t prolonged bedrest

Impaired bed **Mobility** r/t neuromuscular impairment

Risk for **Disuse** syndrome: Risk factor: prolonged immobility

Risk for **Loneliness**: Risk factor: prolonged bedrest

Social isolation r/t prolonged bedrest

Bedsores

See Pressure Ulcer

Bedwetting

See Enuresis; Toilet Training

Bell's Palsy

Acute **Pain** r/t inflammation of facial nerve

Disturbed **Body** image r/t loss of motor control on one side of face

Imbalanced **Nutrition**: less than body requirements r/t difficulty with chewing

Risk for **Injury** (eye): Risk factor: dysfunction of facial nerve

Benign Prostatic Hypertrophy

See BPH (Benign Prostatic Hypertrophy); Prostatic Hypertrophy

Bereavement

Chronic **Sorrow** r/t death of loved one, chronic illness, disability

Grieving r/t loss of significant person

Risk for complicated **Grief**: Risk factor: death of a loved one

Insomnia r/t grief

Risk for **Spiritual** distress: Risk factor: death of a loved one

Biliary Atresia

Anxiety r/t surgical intervention, possible liver transplantation

Imbalanced **Nutrition**: less than body requirements r/t decreased absorption of fat and fat-soluble vitamins, poor feeding

Pruritus r/t inflammation of skin

Risk for impaired **Skin** integrity: Risk factor: pruritus

Risk for ineffective **Breathing** pattern: Risk factors: enlarged liver, development of ascites

Risk for **Injury**: bleeding Risk factors: vitamin K deficiency, altered clotting mechanisms

See Child with Chronic Condition; Cirrhosis (as complication); Hospitalized Child; Terminally Ill Child, Adolescent; Terminally Ill Child, Infant/Toddler; Terminally Ill Child, Preschool Child; Terminally Ill Child, School-Age-Child/Preadolescent; Terminally Ill Child/Death of Child, Parent

Biliary Calculus

See Cholelithiasis

Biliary Obstruction

See Jaundice

Biopsy

Fear r/t outcome of biopsy

Ineffective **Health** maintenance r/t deficient knowledge regarding biopsy site, further needed health care

Bioterrorism

Contamination r/t exposure to bioterrorism

Risk for **Infection**: Risk factor: exposure to harmful biological agent

Risk for **Post-trauma** syndrome: Risk factor: perception of event of bioterrorism

B

Bipolar Disorder I (Most Recent Episode, Depressed or Manic)

Chronic low **Self-esteem** r/t repeated unmet expectations

Disturbed **Energy** field r/t disharmony of mind, body, spirit

Fatigue r/t psychological demands

Ineffective **Coping** r/t complicated grieving

Ineffective **Health** maintenance r/t lack of ability to make good judgments regarding ways to obtain help

Risk for complicated **Grief**: Risk factor: lack of previous resolution of former grieving response

Risk for **Loneliness**: Risk factors: stress, conflict

Risk for **Spiritual** distress: Risk factor: mental illness

Risk-prone health **Behavior** r/t low state of optimism

Self-care deficit: specify r/t depression, cognitive impairment

Social isolation r/t ineffective coping

See Depression (Major Depressive Disorder); Manic Disorder, Bipolar I

Birth Asphyxia

See Asphyxia, Birth

Birth Control

See Contraceptive Method

Bladder Cancer

Urinary retention r/t clots obstructing urethra

See Cancer; TURP (Transurethral Resection of the Prostate)

Bladder Distention

Urinary retention r/t high urethral pressure caused by weak detrusor, inhibition of reflex arc, blockage, strong sphincter

Bladder Training

Disturbed **Body** image r/t difficulty maintaining control of urinary elimination

Functional urinary **Incontinence** r/t altered environment; sensory, cognitive, mobility deficit

Ineffective **Health** maintenance r/t deficient knowledge regarding incontinence self-care

Stress urinary **Incontinence** r/t degenerative change in pelvic muscles and structural supports

Urge urinary **Incontinence** r/t decreased bladder capacity, increased urine concentration, overdistention of bladder

Bladder Training, Child

See Toilet Training

Bleeding Tendency

Ineffective **Protection** r/t abnormal blood profile, drug therapies

Risk for delayed **Surgical** recovery: Risk factor: bleeding tendency

Blepharoplasty

Disturbed **Body** image r/t effects of surgery

Ineffective **Health** maintenance r/t deficient knowledge regarding postoperative care of surgical area

Blindness

Disturbed **Sensory** perception: visual r/t altered sensory reception, transmission, integration

Impaired **Home** maintenance r/t decreased vision

Ineffective **Role** performance r/t alteration in health status (change in visual acuity)

Interrupted **Family** processes r/t shift in health status of family member (change in visual acuity)

Risk for delayed **Development**: Risk factor: vision impairment

Risk for **Injury**: Risk factor: sensory dysfunction

Self-care deficit r/t inability to see to be able to perform activities of daily living

See Vision Impairment

Blood Disorder

Ineffective **Protection** r/t abnormal blood profile

See cause of Blood Disorder

Blood Pressure Alteration

See Hypertension; Hypotension; HTN (Hypertension)

Blood Sugar Control

Risk for unstable blood **Glucose** (See **Glucose,** unstable blood, risk for, Section II)

Blood Transfusion

Anxiety r/t possibility of harm from transfusion

See Anemia

Body Dysmorphic Disorder

Disturbed **Body** image r/t overinvolvement in physical appearance

Body Image Change

Disturbed **Body** image (See **Body** image, disturbed, Section II)

Body Temperature, Altered

Imbalanced **Thermoregulation** (See **Thermoregulation,** imbalanced, Section II)

Bone Marrow Biopsy

Acute **Pain** r/t bone marrow aspiration

Fear r/t unknown outcome of results of biopsy

Ineffective **Health** maintenance r/t deficient knowledge of expectations after procedure, disease treatment after biopsy

See disease necessitating bone marrow biopsy (e.g., Leukemia)

Borderline Personality Disorder

Anxiety r/t perceived threat to self-concept

Defensive **Coping** r/t difficulty with relationships, inability to accept blame for own behavior

Disturbed **Thought** processes r/t poor reality testing

Ineffective **Coping** r/t use of maladjusted defense mechanisms (e.g., projection, denial)

Ineffective family **Therapeutic** regimen management r/t manipulative behavior of client

Powerlessness r/t lifestyle of helplessness

Risk for **Caregiver** role strain: Risk factors: inability of care receiver to accept criticism, care receiver taking advantage of others to meet own needs or having unreasonable expectations

Risk for self-directed **Violence**: Risk factors: feelings of need to punish self, manipulative behavior

Risk for **Self-mutilation**: Risk factors: ineffective coping, feelings of self-hatred

Risk for **Spiritual** distress: Risk factor: poor relationships associated with behaviors attributed to borderline personality disorder

Social isolation r/t immature interests

Boredom

Deficient **Diversional** activity r/t environmental lack of diversional activity

Social isolation r/t altered state of wellness

Botulism

Deficient **Fluid** volume r/t profuse diarrhea

B

Ineffective **Health** maintenance r/t deficient knowledge regarding prevention of botulism, care after episode

Bowel Incontinence

Bowel incontinence r/t decreased awareness of need to defecate, loss of sphincter control, fecal impaction

Bowel Obstruction

Acute **Pain** r/t pressure from distended abdomen

Constipation r/t decreased motility, intestinal obstruction

Deficient **Fluid** volume r/t inadequate fluid volume intake, fluid loss in bowel

Imbalanced **Nutrition**: less than body requirements r/t nausea, vomiting

Bowel Resection

See Abdominal Surgery

Bowel Sounds, Absent or Diminished

Constipation r/t decreased or absent peristalsis

Deficient **Fluid** volume r/t inability to ingest fluids, loss of fluids in bowel

Delayed **Surgical** recovery r/t inability to obtain adequate nutritional status

Bowel Sounds, Hyperactive

Diarrhea r/t increased gastrointestinal motility

Bowel Training

Bowel incontinence r/t loss of control of rectal sphincter

Ineffective **Health** maintenance r/t deficient knowledge regarding treatment of bowel incontinence

Bowel Training, Child

See Toilet Training

BPH (Benign Prostatic Hypertrophy)

Ineffective **Health** maintenance r/t deficient knowledge regarding self-care with prostatic hypertrophy

Insomnia r/t nocturia

Risk for **Infection**: Risk factors: urinary residual after voiding, bacterial invasion of bladder

Risk for urge urinary **Incontinence**: Risk factors: detrusor muscle instability with impaired contractility, involuntary sphincter relaxation

Urinary retention r/t obstruction

See Prostatic Hypertrophy

Bradycardia

Decreased **Cardiac** output r/t slow heart rate supplying inadequate amount of blood for body function

Ineffective **Health** maintenance r/t deficient knowledge of condition, effects of cardiac medications

Ineffective **Tissue** perfusion: cerebral r/t decreased cardiac output secondary to bradycardia, vagal response

Risk for **Injury**: Risk factor: decreased cerebral tissue perfusion

Bradypnea

Ineffective **Breathing** pattern r/t neuromuscular impairment, pain, musculoskeletal impairment, perception or cognitive impairment, anxiety, fatigue or decreased energy, effects of drugs

See cause of Bradypnea

Brain Injury

See Intracranial Pressure, Increased

Brain Surgery

See Craniectomy/Craniotomy

Brain Tumor

Acute **Pain** r/t pressure from tumor

Decreased **Intracranial** adaptive capacity r/t presence of brain tumor

Disturbed **Sensory** perception: specify r/t tumor growth compressing brain tissue

Disturbed **Thought** processes r/t altered circulation, destruction of brain tissue

Fear r/t threat to well-being

Grieving r/t potential loss of physiosocial-psychosocial well-being

Risk for **Injury**: Risk factors: sensory-perceptual alterations, weakness

See Cancer; Chemotherapy; Child with Chronic Condition; Craniectomy/Craniotomy; Hospitalized Child; Radiation Therapy; Terminally Ill Child, Adolescent; Terminally Ill Child, Infant/Toddler; Terminally Ill Child, Preschool Child; Terminally Ill Child, School-Age Child/Preadolescent; Terminally Ill Child/Death of Child, Parent

Braxton Hicks Contractions

Activity intolerance r/t increased perception of contractions with increased gestation

Anxiety r/t uncertainty about beginning labor

Fatigue r/t lack of sleep

Ineffective **Sexuality** pattern r/t fear of contractions

Insomnia r/t contractions when lying down

Stress urinary **Incontinence** r/t increased pressure on bladder with contractions

Breast Biopsy

Fear r/t potential for diagnosis of cancer

Ineffective **Health** maintenance r/t deficient knowledge regarding appropriate postoperative care of breasts

Risk for **Spiritual** distress: Risk factor: fear of diagnosis of cancer

Breast Cancer

Chronic **Sorrow** r/t diagnosis of cancer, loss of body integrity

Death **Anxiety** r/t diagnosis of cancer

Fear r/t diagnosis of cancer

Ineffective **Coping** r/t treatment, prognosis

Risk for **Spiritual** distress: Risk factor: fear of diagnosis of cancer

Sexual dysfunction r/t loss of body part, partner's reaction to loss

See Cancer; Chemotherapy; Mastectomy; Radiation Therapy

Breast Lumps

Fear r/t potential for diagnosis of cancer

Ineffective **Health** maintenance r/t deficient knowledge regarding appropriate care of breasts

Breast Pumping

Ineffective **Health** maintenance r/t deficient knowledge regarding breast milk expression and storage

Risk for impaired **Skin** integrity: Risk factor: high suction

Risk for **Infection**: Risk factors: contaminated breast pump parts, incomplete emptying of breast

Breastfeeding, Effective

Effective **Breastfeeding** (See **Breastfeeding,** effective, Section II)

Breastfeeding, Ineffective

Ineffective **Breastfeeding** (See **Breastfeeding,** ineffective, Section II)

See Painful Breasts, Sore Nipples; Painful Breasts, Engorgement, Infant Feeding Pattern, Ineffective

Breastfeeding, Interrupted

Interrupted **Breastfeeding** (See **Breastfeeding,** interrupted, Section II)

Breath Sounds, Decreased or Absent

See Atelectasis; Pneumothorax

Breathing Pattern Alteration

Ineffective **Breathing** pattern r/t neuromuscular impairment, pain, musculoskeletal impairment, perception or cognitive impairment, anxiety, decreased energy or fatigue

Breech Birth

Anxiety: maternal r/t threat to self, infant

Fear: maternal r/t danger to infant, self

Impaired **Gas** exchange: fetal r/t compressed umbilical cord

Ineffective **Tissue** perfusion r/t compressed umbilical cord

Risk for **Aspiration**: fetal Risk factor: birth of body before head

Risk for delayed **Development**: Risk factor: compressed umbilical cord

Risk for impaired **Tissue** integrity: fetal Risk factor: difficult birth

Risk for impaired **Tissue** integrity: maternal: Risk factor: difficult birth

Bronchitis

Anxiety r/t potential chronic condition

Health-seeking behavior r/t wish to stop smoking

Ineffective **Airway** clearance r/t excessive thickened mucus secretion

Ineffective **Health** maintenance r/t deficient knowledge regarding care of condition

Bronchopulmonary Dysplasia

Activity intolerance r/t imbalance between oxygen supply and demand

Excess **Fluid** volume r/t sodium and water retention

Imbalanced **Nutrition**: less than body requirements r/t poor feeding, increased caloric needs as a result of increased work of breathing

See Child with Chronic Condition; Hospitalized Child; Respiratory Conditions of the Neonate

Bronchoscopy

Risk for **Aspiration**: Risk factor: temporary loss of gag reflex

Risk for **Injury**: Risk factors: complication of pneumothorax, laryngeal edema, hemorrhage (if biopsy done)

Bruits, Carotid

Ineffective **Tissue** perfusion: cerebral r/t interruption of carotid blood flow

Risk for **Injury**: Risk factors: loss of motor, sensory, visual function

Bryant's Traction

See Traction and Casts

Buck's Traction

See Traction and Casts

Buerger's Disease

See Peripheral Vascular Disease

Bulimia

Chronic low **Self-esteem** r/t lack of positive feedback

Defensive **Coping** r/t eating disorder

Diarrhea r/t laxative abuse

Disturbed **Body** image r/t misperception about actual appearance, body weight

Fear r/t food ingestion, weight gain

Imbalanced **Nutrition**: less than body requirements r/t induced vomiting, excessive exercise

Compromised family **Coping** r/t chronically unresolved feelings of guilt, anger, hostility

Noncompliance r/t negative feelings toward treatment regimen

Powerlessness r/t urge to purge self after eating

See Maturational Issues, Adolescent

Bunion

Ineffective **Health** maintenance r/t deficient knowledge regarding appropriate care of feet

Bunionectomy

Impaired physical **Mobility** r/t sore foot

Impaired **Walking** r/t pain associated with surgery

Ineffective **Health** maintenance r/t deficient knowledge regarding postoperative care of feet

Risk for **Infection**: Risk factors: surgical incision, advanced age

Burns

Acute **Pain** r/t burn injury, treatments

Grieving r/t loss of bodily function, loss of future hopes and plans

Deficient **Diversional** activity r/t long-term hospitalization

Delayed **Surgical** recovery r/t ineffective tissue perfusion

Disturbed **Body** image r/t altered physical appearance

Fear r/t pain from treatments, possible permanent disfigurement

Hypothermia r/t impaired skin integrity

Imbalanced **Nutrition**: less than body requirements r/t increased metabolic needs, anorexia, protein and fluid loss

Impaired physical **Mobility** r/t pain, musculoskeletal impairment, contracture formation

Impaired **Skin** integrity r/t injury of skin

Ineffective **Tissue** perfusion: peripheral r/t circumferential burns, impaired arterial/venous circulation

Post-trauma syndrome r/t life-threatening event

Risk for deficient **Fluid** volume: Risk factors: loss from skin surface, fluid shift

Risk for ineffective **Airway** clearance: Risk factors: potential tracheobronchial obstruction, edema

Risk for **Infection**: Risk factors: loss of intact skin, trauma, invasive sites

Risk for **Peripheral** neurovascular dysfunction: Risk factor: eschar formation with circumferential burn

Risk for **Post-trauma** syndrome: Risk factors: perception, duration of event that caused burns

See Hospitalized Child; Safety, Childhood

Bursitis

Acute **Pain** r/t inflammation in joint

Impaired physical **Mobility** r/t inflammation in joint

Bypass Graft

See Coronary Artery Bypass Grafting

C

Cachexia

Adult **Failure** to thrive r/t imbalanced nutrition: less than body requirements

Imbalanced **Nutrition**: less than body requirements r/t inability to ingest food because of biological factors

Ineffective **Protection** r/t inadequate nutrition

Calcium Alteration

See Hypercalcemia; Hypocalcemia

Cancer

Activity intolerance r/t side effects of treatment, weakness from cancer

Chronic **Pain** r/t metastatic cancer

Chronic **Sorrow** r/t chronic illness of cancer

Compromised family **Coping** r/t prolonged disease or disability progression that exhausts supportive ability of significant others

Constipation r/t side effects of medication, altered nutrition, decreased activity

Death **Anxiety** r/t unresolved issues regarding dying

Decisional **Conflict** r/t selection of treatment choices, continuation or discontinuation of treatment, "do not resuscitate" decision

Disturbed **Body** image r/t side effects of treatment, cachexia

Fear r/t serious threat to well-being

Grieving r/t potential loss of significant others, high risk for infertility

Hopelessness r/t loss of control, terminal illness

Imbalanced **Nutrition**: less than body requirements r/t loss of appetite, difficulty swallowing, side effects of chemotherapy, obstruction by tumor

Impaired **Oral** mucous membranes r/t chemotherapy, effects of radiation, oral pH changes, decreased oral secretions

Impaired physical **Mobility** r/t weakness, neuromusculoskeletal impairment, pain

Impaired **Skin** integrity r/t immunological deficit, immobility

Ineffective **Coping** r/t personal vulnerability in situational crisis, terminal illness

Ineffective **Denial** r/t complicated grieving process

Ineffective **Health** maintenance r/t deficient knowledge regarding prescribed treatment

Ineffective **Protection** r/t cancer suppressing immune system

Ineffective **Role** performance r/t change in physical capacity, inability to resume prior role

Insomnia r/t anxiety, pain

Powerlessness r/t treatment, progression of disease

Readiness for enhanced **Spiritual** well-being: desire for harmony with self, others, higher power, God when faced with serious illness

Risk for **Disuse** syndrome: Risk factors: immobility, fatigue

Risk for impaired **Home** maintenance: Risk factor: lack of familiarity with community resources

Risk for **Infection**: Risk factor: inadequate immune system

Risk for **Injury**: Risk factor: bleeding secondary to bone marrow depression

Risk for **Spiritual** distress: Risk factor: physical illness of cancer

Self-care deficit: specify r/t pain, intolerance to activity, decreased strength

Social isolation r/t hospitalization, lifestyle changes

Spiritual distress r/t test of spiritual beliefs

See Chemotherapy; Child with Chronic Condition; Hospitalized Child; Radiation Therapy; Terminally Ill Child, Adolescent; Terminally Ill Child, Infant/Toddler; Terminally Ill Child, Preschool Child; Terminally Ill Child, School-Age Child/Preadolescent; Terminally Ill Child/Death of Child, Parent

Candidiasis, Oral

Impaired **Oral** mucous membranes r/t overgrowth of infectious agent, depressed immune function

Ineffective **Health** maintenance r/t deficient knowledge regarding care of infected mouth

Capillary Refill Time, Prolonged

Impaired **Gas** exchange r/t ventilation perfusion imbalance

Ineffective **Tissue** perfusion: peripheral r/t interruption of arterial or venous flow

See Shock

Carbon Monoxide Poisoning

See Smoke Inhalation

Cardiac Arrest

Post-trauma syndrome r/t sustaining serious life event

See cause of Cardiac Arrest

Cardiac Catheterization

Anxiety r/t invasive procedure, uncertainty of outcome of procedure

Decreased **Cardiac** output r/t ventricular ischemia, dysrhythmia

Ineffective **Health** maintenance r/t deficient knowledge regarding procedure, postprocedure care, treatment and prevention of coronary artery disease

Risk for ineffective **Tissue** perfusion: Risk factors: impaired arterial or venous circulation

Risk for **Injury**: hematoma: Risk factor: invasive procedure

Risk for **Peripheral** neurovascular dysfunction: Risk factor: vascular obstruction

Cardiac Disorders

Decreased **Cardiac** output r/t cardiac disorder

See specific cardiac disorder

Cardiac Disorders in Pregnancy

Activity intolerance r/t cardiac pathophysiology, increased demand because of pregnancy, weakness, fatigue

Anxiety r/t unknown outcomes of pregnancy, family well-being

Compromised family **Coping** r/t prolonged hospitalization or maternal incapacitation that exhausts supportive capacity of significant others

Death **Anxiety** r/t potential danger of condition

Fatigue r/t metabolic, psychological, and emotional demands

Fear r/t potential maternal effects, potential poor fetal or maternal outcome

Ineffective **Coping** r/t personal vulnerability

Ineffective **Health** maintenance r/t deficient knowledge regarding treatment, restrictions with cardiac disorder

Ineffective **Role** performance r/t changes in lifestyle, expectations from disease process with superimposed pregnancy

Interrupted **Family** processes r/t hospitalization, maternal incapacitation, changes in roles

Powerlessness r/t illness-related regimen

Risk for delayed **Development**: Risk factor: poor maternal oxygenation

Risk for disproportionate **Growth**: Risk factor: poor maternal oxygenation

Risk for excess **Fluid** volume: Risk factors: compromised regulatory mechanism with increased afterload, preload, circulating blood volume

Risk for imbalanced **Fluid** volume: Risk factor: sudden changes in circulation after delivery of placenta

Risk for impaired **Gas** exchange: Risk factor: pulmonary edema

Risk for ineffective **Tissue** perfusion: fetal: Risk factor: poor maternal oxygenation

Risk for **Spiritual** distress: Risk factor: fear of diagnosis for self and infant

Situational low **Self-esteem** r/t situational crisis, pregnancy

Social isolation r/t limitations of activity, bed rest or hospitalization, separation from family and friends

Cardiac Dysrhythmia

See Dysrhythmia

Cardiac Output Decrease

Decreased **Cardiac** output r/t cardiac dysfunction

C

Cardiac Tamponade

Decreased **Cardiac** output r/t fluid in pericardial sac

See Pericarditis

Cardiogenic Shock

Decreased **Cardiac** output r/t decreased myocardial contractility, dysrhythmia

See Shock

Caregiver Role Strain

Caregiver role strain (See **Caregiver** role strain, Section II)

Carious Teeth

See Cavities in Teeth

Carotid Endarterectomy

Fear r/t surgery in vital area

Ineffective **Health** maintenance r/t deficient knowledge regarding postoperative care

Risk for ineffective **Airway** clearance: Risk factor: hematoma compressing trachea

Risk for ineffective **Tissue** perfusion: cerebral: Risk factors: hemorrhage, clot formation

Risk for **Injury**: Risk factor: possible hematoma formation

Carpal Tunnel Syndrome

Chronic **Pain** r/t unrelieved pressure on median nerve

Impaired physical **Mobility** r/t neuromuscular impairment

Self-care deficit: bathing, hygiene, dressing, grooming, feeding r/t pain

Carpopedal Spasm

See Hypocalcemia

Casts

Deficient **Diversional** activity r/t physical limitations from cast

Ineffective **Health** maintenance r/t deficient knowledge regarding cast care, personal care with cast

Impaired physical **Mobility** r/t limb immobilization

Impaired **Walking** r/t cast(s) on lower extremities, fracture of bones

Risk for impaired **Skin** integrity: Risk factor: unrelieved pressure on skin

Risk for **Peripheral** neurovascular dysfunction: Risk factor: mechanical compression from cast

Self-care deficit: bathing, hygiene, dressing, grooming, feeding r/t presence of cast(s) on upper extremities

Self-care deficit: toileting r/t presence of cast(s) on lower extremities

Cataract Extraction

Anxiety r/t threat of permanent vision loss, surgical procedure

Disturbed **Sensory** perception: vision r/t edema from surgery

Ineffective **Health** maintenance r/t deficient knowledge regarding postoperative restrictions

Risk for **Injury**: Risk factors: increased intraocular pressure, accommodation to new visual field

See Vision Impairment

Cataracts

Disturbed **Sensory** perception: vision r/t altered sensory input

See Vision Impairment

Catatonic Schizophrenia

Imbalanced **Nutrition**: less than body requirements r/t decrease in outside stimulation, loss of perception of hunger, resistance to instructions to eat

Impaired **Memory** r/t cognitive impairment

Impaired physical **Mobility** r/t cognitive impairment, maintenance of rigid posture, inappropriate or bizarre postures

Impaired verbal **Communication** r/t muteness

Social isolation r/t inability to communicate, immobility

See Schizophrenia

Catheterization, Urinary

Ineffective **Health** maintenance r/t deficient knowledge of normal sensation of catheter in place, care of catheter

Risk for **Infection**: Risk factor: invasive procedure

Cavities in Teeth

Impaired **Dentition** r/t ineffective oral hygiene, barriers to self-care, economic barriers to professional care, nutritional deficits, dietary habits

Cellulitis

Acute **Pain** r/t inflammatory changes in tissues from infection

Impaired **Skin** integrity r/t inflammatory process damaging skin

Ineffective **Health** maintenance r/t lack of knowledge regarding prevention of further incidences of infection

Ineffective **Tissue** perfusion: peripheral r/t edema

Cellulitis, Periorbital

Acute **Pain** r/t edema and inflammation of skin/tissues

Disturbed **Sensory** perception: visual r/t decreased visual fields secondary to edema of eyelids

Hyperthermia r/t infectious process

Impaired **Skin** integrity r/t inflammation or infection of skin, tissues

See Hospitalized Child

Central Line Insertion

Ineffective **Health** maintenance r/t deficient knowledge regarding precautions to take when central line is in place

Risk for **Infection**: Risk factor: invasive procedure

Cerebral Aneurysm

See Craniectomy/Craniotomy; Intracranial Pressure, Increased; Subarachnoid Hemorrhage

Cerebral Palsy

Chronic **Sorrow** r/t presence of chronic disability

Deficient **Diversional** activity r/t physical impairments, limitations on ability to participate in recreational activities

Imbalanced **Nutrition**: less than body requirements r/t spasticity, feeding or swallowing difficulties

Impaired physical **Mobility** r/t spasticity, neuromuscular impairment or weakness

Impaired **Social** interaction r/t impaired communication skills, limited physical activity, perceived differences from peers

Impaired verbal **Communication** r/t impaired ability to articulate or speak words because of facial muscle involvement

Risk for **Falls**: Risk factor: impaired physical mobility

Risk for impaired **Parenting**: Risk factor: caring for child with overwhelming needs resulting from chronic change in health status

Risk for **Injury**: Risk factors: muscle weakness, inability to control spasticity

Risk for **Spiritual** distress: Risk factors: psychological stress associated with chronic illness

Self-care deficit: specify r/t neuromuscular impairments, sensory deficits

See Child with Chronic Condition

Cerebrovascular Accident

See CVA (Cerebrovascular Accident)

C

Cervicitis

Ineffective **Health** maintenance r/t deficient knowledge regarding care and prevention of condition

Ineffective **Sexuality** pattern r/t abstinence during acute stage

Risk for **Infection**: Risk factors: spread of infection, recurrence of infection

Cesarean Delivery

Acute **Pain** r/t surgical incision

Anxiety r/t unmet expectations for childbirth, unknown outcome of surgery

Disturbed **Body** image r/t surgery, unmet expectations for childbirth

Fear r/t perceived threat to own well-being

Impaired physical **Mobility** r/t pain

Ineffective **Health** maintenance r/t deficient knowledge regarding postoperative care

Ineffective **Role** performance r/t unmet expectations for childbirth

Interrupted **Family** processes r/t unmet expectations for childbirth

Risk for deficient **Fluid** volume: Risk factor: increased blood loss from surgery

Risk for imbalanced **Fluid** volume: Risk factor: loss of blood

Risk for **Infection**: Risk factors: surgical incision, stasis of respiratory secretions as a result of general anesthesia

Risk for **Urinary** retention: Risk factor: regional anesthesia

Situational low **Self-esteem** r/t inability to deliver child vaginally

Chemical Dependence

See Alcoholism; Drug Abuse

Chemotherapy

Death **Anxiety** r/t chemotherapy not accomplishing desired results

Delayed **Surgical** recovery r/t compromised immune system

Disturbed **Body** image r/t loss of weight, loss of hair

Fatigue r/t disease process, anemia, drug effects

Imbalanced **Nutrition**: less than body requirements r/t side effects of chemotherapy

Impaired **Oral** mucous membranes r/t effects of chemotherapy

Ineffective **Health** maintenance r/t deficient knowledge regarding action, side effects, way to integrate chemotherapy into lifestyle

Ineffective **Protection** r/t suppressed immune system, decreased platelets

Nausea r/t effects of chemotherapy

Risk for deficient **Fluid** volume: Risk factors: vomiting, diarrhea

Risk for ineffective **Tissue** perfusion: Risk factor: anemia

Risk for **Infection**: Risk factor: immunosuppression

See Cancer

Chest Pain

Acute **Pain** r/t myocardial injury, ischemia

Decreased **Cardiac** output r/t ventricular ischemia

Fear r/t potential threat of death

See Angina Pectoris; MI (Myocardial Infarction)

Chest Tubes

Acute **Pain** r/t presence of chest tubes, injury

Impaired **Gas** exchange r/t decreased functional lung tissue

Ineffective **Breathing** pattern r/t asymmetrical lung expansion secondary to pain

Risk for **Injury**: Risk factor: presence of invasive chest tube

Cheyne-Stokes Respiration

Ineffective **Breathing** pattern r/t critical illness

See cause of Cheyne-Stokes Respiration

CHF (Congestive Heart Failure)

Activity intolerance r/t weakness, fatigue

Constipation r/t activity intolerance

Decreased **Cardiac** output r/t impaired cardiac function

Excess **Fluid** volume r/t impaired excretion of sodium and water

Fatigue r/t disease process

Fear r/t threat to one's own well-being

Impaired **Gas** exchange r/t excessive fluid in interstitial space of lungs, alveoli

Ineffective **Health** maintenance r/t deficient knowledge regarding care of disease

Powerlessness r/t illness-related regimen

See Child with Chronic Condition; Congenital Heart Disease/Cardiac Anomalies; Hospitalized Child

Chickenpox

See Communicable Diseases, Childhood

Child Abuse

Acute **Pain** r/t physical injuries

Chronic low **Self-esteem** r/t lack of positive feedback, excessive negative feedback

Deficient **Diversional** activity r/t diminished or absent environmental or personal stimuli

Delayed **Growth** and development: regression versus delayed r/t diminished or absent environmental stimuli, inadequate caretaking, inconsistent responsiveness by caretaker

Fear r/t threat of punishment for perceived wrongdoing

Imbalanced **Nutrition**: less than body requirements r/t inadequate caretaking

Impaired **Parenting** r/t psychological impairment, physical or emotional abuse of parent, substance abuse, unrealistic expectations of child

Impaired **Skin** integrity r/t altered nutritional state, physical abuse

Ineffective community **Therapeutic** regimen management r/t deficits in community regarding prevention of child abuse

Insomnia r/t hypervigilance, anxiety

Interrupted **Family** process: alcoholism r/t inadequate coping skills

Post-trauma syndrome r/t physical abuse, incest, rape, molestation

Risk for delayed **Development**: Risk factors: shaken baby syndrome, abuse

Risk for disproportionate **Growth**: Risk factor: abuse

Risk for **Poisoning**: Risk factors: inadequate safeguards, lack of proper safety precautions, accessibility of illicit substances because of impaired home maintenance

Risk for **Suffocation**: Risk factors: unattended child, unsafe environment

Risk for **Trauma**: Risk factors: inadequate precautions, cognitive or emotional difficulties

Social isolation: family imposed r/t fear of disclosure of family dysfunction and abuse

Child Neglect

See Child Abuse; Failure to Thrive, Nonorganic

Child with Chronic Condition

Activity intolerance r/t fatigue associated with chronic illness

Chronic low **Self-esteem** r/t actual or perceived differences; peer acceptance; decreased ability to participate in physical, school, and social activities

C

Chronic **Pain** r/t physical, biological, chemical, or psychological factors

Chronic **Sorrow** r/t developmental stages and missed opportunities or milestones that bring comparisons with social or personal norms, unending caregiving as reminder of loss

Compromised family **Coping** r/t prolonged overconcern for child; distortion of reality regarding child's health problem, including extreme denial about its existence or severity

Decisional **Conflict** r/t treatment options, conflicting values

Deficient **Diversional** activity r/t immobility, monotonous environment, frequent or lengthy treatments, reluctance to participate, self-imposed social isolation

Deficient **Knowledge** r/t knowledge or skill acquisition regarding health practices, acceptance of limitations, promotion of maximal potential of child, self-actualization of rest of family

Delayed **Growth** and development r/t regression or lack of progression toward developmental milestones as a result of frequent or prolonged hospitalization, inadequate or inappropriate stimulation, cerebral insult, chronic illness, effects of physical disability, prescribed dependence

Disabled family **Coping** r/t prolonged disease or disability progression that exhausts supportive capacity of significant others

Hopelessness: child r/t prolonged activity restriction, long-term stress, lack of involvement in or passively allowing care as a result of parental overprotection

Imbalanced **Nutrition**: less than body requirements r/t anorexia, fatigue from physical exertion

Imbalanced **Nutrition**: more than body requirements r/t effects of steroid medications on appetite

Impaired **Home** maintenance r/t overtaxed family members (e.g., exhausted, anxious)

Impaired **Social** interaction r/t developmental lag or delay, perceived differences

Ineffective **Coping**: child r/t situational or maturational crises

Ineffective **Health** maintenance r/t exhausting family resources (finances, physical energy, support systems)

Ineffective **Sexuality** pattern: parental r/t disrupted relationship with sexual partner

Insomnia: child or parent r/t time-intensive treatments, exacerbation of condition, 24-hour care needs

Interrupted **Family** processes r/t intermittent situational crisis of illness, disease, hospitalization

Parental role **Conflict** r/t separation from child as a result of chronic illness, home care of child with special needs, interruptions of family life resulting from home care regimen

Powerlessness: child r/t health care environment, illness-related regimen, lifestyle of learned helplessness

Readiness for enhanced family **Coping** r/t impact of crisis on family values, priorities, goals, or relationships; changes in family choices to optimize wellness

Risk for delayed **Development**: Risk factor: chronic illness

Risk for disproportionate **Growth**: Risk factor: chronic illness

Risk for impaired **Parenting**: Risk factors: impaired or disrupted bonding, caring for child with perceived overwhelming care needs

Risk for **Infection**: Risk factor: debilitating physical condition

Social isolation: family r/t actual or perceived social stigmatization, complex care requirements

Childbirth

See Labor, Normal; Postpartum, Normal Care

Chills

Hyperthermia r/t infectious process

Chlamydia Infection

See STD (Sexually Transmitted Disease)

Chloasma

Disturbed **Body** image r/t change in skin color

Choking or Coughing with Feeding

Impaired **Swallowing** r/t neuromuscular impairment

Risk for **Aspiration**: Risk factors: depressed cough and gag reflexes

Cholecystectomy

Acute **Pain** r/t trauma from surgery

Imbalanced **Nutrition**: less than body requirements r/t high metabolic needs, decreased ability to digest fatty foods

Ineffective **Health** maintenance r/t deficient knowledge regarding postoperative care

Risk for deficient **Fluid** volume: Risk factors: restricted intake, nausea, vomiting

Risk for ineffective **Breathing** pattern: Risk factor: proximity of incision to lungs, resulting in pain with deep breathing

See Abdominal Surgery

Cholelithiasis

Acute **Pain** r/t obstruction of bile flow, inflammation in gallbladder

Imbalanced **Nutrition**: less than body requirements r/t anorexia, nausea, vomiting

Ineffective **Health** maintenance r/t deficient knowledge regarding care of disease

Chorioamnionitis

Anxiety r/t threat to self and infant

Grieving r/t guilt about potential loss of ideal pregnancy and birth

Hyperthermia r/t infectious process

Risk for delayed **Growth** and development: Risk factor: risk of preterm birth

Risk for **Infection** transmission from mother to fetus: Risk factor: infection in fetal environment

Situational low **Self-esteem** r/t guilt about threat to infant's health

Chronic Confusion

See Confusion, Chronic

Chronic Lymphocytic Leukemia

See Cancer; Chemotherapy; Leukemia

Chronic Obstructive Pulmonary Disease

See COPD (Chronic Obstructive Pulmonary Disease)

Chronic Pain

See Pain, Chronic

Chronic Renal Failure

See Renal Failure

Chvostek's Sign

See Hypocalcemia

Circumcision

Acute **Pain** r/t surgical intervention

Ineffective **Health** maintenance r/t deficient knowledge (parental) regarding care of surgical area

Risk for deficient **Fluid** volume: Risk factor: hemorrhage

Risk for **Infection**: Risk factor: surgical wound

C

Cirrhosis

Chronic low **Self-esteem** r/t chronic illness

Chronic **Pain** r/t liver enlargement

Chronic **Sorrow** r/t presence of chronic illness

Diarrhea r/t dietary changes, medications

Disturbed **Thought** processes r/t chronic organic disorder with increased ammonia levels, substance abuse

Fatigue r/t malnutrition

Imbalanced **Nutrition**: less than body requirements r/t loss of appetite, nausea, vomiting

Ineffective **Health** maintenance r/t deficient knowledge regarding correlation between lifestyle habits and disease process

Ineffective management of **Therapeutic** regimen r/t denial of severity of illness

Ineffective **Protection** r/t risk of impaired blood coagulation, bleeding from portal hypertension

Nausea r/t irritation to gastrointestinal system

Risk for deficient **Fluid** volume: hemorrhage: Risk factor: abnormal bleeding from esophagus

Risk for impaired **Oral** mucous membranes: Risk factors: altered nutrition, inadequate oral care

Risk for impaired **Skin** integrity: Risk factors: altered nutritional state, altered metabolic state

Risk for **Injury**: Risk factors: substance intoxication, potential delirium tremens

Cleft Lip/Cleft Palate

Acute **Pain** r/t surgical correction, elbow restraints

Chronic **Sorrow** r/t birth of child with congenital defect

Fear: parental r/t special care needs, surgery

Grieving r/t loss of perfect child

Impaired **Oral** mucous membranes r/t surgical correction

Impaired physical **Mobility** r/t imposed restricted activity, use of elbow restraints

Impaired **Skin** integrity r/t incomplete joining of lip, palate ridges

Impaired verbal **Communication** r/t inadequate palate function, possible hearing loss from infected eustachian tubes

Ineffective **Airway** clearance r/t common feeding and breathing passage, postoperative laryngeal, incisional edema

Ineffective **Breastfeeding** r/t infant anomaly

Ineffective **Health** maintenance r/t lack of parental knowledge regarding feeding techniques, wound care, use of elbow restraints

Ineffective **Infant** feeding pattern r/t cleft lip, cleft palate

Risk for **Aspiration**: Risk factor: common feeding and breathing passage

Risk for deficient **Fluid** volume: Risk factor: inability to take liquids in usual manner

Risk for delayed **Development**: Risk factor: inadequate nutrition resulting from difficulty feeding

Risk for disproportionate **Growth**: Risk factor: inability to feed with normal techniques

Risk for disturbed **Body** image: Risk factors: disfigurement, speech impediment

Risk for **Infection**: Risk factors: invasive procedure, disruption of eustachian tube development, aspiration

Clotting Disorder

Fear r/t threat to well-being

Ineffective **Health** maintenance r/t deficient knowledge regarding treatment of disorder

Ineffective **Protection** r/t clotting disorder

Risk for deficient **Fluid** volume: Risk factor: uncontrolled bleeding

See Anticoagulant Therapy; DIC (Disseminated Intravascular Coagulation); Hemophilia

Cocaine Abuse

Disturbed **Thought** processes r/t excessive stimulation of nervous system by cocaine

Ineffective **Breathing** pattern r/t drug effect on respiratory center

Ineffective **Coping** r/t inability to deal with life stresses

See Drug Abuse; Substance Abuse

Cocaine Baby

See Crack Baby; Infant of Substance-Abusing Mother

Codependency

Caregiver role strain r/t codependency

Decisional **Conflict** r/t support system deficit

Ineffective **Coping** r/t inadequate support systems

Ineffective **Denial** r/t unmet self-needs

Impaired verbal **Communication** r/t psychological barriers

Powerlessness r/t lifestyle of helplessness

Cognitive Deficit

Disturbed **Thought** processes r/t neurological impairment

Cold, Viral

Readiness for enhanced **Comfort**: verbalizes desire to enhance comfort (See **Comfort,** readiness for enhanced in Section III)

Ineffective **Health** maintenance r/t deficient knowledge regarding care of viral condition, prevention of further infections

Colectomy

Acute **Pain** r/t recent surgery

Constipation r/t decreased activity, decreased fluid intake

Imbalanced **Nutrition**: less than body requirements r/t high metabolic needs, decreased ability to ingest or digest food

Ineffective **Health** maintenance r/t deficient knowledge regarding procedure, postoperative care

Risk for **Infection**: Risk factor: invasive procedure

See Abdominal Surgery

Colitis

Acute **Pain** r/t inflammation in colon

Deficient **Fluid** volume r/t frequent stools

Diarrhea r/t inflammation in colon

See Crohn's Disease; Inflammatory Bowel Disease

Collagen Disease

See specific disease (e.g., Lupus Erythematosus; JRA [Juvenile Rheumatoid Arthritis]); Congenital Heart Disease/Cardiac Anomalies

Colostomy

Disturbed **Body** image r/t presence of stoma, daily care of fecal material

Ineffective **Health** maintenance r/t deficient knowledge regarding care of stoma, integrating colostomy care into lifestyle

Ineffective **Sexuality** pattern r/t altered body image, self-concept

Risk for **Constipation**: Risk factor: inappropriate diet

Risk for **Diarrhea**: Risk factor: inappropriate diet

Risk for impaired **Skin** integrity: Risk factor: irritation from bowel contents

Risk for **Social** isolation: Risk factor: anxiety about appearance of stoma and possible leakage

C

Colporrhaphy, Anterior

See Vaginal Hysterectomy

Coma

Death **Anxiety**: significant others r/t unknown outcome of coma state

Disturbed **Thought** processes r/t neurological changes

Ineffective family **Therapeutic** regimen management r/t complexity of therapeutic regimen

Interrupted **Family** processes r/t illness or disability of family member

Risk for **Aspiration**: Risk factors: impaired swallowing, loss of cough or gag reflex

Risk for **Disuse** syndrome: Risk factor: altered level of consciousness impairing mobility

Risk for impaired **Oral** mucous membranes: Risk factor: dry mouth

Risk for impaired **Skin** integrity: Risk factor: immobility

Risk for **Injury**: Risk factor: potential seizure activity

Risk for **Spiritual** distress: significant others: Risk factors: loss of ability to relate to loved one, unknown outcome of coma

Self-care deficit: specify r/t neuromuscular impairment

Total urinary **Incontinence** r/t neurological dysfunction

See cause of Coma

Comfort, Loss of

Readiness for enhanced **Comfort** (See **Comfort,** readiness for enhanced, Section II)

Pruritus r/t dry skin, inflammation of skin

Communicable Diseases, Childhood (e.g., Measles, Mumps, Rubella, Chickenpox, Scabies, Lice, Impetigo)

Acute **Pain** r/t impaired skin integrity, edema

Deficient **Diversional** activity r/t imposed isolation from peers, disruption in usual play activities, fatigue, activity intolerance

Ineffective **Health** maintenance r/t nonadherence to appropriate immunization schedules, lack of prevention of transmission of infection

Pruritus r/t inflammation or infection of skin, subdermal organisms

Risk for **Infection**: transmission to others: Risk factor: contagious organisms

See Meningitis/Encephalitis; Respiratory Infections, Acute Childhood; Reye's Syndrome

Communication

Readiness for enhanced **Communication** (See **Communication,** readiness for enhanced, Section II)

Communication Problems

Impaired verbal **Communication** (See **Communication,** impaired verbal, Section II)

Community Coping

Ineffective community **Coping** (See **Coping,** ineffective community, Section II)

Readiness for enhanced community **Coping** r/t community sense of power to manage stressors, social supports available, resources available for problem solving

Community Management of Therapeutic Regimen

Ineffective community **Therapeutic** regimen management r/t inadequate community resources

Compartment Syndrome

Acute **Pain** r/t pressure in compromised body part

Fear r/t possible loss of limb, damage to limb

Ineffective **Tissue** perfusion: peripheral r/t increased pressure within compartment

Compulsion

See Obsessive-Compulsive Disorder

Conduction Disorders (Cardiac)

See Dysrhythmia

Confusion, Acute

Acute **Confusion** r/t older than 70 years of age with hospitalization, alcohol abuse, delirium, dementia, drug abuse

Adult **Failure** to thrive r/t confusion

Confusion, Chronic

Adult **Failure** to thrive r/t confusion

Chronic **Confusion** r/t Alzheimer's disease, Korsakoff's psychosis, multiinfarct dementia, cerebrovascular accident, head injury

Disturbed **Thought** processes r/t organic mental disorder, disruption of cerebral arterial blood flow, chemical imbalance, intoxication

Impaired **Memory** r/t fluid and electrolyte imbalance, neurological disturbances, excessive environmental disturbances, anemia, acute or chronic hypoxia, decreased cardiac output

Confusion, Possible

Risk for acute **Confusion** (See **Confusion,** acute, risk for, Section II)

Congenital Heart Disease/ Cardiac Anomalies

ACYANOTIC

Patent ductus arteriosus, atrial/ventricular septal defect, pulmonary stenosis, endocardial cushion defect, aortic valvular stenosis, coarctation of aorta

CYANOTIC

Tetralogy of Fallot, tricuspid atresia, transposition of great vessels, truncus arteriosus, total anomalous pulmonary venous return, hypoplastic left lung

Activity intolerance r/t fatigue, generalized weakness, lack of adequate oxygenation

Decreased **Cardiac** output r/t cardiac dysfunction

Delayed **Growth** and development r/t inadequate oxygen and nutrients to tissues

Excess **Fluid** volume r/t cardiac defect, side effects of medication

Imbalanced **Nutrition**: less than body requirements r/t fatigue, generalized weakness, inability of infant to suck and feed, increased caloric requirements

Impaired **Gas** exchange r/t cardiac defect, pulmonary congestion

Ineffective **Breathing** pattern r/t pulmonary vascular disease

Risk for deficient **Fluid** volume: Risk factor: side effects of diuretics

Risk for delayed **Development**: Risk factor: inadequate oxygen and nutrients to tissues

Risk for disorganized **Infant** behavior: Risk factor: invasive procedures

Risk for disproportionate **Growth**: Risk factor: inadequate oxygen and nutrients to tissues

Risk for ineffective **Thermoregulation**: Risk factor: neonatal age

Risk for **Poisoning**: Risk factor: potential toxicity of cardiac medications

See Child with Chronic Condition; Hospitalized Child

C

Congestive Heart Failure

See CHF (Congestive Heart Failure)

Conjunctivitis

Acute **Pain** r/t inflammatory process

Disturbed **Sensory** perception r/t change in visual acuity resulting from inflammation

Consciousness, Altered Level of

Acute **Confusion** r/t alcohol abuse, delirium, dementia, drug abuse

Adult **Failure** to thrive r/t altered level of consciousness

Chronic **Confusion** r/t multiinfarct dementia, Korsakoff's psychosis, head injury, Alzheimer's disease, cerebrovascular accident

Decreased **Intracranial** adaptive capacity r/t brain injury

Disturbed **Thought** processes r/t neurological changes

Impaired **Memory** r/t neurological disturbances

Ineffective **Tissue** perfusion: cerebral r/t increased intracranial pressure, decreased cerebral perfusion

Risk for **Aspiration**: Risk factors: impaired swallowing, loss of cough or gag reflex

Risk for **Disuse** syndrome: Risk factors: impaired mobility resulting from altered level of consciousness

Risk for impaired **Oral** mucous membranes: Risk factor: dry mouth

Risk for impaired **Skin** integrity: Risk factor: immobility

Self-care deficit: specify r/t neuromuscular impairment

Total urinary **Incontinence** r/t neurological dysfunction

See cause of Altered Level of Consciousness

Constipation

Constipation (See **Constipation,** Section II)

Constipation, Perceived

Perceived **Constipation** (See **Constipation,** perceived, Section II)

Constipation, Risk for

Risk for **Constipation** (See **Constipation,** risk for, Section II)

Contamination

Contamination (See **Contamination,** Section II)

Risk for **Contamination** (See **Contamination,** risk for, Section II)

Continent Ileostomy (Kock Pouch)

Imbalanced **Nutrition**: less than body requirements r/t malabsorption

Ineffective **Coping** r/t stress of disease, exacerbations caused by stress

Ineffective **Health** maintenance r/t deficient knowledge regarding postoperative care

Risk for **Injury**: Risk factors: failure of valve, stomal cyanosis, intestinal obstruction

See Abdominal Surgery

Contraceptive Method

Decisional **Conflict**: method of contraception r/t unclear personal values or beliefs, lack of experience or interference with decision making, lack of relevant information, support system deficit

Health-seeking behaviors r/t requesting information about available and appropriate birth control methods

Ineffective **Sexuality** pattern r/t fear of pregnancy

Conversion Disorder

Anxiety r/t unresolved conflict

Disturbed personal **Identity** r/t overwhelming stress

Hopelessness r/t long-term stress

Risk-prone health **Behavior** r/t multiple stressors

Impaired physical **Mobility** r/t physical conversion symptom

Impaired **Social** interaction r/t altered thought process

Ineffective **Coping** r/t personal vulnerability

Ineffective **Role** performance r/t physical conversion system

Powerlessness r/t lifestyle of helplessness

Risk for **Injury**: Risk factors: physical conversion symptom

Self-esteem disturbance r/t unsatisfactory or inadequate interpersonal relationships

Convulsions

Anxiety r/t concern over controlling convulsions

Impaired **Memory** r/t neurological disturbance

Ineffective **Health** maintenance r/t deficient knowledge regarding need for medication and care during seizure activity

Risk for **Aspiration**: Risk factor: impaired swallowing

Risk for delayed **Development**: Risk factor: seizures

Risk for **Injury**: Risk factor: seizure activity

See Seizure Disorders, Adult; Seizure Disorders, Childhood

COPD (Chronic Obstructive Pulmonary Disease)

Activity intolerance r/t imbalance between oxygen supply and demand

Interrupted **Family** processes r/t role changes

Anxiety r/t breathlessness, change in health status

Chronic low **Self-esteem** r/t chronic illness

Chronic **Sorrow** r/t presence of chronic illness

Death **Anxiety** r/t seriousness of medical condition, difficulty being able to "catch breath," feeling of suffocation

Health-seeking behaviors r/t wishes to stop smoking

Imbalanced **Nutrition**: less than body requirements r/t decreased intake because of dyspnea, unpleasant taste in mouth left by medications

Impaired **Gas** exchange r/t ventilation-perfusion inequality

Impaired **Social** interaction r/t social isolation because of oxygen use, activity intolerance

Ineffective **Airway** clearance r/t bronchoconstriction, increased mucus, ineffective cough, infection

Ineffective **Health** maintenance r/t deficient knowledge regarding care of disease

Noncompliance r/t reluctance to accept responsibility for changing detrimental health practices

Powerlessness r/t progressive nature of disease

Risk for **Infection**: Risk factor: stasis of respiratory secretions

Self-care deficit: specify: r/t fatigue from the increased work of breathing

Sleep deprivation r/t breathing difficulties when lying down

Coping

Readiness for enhanced **Coping** (See **Coping,** readiness for enhanced, Section II)

C

Coping Problems

Defensive **Coping** (See **Coping**, defensive, Section II)

Ineffective **Coping** (See **Coping**, ineffective, Section II)

See Community Coping; Family Problems

Corneal Reflex, Absent

Risk for **Injury**: Risk factors: accidental corneal abrasion, drying of cornea

Corneal Transplant

Risk for **Infection**: Risk factors: invasive procedure, surgery

Readiness for enhanced **Therapeutic** regimen management: describes need to rest and avoid strenuous activities during healing phase

Coronary Artery Bypass Grafting

Acute **Pain** r/t traumatic surgery

Decreased **Cardiac** output r/t dysrhythmia, depressed cardiac function, increased systemic vascular resistance

Deficient **Fluid** volume r/t intraoperative fluid loss, use of diuretics in surgery

Fear r/t outcome of surgical procedure

Ineffective **Health** maintenance r/t deficient knowledge regarding postprocedure care, lifestyle adjustment after surgery

Risk for perioperative positioning **Injury**: Risk factors: hypothermia, extended supine position

Costovertebral Angle Tenderness

See Kidney Stone; Pyelonephritis

Cough, Effective/Ineffective

Ineffective **Airway** clearance r/t decreased energy, fatigue, normal aging changes

See Bronchitis; COPD (Chronic Obstructive Pulmonary Disease); Pulmonary Edema

Crack Abuse

See Cocaine Abuse; Drug Abuse; Substance Abuse

Crack Baby

Disorganized **Infant** behavior r/t prematurity, pain, lack of attachment

Risk for impaired parent/child **Attachment**: Risk factors: parent's inability to meet infant's needs, substance abuse

See Infant of Substance-Abusing Mother

Crackles in Lungs, Coarse

Ineffective **Airway** clearance r/t excessive secretions in airways, ineffective cough

See cause of Coarse Crackles

Crackles in Lungs, Fine

Ineffective **Breathing** pattern r/t fatigue, surgery, decreased energy

See Bronchitis or Pneumonia (if from pulmonary infection); CHF (Congestive Heart Failure) (if cardiac in origin); Infection

Craniectomy/Craniotomy

Acute **Pain** r/t recent surgery, headache

Adult **Failure** to thrive r/t altered cerebral tissue perfusion

Decreased **Intracranial** adaptive capacity r/t brain injury, intracranial hypertension

Fear r/t threat to well-being

Impaired **Memory** r/t neurological surgery

Ineffective **Tissue** perfusion: cerebral r/t cerebral edema, decreased cerebral perfusion, increased intracranial pressure

Risk for disturbed **Thought** processes: Risk factor: neurophysiological changes

Risk for **Injury**: Risk factor: potential confusion

See Coma (if relevant)

Crepitation, Subcutaneous

See Pneumothorax

Crisis

Anxiety r/t threat to or change in environment, health status, interaction patterns, situation, self-concept, or role functioning; threat of death of self or significant other

Compromised family **Coping** r/t situational or developmental crisis

Death **Anxiety** r/t feelings of hopelessness associated with crisis

Disturbed **Energy** field r/t disharmony caused by crisis

Fear r/t crisis situation

Grieving r/t potential significant loss

Ineffective **Coping** r/t situational or maturational crisis

Risk for **Spiritual** distress: Risk factors: physical or psychological stress, natural disasters, situational losses, maturational losses

Situational low **Self-esteem** r/t perception of inability to handle crisis

Spiritual distress r/t intense suffering

Crohn's Disease

Acute **Pain** r/t increased peristalsis

Anxiety r/t change in health status

Diarrhea r/t inflammatory process

Imbalanced **Nutrition**: less than body requirements r/t diarrhea, altered ability to digest and absorb food

Ineffective **Coping** r/t repeated episodes of diarrhea

Ineffective **Health** maintenance r/t deficient knowledge regarding management of disease

Powerlessness r/t chronic disease

Risk for deficient **Fluid** volume: Risk factor: abnormal fluid loss with diarrhea

Croup

See Respiratory Infections, Acute Childhood

Cryosurgery for Retinal Detachment

See Retinal Detachment

Cushing's Syndrome

Activity intolerance r/t fatigue, weakness

Disturbed **Body** image r/t change in appearance from disease process

Excess **Fluid** volume r/t failure of regulatory mechanisms

Ineffective **Health** maintenance r/t deficient knowledge regarding needed care

Risk for **Infection**: Risk factors: suppression of immune system caused by increased cortisol levels

Risk for **Injury**: Risk factors: decreased muscle strength, osteoporosis

Sexual dysfunction r/t loss of libido

CVA (Cerebrovascular Accident)

Adult **Failure** to thrive r/t neurophysiological changes

Anxiety r/t situational crisis, change in physical or emotional condition

Caregiver role strain r/t cognitive problems of care receiver, need for significant home care

Chronic **Confusion** r/t neurological changes

Constipation r/t decreased activity

Disturbed **Body** image r/t chronic illness, paralysis

Disturbed **Sensory** perception: visual, tactile, kinesthetic r/t neurological deficit

Disturbed **Thought** processes r/t neurophysiological changes

Grieving r/t loss of health

Impaired **Home** maintenance r/t neurological disease affecting ability to perform activities of daily living

C

Impaired **Memory** r/t neurological disturbances

Impaired physical **Mobility** r/t loss of balance and coordination

Impaired **Social** interaction r/t limited physical mobility, limited ability to communicate

Impaired **Swallowing** r/t neuromuscular dysfunction

Impaired **Transfer** ability r/t limited physical mobility

Impaired verbal **Communication** r/t pressure damage, decreased circulation to brain in speech center informational sources

Impaired **Walking** r/t loss of balance and coordination

Ineffective **Coping** r/t disability

Ineffective **Health** maintenance r/t deficient knowledge regarding self-care after CVA

Interrupted **Family** process r/t illness, disability of family member

Reflex **Incontinence** r/t loss of feeling to void

Risk for **Aspiration**: Risk factors: impaired swallowing, loss of gag reflex

Risk for **Disuse** syndrome: Risk factor: paralysis

Risk for impaired **Skin** integrity: Risk factor: immobility

Risk for **Injury**: Risk factor: disturbed sensory perception

Self-care deficit: specify r/t decreased strength and endurance, paralysis

Total urinary **Incontinence** r/t neurological dysfunction

Unilateral **Neglect** r/t disturbed perception from neurological damage

Cyanosis, Central with Cyanosis of Oral Mucous Membranes

Impaired **Gas** exchange r/t alveolar-capillary membrane changes

Cyanosis, Peripheral with Cyanosis of Nail Beds

Ineffective **Tissue** perfusion r/t interruption of arterial flow, severe vasoconstriction, cold temperatures

Risk for **Peripheral** neurovascular dysfunction: Risk factor: condition causing disruption in circulation

Cystic Fibrosis

Activity intolerance r/t imbalance between oxygen supply and demand

Anxiety r/t dyspnea, oxygen deprivation

Chronic **Sorrow** r/t presence of chronic disease

Disturbed **Body** image r/t changes in physical appearance, treatment of chronic lung disease (clubbing, barrel chest, home oxygen therapy)

Imbalanced **Nutrition**: less than body requirements r/t anorexia; decreased absorption of nutrients, fat; increased work of breathing

Impaired **Gas** exchange r/t ventilation-perfusion imbalance

Impaired **Home** maintenance r/t extensive daily treatment, medications necessary for health, mist or oxygen tents

Ineffective **Airway** clearance r/t increased production of thick mucus

Risk for **Caregiver** role strain: Risk factors: illness severity of care receiver, unpredictable course of illness

Risk for deficient **Fluid** volume: Risk factors: decreased fluid intake, increased work of breathing

Risk for **Infection**: Risk factors: thick, tenacious mucus; harboring of bacterial organisms; immunocompromised state

Risk for **Spiritual** distress: Risk factor: presence of chronic disease

See Child with Chronic Condition; Hospitalized Child; Terminally Ill Child, Adolescent; Terminally Ill Child, Infant/Toddler; Terminally Ill Child, Preschool Child; Terminally Ill Child, School-Age Child/Preadolescent;

Terminally Ill Child/Death of Child, Parent

Cystitis

Acute **Pain**: dysuria r/t inflammatory process in bladder

Impaired **Urinary** elimination: frequency r/t urinary tract infection

Ineffective **Health** maintenance r/t deficient knowledge regarding methods to treat and prevent urinary tract infections

Risk for urge urinary **Incontinence**: Risk factor: infection in bladder

Cystocele

Ineffective **Health** maintenance r/t deficient knowledge regarding personal care, Kegel exercises to strengthen perineal muscles

Stress urinary **Incontinence** r/t prolapsed bladder

Urge urinary **Incontinence** r/t prolapsed bladder

Cystoscopy

Ineffective **Health** maintenance r/t deficient knowledge regarding postoperative care

Risk for **Infection**: Risk factor: invasive procedure

Urinary retention r/t edema in urethra obstructing flow of urine

D

Deafness

Disturbed **Sensory** perception: auditory r/t alteration in sensory reception, transmission, integration

Impaired verbal **Communication** r/t impaired hearing

Risk for delayed **Development** r/t impaired hearing

Risk for **Injury** r/t alteration in sensory perception

Death

Risk for sudden infant **Death** syndrome (SIDS) (See **Death** syndrome, sudden infant, risk for, Section II)

Death, Oncoming

Grieving r/t loss of significant other

Compromised family **Coping** r/t client's inability to provide support to family

Death **Anxiety** r/t unresolved issues surrounding dying

Fear r/t threat of death

Ineffective **Coping** r/t personal vulnerability

Powerlessness r/t effects of illness, oncoming death

Readiness for enhanced **Spiritual** well-being: desire of client and family to be in harmony with each other and higher power, God

Social isolation r/t altered state of wellness

Spiritual distress r/t intense suffering

See Terminally Ill Child, Adolescent; Terminally Ill Child, Infant/Toddler; Terminally Ill Child, Preschool Child; Terminally Ill Child, School-Age Child/Preadolescent; Terminally Ill Child/Death of Child, Parent

Decisions, Difficulty Making

Decisional **Conflict** r/t support system deficit, perceived threat to value system, multiple or divergent sources of information, lack of relevant information, unclear personal values or beliefs

Readiness for enhanced **Decision** making (See **Decision** making, readiness for enhanced, Section II)

Decubitus Ulcer

See Pressure Ulcer

Deep Vein Thrombosis

See DVT (Deep Vein Thrombosis)

D

Defensive Behavior

Defensive **Coping** r/t nonacceptance of blame, denial of problems or weakness

Ineffective **Denial** r/t inability to face situation realistically

Dehiscence, Abdominal

Acute **Pain** r/t stretching of abdominal wall

Delayed **Surgical** recovery r/t altered circulation, malnutrition, opening in incision

Fear r/t threat of death, severe dysfunction

Impaired **Skin** integrity r/t altered circulation, malnutrition, opening in incision

Impaired **Tissue** integrity r/t exposure of abdominal contents to external environment

Risk for imbalanced **Fluid** volume: Risk factor: altered circulation associated with opening of wound and exposure of abdominal contents

Risk for **Infection**: Risk factor: loss of skin integrity

Dehydration

Deficient **Fluid** volume r/t active fluid volume loss

Impaired **Oral** mucous membranes r/t decreased salivation, fluid deficit

Ineffective **Health** maintenance r/t deficient knowledge regarding treatment and prevention of dehydration

See cause of Dehydration

Delirium

Acute **Confusion** r/t effects of medication, response to hospitalization, alcohol abuse, substance abuse, sensory deprivation or overload

Adult **Failure** to thrive r/t delirium

Disturbed **Thought** processes r/t head trauma, altered metabolic state, substance abuse, sleep deprivation, sensory deprivation or overload

Impaired **Memory** r/t delirium

Risk for **Injury**: Risk factor: altered level of consciousness

Sleep deprivation r/t nightmares

Delirium Tremens (DT)

See Alcohol Withdrawal

Delivery

See Labor, Normal

Delusions

Acute **Confusion** r/t alcohol abuse, delirium, dementia, drug abuse

Adult **Failure** to thrive r/t delusional state

Anxiety r/t content of intrusive thoughts

Disturbed **Thought** processes r/t mental disorder

Impaired verbal **Communication** r/t psychological impairment, delusional thinking

Ineffective **Coping** r/t distortion and insecurity of life events

Risk for other-directed **Violence**: Risk factor: delusional thinking

Risk for self-directed **Violence**: Risk factor: delusional thinking

Dementia

Adult **Failure** to thrive r/t depression, apathy

Chronic **Confusion** r/t neurological dysfunction

Chronic **Sorrow** r/t chronic mental illness

Imbalanced **Nutrition**: less than body requirements r/t psychological impairment

Impaired **Environmental** interpretation syndrome r/t dementia

Impaired **Home** maintenance r/t inadequate support system

Impaired physical **Mobility** r/t neuromuscular impairment

Insomnia r/t neurological impairment, naps during the day

Interrupted **Family** process r/t disability of family member

Risk for **Caregiver** role strain: Risk factors: number of caregiving tasks, duration of caregiving required

Risk for **Falls**: Risk factor: diminished mental status

Risk for impaired **Skin** integrity: Risk factors: altered nutritional status, immobility

Risk for **Injury**: Risk factors: confusion, decreased muscle coordination

Self-care deficit: specify r/t psychological or neuromuscular impairment

Total urinary **Incontinence** r/t neuromuscular impairment

Denial of Health Status

Ineffective **Denial** r/t lack of perception about health status effects of illness

Ineffective management of **Therapeutic** regimen r/t denial of seriousness of health situation

Dental Caries

Impaired **Dentition** r/t ineffective oral hygiene, barriers to self-care, economic barriers to professional care, nutritional deficits, dietary habits

Ineffective **Health** maintenance r/t lack of knowledge regarding prevention of dental disease

Dentition Problems

See Dental Caries

Depression (Major Depressive Disorder)

Adult **Failure** to thrive r/t depression

Chronic low **Self-esteem** r/t repeated unmet expectations

Chronic **Sorrow** r/t unresolved grief

Constipation r/t inactivity, decreased fluid intake

Death **Anxiety** r/t feelings of lack of self-worth

Disturbed **Energy** field r/t disharmony

Insomnia r/t inactivity

Risk for complicated **Grieving**: Risk factor: lack of previous resolution of former grieving response

Fatigue r/t psychological demands

Hopelessness r/t feeling of abandonment, long-term stress

Impaired **Environmental** interpretation syndrome r/t severe mental functional impairment

Ineffective **Coping** r/t grieving

Ineffective **Health** maintenance r/t lack of ability to make good judgments regarding ways to obtain help

Powerlessness r/t pattern of helplessness

Risk for **Suicide**: Risk factor: panic state

Self-care deficit: specify r/t depression, cognitive impairment

Sexual dysfunction r/t loss of sexual desire

Social isolation r/t ineffective coping

Dermatitis

Anxiety r/t situational crisis imposed by illness

Impaired **Skin** integrity r/t side effect of medication, allergic reaction

Ineffective **Health** maintenance r/t deficient knowledge regarding methods to decrease inflammation

Pruritus r/t inflammation of skin

See Itching

Despondency

Hopelessness r/t long-term stress

See Depression

Destructive Behavior Toward Others

Risk-prone health **Behavior** r/t intense emotional state

Ineffective **Coping** r/t situational crises,

maturational crises, personal vulnerability

Risk for other-directed **Violence** (See **Violence,** other-directed, risk for, Section II)

D

Developmental Concerns

Delayed **Growth** and development (See **Growth** and development, delayed, Section II)

INDIVIDUAL/ENVIRONMENTAL/ CAREGIVER

Risk for delayed **Development** (See **Development,** delayed, risk for, Section II)

See Growth and Development Lag

Diabetes in Pregnancy

See Gestational Diabetes (Diabetes in Pregnancy)

Diabetes Insipidus

Deficient **Fluid** volume r/t inability to conserve fluid

Ineffective **Health** maintenance r/t deficient knowledge regarding care of disease, importance of medications

Diabetes Mellitus

Adult **Failure** to thrive r/t undetected disease process

Disturbed **Sensory** perception r/t ineffective tissue perfusion

Imbalanced **Nutrition**: less than body requirements r/t inability to use glucose (type 1 [insulin-dependent] diabetes)

Imbalanced **Nutrition**: more than body requirements r/t excessive intake of nutrients (type 2 diabetes)

Ineffective **Health** maintenance r/t deficient knowledge regarding care of diabetic condition

Ineffective management of **Therapeutic** regimen r/t complexity of therapeutic regimen

Ineffective **Tissue** perfusion: peripheral r/t impaired arterial circulation

Noncompliance r/t restrictive lifestyle; changes in diet, medication, exercise

Powerlessness r/t perceived lack of personal control

Risk for disturbed **Thought** processes: Risk factors: hypoglycemia, hyperglycemia

Risk for impaired **Skin** integrity: Risk factor: loss of pain perception in extremities

Risk for **Infection**: Risk factors: hyperglycemia, impaired healing, circulatory changes

Risk for **Injury**: Risk factors: hypoglycemia or hyperglycemia from failure to consume adequate calories, failure to take insulin

Risk for unstable blood **Glucose** (See **Glucose,** unstable blood, risk for, Section II)

Sexual dysfunction r/t neuropathy associated with disease

Diabetes Mellitus, Juvenile (IDDM Type 1)

Acute **Pain** r/t insulin injections, peripheral blood glucose testing

Disturbed **Body** image r/t imposed deviations from biophysical and psychosocial norm, perceived differences from peers

Imbalanced **Nutrition**: less than body requirements r/t inability of body to adequately metabolize and use glucose and nutrients, increased caloric needs of child to promote growth and physical activity participation with peers

Impaired **Adjustment** r/t inability to participate in normal childhood activities

Ineffective **Health** maintenance r/t parental/child deficient knowledge regarding dietary management, medication administration, physical activity, and interaction between the three; daily changes in diet, medications, illness, stress, activity associated with child's growth spurts and needs; need to instruct other caregivers and teachers regarding signs and symptoms of hypoglycemia or hyperglycemia and treatment

Noncompliance r/t disturbed body image, impaired adjustment attributable to adolescent maturational crises

See Diabetes Mellitus; Child with Chronic Condition; Hospitalized Child

Diabetic Coma

Deficient **Fluid** volume r/t hyperglycemia resulting in polyuria

Disturbed **Thought** processes r/t hyperglycemia, presence of excessive metabolic acids

Ineffective management of **Therapeutic** regimen r/t lack of understanding of preventive measures, adequate blood sugar control

Risk for **Infection**: Risk factors: hyperglycemia, changes in vascular system

Risk for unstable blood **Glucose** (See **Glucose,** unstable blood, risk for, Section II)

See Diabetes Mellitus

Diabetic Ketoacidosis

See Ketoacidosis, Diabetic

Diabetic Retinopathy

Disturbed **Sensory** perception r/t change in sensory reception

Grieving r/t loss of vision

Ineffective **Health** maintenance r/t deficient knowledge regarding preserving vision with treatment if possible, use of low-vision aids

See Vision Impairment

Dialysis

See Hemodialysis; Peritoneal Dialysis

Diaphragmatic Hernia

See Hiatal Hernia

Diarrhea

Diarrhea r/t infection, change in diet, gastrointestinal disorders, stress, medication effect, impaction

DIC (Disseminated Intravascular Coagulation)

Deficient **Fluid** volume: hemorrhage r/t depletion of clotting factors

Fear r/t threat to well-being

Ineffective **Protection** r/t abnormal clotting mechanism

Risk for ineffective **Tissue** perfusion: peripheral: Risk factors: hypovolemia from profuse bleeding, formation of microemboli in vascular system

Digitalis Toxicity

Decreased **Cardiac** output r/t drug toxicity affecting cardiac rhythm, rate

Ineffective management of **Therapeutic** regimen r/t deficient knowledge regarding action, appropriate method of administration of digitalis

Dignity, Loss of

Risk for compromised human **Dignity** (See **Dignity,** compromised human, risk for, Section II)

Dilation and Curettage (D&C)

Acute **Pain** r/t uterine contractions

Ineffective **Health** maintenance r/t deficient knowledge regarding postoperative self-care

Risk for deficient **Fluid** volume: hemorrhage: Risk factor: excessive blood loss during or after procedure

Risk for ineffective **Sexuality** pattern: Risk factors: painful coitus, fear associated with surgery on genital area

Risk for **Infection**: Risk factor: surgical procedure

D

Discharge Planning

Deficient **Knowledge**: Risk factor: lack of exposure to information for home care

Impaired **Home** maintenance r/t family member's disease or injury interfering with home maintenance

Ineffective **Health** maintenance r/t lack of material sources

Discomforts of Pregnancy

Acute **Pain**: headache r/t hormonal changes of pregnancy

Acute **Pain**: leg cramps r/t nerve compression, calcium/phosphorus/potassium imbalance

Constipation r/t decreased gastrointestinal tract motility, pressure from enlarged uterus, supplementary iron

Disturbed **Body** image r/t pregnancy-induced body changes

Fatigue r/t hormonal, metabolic, body changes

Insomnia r/t psychological stress, fetal movement, muscular cramping, urinary frequency, shortness of breath

Nausea r/t hormone effect

Readiness for enhanced **Comfort**: Headache: hormonal changes of pregnancy

Risk for **Constipation**: Risk factors: decreased intestinal motility, inadequate fiber in diet

Risk for **Injury**: Risk factors: faintness and/or syncope caused by vasomotor lability or postural hypotension, venous stasis in lower extremities

Risk for urge urinary **Incontinence**: Risk factors: hormone effect, pressure on bladder from growing uterus

Stress urinary **Incontinence**: Risk factors: enlarged uterus, fetal movement

Dislocation

Acute **Pain** r/t dislocation of a joint

Risk for **Injury**: Risk factor: unstable joint

Self-care deficit: specify r/t inability to use a joint

Dissecting Aneurysm

Fear r/t threat to well-being

See Abdominal Surgery; Aneurysm, Abdominal Surgery

Disseminated Intravascular Coagulation

See DIC (Disseminated Intravascular Coagulation)

Dissociative Identity Disorder (Not Otherwise Specified)

Anxiety r/t psychosocial stress

Disturbed personal **Identity** r/t inability to distinguish self caused by multiple personality disorder, depersonalization, disturbance in memory

Disturbed **Sensory** perception: kinesthetic r/t underdeveloped ego

Disturbed **Thought** processes r/t repressed anxiety

Impaired **Memory** r/t altered state of consciousness

Ineffective **Coping** r/t personal vulnerability in crisis of accurate self-perception

See Multiple Personality Disorder (Dissociative Identity Disorder)

Distress

Anxiety r/t situational crises, maturational crises

Death **Anxiety** r/t denial of one's own mortality or impending death

Disturbed **Energy** field r/t disruption in flow of energy as result of pain, depression, fatigue, anxiety, stress

Disuse Syndrome, Potential to Develop

Risk for **Disuse** syndrome: Risk factors: paralysis, mechanical immobilization, prescribed immobilization, severe pain, altered level of consciousness

Diversional Activity, Lack of

Deficient **Diversional** activity r/t environmental lack of diversional activity as in frequent hospitalizations, lengthy treatments

Diverticulitis

Acute **Pain** r/t inflammation of bowel

Constipation r/t dietary deficiency of fiber and roughage

Deficient **Knowledge** r/t diet needed to control disease, medication regimen

Diarrhea r/t increased intestinal motility caused by inflammation

Imbalanced **Nutrition**: less than body requirements r/t loss of appetite

Risk for deficient **Fluid** volume: Risk factor: diarrhea

Dizziness

Decreased **Cardiac** output r/t dysfunctional electrical conduction

Impaired physical **Mobility** r/t dizziness

Ineffective **Tissue** perfusion: cerebral r/t interruption of cerebral arterial blood flow

Risk for **Falls**: Risk factor: difficulty maintaining balance

Domestic Violence

Anxiety r/t threat to self-concept, situational crisis of abuse

Caregiver role strain r/t chronic illness, self-care deficits, lack of respite care, extent of caregiving required

Compromised family **Coping** r/t abusive patterns

Defensive **Coping** r/t low self-esteem

Impaired verbal **Communication** r/t psychological barriers of fear

Insomnia r/t psychological stress

Interrupted **Family** processes: alcoholism r/t inadequate coping skills

Post-trauma syndrome r/t history of abuse

Powerlessness r/t lifestyle of helplessness

Risk for **Post-trauma** syndrome r/t inadequate social support

Risk for self-directed **Violence** r/t history of abuse

Self-esteem disturbance r/t negative family interactions

Down Syndrome

See Child with Chronic Condition; Mental Retardation

Dress Self (Inability to)

Dressing or grooming **Self-care** deficit r/t intolerance to activity, decreased strength and endurance, pain, discomfort, perceptual or cognitive impairment, neuromuscular impairment, musculoskeletal impairment, depression, severe anxiety

Dribbling of Urine

Overflow urinary **Incontinence** r/t degenerative changes in pelvic muscles and urinary structures

Stress urinary **Incontinence** r/t degenerative changes in pelvic muscles and urinary structures

Drooling

Impaired **Swallowing** r/t neuromuscular impairment, mechanical obstruction

Risk for **Aspiration** r/t impaired swallowing

Drug Abuse

Anxiety r/t threat to self-concept, lack of control of drug use

Disturbed **Sensory** perception: specify r/t substance intoxication

Disturbed **Thought** processes r/t mind-altering effects of drugs

Imbalanced **Nutrition**: less than body requirements r/t poor eating habits

Impaired **Social** interaction r/t disturbed thought processes from drug abuse

Ineffective **Coping** r/t situational crisis

Insomnia r/t effects of medications

Noncompliance r/t denial of illness

Powerlessness r/t feeling unable to change patterns of abuse

Risk for **Injury**: Risk factors: hallucinations, drug effects

Risk for **Violence**: Risk factor: poor impulse control

Risk-prone health **Behavior**: r/t failure to change destructive behavior

Sexual dysfunction r/t actions and side effects of drug abuse

Sleep deprivation r/t prolonged psychological discomfort

Spiritual distress r/t separation from religious, cultural ties

See Cocaine Abuse; Substance Abuse

Drug Withdrawal

Acute **Confusion** r/t effects of substance withdrawal

Anxiety r/t physiological withdrawal

Disturbed **Sensory** perception: specify r/t substance intoxication

Imbalanced **Nutrition**: less than body requirements r/t poor eating habits

Ineffective **Coping** r/t situational crisis, withdrawal

Insomnia r/t effects of medications

Noncompliance r/t denial of illness

Risk for **Injury**: Risk factor: hallucinations

Risk for **Violence**: Risk factor: poor impulse control

See Drug Abuse

Dry Eye

See Conjunctivitis; Keratoconjunctivitis Sicca

DT (Delirium Tremens)

See Alcohol Withdrawal

DVT (Deep Vein Thrombosis)

Acute **Pain** r/t vascular inflammation, edema

Constipation r/t inactivity, bedrest

Delayed **Surgical** recovery r/t impaired physical mobility

Impaired physical **Mobility** r/t pain in extremity, forced bed rest

Ineffective **Health** maintenance r/t deficient knowledge regarding self-care needs, treatment regimen, outcome

Ineffective **Tissue** perfusion: peripheral r/t interruption of venous blood flow

See Anticoagulant Therapy

Dying Client

See Terminally Ill Adult, Terminally Ill Adolescent; Terminally Ill Child, Infant/Toddler; Terminally Ill Child, Preschool Child; Terminally Ill Child, School-Age Child/Preadolescent; Terminally Ill Child/Death of Child, Parent

Dysfunctional Eating Pattern

Imbalanced **Nutrition**: less than body requirements r/t psychological factors

Risk for imbalanced **Nutrition**: more than body requirements: Risk factor: observed use of food as reward or comfort measure

See Anorexia Nervosa; Bulimia; Maturational Issues, Adolescent

Dysfunctional Family Unit

See Family Problems

Dysfunctional Ventilatory Weaning

Dysfunctional **Ventilatory** weaning response r/t physical, psychological, situational factors

Dysmenorrhea

Ineffective **Health** maintenance r/t deficient knowledge regarding prevention and treatment of painful menstruation

Nausea r/t prostaglandin effect

Acute **Pain** r/t cramping from hormonal effects

Dyspareunia

Sexual dysfunction r/t lack of lubrication during intercourse, alteration in reproductive organ function

Dyspepsia

Acute **Pain** r/t gastrointestinal disease, consumption of irritating foods

Anxiety r/t pressures of personal role

Ineffective **Health** maintenance r/t deficient knowledge regarding treatment of disease

Dysphagia

Impaired **Swallowing** r/t neuromuscular impairment

Risk for **Aspiration**: Risk factor: loss of gag or cough reflex

Dysphasia

Impaired **Social** interaction r/t difficulty in communicating

Impaired verbal **Communication** r/t decrease in circulation to brain

Dyspnea

Activity intolerance r/t imbalance between oxygen supply and demand

Anxiety r/t ineffective breathing pattern

Fear r/t threat to state of well-being, potential death

Impaired **Gas** exchange r/t alveolar-capillary damage

Ineffective **Breathing** pattern r/t compromised cardiac or pulmonary function, decreased lung expansion, neurological impairment affecting respiratory center, extreme anxiety

Insomnia r/t difficulty breathing, positioning required for effective breathing

Sleep deprivation r/t ineffective breathing pattern

Dysrhythmia

Activity intolerance r/t decreased cardiac output

Anxiety/Fear r/t threat of death, change in health status

Decreased **Cardiac** output r/t altered electrical conduction

Ineffective **Health** maintenance r/t deficient knowledge regarding self-care with disease

Ineffective **Tissue** perfusion: cerebral r/t interruption of cerebral arterial flow as a result of decreased cardiac output

Dysthymic Disorder

Chronic low **Self-esteem** r/t repeated unmet expectations

Ineffective **Coping** r/t impaired social interaction

Ineffective **Health** maintenance r/t inability to make good judgments regarding ways to obtain help

Ineffective **Sexuality** pattern r/t loss of sexual desire

Insomnia r/t anxious thoughts

Social isolation r/t ineffective coping

See Depression (Major Depressive Disorder)

Dystocia

Acute **Pain** r/t difficult labor, medical interventions

Anxiety r/t difficult labor, deficient knowledge regarding normal labor pattern

Fatigue r/t prolonged labor

Grieving r/t loss of ideal labor experience

Ineffective **Coping** r/t situational crisis

Powerlessness r/t perceived inability to control outcome of labor

Risk for deficient **Fluid** volume: Risk factor: hemorrhage secondary to uterine atony

Risk for delayed **Development**: Risk factor: difficult labor and birth

Risk for disproportionate **Growth**: Risk factor: difficult labor and birth

Risk for impaired **Tissue** integrity: maternal and fetal: Risk factor: difficult labor

Risk for ineffective **Tissue** perfusion: cerebral (fetal): Risk factor: difficult labor and birth

Risk for **Infection**: Risk factor: prolonged rupture of membranes

Risk for **Post-trauma** syndrome: Risk factor: sudden emergency during delivery of infant

Situational low **Self-esteem** r/t perceived inability to have normal labor and delivery

Dysuria

Impaired **Urinary** elimination r/t urinary tract infection

Risk for urge urinary **Incontinence**: Risk factors: detrusor hyperreflexia from cystitis, urethritis

E

E. Coli Infection

Deficient **Knowledge** r/t how to prevent disease; care of self with serious illness

Fear r/t serious illness, unknown outcome

See Gastroenteritis; Gastroenteritis, Child; Hospitalized Child

Ear Surgery

Acute **Pain** r/t edema in ears from surgery

Disturbed **Sensory** perception: hearing r/t invasive surgery of ears, dressings

Ineffective **Health** maintenance r/t deficient knowledge regarding postoperative restrictions, expectations, care

Risk for delayed **Development**: Risk factor: hearing impairment

Risk for **Falls**: Risk factor: dizziness from excessive stimuli to vestibular apparatus

See Hospitalized Child

Earache

Acute **Pain** r/t trauma, edema, infection

Disturbed **Sensory** perception: auditory r/t altered sensory reception, transmission, integration

Eclampsia

Fear r/t threat of well-being to self and fetus

Interrupted **Family** processes r/t unmet expectations for pregnancy and childbirth

Risk for **Aspiration**: Risk factor: seizure activity

Risk for delayed **Development**: Risk factor: uteroplacental insufficiency

Risk for disproportionate **Growth**: Risk factor: uteroplacental insufficiency

Risk for excess **Fluid** volume: Risk factor: decreased urine output as a result of renal dysfunction

Risk for imbalanced **Fluid** volume: Risk factors: retained fluid, decreased renal activity

Risk for ineffective **Tissue** perfusion: fetal: Risk factor: uteroplacental insufficiency

Risk for **Injury**: maternal: Risk factor: seizure activity

ECT (Electroconvulsive Therapy)

Decisional **Conflict** r/t lack of relevant information

Fear r/t real or imagined threat to well-being

Impaired **Memory** r/t effects of treatment

See Depression (Major Depressive Disorder)

Ectopic Pregnancy

Acute **Pain** r/t stretching or rupture of implantation site

Chronic **Sorrow** r/t loss of pregnancy, potential loss of fertility

Death Anxiety r/t emergency condition, hemorrhage

Deficient **Fluid** volume r/t loss of blood

Disturbed **Body** image r/t negative feelings about body and reproductive functioning

Fear r/t threat to self, surgery, implications for future pregnancy

Ineffective **Role** performance r/t loss of pregnancy

Risk for ineffective **Coping**: Risk factor: loss of pregnancy

Risk for **Infection**: Risk factor: traumatized tissue, blood loss

Risk for interrupted **Family** processes: Risk factor: situational crisis

Risk for **Spiritual** distress: Risk factor: grief process

Situational low **Self-esteem** r/t loss of pregnancy, inability to carry pregnancy to term

Eczema

Acute **Pain**: pruritus r/t inflammation of skin

Disturbed **Body** image r/t change in appearance from inflamed skin

Impaired **Skin** integrity r/t side effect of medication, allergic reaction

Ineffective **Health** maintenance r/t deficient knowledge regarding how to decrease inflammation and prevent further outbreaks

ED (Erectile Dysfunction)

See Erectile Dysfunction (ED); Impotence

Edema

Excess **Fluid** volume r/t excessive fluid intake, cardiac dysfunction, renal dysfunction, loss of plasma proteins

Ineffective **Health** maintenance r/t deficient knowledge regarding treatment of edema

Risk for impaired **Skin** integrity: Risk factors: impaired circulation, fragility of skin

See cause of Edema

Elder Abuse

See Abuse, Spouse, Parent, or Significant Other

Elderly

See Aging

Electroconvulsive Therapy

See ECT (Electroconvulsive Therapy)

Emaciated Person

Adult **Failure** to thrive r/t imbalanced nutrition: less than body requirements

Imbalanced **Nutrition**: less than body requirements r/t inability to ingest food, digest food, absorb nutrients because of biological, psychological, economic factors

Embolectomy

Fear r/t threat of great bodily harm from embolus

Ineffective **Tissue** perfusion: specify r/t presence of embolus

Risk for deficient **Fluid** volume: hemorrhage: Risk factors: postoperative complication, surgical area

See Surgery, Postoperative Care

Emboli

See Pulmonary Embolism

E

Emesis

Nausea (See **Nausea,** Section II)

See Vomiting

Emotional Problems

See Coping Problems

Empathy

Health-seeking behaviors r/t desire to attain maximal level of health

Readiness for enhanced community **Coping** r/t social supports, being available for problem solving

Readiness for enhanced family **Coping** r/t basic needs met, desire to move to higher level of health

Readiness for enhanced **Spiritual** well-being: desire to establish interconnectedness through spirituality

Emphysema

See COPD (Chronic Obstructive Pulmonary Disease)

Emptiness

Chronic **Sorrow** r/t unresolved grief

Social isolation r/t inability to engage in satisfying personal relationships

Spiritual distress r/t separation from religious or cultural ties

Encephalitis

See Meningitis/Encephalitis

Endocardial Cushion Defect

See Congenital Heart Disease/Cardiac Anomalies

Endocarditis

Activity intolerance r/t reduced cardiac reserve, prescribed bedrest

Acute **Pain** r/t biological injury, inflammation

Decreased **Cardiac** output r/t inflammation of lining of heart and change in structure of valve leaflets, increased myocardial workload

Ineffective **Health** maintenance r/t deficient knowledge regarding treatment of disease, preventive measures against further incidence of disease

Ineffective **Tissue** perfusion: cardiopulmonary, peripheral r/t high risk for development of emboli

Risk for imbalanced **Nutrition**: less than body requirements: Risk factors: fever, hypermetabolic state associated with fever

Endometriosis

Acute **Pain** r/t onset of menses with distention of endometrial tissue

Grieving r/t possible infertility

Ineffective **Health** maintenance r/t deficient knowledge about disease condition, medications, other treatments

Nausea r/t prostaglandin effect

Sexual dysfunction r/t painful coitus

Endometritis

Acute **Pain** r/t infectious process in reproductive tract

Anxiety r/t prolonged hospitalization, fear of unknown

Hyperthermia r/t infectious process

Ineffective **Health** maintenance r/t deficient knowledge regarding condition, treatment, antibiotic regimen

Enuresis

Ineffective **Health** maintenance r/t unachieved developmental task, neuromuscular immaturity, diseases of urinary system

See Toilet Training

Environmental Interpretation Problems

Adult **Failure** to thrive r/t impaired environmental interpretation syndrome

Chronic **Confusion** r/t impaired environmental interpretation syndrome

Disturbed **Thought** processes r/t lack of orientation to person, place, time, circumstances

Impaired **Environmental** interpretation syndrome r/t dementia, Parkinson's disease, Huntington's disease, depression, alcoholism

Impaired **Memory** r/t environmental disturbances

Risk for **Injury**: Risk factor: lack of orientation to person, place, time, circumstances

Epididymitis

Acute **Pain** r/t inflammation in scrotal sac

Anxiety r/t situational crisis, pain, threat to future fertility

Ineffective **Health** maintenance r/t deficient knowledge regarding treatment for pain and infection

Ineffective **Sexuality** pattern r/t edema of epididymis and testes

Epiglottitis

See Respiratory Infections, Acute Childhood (Croup, Epiglottis, Pertussis, Pneumonia, Respiratory Syncytial Virus)

Epilepsy

Anxiety r/t threat to role functioning

Impaired **Memory** r/t seizure activity

Ineffective **Health** maintenance r/t deficient knowledge regarding seizures and seizure control

Ineffective **Therapeutic** regimen management r/t deficient knowledge regarding seizure control

Risk for **Aspiration**: Risk factors: impaired swallowing, excessive secretions

Risk for delayed **Development**: Risk factor: seizure disorder

Risk for disturbed **Thought** processes: Risk factor: excessive, uncontrolled neurological stimuli

Risk for **Injury**: Risk factor: environmental factors during seizure

See Seizure Disorders, Adult; Seizure Disorders, Childhood

E

Episiotomy

Acute **Pain** r/t tissue trauma

Anxiety r/t fear of pain

Disturbed **Body** image r/t fear of resuming sexual relations

Impaired physical **Mobility** r/t pain, swelling, tissue trauma

Impaired **Skin** integrity r/t perineal incision

Risk for **Infection**: Risk factor: tissue trauma

Sexual dysfunction r/t altered body structure, tissue trauma

Epistaxis

Fear r/t large amount of blood loss

Risk for deficient **Fluid** volume: Risk factor: excessive fluid loss

Epstein-Barr Virus

See Mononucleosis

Erectile Dysfunction (ED)

Readiness for enhanced **Knowledge** of treatment information for erectile dysfunction

Self-esteem disturbance r/t physiological crisis, inability to practice usual sexual activity

Sexual dysfunction r/t altered body function

See Impotence

Esophageal Varices

Deficient **Fluid** volume: hemorrhage r/t portal hypertension, distended variceal vessels that can easily rupture

Fear r/t threat of death

See Cirrhosis

Esophagitis

Acute **Pain** r/t inflammation of esophagus

Ineffective **Health** maintenance r/t deficient knowledge regarding treatment of disease

F

ETOH Withdrawal

See Alcohol Withdrawal

Evisceration

See Dehiscence, Abdominal

Exposure to Hot or Cold Environment

Risk for imbalanced **Body** temperature: Risk factor: exposure

External Fixation

Disturbed **Body** image r/t trauma, change to affected part

Risk for **Infection**: Risk factor: pressure of pins on skin surface

See Fracture

Eye Surgery

Anxiety r/t possible loss of vision

Disturbed **Sensory** perception: visual r/t surgical procedure

Ineffective **Health** maintenance r/t deficient knowledge regarding postoperative activity, medications, eye care

Risk for **Injury**: Risk factor: impaired vision

Self-care deficit r/t impaired vision

See Hospitalized Child; Vision Impairment

F

Failure to Thrive, Adult

Adult **Failure** to thrive r/t depression, apathy, fatigue

Failure to Thrive, Nonorganic

Chronic low **Self-esteem**: parental r/t feelings of inadequacy, support system deficiencies, inadequate role model

Delayed **Growth** and development r/t parental deficient knowledge, lack of stimulation, nutritional deficit, long-term hospitalization

Disorganized **Infant** behavior r/t lack of boundaries

Imbalanced **Nutrition**: less than body requirements r/t inadequate type or amounts of food for infant, inappropriate feeding techniques

Impaired **Parenting** r/t lack of parenting skills, inadequate role modeling

Insomnia r/t inconsistency of caretaker; lack of quiet, consistent environment

Risk for delayed **Development**: Risk factor: failure to thrive

Risk for disproportionate **Growth**: Risk factor: failure to thrive

Risk for impaired parent/child **Attachment**: Risk factor: inability of parents to meet infant's needs

Social isolation r/t limited support systems, self-imposed situation

Falls, Risk for

Risk for **Falls** (See **Falls,** risk for, Section II)

Family Problems

Compromised family **Coping** (See **Coping,** compromised family, Section II)

Disabled family **Coping** (See **Coping,** disabled family, Section II)

Ineffective family **Therapeutic** regimen management r/t complexity of health care system, complexity of therapeutic regimen, decisional conflicts, economic difficulties, excessive demands made on individual or family, family conflict

Interrupted **Family** processes r/t situation transition and/or crises, developmental transition and/or crises

Readiness for enhanced family **Coping** r/t needs sufficiently gratified, adaptive tasks effectively addressed to enable goals of self-actualization to surface

Family Process

Readiness for enhanced **Family** processes (See **Family** processes, readiness for enhanced, Section II)

Fatigue

Disturbed **Energy** field r/t disharmony

Fatigue (See **Fatigue,** Section II)

Fear

Death Anxiety r/t fear of death

Fear r/t identifiable physical or psychological threat to person

Febrile Seizures

See Seizure Disorders, Childhood

Fecal Impaction

See Impaction of Stool

Fecal Incontinence

Bowel incontinence r/t neurological impairment, gastrointestinal disorders, anorectal trauma

Feeding Problems, Newborn

Disorganized **Infant** behavior r/t prematurity, immature neurological system

Impaired **Swallowing** r/t prematurity

Ineffective **Breastfeeding** r/t prematurity, infant anomaly, maternal breast anomaly, previous breast surgery, previous history of breastfeeding failure, infant receiving supplemental feedings with artificial nipple, poor infant sucking reflex, nonsupportive partner and family, deficient knowledge, maternal anxiety or ambivalence

Ineffective **Infant** feeding pattern r/t prematurity, neurological impairment or delay, oral hypersensitivity, prolonged nothing-by-mouth status

Interrupted **Breastfeeding** r/t maternal or infant illness, prematurity, maternal employment, contraindications to breastfeeding, need to abruptly wean infant

Risk for delayed **Development**: Risk factor: inadequate nutrition

Risk for disproportionate **Growth**: Risk factor: feeding problems

Risk for imbalanced **Fluid** volume: Risk factor: inability to take in adequate amount of fluids

Femoral Popliteal Bypass

Acute **Pain** r/t surgical trauma, edema in surgical area

Anxiety r/t threat to or change in health status

Ineffective **Tissue** perfusion: peripheral r/t impaired arterial circulation

Risk for deficient **Fluid** volume: hemorrhage: Risk factor: abnormal blood loss

Risk for **Infection**: Risk factor: invasive procedure

Risk for **Peripheral** neurovascular dysfunction: Risk factor: vascular surgery, emboli

Fetal Alcohol Syndrome

See Infant of Substance-Abusing Mother

Fetal Distress/Nonreassuring Fetal Heart Rate Pattern

Fear r/t threat to fetus

Ineffective **Tissue** perfusion: fetal r/t interruption of umbilical cord blood flow

Ineffective **Tissue** perfusion: placental r/t small or old placenta, interference with gas exchange transplacentally

Fever

Hyperthermia r/t infectious process, damage to hypothalamus, exposure to hot environment, medications, anesthesia, inability or decreased ability to perspire

F

Fibrocystic Breast Disease

See Breast Lumps

Filthy Home Environment

Impaired **Home** maintenance (See **Home** maintenance, impaired, Section II)

F

Financial Crisis in the Home Environment

Impaired **Home** maintenance r/t insufficient finances

Fistulectomy

See Hemorrhoidectomy (same nursing care)

Flail Chest

Anxiety r/t difficulty breathing

Impaired spontaneous **Ventilation** r/t paradoxical respirations

Ineffective **Breathing** pattern r/t chest trauma

Flashbacks

Post-trauma syndrome r/t catastrophic event

Flat Affect

Adult **Failure** to thrive r/t apathy

Hopelessness r/t prolonged activity restriction creating isolation, failing or deteriorating physiological condition, long-term stress, abandonment, lost belief in transcendent values or higher power or God

Risk for **Loneliness**: Risk factors: social isolation, lack of interest in surroundings

See Depression (Major Depressive Disorder); Dysthymic Disorder

Flesh-Eating Bacteria

See Necrotizing Fasciitis

Fluid Balance

Readiness for enhanced **Fluid** balance (See **Fluid** balance, readiness for enhanced, Section II)

Fluid Volume Deficit

Deficient **Fluid** volume r/t active fluid loss, failure of regulatory mechanisms

Fluid Volume Excess

Excess **Fluid** volume r/t compromised regulatory mechanism, excess sodium intake

Fluid Volume Imbalance, Risk for

Risk for imbalanced **Fluid** volume: Risk factor: major invasive surgeries

Foodborne Illness

Deficient **Fluid** volume r/t active fluid loss

Deficient **Knowledge** r/t care of self with serious illness, prevention of further incidences of foodborne illness

Diarrhea r/t infectious material in gastrointestinal tract

Nausea r/t contamination irritating stomach

See Gastroenteritis; Gastroenteritis, Child; Hospitalized Child; E. coli Infection

Foreign Body Aspiration

Impaired **Home** maintenance r/t inability to maintain orderly and clean surroundings

Ineffective **Airway** clearance r/t obstruction of airway

Ineffective **Health** maintenance r/t parental deficient knowledge regarding high-risk items

Risk for **Suffocation**: Risk factor: inhalation of small object

See Safety, Childhood

Formula Feeding

Grieving: maternal r/t loss of desired breastfeeding experience

Ineffective **Health** maintenance r/t maternal deficient knowledge regarding formula feeding

Risk for **Constipation**: infant: Risk factor: iron-fortified formula

Risk for **Infection**: infant: Risk factors: lack of passive maternal immunity, supine feeding position

Fracture

Acute **Pain** r/t muscle spasm, edema, trauma

Deficient **Diversional** activity r/t immobility

Impaired physical **Mobility** r/t limb immobilization

Impaired **Walking** r/t limb immobility

Ineffective **Health** maintenance r/t deficient knowledge regarding care of fracture

Risk for impaired **Skin** integrity: Risk factors: immobility, presence of cast

Risk for ineffective **Tissue** perfusion: Risk factors: immobility, presence of cast

Risk for **Peripheral** neurovascular dysfunction: Risk factors: mechanical compression, treatment of fracture

Fractured Hip

See Hip Fracture

Frequency of Urination

Impaired **Urinary** elimination r/t anatomical obstruction, sensory-motor impairment, urinary tract infection

Stress urinary **Incontinence** r/t degenerative change in pelvic muscles and structural support

Urge urinary **Incontinence** r/t decreased bladder capacity, irritation of bladder stretch receptors causing spasm, alcohol, caffeine, increased fluids, increased urine concentration, overdistended bladder

Urinary retention r/t high urethral pressure caused by weak detrusor, inhibition of reflex arc, strong sphincter, blockage

Frostbite

Acute **Pain** r/t decreased circulation from prolonged exposure to cold

Impaired **Skin** integrity r/t freezing of skin

Impaired **Tissue** integrity r/t freezing of skin

Ineffective **Tissue** perfusion r/t damage to extremities from prolonged exposure to cold

See Hypothermia

Frothy Sputum

See CHF (Congestive Heart Failure); Pulmonary Edema; Seizure Disorders, Adult; Seizure Disorders, Childhood

Fusion, Lumbar

Acute **Pain** r/t discomfort at bone donor site, surgical operation

Anxiety r/t fear of surgical procedure, possible recurring problems

Impaired physical **Mobility** r/t limitations from surgical procedure, presence of brace

Ineffective **Health** maintenance r/t deficient knowledge regarding postoperative mobility restrictions, body mechanics

Risk for **Injury**: Risk factor: improper body mechanics

Risk for perioperative positioning **Injury**: Risk factor: immobilization

G

Gag Reflex, Depressed or Absent

Impaired **Swallowing** r/t neuromuscular impairment

Risk for **Aspiration**: Risk factors: depressed cough or gag reflex

Gallop Rhythm

Decreased **Cardiac** output r/t decreased contractility of heart

Gallstones

See Cholelithiasis

Gangrene

G

Delayed **Surgical** recovery r/t obstruction of arterial flow

Fear r/t possible loss of extremity

Ineffective **Tissue** perfusion: peripheral r/t obstruction of arterial flow

Gas Exchange, Impaired

Impaired **Gas** exchange r/t ventilation-perfusion imbalance

Gastric Surgery

Risk for **Injury**: Risk factor: inadvertent insertion of nasogastric tube through gastric incision line

See Abdominal Surgery

Gastric Ulcer

See GI Bleed (Gastrointestinal Bleeding); Ulcer, Peptic

Gastritis

Acute **Pain** r/t inflammation of gastric mucosa

Imbalanced **Nutrition**: less than body requirements r/t vomiting, inadequate intestinal absorption of nutrients, restricted dietary regimen

Risk for deficient **Fluid** volume: Risk factors: excessive loss from gastrointestinal tract as a result of vomiting, decreased intake

Gastroenteritis

Acute **Pain** r/t increased peristalsis causing cramping

Deficient **Fluid** volume r/t excessive loss from gastrointestinal tract from diarrhea, vomiting

Diarrhea r/t infectious process involving intestinal tract

Imbalanced **Nutrition**: less than body requirements r/t vomiting, inadequate intestinal absorption of nutrients, restricted dietary intake

Ineffective **Health** maintenance r/t deficient knowledge regarding treatment of disease

Nausea r/t irritation to gastrointestinal system

See Gastroenteritis, Child

Gastroenteritis, Child

Impaired **Skin** integrity: diaper rash r/t acidic excretions on perineal tissues

Ineffective **Health** maintenance r/t lack of parental knowledge regarding fluid and dietary changes

See Gastroenteritis; Hospitalized Child

Gastroesophageal Reflux: Child

Acute **Pain** r/t irritation of esophagus from gastric acids

Anxiety: parental r/t possible need for surgical intervention (Nissen fundoplication, gastrostomy tube)

Deficient **Fluid** volume r/t persistent vomiting

Imbalanced **Nutrition**: less than body requirements r/t poor feeding, vomiting

Ineffective **Airway** clearance r/t reflux of gastric contents into esophagus and tracheal or bronchial tree

Ineffective **Health** maintenance r/t deficient knowledge regarding antireflux regimen (e.g., positioning, oral or enteral feeding techniques, medications), possible home apnea monitoring

Risk for **Aspiration**: Risk factor: entry of gastric contents in tracheal or bronchial tree

Risk for impaired **Parenting**: Risk factors: disruption in bonding as a result of irritable or inconsolable infant

See Child with Chronic Condition; Hospitalized Child

Gastrointestinal Hemorrhage

See GI Bleed (Gastrointestinal Bleeding)

Gastroschisis/Omphalocele

Grieving r/t threatened loss of infant, loss of perfect birth or infant because of serious medical condition

Impaired **Gas** exchange r/t effects of anesthesia, subsequent atelectasis

Ineffective **Airway** clearance r/t complications of anesthetic effects

Risk for deficient **Fluid** volume: Risk factors: inability to feed because of condition, subsequent electrolyte imbalance

Risk for **Infection**: Risk factor: disrupted skin integrity with exposure of abdominal contents

Risk for **Injury**: Risk factors: disrupted skin integrity, ineffective protection

Gastrostomy

Risk for impaired **Skin** integrity: Risk factor: presence of gastric contents on skin

See Tube Feeding

Genital Herpes

See Herpes Simplex II

Genital Warts

See STD (Sexually Transmitted Disease)

Gestational Diabetes (Diabetes in Pregnancy)

Anxiety r/t threat to self and/or fetus

Impaired fetal **Nutrition**: more than body requirements r/t excessive glucose uptake

Impaired **Nutrition**: less than body requirements r/t decreased insulin production and glucose uptake in cells

Ineffective **Health** maintenance: maternal r/t deficient knowledge regarding care of diabetic condition in pregnancy

Powerlessness r/t lack of control over outcome of pregnancy

Risk for delayed **Development**: fetal: Risk factor: endocrine disorder of mother

Risk for disproportionate **Growth**: fetal: Risk factor: endocrine disorder of mother

Risk for impaired **Tissue** integrity: fetal: Risk factors: macrosomia, congenital defects, birth injury

Risk for impaired **Tissue** integrity: maternal: Risk factor: delivery of large infant

See Diabetes Mellitus

GI Bleed (Gastrointestinal Bleeding)

Acute **Pain** r/t irritated mucosa from acid secretion

Deficient **Fluid** volume r/t gastrointestinal bleeding

Fatigue r/t loss of circulating blood volume, decreased ability to transport oxygen

Fear r/t threat to well-being, potential death

Imbalanced **Nutrition**: less than body requirements r/t nausea, vomiting

Risk for ineffective **Coping**: Risk factors: personal vulnerability in crisis, bleeding, hospitalization

Gingivitis

Impaired **Dentition** r/t ineffective oral hygiene, barriers to self-care

Impaired **Oral** mucous membrane r/t ineffective oral hygiene

Glaucoma

Deficient **Knowledge** r/t treatment and self-care for disease

Disturbed **Sensory** perception: visual r/t increased intraocular pressure

See Vision Impairment

G

Glomerulonephritis

Acute **Pain** r/t edema of kidney

Excess **Fluid** volume r/t renal impairment

Imbalanced **Nutrition**: less than body requirements r/t anorexia, restrictive diet

Ineffective **Health** maintenance r/t deficient knowledge regarding care of disease

Gonorrhea

Acute **Pain** r/t inflammation of reproductive organs

Ineffective **Health** maintenance r/t deficient knowledge regarding treatment and prevention of disease

Risk for **Infection**: Risk factor: spread of organism throughout reproductive organs

See STD (Sexually Transmitted Disease)

Gout

Chronic **Pain** r/t inflammation of affected joint

Impaired physical **Mobility** r/t musculoskeletal impairment

Ineffective **Health** maintenance r/t deficient knowledge regarding medications and home care

Grand Mal Seizure

See Seizure Disorders, Adult; Seizure Disorders, Childhood

Grandiosity

Defensive **Coping** r/t inaccurate perception of self and abilities

Grandparents Raising Grandchildren

Anxiety r/t change in role status

Compromised family **Coping** r/t family role changes

Decisional **Conflict** r/t support system deficit

Ineffective family **Therapeutic** regimen management r/t excessive demands on individual or family

Ineffective **Role** performance r/t role transition

Interrupted **Family** processes r/t family roles shift

Parental role **Conflict** r/t change in parental role

Readiness for enhanced **Parenting**: physical and emotional needs of children are met

Risk for impaired **Parenting**: Risk factor: role strain

Risk for **Powerlessness**: Risk factors: role strain, situational crisis, aging

Risk for **Spiritual** distress: Risk factor: life change

Graves' Disease

See Hyperthyroidism

Grieving

Grieving r/t anticipated or actual significant loss, change in life status, style, or function

Grieving, Complicated

Complicated **Grieving** r/t expected or sudden death of a significant other, emotional instability, lack of social support

Risk for complicated **Grieving**: Risk factors: death of a significant other, emotional instability, lack of social support

Groom Self (Inability to)

Dressing/grooming **Self-care** deficit (See **Self-care** deficit, dressing/grooming, Section II)

Growth and Development Lag

Delayed **Growth** and development (See **Growth** and development, delayed, Section II)

PRENATAL/INDIVIDUAL/ ENVIRONMENTAL

Risk for disproportionate **Growth** (See disproportionate **Growth,** risk for, Section II)

See Developmental Concerns

Guillain-Barré Syndrome

Impaired spontaneous **Ventilation** r/t weak respiratory muscles

See Neurological Disorders

Guilt

Chronic **Sorrow** r/t unresolved grieving

Grieving r/t potential loss of significant person, animal, prized material possession

Risk for complicated **Grief**: Risk factors: actual loss of significant person, animal, prized material possession

Readiness for enhanced **Spiritual** well-being: desire to be in harmony with self, others, higher power or God

Risk for **Post-trauma** syndrome: Risk factor: exaggerated sense of responsibility for traumatic event

Self-esteem disturbance r/t unmet expectations of self

Hair Loss

Disturbed **Body** image r/t psychological reaction to loss of hair

Imbalanced **Nutrition**: less than body requirements r/t inability to ingest food because of biological, psychological, economic factors

Halitosis

Impaired **Dentition** r/t ineffective oral hygiene

Impaired **Oral** mucous membranes r/t ineffective oral hygiene

Hallucinations

Acute **Confusion** r/t alcohol abuse, delirium, dementia, mental illness, drug abuse

Adult **Failure** to thrive r/t altered mental status

Anxiety r/t threat to self-concept

Disturbed **Thought** processes r/t inability to control bizarre thoughts

Ineffective **Coping** r/t distortion and insecurity of life events

Risk for other-directed **Violence**: Risk factors: catatonic excitement, manic excitement, rage or panic reactions, response to violent internal stimuli

Risk for self-directed **Violence**: Risk factors: catatonic excitement, manic excitement, rage or panic reactions, response to violent internal stimuli

Risk for **Self-mutilation**: Risk factor: command hallucinations

Head Injury

Acute **Confusion** r/t brain injury

Decreased **Intracranial** adaptive capacity r/t brain injury

Disturbed **Sensory** perception r/t pressure damage to sensory centers in brain

Disturbed **Thought** processes r/t pressure damage to brain

Ineffective **Breathing** pattern r/t pressure damage to breathing center in brainstem

Ineffective **Tissue** perfusion: cerebral r/t effects of increased intracranial pressure

See Neurological Disorders

Headache

Acute **Pain** r/t lack of knowledge of pain control techniques or methods to prevent headaches

Disturbed **Energy** field r/t disharmony

Ineffective management of **Therapeutic** regimen r/t lack of knowledge, identification, elimination of aggravating factors

Health Maintenance Problems

Ineffective **Health** maintenance (See **Health** maintenance, ineffective, Section II)

Health-Seeking Person

Health-seeking behaviors r/t expressed desire for increased control of own personal health

H

Hearing Impairment

Disturbed **Sensory** perception: auditory r/t altered state of auditory system

Impaired verbal **Communication** r/t inability to hear own voice

Social isolation r/t difficulty with communication

Heart Failure

See CHF (Congestive Heart Failure)

Heart Surgery

See Coronary Artery Bypass Grafting

Heartburn

Acute **Pain**: heartburn r/t gastroesophageal reflux

Ineffective **Health** maintenance r/t deficient knowledge regarding information about factors that cause esophageal reflex

Nausea r/t gastrointestinal irritation

Risk for imbalanced **Nutrition**: less than body requirements: Risk factor: pain after eating

Heat Stroke

Deficient **Fluid** volume r/t profuse diaphoresis

Disturbed **Thought** processes r/t hyperthermia, increased oxygen needs

Hyperthermia r/t vigorous activity, hot environment

Hematemesis

See GI Bleed (Gastrointestinal Bleeding)

Hematological Disorder

Ineffective **Protection** r/t abnormal blood profile

See cause of Hematological Disorder

Hematuria

See UTI (Urinary Tract Infection); Kidney Stone

Hemianopia

Anxiety r/t change in vision

Disturbed **Sensory** perception r/t altered sensory reception, transmission, integration

Risk for **Injury**: Risk factor: disturbed sensory perception

Unilateral **Neglect** r/t effects of disturbed perceptual abilities

Hemiplegia

Anxiety r/t change in health status

Disturbed **Body** image r/t functional loss of one side of body

Impaired physical **Mobility** r/t loss of neurological control of involved extremities

Impaired **Transfer** ability r/t partial paralysis

Impaired **Walking** r/t loss of neurological control of involved extremities

Risk for impaired **Skin** integrity: Risk factors: alteration in sensation, immobility

Risk for **Injury**: Risk factor: impaired mobility

Self-care deficit: specify: r/t neuromuscular impairment

Unilateral **Neglect** r/t effects of disturbed perceptual abilities

See CVA (Cerebrovascular Accident)

Hemodialysis

Excess **Fluid** volume r/t renal disease with minimal urine output

Ineffective **Coping** r/t situational crisis

Ineffective **Health** maintenance r/t deficient knowledge regarding hemodialysis procedure, restrictions, blood access care

Interrupted **Family** processes r/t changes in role responsibilities as a result of therapy regimen

Noncompliance: dietary restrictions r/t denial of chronic illness

Powerlessness r/t treatment regimen

Risk for **Caregiver** role strain: Risk factor: complexity of care receiver treatment

Risk for deficient **Fluid** volume: Risk factor: excessive removal of fluid during dialysis

Risk for **Infection**: Risk factors: exposure to blood products, risk for developing hepatitis B or C

Risk for **Injury**: clotting of blood access: Risk factor: abnormal surface for blood flow

See Renal Failure; Renal Failure, Acute/Chronic, Child

Hemodynamic Monitoring

Risk for **Infection**: Risk factor: invasive procedure

Risk for **Injury**: Risk factors: inadvertent wedging of catheter, dislodgement of catheter, disconnection of catheter with embolism

Hemolytic Uremic Syndrome

Deficient **Fluid** volume r/t vomiting, diarrhea

Nausea r/t effects of uremia

Risk for impaired **Skin** integrity: Risk factor: diarrhea

Risk for **Injury**: Risk factors: decreased platelet count, seizure activity

See Hospitalized Child; Renal Failure, Acute/Chronic, Child

Hemophilia

Acute **Pain** r/t bleeding into body tissues

Fear r/t high risk for AIDS infection from contaminated blood products

Impaired physical **Mobility** r/t pain from acute bleeds, imposed activity restrictions

Ineffective **Health** maintenance r/t knowledge and skill acquisition regarding home administration of intravenous clotting factors, protection from injury

Ineffective **Protection** r/t deficient clotting factors

Risk for **Injury**: Risk factors: deficient clotting factors, child's developmental level, age-appropriate play, inappropriate use of toys or sports equipment

See Child with Chronic Condition; Hospitalized Child; Maturational Issues, Adolescent

Hemoptysis

Fear r/t serious threat to well-being

Risk for deficient **Fluid** volume: Risk factor: excessive loss of blood

Risk for ineffective **Airway** clearance: Risk factor: obstruction of airway with blood and mucus

Hemorrhage

Deficient **Fluid** volume r/t massive blood loss

Fear r/t threat to well-being

See cause of Hemorrhage; Hypovolemic Shock

Hemorrhoidectomy

Acute **Pain** r/t surgical procedure

Anxiety r/t embarrassment, need for privacy

Constipation r/t fear of pain with defecation

Ineffective **Health** maintenance r/t defi-

H

cient knowledge regarding pain relief, use of stool softeners, dietary changes

Risk for deficient **Fluid** volume: hemorrhage: Risk factor: inadequate clotting

Urinary retention r/t pain, anesthetic effect

Hemorrhoids

Constipation r/t painful defecation, poor bowel habits

Ineffective **Health** maintenance r/t deficient knowledge regarding care of condition

Pruritus r/t inflammation of skin and tissues with hemorrhoids

Hemothorax

Deficient **Fluid** volume r/t blood in pleural space

See Pneumothorax

Hepatitis

Activity intolerance r/t weakness or fatigue caused by infection

Acute **Pain** r/t edema of liver, bile irritating skin

Deficient **Diversional** activity r/t isolation

Fatigue r/t infectious process, altered body chemistry

Imbalanced **Nutrition**: less than body requirements r/t anorexia, impaired use of proteins and carbohydrates

Ineffective **Health** maintenance r/t deficient knowledge regarding disease process and home management

Risk for deficient **Fluid** volume: Risk factor: excessive loss of fluids from vomiting and diarrhea

Social isolation r/t treatment-imposed isolation

Hernia

See Hiatal Hernia; Inguinal Hernia Repair

Herniated Disk

See Low Back Pain

Herniorrhaphy

See Inguinal Hernia Repair

Herpes in Pregnancy

Acute **Pain** r/t active herpes lesion

Fear r/t threat to fetus, impending surgery

Impaired **Tissue** integrity r/t active herpes lesion

Impaired **Urinary** elimination r/t pain with urination

Ineffective **Health** maintenance r/t deficient knowledge regarding treatment of disease, protection of fetus

Risk for **Infection** transmission: Risk factors: transplacental transfer during primary herpes, exposure to active herpes during birth process

Situational low **Self-esteem** r/t threat to fetus as a result of disease process

Herpes Simplex I

Impaired **Oral** mucous membranes r/t inflammatory changes in mouth

Herpes Simplex II

Acute **Pain** r/t active herpes lesion

Impaired **Tissue** integrity r/t active herpes lesion

Impaired **Urinary** elimination r/t pain with urination

Ineffective **Health** maintenance r/t deficient knowledge regarding treatment, prevention, spread of disease

Sexual dysfunction r/t disease process

Situational low **Self-esteem** r/t expressions of shame or guilt

Herpes Zoster

See Shingles

HHNC (Hyperosmolar Hyperglycemic Nonketotic Coma)

See Hyperosmolar Hyperglycemic Nonketotic Coma (HHNC)

Hiatal Hernia

Acute **Pain** r/t gastroesophageal reflux

Imbalanced **Nutrition**: less than body requirements r/t pain after eating

Ineffective **Health** maintenance r/t deficient knowledge regarding care of disease

Nausea r/t effects of gastric contents in esophagus

Hip Fracture

Acute **Confusion** r/t sensory overload, sensory deprivation, medication side effects

Acute **Pain** r/t injury, surgical procedure

Constipation r/t immobility, narcotics, anesthesia

Fear r/t outcome of treatment, future mobility, present helplessness

Impaired physical **Mobility** r/t surgical incision, temporary absence of weight bearing

Impaired **Transfer** ability r/t immobilization of hip

Impaired **Walking** r/t temporary absence of weight bearing

Powerlessness r/t health care environment

Risk for deficient **Fluid** volume: hemorrhage: Risk factors: postoperative complication, surgical blood loss

Risk for impaired **Skin** integrity: Risk factor: immobility

Risk for **Infection**: Risk factor: invasive procedure

Risk for **Injury**: Risk factors: dislodged prosthesis, unsteadiness when ambulating

Risk for perioperative positioning **Injury**: Risk factors: immobilization, muscle weakness, emaciation

Self-care deficit: specify r/t musculoskeletal impairment

Hip Replacement

See Total Joint Replacement

Hirschsprung's Disease

Acute **Pain** r/t distended colon, incisional postoperative pain

Constipation: bowel obstruction r/t inhibited peristalsis as a result of congenital absence of parasympathetic ganglion cells in distal colon

Grieving r/t loss of perfect child, birth of child with congenital defect even though child expected to be normal within 2 years

Imbalanced **Nutrition**: less than body requirements r/t anorexia, pain from distended colon

Impaired **Skin** integrity r/t stoma, potential skin care problems associated with stoma

Ineffective **Health** maintenance r/t parental deficient knowledge regarding temporary stoma care, dietary management, treatment for constipation or diarrhea

See Hospitalized Child

Hirsutism

Disturbed **Body** image r/t excessive hair

Hitting Behavior

Acute **Confusion** r/t dementia, alcohol abuse, drug abuse, delirium

Risk for other-directed **Violence** (See **Violence,** other-directed, risk for, Section II)

HIV (Human Immunodeficiency Virus)

Fear r/t possible death

Ineffective **Protection** r/t depressed immune system

See AIDS (Acquired Immune Deficiency Syndrome)

Hodgkin's Disease

See Anemia; Cancer; Chemotherapy

Home Maintenance Problems

Impaired **Home** maintenance (See **Home** maintenance, impaired, Section II)

Homelessness

Impaired **Home** maintenance r/t impaired cognitive or emotional functioning, inadequate support system, insufficient finances

Powerlessness r/t interpersonal interactions

Risk for **Trauma**: Risk factor: being in high-crime neighborhood

Hope

Readiness for enhanced **Hope** (See **Hope,** readiness for enhanced, Section II)

Hopelessness

Hopelessness (See **Hopelessness,** Section II)

Hospitalized Child

Activity intolerance r/t fatigue associated with acute illness

Acute **Pain** r/t treatments, diagnostic or therapeutic procedures

Anxiety: separation (child) r/t familiar surroundings and separation from family and friends

Compromised family **Coping** r/t possible prolonged hospitalization that exhausts supportive capacity of significant people

Deficient **Diversional** activity r/t immobility, monotonous environment, frequent or lengthy treatments, reluctance to participate, therapeutic isolation, separation from peers

Delayed **Growth** and development r/t regression or lack of progression toward developmental milestones as a result of frequent or prolonged hospitalization, inadequate or inappropriate stimulation, cerebral insult, chronic illness, effects of physical disability, prescribed dependence

Fear r/t deficient knowledge or maturational level with fear of unknown, mutilation, painful procedures, surgery

Hopelessness: child r/t prolonged activity restriction, uncertain prognosis

Ineffective **Coping**: parent r/t possible guilt regarding hospitalization of child, parental inadequacies

Insomnia: child or parent r/t 24-hour care needs of hospitalization

Interrupted **Family** processes r/t situational crisis of illness, disease, hospitalization

Powerlessness: child r/t health care environment, illness-related regimen

Readiness for enhanced family **Coping** r/t impact of crisis on family values, priorities, goals, relationships in family

Risk for impaired parent/child **Attachment**: Risk factor: separation

Risk for delayed **Growth** and development: regression: Risk factors: disruption of normal routine, unfamiliar environment or caregivers, developmental vulnerability of young children

Risk for imbalanced **Nutrition**: less than body requirements: Risk factors: anorexia, absence of familiar foods, cultural preferences

Risk for **Injury**: Risk factors: unfamiliar environment, developmental age, lack of parental knowledge regarding safety (e.g., side rails, IV site/pole)

See Child with Chronic Condition

Hostile Behavior

Risk for other-directed **Violence**: Risk factor: antisocial personality disorder

HTN (Hypertension)

Disturbed **Energy** field r/t pain, discomfort

Imbalanced **Nutrition**: more than body requirements r/t lack of knowledge of relationship between diet and disease process

Ineffective **Health** maintenance r/t deficient knowledge regarding treatment and control of disease process

Noncompliance r/t side effects of treatments, lack of understanding regarding importance of controlling hypertension

Human Immunodeficiency Virus (HIV)

See AIDS (Acquired Immune Deficiency Syndrome); HIV (Human Immunodeficiency Virus)

Humiliating Experience

Risk for compromised human **Dignity** (See **Dignity**, compromised human, risk for, Section II)

Huntington's Disease

Decisional **Conflict** r/t whether to have children

See Neurological Disorders

Hydrocele

Acute **Pain** r/t severely enlarged hydrocele

Ineffective **Sexuality** pattern r/t recent surgery on area of scrotum

Hydrocephalus

Decisional **Conflict** r/t unclear or conflicting values regarding selection of treatment modality

Delayed **Growth** and development r/t sequelae of increased intracranial pressure

Imbalanced **Nutrition**: less than body requirements r/t inadequate intake as a result of anorexia, nausea, vomiting, feeding difficulties

Impaired **Skin** integrity r/t impaired physical mobility, mechanical irritation

Ineffective **Tissue** perfusion: cerebral r/t interrupted flow, hypervolemia of cerebral ventricles

Interrupted **Family** processes r/t situational crisis

Risk for delayed **Development**: Risk factor: sequelae of increased intracranial pressure

Risk for disproportionate **Growth**: Risk factor: sequelae of increased intracranial pressure

Risk for **Infection**: Risk factor: sequelae of invasive procedure (shunt placement)

See Normal Pressure Hydrocephalous (NPH); Child with Chronic Condition; Hospitalized Child; Mental Retardation (if appropriate); Premature Infant (Child); Premature Infant (Parent)

Hygiene, Inability to Provide Own

Adult **Failure** to thrive r/t depression, apathy as evidenced by inability to perform self-care

Self-care deficit: bathing/hygiene (See **Self-care** deficit, bathing/hygiene, Section II)

Hyperactive Syndrome

Compromised family **Coping** r/t unsuccessful strategies to control excessive activity, behaviors, frustration, anger

Decisional **Conflict** r/t multiple or divergent sources of information regarding education, nutrition, medication regimens; willingness to change own food habits; limited resources

Impaired **Social** interaction r/t impulsive and overactive behaviors, concomitant emotional difficulties, distractibility and excitability

Ineffective **Role** performance: parent r/t stressors associated with dealing with hyperactive child, perceived or projected blame for causes of child's behavior, unmet needs for support or care, lack of energy to provide for those needs

Parental role **Conflict**: when siblings present r/t increased attention toward hyperactive child

Risk for delayed **Development**: Risk factor: behavior disorders

Risk for impaired **Parenting**: Risk factor: disruptive or uncontrollable behaviors of child

Risk for other-directed **Violence**: parent or child: Risk factors: frustration with disruptive behavior, anger, unsuccessful relationships

Self-esteem disturbance r/t inability to achieve socially acceptable behaviors; frustration; frequent reprimands, punishment, or scolding for uncontrolled activity and behaviors; mood fluctuations and restlessness; inability to succeed academically; lack of peer support

Hyperalimentation

See TPN (Total Parenteral Nutrition)

Hyperbilirubinemia

Anxiety: parent r/t threat to infant, unknown future

Disturbed **Sensory** perception: visual (infant) r/t use of eye patches for protection of eyes during phototherapy

Imbalanced **Nutrition**: less than body requirements (infant) r/t disinterest in feeding because of jaundice-related lethargy

Parental role **Conflict** r/t interruption of family life because of care regimen

Risk for disproportionate **Growth**: infant: Risk factor: disinterest in feeding because of jaundice-related lethargy

Risk for **Imbalanced** body temperature: infant: Risk factor: phototherapy

Risk for **Injury**: infant: Risk factors: kernicterus, phototherapy lights

Hypercalcemia

Decreased **Cardiac** output r/t bradydysrhythmia

Disturbed **Thought** processes r/t elevated calcium levels that cause paranoia, decreased level of consciousness

Imbalanced **Nutrition**: less than body requirements r/t gastrointestinal manifestations of hypercalcemia (nausea, anorexia, ileus)

Impaired physical **Mobility** r/t decreased tone in smooth and striated muscle

Risk for **Trauma**: Risk factors: risk for fractures

Hypercapnia

Fear r/t difficulty breathing

Impaired **Gas** exchange r/t ventilation perfusion imbalance

Hyperemesis Gravidarum

Anxiety r/t threat to self and infant, hospitalization

Deficient **Fluid** volume r/t vomiting

Imbalanced **Nutrition**: less than body requirements r/t vomiting

Impaired **Home** maintenance r/t chronic nausea, inability to function

Nausea r/t hormonal changes of pregnancy

Powerlessness r/t health care regimen

Social isolation r/t hospitalization

Hyperglycemia

Ineffective management of **Therapeutic** regimen r/t complexity of therapeutic regimen, decisional conflicts, economic difficulties, unsupportive family, insufficient cues to action, deficient knowledge, mistrust, lack of acknowledgment of seriousness of condition

Risk for unstable blood **Glucose** (See **Glucose,** unstable blood, risk for, Section II)

See Diabetes Mellitus

Hyperkalemia

Decreased **Cardiac** output r/t possible dysrhythmia

Risk for **Activity** intolerance: Risk factor: muscle weakness

Risk for excess **Fluid** volume: Risk factor: untreated renal failure

Hypernatremia

Risk for deficient **Fluid** volume: Risk factors: abnormal water loss, inadequate water intake

Hyperosmolar Hyperglycemic Nonketotic Coma (HHNC)

Deficient **Fluid** volume r/t polyuria, inadequate fluid intake

Disturbed **Thought** processes r/t dehydration, electrolyte imbalance

Risk for **Injury**: seizures: Risk factors: hyperosmolar state, electrolyte imbalance

See Diabetes Mellitus; Diabetes Mellitus, Juvenile

Hyperphosphatemia

Deficient **Knowledge** r/t dietary changes needed to control phosphate levels

See Renal Failure

Hypersensitivity to Slight Criticism

Defensive **Coping** r/t situational crisis, psychological impairment, substance abuse

Hypertension

Imbalanced **Nutrition**: more than body requirements r/t lack of knowledge of relation between diet and disease process

Ineffective **Health** maintenance r/t deficient knowledge regarding treatment and control of disease process

Noncompliance r/t side effects of treatment

Hyperthermia

Hyperthermia (See **Hyperthermia,** Section II)

Hyperthyroidism

Activity intolerance r/t increased oxygen demands from increased metabolic rate

Anxiety r/t increased stimulation, loss of control

Diarrhea r/t increased gastric motility

Imbalanced **Nutrition**: less than body requirements r/t increased metabolic rate, increased gastrointestinal activity

Ineffective **Health** maintenance r/t deficient knowledge regarding medications, methods of coping with stress

Insomnia r/t anxiety, excessive sympathetic discharge

Risk for **Injury**: eye damage: Risk factor: exophthalmos

Hyperventilation

Ineffective **Breathing** pattern r/t anxiety, acid-base imbalance

Hypocalcemia

Activity intolerance r/t neuromuscular irritability

Imbalanced **Nutrition**: less than body requirements r/t effects of vitamin D deficiency, renal failure, malabsorption, laxative use

Ineffective **Breathing** pattern r/t laryngospasm

Hypoglycemia

Disturbed **Thought** processes r/t insufficient blood glucose to brain

Imbalanced **Nutrition**: less than body requirements r/t imbalance of glucose and insulin level

Ineffective **Health** maintenance r/t deficient knowledge regarding disease process, self-care

Risk for unstable blood **Glucose** (See

Glucose, unstable blood, risk for, Section II)

See Diabetes Mellitus; Diabetes Mellitus, Juvenile

Hypokalemia

Activity intolerance r/t muscle weakness

Decreased **Cardiac** output r/t possible dysrhythmia from electrolyte imbalance

H

Hypomagnesemia

Imbalanced **Nutrition**: less than body requirements r/t deficient knowledge of nutrition, alcoholism

See Alcoholism

Hypomania

Insomnia r/t psychological stimulus

See Manic Disorder, Bipolar I

Hyponatremia

Disturbed **Thought** processes r/t electrolyte imbalance

Excess **Fluid** volume r/t excessive intake of hypotonic fluids

Risk for **Injury**: Risk factors: seizures, new onset of confusion

Hypoplastic Left Lung

See Congenital Heart Disease/Cardiac Anomalies

Hypotension

Decreased **Cardiac** output r/t decreased preload, decreased contractility

Ineffective **Tissue** perfusion: cerebral/cardiopulmonary or peripheral r/t hypovolemia, decreased contractility, decreased afterload

Risk for deficient **Fluid** volume: Risk factor: excessive fluid loss

See cause of Hypotension

Hypothermia

Hypothermia (See **Hypothermia**, Section II)

Hypothyroidism

Activity intolerance r/t muscular stiffness, shortness of breath on exertion

Constipation r/t decreased gastric motility

Disturbed **Thought** processes r/t altered metabolic process

Imbalanced **Nutrition**: more than body requirements r/t decreased metabolic process

Impaired **Gas** exchange r/t possible respiratory depression

Impaired **Skin** integrity r/t edema, dry or scaly skin

Ineffective **Health** maintenance r/t deficient knowledge regarding disease process and self-care

Hypovolemic Shock

Deficient **Fluid** volume r/t trauma, third spacing, loss of fluid from body

See Shock

Hypoxia

Acute **Confusion** r/t decreased oxygen supply to brain

Disturbed **Thought** processes r/t decreased oxygen supply to brain

Fear r/t breathlessness

Impaired **Gas** exchange r/t altered oxygen supply, inability to transport oxygen

Hysterectomy

Acute **Pain** r/t surgical injury

Constipation r/t opioids, anesthesia, bowel manipulation during surgery

Ineffective **Coping** r/t situational crisis of surgery

Grieving r/t change in body image, loss of reproductive status

Ineffective **Health** maintenance r/t deficient knowledge regarding precautions and self-care after surgery

Risk for **Constipation**: Risk factors: narcotics, anesthesia, bowel manipulation during surgery

Risk for deficient **Fluid** volume: Risk factors: abnormal blood loss, hemorrhage

Risk for ineffective **Tissue** perfusion: Risk factor: thromboembolism

Risk for urge urinary **Incontinence**: Risk factors: edema in area, anesthesia, narcotics, pain

Sexual dysfunction r/t disturbance in self-concept

Urinary retention r/t edema in area, anesthesia, opioids, pain

See Surgery, Perioperative; Surgery, Preoperative; Surgery, Postoperative

I

IBS (Irritable Bowel Syndrome)

Chronic **Pain** r/t spasms, increased motility of bowel

Constipation r/t low-residue diet, stress

Diarrhea r/t increased motility of intestines associated with stress

Ineffective **Health** maintenance r/t deficient knowledge regarding self-care with IBS

Ineffective **Therapeutic** regimen management r/t deficient knowledge, powerlessness

Readiness for enhanced **Therapeutic** regimen management: r/t expressed desire to manage illness and prevent onset of symptoms

ICD (Implantable Cardioverter/Defibrillator)

Ineffective **Health** maintenance r/t deficient knowledge regarding self-care, action of internal cardiac defibrillator

Decreased **Cardiac** output r/t possible dysrhythmia

IDDM (Insulin-Dependent Diabetes)

See Diabetes Mellitus

Identity Disturbance

Disturbed personal **Identity** r/t situational crisis, psychological impairment, chronic illness, pain

Readiness for enhanced **Coping** r/t seeking social support

Spiritual distress r/t expression of alienation from others

Idiopathic Thrombocytopenic Purpura

See ITP (Idiopathic Thrombocytopenic Purpura)

Ileal Conduit

Deficient **Knowledge** r/t care of stoma

Disturbed **Body** image r/t presence of stoma

Ineffective **Sexuality** pattern r/t altered body function and structure

Ineffective **Therapeutic** regimen management r/t new skills required to care for appliance and self

Readiness for enhanced **Therapeutic** regimen management: r/t expressed desire to care for stoma

Risk for impaired **Skin** integrity: Risk factor: difficulty obtaining tight seal of appliance

Risk for latex **Allergy** response: Risk factor: repeated exposures to latex associated with treatment and management of disease

Social isolation r/t alteration in physical appearance, fear of accidental spill of ostomy contents

Ileostomy

Constipation r/t dietary changes, change in intestinal motility

Deficient **Knowledge** r/t limited practice of stoma care, dietary modifications

Diarrhea r/t dietary changes, alteration in intestinal motility

Disturbed **Body** image r/t presence of stoma

Ineffective **Sexuality** pattern r/t altered body function and structure

Ineffective **Therapeutic** regimen management r/t new skills required to care for appliance and self

Risk for impaired **Skin** integrity: Risk factors: difficulty obtaining tight seal of appliance, caustic drainage

Social isolation r/t alteration in physical appearance, fear of accidental spill of ostomy contents

Ileus

Acute **Pain** r/t pressure, abdominal distention

Constipation r/t decreased gastric motility

Deficient **Fluid** volume r/t loss of fluids from vomiting, fluids trapped in bowel

Nausea r/t gastrointestinal irritation

Immobility

Adult **Failure** to thrive r/t limited physical mobility

Constipation r/t immobility

Disturbed **Thought** processes r/t sensory deprivation from immobility

Impaired physical **Mobility** r/t medically imposed bedrest

Impaired **Transfer** ability r/t limited physical mobility

Impaired **Walking** r/t limited physical mobility

Ineffective **Breathing** pattern r/t inability to deep breathe in supine position

Ineffective **Tissue** perfusion: peripheral r/t interruption of venous flow

Powerlessness r/t forced immobility from health care environment

Risk for **Disuse** syndrome: Risk factor: immobilization

Risk for impaired **Skin** integrity: Risk factors: pressure on immobile parts, shearing forces when moved

Immunization

Readiness for enhanced **Immunization** status (See **Immunization** status, readiness for enhanced, Section II)

Immunosuppression

Ineffective **Protection** r/t medications, treatments, or pathology suppressing immune system function

Risk for **Infection**: Risk factor: immunosuppression

Impaction of Stool

Constipation r/t decreased fluid intake, less than adequate amounts of fiber and bulk-forming foods in diet, medication effect, or immobility

Imperforate Anus

Anxiety r/t ability to care for newborn

Deficient **Knowledge** r/t home care for newborn

Impaired **Skin** integrity r/t pruritus

Risk for impaired **Skin** integrity: Risk factor: presence of stool at surgical repair site

Impetigo

Ineffective **Health** maintenance r/t parental deficient knowledge regarding care of impetigo

See Communicable Diseases, Childhood

Implantable Cardioverter/Defibrillator

See ICD (Implantable Cardioverter/Defibrillator)

Impotence

Readiness for enhanced **Knowledge**: treatment information for erectile dysfunction

Self-esteem disturbance r/t physiological crisis, inability to practice usual sexual activity

Sexual dysfunction r/t altered body function

See Erectile Dysfunction

Inactivity

Activity intolerance r/t imbalance between oxygen supply and demand, sedentary lifestyle, weakness, immobility

Impaired physical **Mobility** r/t intolerance to activity, decreased strength and endurance, depression, severe anxiety, musculoskeletal impairment, perceptual or cognitive impairment, neuromuscular impairment, pain, discomfort

Risk for **Constipation**: Risk factor: insufficient physical activity

Incompetent Cervix

See Premature Dilation of the Cervix (Incompetent Cervix)

Incontinence of Stool

Bowel incontinence r/t decreased awareness of need to defecate, loss of sphincter control

Deficient **Knowledge** r/t lack of information on normal bowel elimination

Disturbed **Body** image r/t inability to control elimination of stool

Risk for impaired **Skin** integrity: Risk factor: presence of stool

Situational low **Self-esteem** r/t inability to control elimination of stool

Toileting **Self-care** deficit r/t toileting needs

Incontinence of Urine

Functional urinary **Incontinence** r/t altered environment; sensory, cognitive, or mobility deficits

Overflow urinary **Incontinence** r/t relaxation of pelvic muscles and changes in urinary structures

Reflex urinary **Incontinence** r/t neurological impairment

Risk for impaired **Skin** integrity: Risk factor: presence of urine

Toileting **Self-care** deficit r/t neuromuscular dysfunction

Situational low **Self-esteem** r/t inability to control passage of urine

Stress urinary **Incontinence** (See **Incontinence,** stress urinary, Section II)

Total urinary **Incontinence** (See **Incontinence,** total urinary, Section II)

Urge urinary **Incontinence** (See **Incontinence,** urge urinary, Section II)

Indigestion

Imbalanced **Nutrition**: less than body requirements r/t discomfort when eating

Nausea r/t gastrointestinal irritation

Induction of Labor

Anxiety r/t medical interventions

Decisional **Conflict** r/t perceived threat to idealized birth

Ineffective **Coping** r/t situational crisis of medical intervention in birthing process

Readiness for enhanced **Family** processes: family support during induction of labor

Risk for **Injury**: maternal and fetal: Risk factors: hypertonic uterus, potential prematurity of newborn

Self-esteem disturbance r/t inability to carry out normal labor

Infant Apnea

See Premature Infant (Child); Respiratory Conditions of the Neonate; SIDS (Sudden Infant Death Syndrome)

I

Infant Behavior

Disorganized **Infant** behavior r/t pain, oral/motor problems, feeding intolerance, environmental overstimulation, lack of containment or boundaries, prematurity, invasive or painful procedures

Readiness for enhanced organized **Infant** behavior r/t prematurity, pain

Risk for disorganized **Infant** behavior: Risk factors: pain, oral/motor problems, environmental overstimulation, lack of containment or boundaries

I

Infant Feeding Pattern, Ineffective

Ineffective **Infant** feeding pattern r/t prematurity, neurological impairment or delay, oral hypersensitivity, prolonged nothing-by-mouth order

Infant of Diabetic Mother

Deficient **Fluid** volume r/t increased urinary excretion and osmotic diuresis

Delayed **Growth** and development r/t prolonged and severe postnatal hypoglycemia

Imbalanced **Nutrition**: less than body requirements r/t hypotonia, lethargy, poor sucking, postnatal metabolic changes from hyperglycemia to hypoglycemia and hyperinsulinism

Risk for decreased **Cardiac** output: Risk factor: increased incidence of cardiomegaly

Risk for delayed **Development**: Risk factors: prolonged and severe postnatal hypoglycemia

Risk for disproportionate **Growth**: Risk factors: prolonged and severe postnatal hypoglycemia

Risk for impaired **Gas** exchange: Risk factors: increased incidence of cardiomegaly, prematurity

See Premature Infant (Child); Respiratory Conditions of the Neonate

Infant of Substance-Abusing Mother (Fetal Alcohol Syndrome, Crack Baby, Other Drug Withdrawal Infants)

Delayed **Growth** and development r/t effects of maternal use of drugs, effects of neurological impairment, decreased attentiveness to environmental stimuli or inadequate stimuli

Diarrhea r/t effects of withdrawal, increased peristalsis from hyperirritability

Disturbed **Sensory** perception r/t hypersensitivity to environmental stimuli

Imbalanced **Nutrition**: less than body requirements r/t feeding problems; uncoordinated or ineffective suck and swallow; effects of diarrhea, vomiting, or colic associated with maternal substance abuse

Impaired **Parenting** r/t impaired or absent attachment behaviors, inadequate support systems

Ineffective **Airway** clearance r/t pooling of secretions from the lack of adequate cough reflex, effects of viral or bacterial lower airway infection as a result of altered protective state

Ineffective **Infant** feeding pattern r/t uncoordinated or ineffective sucking reflex

Ineffective **Protection** r/t effects of maternal substance abuse

Insomnia r/t hyperirritability or hypersensitivity to environmental stimuli

Interrupted **Breastfeeding** r/t use of drugs or alcohol by mother

Risk for delayed **Development**: Risk factor: substance abuse

Risk for disproportionate **Growth**: Risk factor: substance abuse

Risk for **Infection**: skin, meningeal, respiratory: Risk factor: effects of withdrawal

See Cerebral Palsy; Child with Chronic Condition; Crack Baby; Failure to Thrive, Nonorganic; Hospitalized Child; Hyperactive Syndrome;

Premature Infant (Child); SIDS (Sudden Infant Death Syndrome)

Infantile Polyarteritis

See Kawasaki Disease

Infantile Spasms

See Seizure Disorders, Childhood

Infection

Hyperthermia r/t increased metabolic rate

Ineffective **Protection** r/t inadequate nutrition, abnormal blood profiles, drug therapies, treatments

Infection, Potential for

Risk for **Infection** (See **Infection,** risk for, Section II)

Infertility

Chronic **Sorrow** r/t inability to conceive a child

Ineffective **Therapeutic** regimen management r/t deficient knowledge about infertility

Powerlessness r/t infertility

Spiritual distress r/t inability to conceive a child

Inflammatory Bowel Disease (Child and Adult)

Acute **Pain** r/t abdominal cramping and anal irritation

Deficient **Fluid** volume r/t frequent and loose stools

Diarrhea r/t effects of inflammatory changes of the bowel

Imbalanced **Nutrition**: less than body requirements r/t anorexia, decreased absorption of nutrients from gastrointestinal tract

Impaired **Skin** integrity r/t frequent stools, development of anal fissures

Ineffective **Coping** r/t repeated episodes of diarrhea

Social isolation r/t diarrhea

See Child with Chronic Condition; Crohn's Disease; Hospitalized Child; Maturational Issues, Adolescent

Influenza

Acute **Pain** r/t inflammatory changes in joints

Deficient **Fluid** volume r/t inadequate fluid intake

Hyperthermia r/t infectious process

Ineffective **Health** maintenance r/t deficient knowledge regarding self-care

Ineffective **Therapeutic** regimen management r/t lack of knowledge regarding preventive immunizations

Readiness for enhanced **Knowledge**: about information to prevent or treat influenza

Inguinal Hernia Repair

Acute **Pain** r/t surgical procedure

Impaired physical **Mobility** r/t pain at surgical site and fear of causing hernia to rupture

Risk for **Infection**: Risk factor: surgical procedure

Urinary retention r/t possible edema at surgical site

Injury

Risk for **Falls**: Risk factors: orthostatic hypertension, impaired physical mobility, diminished mental status

Risk for **Injury**: Risk factor: environmental conditions interacting with client's adaptive and defensive resources

Insomnia

Insomnia (See **Insomnia,** Section II)

Insulin Shock

See Hypoglycemia

Intermittent Claudication

Acute **Pain** r/t decreased circulation to extremities with activity

Deficient **Knowledge** r/t lack of knowledge of cause and treatment of peripheral vascular diseases

Ineffective **Tissue** perfusion: peripheral r/t interruption of arterial flow

Readiness for enhanced **Knowledge**: prevention of pain and impaired circulation

Risk for **Injury**: Risk factor: tissue hypoxia

Risk for **Peripheral** neurovascular dysfunction: Risk factor: disruption in arterial flow

See Peripheral Vascular Disease

Internal Cardioverter/Defibrillator

See ICD (Implantable Cardioverter/Defibrillator)

Internal Fixation

Impaired **Walking** r/t repair of fracture

Risk for **Infection**: Risk factors: traumatized tissue, broken skin

See Fracture

Interstitial Cystitis

Acute **Pain** r/t inflammatory process

Impaired **Urinary** elimination r/t inflammation of bladder

Risk for **Infection**: Risk factor: suppressed inflammatory response

Intervertebral Disk Excision

See Laminectomy

Intestinal Obstruction

See Ileus

Intoxication

Acute **Confusion** r/t alcohol abuse

Anxiety r/t loss of control of actions

Disturbed **Sensory** perception r/t neurochemical imbalance in brain

Disturbed **Thought** processes r/t effect of substance on central nervous system

Impaired **Memory** r/t effects of alcohol on mind

Ineffective **Coping** r/t use of mind-altering substances as a means of coping

Risk for **Falls**: Risk factor: diminished mental status

Risk for other-directed **Violence**: Risk factor: inability to control thoughts and actions

Intraaortic Balloon Counterpulsation

Anxiety r/t device providing cardiovascular assistance

Compromised family **Coping** r/t seriousness of significant other's medical condition

Decreased **Cardiac** output r/t failing heart needing counterpulsation

Impaired physical **Mobility** r/t restriction of movement because of mechanical device

Risk for **Peripheral** neurovascular dysfunction: Risk factors: vascular obstruction of balloon catheter, thrombus formation, emboli, edema

Intracranial Pressure, Increased

Acute **Confusion** r/t increased intracranial pressure

Adult **Failure** to thrive r/t undetected changes from increased intracranial pressure

Decreased **Intracranial** adaptive capacity r/t sustained increase in intracranial pressure

Disturbed **Sensory** perception r/t pressure damage to sensory centers in brain

Disturbed **Thought** processes r/t pressure damage to brain

Impaired **Memory** r/t neurological disturbance

Ineffective **Breathing** pattern r/t pressure damage to breathing center in brainstem

Ineffective **Tissue** perfusion: cerebral r/t effects of increased intracranial pressure

See cause of Increased Intracranial Pressure

Intrauterine Growth Retardation

Anxiety: maternal r/t threat to fetus

Delayed **Growth** and development r/t insufficient supply of oxygen and nutrients

Imbalanced **Nutrition**: less than body requirements r/t insufficient placenta

Impaired **Gas** exchange r/t insufficient placental perfusion

Ineffective **Coping**: maternal r/t situational crisis, threat to fetus

Risk for delayed **Development**: Risk factor: insufficient supply of oxygen and nutrients

Risk for disproportionate **Growth**: Risk factor: insufficient supply of oxygen and nutrients

Risk for **Injury**: Risk factor: insufficient supply of oxygen and nutrients

Risk for **Powerlessness**: Risk factor: unknown outcome of fetus

Situational low **Self-esteem**: maternal r/t guilt about threat to fetus

Spiritual distress r/t unknown outcome of fetus

Intubation, Endotracheal or Nasogastric

Acute **Pain** r/t presence of tube

Disturbed **Body** image r/t altered appearance with mechanical devices

Imbalanced **Nutrition**: less than body requirements r/t inability to ingest food because of the presence of tubes

Impaired **Oral** mucous membrane r/t presence of tubes

Impaired verbal **Communication** r/t endotracheal tube

Irregular Pulse

See Dysrhythmia

Irritable Bowel Syndrome

See IBS (Irritable Bowel Syndrome)

Isolation

Social isolation (See **Social** isolation, Section II)

Itching

Risk for **Infection**: Risk factor: potential break in skin

Pruritus r/t inflammation of the skin

ITP (Idiopathic Thrombocytopenic Purpura)

Deficient **Diversional** activity r/t activity restrictions, safety precautions

Ineffective **Protection** r/t decreased platelet count

Risk for **Injury**: Risk factors: decreased platelet count, developmental level, age-appropriate play

See Hospitalized Child

J

Jaundice

Disturbed **Thought** processes r/t toxic blood metabolites

Pruritus r/t toxic metabolites excreted in the skin

Risk for impaired **Liver** function: Risk factor: possible viral infection

Risk for impaired **Skin** integrity: Risk factors: pruritus, itching

See Cirrhosis; Hepatitis

Jaundice, Neonatal

Readiness for enhanced **Therapeutic** regimen management: r/t expresses desire to manage treatment: assessment of jaundice when infant is discharged from the hospital, when to call the physician, and possible preventive measures such as frequent breastfeeding

See Hyperbilirubinemia

Jaw Pain and Heart Attacks

See Angina Pectoris; Chest Pain; MI (Myocardial Infarction)

Jaw Surgery

Acute **Pain** r/t surgical procedure

Deficient **Knowledge** r/t emergency care for wired jaws (e.g., cutting bands and wires), oral care

Imbalanced **Nutrition**: less than body requirements r/t jaws wired closed

Impaired **Swallowing** r/t edema from surgery

Risk for **Aspiration**: Risk factor: wired jaws

Jet Lag Prevention

Readiness for enhanced **Knowledge** r/t getting adequate sleep before travel, drinking extra water, avoiding caffeine and alcohol, engaging in regular exercise (but not at bedtime)

Jittery

Anxiety r/t unconscious conflict about essential values and goals, threat to or change in health status

Death Anxiety r/t unresolved issues relating to end of life

Risk for **Post-trauma** syndrome: Risk factors: occupation, survivor's role in event, inadequate social support

Jock Itch

Impaired **Skin** integrity r/t moisture and irritating or tight-fitting clothing

Ineffective **Therapeutic** regimen management r/t prevention and treatment

See Itching

Joint Dislocation

See Dislocation

Joint Inflammation

See Arthritis; JRA (Juvenile Rheumatoid Arthritis)

Joint Pain

See Arthritis; Bursitis; JRA (Juvenile Rheumatoid Arthritis); Osteoarthritis; Rheumatoid Arthritis

Joint Replacement

Risk for **Peripheral** neurovascular dysfunction: Risk factor: orthopedic surgery

See Total Joint Replacement

JRA (Juvenile Rheumatoid Arthritis)

Acute **Pain** r/t swollen or inflamed joints, restricted movement, physical therapy

Delayed **Growth** and development r/t effects of physical disability, chronic illness

Fatigue r/t chronic inflammatory disease

Impaired physical **Mobility** r/t pain, restricted joint movement

Risk for compromised human **Dignity**: Risk factors: perceived intrusion by clinicians, invasion of privacy

Risk for impaired **Skin** integrity: Risk factors: splints, adaptive devices

Risk for **Injury**: Risk factors: impaired physical mobility, splints, adaptive devices, increased bleeding potential from antiinflammatory medications

Risk for situational low **Self-esteem**: Risk factor: disturbed body image

Self-care deficits: feeding, bathing/hygiene, dressing, grooming, toileting r/t restricted joint movement, pain

See Child with Chronic Condition; Hospitalized Child

Juvenile Onset Diabetes

See Diabetes Mellitus, Juvenile

Kaposi's Sarcoma

Risk for Complicated **Grieving**: Risk factor: loss of social support

Risk for compromised human **Dignity**: Risk factor: use of undefined medical terms

Risk for impaired **Religiosity**: Risk factors: illness/hospitalization, ineffective coping

See AIDS (Acquired Immune Deficiency Syndrome)

Kawasaki Disease (Formerly Mucocutaneous Lymph Node Syndrome)

Acute **Pain** r/t enlarged lymph nodes; erythematous skin rash that progresses to desquamation, peeling, denuding of skin

Anxiety: parental r/t progression of disease, complications of arthritis, and cardiac involvement

Hyperthermia r/t inflammatory disease process

Imbalanced **Nutrition**: less than body requirements r/t impaired oral mucous membranes

Impaired **Oral** mucous membranes r/t inflamed mouth and pharynx; swollen lips that become dry, cracked, fissured

Impaired **Skin** integrity r/t inflammatory skin changes

See Hospitalized Child

Kegel Exercise

Health-seeking behavior r/t desire for information to relieve incontinence

Risk for urge urinary **Incontinence**: Risk factors: effects of alcohol, caffeine, decreased bladder capacity, irritation of bladder stretch receptors causing spasm, increased urine concentration, overdistention of bladder

Stress urinary **Incontinence** r/t degenerative change in pelvic muscles

Urge urinary **Incontinence** r/t decreased bladder capacity

Keloids

Disturbed **Body** image r/t presence of scar tissue at site of a healed skin injury

Readiness for enhanced **Therapeutic** regimen management: desire to have information to decrease discoloration of skin from sun exposure

Keratoconjunctivitis Sicca

Risk for **Infection** r/t dry eyes

See Conjunctivitis

Keratoplasty

See Corneal Transplant

Ketoacidosis, Diabetic

Deficient **Fluid** volume r/t excess excretion of urine, nausea, vomiting, increased respiration

Imbalanced **Nutrition**: less than body requirements r/t body's inability to use nutrients

Impaired **Memory** r/t fluid and electrolyte imbalance

Ineffective **Therapeutic** regimen management r/t denial of illness, lack of understanding of preventive measures, and adequate blood sugar control

Noncompliance: diabetic regimen r/t ineffective coping with chronic disease

Risk for **Powerlessness**: Risk factor: illness-related regimen

Risk for unstable **Glucose** Level: Risk factor: deficient knowledge of diabetes management (e.g., action plan)

See Diabetes Mellitus

Ketoacidosis: Alcoholic

See Alcohol Withdrawal; Alcoholism

Keyhole Heart Surgery

See MIDCAB (Minimally Invasive Direct Coronary Artery Bypass)

Kidney Failure

See Renal Failure

Kidney Stone

Acute **Pain** r/t obstruction from renal calculi

Deficient **Knowledge** r/t fluid requirements and dietary restrictions

Impaired **Urinary** elimination: urgency and frequency r/t anatomical obstruction, irritation caused by stone

Overflow urinary **Incontinence** r/t bladder outlet obstruction

Risk for deficient **Fluid** volume: Risk factors: nausea, vomiting

Risk for **Infection**: Risk factor: obstruction of urinary tract with stasis of urine

Kidney Transplant

Decisional **Conflict** r/t acceptance of donor kidney

Ineffective **Protection** r/t immunosuppressive therapy

Readiness for enhanced **Decision** making: expresses desire to enhance understanding of choices

Readiness for enhanced **Family** processes: adapting to life without dialysis

Readiness for enhanced **Spiritual** well-being: heightened coping, living without dialysis

Readiness for enhanced **Therapeutic** regimen management: desire to manage the treatment and prevention of complications post transplant

See Nephrectomy; Renal Failure; Renal Transplantation, Donor; Renal Transplantation, Recipient; Surgery, Perioperative Care; Surgery, Postoperative Care; Surgery, Preoperative Care

Kidney Tumor

See Wilms' Tumor

Kissing Disease

See Mononucleosis

Knee Replacement

See Total Joint Replacement

Knowledge

Readiness for enhanced **Knowledge** (See **Knowledge**, readiness for enhanced, Section II)

Knowledge, Deficient

Deficient **Knowledge** (See **Knowledge**, deficient, Section II)

Ineffective **Health** maintenance r/t lack of or significant alteration in communication skills (written, verbal, and/or gestural)

Ineffective **Therapeutic** regimen management r/t complexity of therapeutic regimen

Kock Pouch

See Continent Ileostomy (Kock Pouch)

Korsakoff's Syndrome

Acute **Confusion** r/t alcohol abuse

Dysfunctional **Family** processes: alcoholism r/t possible cause of syndrome

Impaired **Memory** r/t neurological changes

Risk for **Falls**: Risk factor: cognitive impairment

Risk for imbalanced **Nutrition**: less than body requirements: Risk factor: lack of adequate balanced intake

Risk for impaired **Liver** function: Risk factor: substance abuse (alcohol)

Risk for **Injury**: Risk factors: sensory dysfunction, lack of coordination when ambulating

L

Labor, Induction of

See Induction of Labor

Labor, Normal

Acute **Pain** r/t uterine contractions, stretching of cervix and birth canal

Anxiety r/t fear of the unknown, situational crisis

Deficient **Knowledge** r/t lack of preparation for labor

Fatigue r/t childbirth

Health-seeking behaviors healthy outcome of pregnancy, prenatal care, and childbirth education

Impaired **Tissue** integrity r/t passage of infant through birth canal, episiotomy

Readiness for enhanced family **Coping** r/t significant other providing support during labor

Readiness for enhanced **Power**: expresses readiness to enhance participation in choices regarding treatment during labor

Risk for deficient **Fluid** volume: Risk factor: excessive loss of blood

Risk for **Infection**: Risk factors: multiple vaginal examinations, tissue trauma, prolonged rupture of membranes

Risk for **Injury**: Risk factor: fetal, r/t hypoxia

Risk for **Post-trauma** syndrome: Risk factors: trauma or violence associated with labor pains, birth process, medical or surgical interventions, history of sexual abuse

Risk for **Powerlessness**: Risk factor: labor process

Labyrinthitis

Risk for **Injury** r/t dizziness

Ineffective **Therapeutic** regimen management r/t delay in seeking treatment for respiratory and ear infections

Readiness for enhanced **Therapeutic** regimen management: management of episodes

Lactation

See Breastfeeding, Effective; Breastfeeding, Ineffective; Breastfeeding, Interrupted

Lactic acidosis

Decreased **Cardiac** output r/t altered heart rate/rhythm, preload, and contractility

See Ketoacidosis, Diabetic

Lactose Intolerance

Readiness for enhanced **Knowledge** r/t interest in identifying lactose intolerance, treatment, and substitutes for milk products

See Abdominal Distention; Diarrhea

Laminectomy

Acute **Pain** r/t localized inflammation and edema

Anxiety r/t change in health status, surgical procedure

Deficient **Knowledge** r/t appropriate postoperative and postdischarge activities

Disturbed **Sensory** perception: tactile r/t possible edema or nerve injury

Impaired physical **Mobility** r/t neuromuscular impairment

Risk for impaired **Tissue** perfusion: Risk factors: edema, hemorrhage, embolism

Risk for perioperative positioning **Injury**: Risk factor: prone position

Urinary retention r/t competing sensory impulses, effects of narcotics or anesthesia

See Scoliosis; Surgery, Perioperative; Surgery, Postoperative; Surgery, Preoperative

Laparoscopic Laser Cholecystectomy

See Cholecystectomy; Laser Surgery

Laparoscopy

Acute **Pain**: shoulder r/t gas irritating the diaphragm

Urge urinary **Incontinence** r/t pressure on the bladder from gas

Laparotomy

L

See Abdominal Surgery

Laryngectomy

Grieving r/t loss of voice, fear of death

Chronic **Sorrow** r/t change in body image

Death **Anxiety** r/t unknown results of surgery

Disturbed **Body** image r/t change in body structure and function

Imbalanced **Nutrition**: less than body requirements r/t absence of oral feeding, difficulty swallowing, increased need for fluids

Impaired **Oral** mucous membranes r/t absence of oral feeding

Impaired **Swallowing** r/t edema, laryngectomy tube

Impaired verbal **Communication** r/t removal of larynx

Ineffective **Airway** clearance r/t surgical removal of glottis, decreased humidification of air

Ineffective **Health** maintenance r/t deficient knowledge regarding self-care with laryngectomy

Interrupted **Family** processes r/t surgery, serious condition of family member, difficulty communicating

Risk for complicated **Grieving**: Risk factors: loss, major life event

Risk for compromised human **Dignity**: Risk factor: loss of control of body function

Risk for **Infection**: Risk factors: invasive procedure, surgery

Risk for **Powerlessness**: Risk factors: chronic illness, change in communication

Risk for situational low **Self-esteem**: Risk factor: disturbed body image

Laser Surgery

Acute **Pain** r/t heat from laser

Constipation r/t laser intervention in vulval and perianal areas

Deficient **Knowledge** r/t preoperative and postoperative care associated with laser procedure

Risk for **Infection**: Risk factor: delayed heating reaction of tissue exposed to laser

Risk for **Injury**: Risk factor: accidental exposure to laser beam

LASIK Eye Surgery (Laser-Assisted in Situ Keratomileusis)

Decisional **Conflict** r/t decision to have the surgery

Readiness for enhanced **Therapeutic** regimen management: surgical procedure pre- and postoperative teaching and expectations

Latex Allergy

Latex **Allergy** response (See **Allergy** response, latex, Section II)

Readiness for enhanced **Knowledge** of prevention and treatment of exposure to latex products

Risk for latex **Allergy** response (See **Allergy** response, latex, risk for, Section II)

Laxative Abuse

Perceived **Constipation** r/t health belief, faulty appraisal, impaired thought processes

Lead Poisoning

Contamination r/t flaking, peeling paint in presence of young children

Impaired **Home** maintenance r/t presence of lead paint

Risk for delayed **Development**: Risk factor: lead poisoning

Legionnaires' Disease

Contamination r/t contaminated water in air-conditioning systems

Ineffective community **Therapeutic** regimen management r/t contaminated air systems in large buildings

See Pneumonia

Lens Implant

See Cataract Extraction; Vision Impairment

Lethargy/Listlessness

Adult **Failure** to thrive r/t apathy

Insomnia r/t internal or external stressors

Fatigue r/t decreased metabolic energy production

Ineffective **Tissue** perfusion: cerebral r/t lack of oxygen supply to brain

See cause of Lethargy/Listlessness

Leukemia

Ineffective **Protection** r/t abnormal blood profile

Risk for deficient **Fluid** volume: Risk factors: nausea, vomiting, bleeding, side effects of treatment

Risk for **Infection**: Risk factor: ineffective immune system

See Cancer; Chemotherapy

Leukopenia

Ineffective **Protection** r/t leukopenia

Risk for **Infection** r/t low white blood cell count

Level of Consciousness, Decreased

See Confusion, Acute; Confusion, Chronic

Lice

Pruritus r/t inflammation

Impaired **Home** maintenance r/t close unsanitary, overcrowded conditions

Readiness for enhanced **Therapeutic** regimen management: r/t preventing and treating infestation

See Communicable Diseases, Childhood

Lifestyle, sedentary

Sedentary **Lifestyle** (See **Lifestyle,** sedentary, Section II)

Lightheadedness

See Dizziness; Vertigo

Limb Reattachment Procedures

Anxiety r/t unknown outcome of reattachment procedure, use and appearance of limb

Disturbed **Body** image r/t unpredictability of function and appearance of reattached body part

Grieving r/t unknown outcome of reattachment procedure

Risk for deficient **Fluid** volume: hemorrhage: Risk factor: severed vessels

Risk for impaired **Religiosity**: Risk factors: suffering, hospitalization

Risk for perioperative positioning **Injury**: Risk factor: immobilization

Risk for **Peripheral** neurovascular dysfunction: Risk factors: trauma, orthopedic and neurovascular surgery, compression of nerves and blood vessels

Risk for **Powerlessness**: Risk factor: unknown outcome of procedure

Spiritual distress r/t anxiety about condition

Stress overload r/t multiple coexisting stressors, physical demands

See Surgery, Postoperative Care

Liposuction

Disturbed **Body** image r/t dissatisfaction with unwanted fat deposits in body

Readiness for enhanced **Decision** making r/t expressed desire to make decision regarding liposuction

Readiness for enhanced **Self-concept** r/t satisfaction with new body image

See Surgery, Perioperative Care; Surgery, Postoperative Care; Surgery, Preoperative Care

L

Lithotripsy

Readiness for enhanced **Therapeutic** regimen management: expresses desire for information related to procedure and after care and prevention of stones

See Kidney Stone

Liver Biopsy

Anxiety r/t procedure and results

Risk for deficient **Fluid** volume r/t hemorrhage from biopsy site

Risk for **Powerlessness** r/t inability to control outcome of procedure

Liver Disease

See Cirrhosis; Hepatitis

Liver Function

Risk for impaired **Liver** function: Risk factors (See **Liver** function, risk for impaired, Section II)

Liver Transplant

Decisional **Conflict** r/t acceptance of donor liver

Ineffective **Protection** r/t immunosuppressive therapy

Readiness for enhanced **Family** processes: change in physical needs of family member

Readiness for enhanced **Spiritual** well-being: heightened coping

Readiness for enhanced **Therapeutic** regimen management: desire to manage the treatment and prevention of complications posttransplant

Risk for impaired **Liver** function: Risk factors: possible rejection, infection

See Surgery, Perioperative Care; Surgery, Postoperative Care; Surgery, Preoperative Care

Living Will

Moral distress r/t end-of-life decisions

Readiness for enhanced **Decision Making**: expresses desire to enhance understanding of choices for decision making

Readiness for enhanced **Religiosity** r/t request to meet with religious leaders or facilitators

Readiness for enhanced **Spiritual** well-being r/t acceptance of and preparation for end of life

See Advance Directives

Lobectomy

See Thoracotomy

Loneliness

Readiness for enhanced **Hope** r/t expresses desire to enhance interconnectedness with others

Risk for impaired **Religiosity**: Risk factor: lack of social interaction

Risk for **Loneliness**: Risk factors (See **Loneliness,** risk for, Section II)

Risk for situational low **Self-esteem**: Risk factors: failure, rejection

Spiritual distress r/t loneliness, social alienation

Loose Stools

Diarrhea r/t increased gastric motility

See cause of Loose Stools

Loss of Bladder Control

See Incontinence of Urine

Loss of Bowel Control

See Incontinence of Stool

Lou Gehrig's Disease

See ALS (Amyotrophic Lateral Sclerosis)

Low Back Pain

Chronic **Pain** r/t degenerative processes, musculotendinous strain, injury, inflammation, congenital deformities

Impaired physical **Mobility** r/t back pain

Ineffective **Health** maintenance r/t deficient knowledge regarding self-care with back pain

Readiness for enhanced **Therapeutic** regimen management: expressed desire for information to manage pain

Risk for **Powerlessness**: Risk factor: living with chronic pain

Urinary retention r/t possible spinal cord compression

Lumbar Puncture

Acute **Pain**: headache r/t possible loss of cerebrospinal fluid

Anxiety r/t invasive procedure and unknown results

Deficient **Knowledge** r/t information about procedure

Risk for **Infection**: Risk factor: invasive procedure

Lumpectomy

Decisional **Conflict** r/t treatment choices

Readiness for enhanced **Knowledge** r/t preoperative and postoperative care

Readiness for enhanced **Spiritual** well-being r/t hope of benign diagnosis

See Cancer

Lung Cancer

See Cancer; Chemotherapy; Radiation Therapy; Thoracotomy

Lupus Erythematosus

Acute **Pain** r/t inflammatory process

Chronic **Sorrow** r/t presence of chronic illness

Disturbed **Body** image r/t change in skin, rash, lesions, ulcers, mottled erythema

Fatigue r/t increased metabolic requirements

Impaired **Religiosity** r/t ineffective coping with disease

Ineffective **Health** maintenance r/t deficient knowledge regarding medication, diet, activity

Powerlessness r/t unpredictability of course of disease

Risk for impaired **Skin** integrity: Risk factors: chronic inflammation, edema, altered circulation

Spiritual distress r/t chronicity of disease, unknown etiology

Lyme Disease

Acute **Pain** r/t inflammation of joints, urticaria, rash

Deficient **Knowledge** r/t lack of information concerning disease, prevention, treatment

Fatigue r/t increased energy requirements

Risk for decreased **Cardiac** output: Risk factor: dysrhythmia

Risk for **Powerlessness**: Risk factor: possible chronic condition

Lymphedema

Deficient **Knowledge** r/t management of condition

Disturbed **Body** image r/t change in appearance of body part with edema

Excess **Fluid** volume r/t compromised

regulatory system; inflammation, obstruction, or removal of lymph glands

Risk for situational low **Self-esteem** r/t disturbed body image

Lymphoma

See Cancer

Macular Degeneration

Compromised **Family** coping r/t deteriorating vision of family member

Disturbed **Sensory** perception: visual r/t blurred, distorted, dim, or absent central vision

Effective management of **Therapeutic** regimen: appropriate choices of daily activities for meeting the goals of a treatment program

Hopelessness r/t deteriorating vision

Ineffective **Coping** r/t visual loss

Risk for **Falls**: Risk factor: visual difficulties

Risk for impaired **Religiosity**: Risk factor: possible lack of transportation

Risk for **Injury**: Risk factor: inability to distinguish traffic lights

Risk for **Powerlessness**: Risk factor: deteriorating vision

Risk prone health **Behavior** r/t deteriorating vision

Sedentary **Lifestyle** r/t visual loss

Social isolation r/t inability to drive because of visual changes

Magnetic Resonance Imaging

See MRI (Magnetic Resonance Imaging)

Major Depressive Disorder

Interrupted **Family** processes r/t change in health status of family member

Risk for **Loneliness**: Risk factors: social isolation associated with feelings of sadness, hopelessness

See Depression (Major Depressive Disorder)

Malabsorption Syndrome

Deficient **Knowledge** r/t lack of information about diet and nutrition

Diarrhea r/t lactose intolerance, gluten sensitivity, resection of small bowel

Imbalanced **Nutrition**: less than body requirements r/t inability of body to absorb nutrients because of biological factors

Risk for deficient **Fluid** volume: Risk factor: diarrhea

Risk for disproportionate **Growth**: Risk factor: malnutrition from malabsorption

See Abdominal Distention

Maladaptive Behavior

See Crisis; Post-trauma Syndrome; Suicide Attempt

Malaise

See Fatigue

Malaria

Contamination r/t geographic area

Readiness for enhanced community **Coping**: Uses resources available for problem solving

Readiness for enhanced **Immunization** status: expresses desire to enhance immunization status and knowledge of immunization standards

Risk for **Contamination**: Risk factors: increased environmental exposure (not wearing protective clothing, not using insecticide or repellant on skin and in room in areas where infected mosquitoes are present); inadequate defense mechanisms (inappropriate use of prophylactic regimen)

See Anemia

Malignancy

See Cancer

Malignant Hypertension (Arteriolar Nephrosclerosis)

Decreased **Cardiac** output r/t altered afterload, altered contractility

Disturbed **Sensory** perception: visual r/t altered sensory reception from papilledema

Excess **Fluid** volume r/t decreased renal function

Fatigue r/t disease state, increased blood pressure

Readiness for enhanced **Therapeutic** regimen: management expresses desire to manage the illness, high blood pressure

Risk for acute **Confusion**: Risk factors: increased blood urea nitrogen or creatine levels

Risk for imbalanced **Fluid** volume: Risk factors: hypertension, altered renal function

Malignant Hyperthermia

Effective **Therapeutic** regimen management: verbalizes desire to manage the treatment of illness; informs health care providers of anesthesia problems

Hyperthermia r/t anesthesia reaction associated with inherited condition

Malnutrition

Adult **Failure** to thrive r/t undetected malnutrition

Deficient **Knowledge** r/t misinformation about normal nutrition, social isolation, lack of food preparation facilities

Imbalanced **Nutrition**: less than body requirements r/t inability to ingest food, digest food, or absorb nutrients because of biological, psychological, or economic factors; institutionalization (i.e., lack of menu choices)

Ineffective **Protection** r/t inadequate nutrition

Ineffective **Therapeutic** regimen management r/t economic difficulties

Risk for disproportionate **Growth**: Risk factor: malnutrition

Risk for **Powerlessness**: Risk factor: possible inability to provide adequate nutrition

Mammography

Effective **Therapeutic** regimen management: verbalizes desire to manage prevention of sequelae; follows guidelines for mammograms

Health-seeking behaviors: information regarding mammograms

Manic Disorder, Bipolar I

Anxiety r/t change in role function

Deficient **Fluid** volume r/t decreased intake

Disturbed **Thought** processes r/t mania

Imbalanced **Nutrition**: less than body requirements r/t lack of time and motivation to eat, constant movement

Impaired **Home** maintenance r/t altered psychological state, inability to concentrate

Ineffective **Coping** r/t situational crisis

Ineffective **Denial** r/t fear of inability to control behavior

Ineffective **Role** performance r/t impaired social interactions

Interrupted **Family** processes r/t family member's illness

Ineffective **Therapeutic** regimen management r/t lack of social supports

Ineffective **Therapeutic** regimen management: families r/t unpredictability of client, excessive demands on family, chronicity of condition

Insomnia r/t constant anxious thoughts

Noncompliance r/t denial of illness

Readiness for enhanced **Hope** r/t expresses desire to enhance problem-solving goals

Risk for **Caregiver** role strain r/t unpredictability of condition

Risk for impaired **Religiosity**: Risk factor: depression

Risk for **Powerlessness**: Risk factor: inability to control changes in mood

Risk for self- or other-directed **Violence**: Risk factors: hallucinations, delusions

Risk for **Spiritual** distress: Risk factor: depression

Risk for **Suicide**: Risk factor: bipolar disorder

Sleep deprivation r/t hyperagitated state

Manipulation of Organs, Surgical Incision

Deficient **Knowledge** r/t lack of exposure to information regarding care after surgery and at home

Risk for **Infection**: Risk factor: presence of urinary catheter

Urinary retention r/t swelling of urinary meatus

Manipulative Behavior

Defensive **Coping** r/t superior attitude toward others

Impaired **Social** interaction r/t self-concept disturbance

Ineffective **Coping** r/t inappropriate use of defense mechanisms

Risk for **Loneliness**: Risk factor: inability to interact appropriately with others

Risk for **Self-mutilation**: Risk factor: inability to cope with increased psychological or physiological tension in healthy manner

Risk for situational low **Self-esteem** Risk factor: history of learned helplessness

Self-mutilation r/t use of manipulation to obtain nurturing relationship with others

Marasmus

See Failure to Thrive, Nonorganic

Marfan Syndrome

Decreased **Cardiac** output r/t dilation of the aortic root, dissection or rupture of the aorta

Disturbed **Sensory** perception; visual r/t myopia associated with Marfan syndrome

Effective **Therapeutic** regimen management: Verbalizes desire to manage the treatment of illness and intent to reduce risk factors for progression of illness

Readiness for enhanced **Therapeutic** regimen management: Describes reduction of risk factors

See Mitral Valve Prolapse; Scoliosis

Marshall-Marchetti-Krantz Operation

PREOPERATIVE

Stress urinary **Incontinence** r/t weak pelvic muscles and pelvic supports

POSTOPERATIVE

Acute **Pain** r/t manipulation of organs, surgical incision

Deficient **Knowledge** r/t lack of exposure to information regarding care after surgery and at home

Risk for **Infection** r/t presence of urinary catheter

Urinary retention r/t swelling of urinary meatus

Mastectomy

Acute **Pain** r/t surgical procedure

Chronic **Sorrow** r/t disturbed body image, unknown long-term health status

Death **Anxiety** r/t threat of mortality associated with breast cancer

Deficient **Knowledge** r/t self-care activities

Disturbed **Body** image r/t loss of sexually significant body part

Fear r/t change in body image, prognosis

Nausea r/t chemotherapy

Risk for impaired physical **Mobility**: Risk factors: nerve or muscle damage, pain

Risk for **Post-trauma** syndrome: Risk factors: loss of body part, surgical wounds

Risk for **Powerlessness**: Risk factor: fear of unknown outcome of procedure

Sexual dysfunction r/t change in body image, fear of loss of femininity

Spiritual distress r/t change in body image

See Cancer; Modified Radical Mastectomy; Surgery, Perioperative; Surgery, Postoperative; Surgery, Preoperative

Mastitis

Acute **Pain** r/t infectious disease process, swelling of breast tissue

Anxiety r/t threat to self, concern over safety of milk for infant

Deficient **Knowledge** r/t antibiotic regimen, comfort measures

Ineffective **Breastfeeding** r/t breast pain, conflicting advice from health care providers

Ineffective **Role** performance r/t change in capacity to function in expected role

Maternal Infection

Ineffective **Protection** r/t invasive procedures, traumatized tissue

See Postpartum, Normal Care

Maturational Issues, Adolescent

Deficient **Knowledge**: potential for enhanced health maintenance r/t information misinterpretation, lack of education regarding age-related factors

Impaired **Social** interaction r/t ineffective, unsuccessful, or dysfunctional interaction with peers

Ineffective **Coping** r/t maturational crises

Interrupted **Family** processes r/t developmental crises of adolescence resulting from challenge of parental authority and values, situational crises from change in parental marital status

Readiness for enhanced **Communication**: expressing willingness to communicate with parental figures

Risk for **Injury/Trauma**: Risk factor: thrill-seeking behaviors

Risk for situational low **Self-esteem**: Risk factor: developmental changes

Risk-prone health **Behavior** r/t inadequate comprehension, negative attitude toward health care

Social isolation r/t perceived alteration in physical appearance, social values not accepted by dominant peer group

See Sexuality, Adolescent; Substance Abuse (if relevant)

Maze III Procedure

See Open Heart Surgery; Dysrhythmia

Measles (Rubeola)

See Communicable Diseases, Childhood

Meconium Aspiration

See Respiratory Conditions of the Neonate

Melanoma

Acute **Pain** r/t surgical incision

Disturbed **Body** image r/t altered pigmentation, surgical incision

Fear r/t threat to well-being

Ineffective **Health** maintenance r/t deficient knowledge regarding self-care and treatment of melanoma

See Cancer

Melena

Fear r/t presence of blood in feces

Risk for deficient **Fluid** volume: Risk factor: hemorrhage

See GI Bleed (Gastrointestinal Bleeding)

Memory Deficit

Impaired **Memory** (See **Memory**, impaired, Section II)

Ménière's Disease

Effective management of **Therapeutic** regimen; prompt treatment of ear infection

Readiness for enhanced **Therapeutic** regimen management: expresses desire to manage illness

Risk for **Injury**: r/t symptoms from disease

See Dizziness; Nausea; Vertigo

M

Meningitis/Encephalitis

Acute **Pain** r/t biological injury

Decreased **Intracranial** adaptive capacity r/t sustained increase in intracranial pressure of 10 to 15 mm Hg

Delayed **Growth** and development r/t effects of physical disability

Disturbed **Sensory** perception: hearing r/t central nervous system infection, ear infection

Disturbed **Sensory** perception: kinesthetic r/t central nervous system infection

Disturbed **Sensory** perception: visual r/t photophobia attributable to central nervous system infection

Disturbed **Thought** processes r/t inflammation of brain, fever

Excess **Fluid** volume r/t increased intracranial pressure, syndrome of inappropriate secretion of antidiuretic hormone

Impaired **Mobility** r/t neuromuscular or central nervous system insult

Ineffective **Airway** clearance r/t seizure activity

Ineffective **Tissue** perfusion: cerebral r/t inflamed cerebral tissues and meninges, increased intracranial pressure

Readiness for enhanced **Immunization** status r/t expresses desire to enhance immunization status and knowledge of immunization standards

Risk for acute **Confusion** r/t infection of brain

Risk for **Aspiration**: Risk factor: seizure activity

Risk for **Falls**: Risk factor: neuromuscular dysfunction

Risk for **Injury**: Risk factor: seizure activity

See Hospitalized Child

Meningocele

See Neural Tube Defects

Menopause

Health-seeking behavior: expresses desire for increased control of health practice

Impaired **Memory** r/t change in hormonal levels

Ineffective **Sexuality** pattern r/t altered body structure, lack of physiological lubrication, lack of knowledge of artificial lubrication

Ineffective **Thermoregulation** r/t changes in hormonal levels

Readiness for enhanced **Spiritual** well-being r/t desire for harmony of mind, body, and spirit

Readiness for enhanced **Therapeutic** regimen management: verbalized desire to manage menopause

Readiness for enhanced **Self-care**: expresses satisfaction with body image

Risk for imbalanced **Nutrition**: more than body requirements: Risk factor: change in metabolic rate caused by fluctuating hormone levels

Risk for **Powerlessness**: Risk factor: changes associated with menopause

Risk for situational low **Self-esteem**: Risk factors: developmental changes: menopause

Risk for urge urinary **Incontinence**: Risk

factor: changes in hormonal levels affecting bladder function

Menorrhagia

Fear r/t loss of large amounts of blood

Risk for deficient **Fluid** volume r/t excessive loss of menstrual blood

Mental Illness

Chronic **Sorrow** r/t presence of mental illness

Compromised family **Coping** r/t lack of available support from client

Defensive **Coping** r/t psychological impairment, substance abuse

Disabled family **Coping** r/t chronically unexpressed feelings of guilt, anxiety, hostility, or despair

Disturbed **Thought** processes: inaccurate interpretation of environment, inappropriate thinking

Ineffective community **Therapeutic** regimen management: insufficient health care resources/programs

Ineffective **Coping** r/t situational crisis, coping with mental illness

Ineffective **Denial** r/t refusal to acknowledge abuse problem, fear of the social stigma of disease

Ineffective family **Therapeutic** regimen management r/t chronicity of condition, unpredictability of client, unknown prognosis

Risk for **Loneliness**: Risk factor: social isolation

Risk for **Powerlessness**: Risk factor: lifestyle of helplessness

Stress overload r/t multiple coexisting stressors

Mental Retardation

Delayed **Growth** and development r/t cognitive or perceptual impairment, developmental delay

Grieving r/t loss of perfect child, birth of child with congenital defect or subsequent head injury

Impaired **Home** maintenance r/t insufficient support systems

Impaired **Swallowing** r/t neuromuscular impairment

Impaired verbal **Communication** r/t developmental delay

Interrupted **Family** processes r/t crisis of diagnosis and situational transition

Readiness for enhanced family **Coping**: adaptation and acceptance of child's condition and needs

Risk for delayed **Development**: Risk factor: cognitive or perceptual impairment

Risk for disproportionate **Growth**: Risk factor: mental retardation

Risk for impaired **Religiosity**: Risk factor: social isolation

Risk for **Self-mutilation**: Risk factors: separation anxiety, depersonalization

Self-care deficit: bathing, hygiene, dressing, grooming, feeding, toileting r/t perceptual or cognitive impairment

Self-mutilation r/t inability to express tension verbally

Spiritual distress r/t chronic condition of child with special needs

Stress overload r/t intense, repeated stressor (chronic condition)

See Child with Chronic Condition; Safety, Childhood

Metabolic Acidosis

See Ketoacidosis, Diabetic; Ketoacidosis, Alcoholic

Metabolic Alkalosis

Deficient **Fluid** volume r/t fluid volume loss, vomiting, gastric suctioning, failure of regulatory mechanisms

Metastasis

See Cancer

M

MI (Myocardial Infarction)

Acute **Pain** r/t myocardial tissue damage from inadequate blood supply

Anxiety r/t threat of death, possible change in role status

Constipation r/t decreased peristalsis from decreased physical activity, medication effect, change in diet

Death **Anxiety** r/t seriousness of medical condition

Decreased **Cardiac** output r/t ventricular damage, ischemia, dysrhythmias

Fear r/t threat to well-being

Ineffective **Denial** r/t fear, deficient knowledge about heart disease

Ineffective family **Coping** r/t spouse or significant other's fear of partner loss

Ineffective **Health** maintenance r/t deficient knowledge regarding self-care and treatment

Ineffective **Sexuality** pattern r/t fear of chest pain, possibility of heart damage

Ineffective **Therapeutic** regimen management r/t knowledge deficit

Interrupted **Family** processes r/t crisis, role change

Readiness for enhanced **Knowledge**: expresses an interest in learning about condition

Risk for **Powerlessness**: Risk factor: acute illness

Risk for **Spiritual** distress: Risk factors: physical illness: MI

Situational low **Self-esteem** r/t crisis of MI

MIDCAB (Minimally Invasive Direct Coronary Artery Bypass)

Readiness for enhanced **Therapeutic** regimen management: pre- and postoperative care associated with the surgery

Risk for **Infection**: Risk factor: large breasts on incision line

See Angioplasty, Coronary; Coronary Artery Bypass Grafting

Midlife Crisis

Ineffective **Coping** r/t inability to deal with changes associated with aging

Powerlessness r/t lack of control over life situation

Readiness for enhanced **Spiritual** well-being: desire to find purpose and meaning to life

Spiritual distress r/t questioning beliefs or value system

Migraine Headache

Acute **Pain**: headache r/t vasodilation of cerebral and extracerebral vessels

Disturbed **Energy** field r/t pain, disruption of normal flow of energy

Ineffective **Health** maintenance r/t deficient knowledge regarding prevention and treatment of headaches

Readiness for enhanced **Therapeutic** regimen management: expressed desire to manage the illness

Milk Intolerance

See Lactose Intolerance

Minimally Invasive Heart Surgery

See MIDCAB (Minimally Invasive Direct Coronary Artery Bypass); OPCAB (Off-Pump Coronary Artery Bypass)

Miscarriage

See Pregnancy Loss

Mitral Stenosis

Activity intolerance r/t imbalance between oxygen supply and demand

Anxiety r/t possible worsening of symptoms, activity intolerance, fatigue

Decreased **Cardiac** output r/t incompetent heart valves, abnormal forward or backward blood flow, flow into a dilated chamber, flow through an abnormal passage between chambers

Fatigue r/t reduced cardiac output

Ineffective **Health** maintenance r/t deficient knowledge regarding self-care with disorder

Mitral Valve Prolapse

Acute **Pain** r/t mitral valve regurgitation

Anxiety r/t symptoms of condition: palpitations, chest pain

Effective management of **Therapeutic** regimen: verbalizes desire to manage prevention of sequelae

Fatigue r/t abnormal catecholamine regulation, decreased intravascular volume

Fear r/t lack of knowledge about mitral valve prolapse, feelings of having a heart attack

Ineffective **Health** maintenance r/t deficient knowledge regarding methods to relieve pain and treat dysrhythmia and shortness of breath, need for prophylactic antibiotics before invasive procedures

Ineffective **Tissue** perfusion: cerebral r/t postural hypotension

Readiness for enhanced **Knowledge**: expresses an interest in learning about condition

Risk for **Infection**: Risk factor: invasive procedures

Risk for **Powerlessness**: Risk factor: unpredictability of onset of symptoms

Mobility, Impaired Bed

Impaired bed **Mobility** (See **Mobility,** impaired bed, Section II)

Mobility, Impaired Physical

Impaired physical **Mobility** (See **Mobility,** impaired physical, Section II)

Risk for **Falls** r/t impaired physical mobility

Mobility, Impaired Wheelchair

Impaired wheelchair **Mobility** (See **Mobility,** impaired wheelchair, Section II)

Modified Radical Mastectomy

Decisional **Conflict** r/t treatment of choice

Readiness for enhanced **Communication**: willingness to enhance communication

See Mastectomy

Mononucleosis

Activity intolerance r/t generalized weakness

Acute **Pain** r/t enlargement of lymph nodes, oropharyngeal edema

Fatigue r/t disease state, stress

Hyperthermia r/t infectious process

Impaired **Swallowing** r/t enlargement of lymph nodes, oropharyngeal edema

Ineffective **Health** maintenance r/t deficient knowledge concerning transmission and treatment of disease

Risk for **Injury**: Risk factor: possible rupture of spleen

Risk for **Loneliness**: Risk factor: social isolation

Mood Disorders

Caregiver role strain r/t symptoms associated with disorder of care receiver

Readiness for enhanced **Communication**: expresses feelings

Risk for situational low **Self-esteem**: Risk factor: unpredictable changes in mood

Risk-prone health **Behavior** r/t hopelessness, altered locus of control

Social isolation r/t alterations in mental status

See Specific Disorder: Depression; Dysthymic Disorder; Hypomania; Manic Disorder, Bipolar I

Moon Face

Disturbed **Body** image r/t change in appearance from disease and medication

Risk for situational low **Self-esteem**: Risk factor: change in body image

See Cushing's Syndrome

Moral/Ethical Dilemmas

Decisional **Conflict** r/t questioning personal values and belief, which alter decision

Moral Distress r/t conflicting information guiding moral or ethical decision making

Readiness for enhanced **Decision** making: expresses desire to enhance congruency of decisions with personal values and goals

Readiness for enhanced **Religiosity**: requests assistance in expanding religious options

Readiness for enhanced **Spiritual** well-being: request for interaction with others regarding difficult decisions

Risk for **Powerlessness**: Risk factor: lack of knowledge to make a decision

Risk for **Spiritual** distress: Risk factor: moral or ethical crisis

Morning Sickness

See Hyperemesis Gravidarum; Pregnancy, Normal

Mottling of Peripheral Skin

Ineffective **Tissue** perfusion: peripheral r/t interruption of arterial flow, decreased circulating blood volume

Mourning

See Grieving

Mouth Lesions

See Mucous Membranes, Impaired Oral

MRI (Magnetic Resonance Imaging)

Anxiety r/t fear of being in closed spaces

Deficient **Knowledge** r/t unfamiliarity with information resources; exam information

Readiness for enhanced **Knowledge**: expresses interest in learning about exam

Readiness for enhanced **Therapeutic** regimen management: describes reduction of risk factors associated with exam

Mucocutaneous Lymph Node Syndrome

See Kawasaki Syndrome

Mucous Membranes, Impaired Oral

Impaired **Oral** mucous membranes (See **Oral** mucous membranes, impaired, Section II)

Multiinfarct Dementia

See Dementia

Multiple Gestation

Anxiety r/t uncertain outcome of pregnancy

Death **Anxiety** r/t maternal complications associated with multiple gestation

Deficient **Knowledge** r/t caring for more than one infant

Fatigue r/t physiological demands of a multifetal pregnancy and/or care of more than one infant

Imbalanced **Nutrition**: less than body requirements r/t physiological demands of a multifetal pregnancy

Impaired **Home** maintenance r/t fatigue

Impaired physical **Mobility** r/t increased uterine size

Impaired **Transfer** ability r/t enlarged uterus

Insomnia r/t impairment of normal sleep pattern; parental responsibilities

Readiness for enhanced **Family** processes: family adapting to change with more than one infant

Risk for **Constipation**: Risk factor: enlarged uterus

Risk for delayed **Development**: fetus: Risk factor: multiple gestation

Risk for disproportionate **Growth**: fetus: Risk factor: multiple gestation

Risk for ineffective **Breastfeeding**: Risk factors: lack of support, physical demands of feeding more than one infant

Stress overload r/t multiple coexisting stressors, family demands

Stress urinary **Incontinence** r/t increased pelvic pressure

Multiple Personality Disorder (Dissociative Identity Disorder)

Anxiety r/t loss of control of behavior and feelings

Chronic low **Self-esteem** r/t rejection, failure

Defensive **Coping** r/t unresolved past traumatic events, severe anxiety

Disturbed **Body** image r/t psychosocial changes

Disturbed personal **Identity** r/t severe child abuse

Hopelessness r/t long-term stress

Ineffective **Coping** r/t history of abuse

Readiness for enhanced **Communication**: willingness to discuss problems associated with condition

Risk for **Self-mutilation**: Risk factor: need to act out to relieve stress

See Dissociative Identity Disorder (Not Otherwise Specified)

Multiple Sclerosis (MS)

Chronic **Sorrow** r/t loss of physical ability

Disturbed **Energy** field r/t disruption in energy flow resulting from disharmony between mind and body

Disturbed **Sensory** perception: specify r/t pathology in sensory tracts

Impaired physical **Mobility** r/t neuromuscular impairment

Ineffective **Airway** clearance r/t decreased energy or fatigue

Powerlessness r/t progressive nature of disease

Readiness for enhanced **Self-care**: expresses desire to enhance knowledge of strategies and responsibility for self-care

Readiness for enhanced **Spiritual** well-being: struggling with chronic debilitating condition

Readiness for enhanced **Therapeutic** regimen management: expresses a desire to manage condition

Risk for **Disuse** syndrome: Risk factor: physical immobility

Risk for imbalanced **Nutrition**: less than body requirements: Risk factors: impaired swallowing, depression

Risk for impaired **Religiosity**: Risk factor: illness

Risk for **Injury**: Risk factors: altered mobility, sensory dysfunction

Risk for latex **Allergy** response: Risk factor: possible repeated exposures to latex associated with intermittent catheterizations

Risk for **Powerlessness**: Risk factor: chronic illness

Self-care deficit: specify r/t neuromuscular impairment

Sexual dysfunction r/t biopsychosocial alteration of sexuality

Spiritual distress r/t perceived hopelessness of diagnosis

Urinary retention r/t inhibition of the reflex arc

See Neurological Disorders

Mumps

See Communicable Diseases, Childhood

Murmurs

Decreased **Cardiac** output r/t altered preload/afterload

Muscular Atrophy/Weakness

Risk for **Disuse** syndrome: Risk factor: impaired physical mobility

Risk for **Falls**: Risk factor: impaired physical mobility

Muscular Dystrophy (MD)

Activity intolerance r/t fatigue

Constipation r/t immobility

Decreased **Cardiac** output r/t effects of congestive heart failure

Disturbed **Energy** field r/t illness

Fatigue r/t increased energy requirements to perform activities of daily living

Imbalanced **Nutrition**: less than body requirements r/t impaired swallowing or chewing

Imbalanced **Nutrition**: more than body requirements r/t inactivity

Impaired **Mobility** r/t muscle weakness and development of contractures

Impaired **Transfer** ability r/t muscle weakness

Impaired **Walking** r/t muscle weakness

Ineffective **Airway** clearance r/t muscle weakness and decreased ability to cough

Readiness for enhanced **Self-concept**: acceptance of strength and abilities

Risk for **Aspiration**: Risk factor: impaired swallowing

Risk for **Disuse** syndrome: Risk factor: complications of immobility

Risk for **Falls**: Risk factor: muscle weakness

Risk for impaired **Gas** exchange: Risk factor: ineffective airway clearance and ineffective breathing pattern caused by muscle weakness

Risk for impaired **Religiosity**: Risk factor: illness

Risk for impaired **Skin** integrity: Risk factors: immobility, braces, or adaptive devices

Risk for ineffective **Breathing** pattern: Risk factor: muscle weakness

Risk for **Infection**: Risk factor: pooling of pulmonary secretions as a result of immobility and muscle weakness

Risk for **Injury**: Risk factor: muscle weakness and unsteady gait

Risk for **Powerlessness**: Risk factor: chronic condition

Risk for situational low **Self-esteem**: Risk factor: presence of chronic condition

Self-care deficits: feeding, bathing, dressing, toileting r/t muscle weakness and fatigue

See Child with Chronic Condition; Hospitalized Child

MVA (Motor Vehicle Accident)

See Fracture; Head Injury; Injury; Pneumothorax

Myasthenia Gravis

Fatigue r/t paresthesia, aching muscles

Imbalanced **Nutrition**: less than body requirements r/t difficulty eating and swallowing

Impaired physical **Mobility** r/t defective transmission of nerve impulses at the neuromuscular junction

Impaired **Swallowing** r/t neuromuscular impairment

Ineffective **Airway** clearance r/t decreased ability to cough and swallow

Ineffective **Therapeutic** regimen management r/t lack of knowledge of treatment, uncertainty of outcome

Interrupted **Family** processes r/t crisis of dealing with diagnosis

Readiness for enhanced **Spiritual** well-being: heightened coping with serious illness

Risk for **Caregiver** role strain: Risk factor: severity of illness of client

Risk for impaired **Religiosity**: Risk factor: illness

See Neurological Disorders

Mycoplasma Pneumonia

See Pneumonia

Myelocele

See Neural Tube Defects

Myelogram, Contrast

Acute **Pain** r/t irritation of nerve roots

Risk for deficient **Fluid** volume: Risk factor: possible dehydration

Risk for ineffective **Tissue** perfusion: cerebral: Risk factors: hypotension, loss of cerebrospinal fluid

Urinary retention r/t pressure on spinal nerve roots

Myelomeningocele

See Neural Tube Defects

Myocardial Infarction

See MI (Myocardial Infarction)

Myocarditis

Activity intolerance r/t reduced cardiac reserve and prescribed bed rest

Decreased **Cardiac** output r/t altered preload/afterload

Deficient **Knowledge** r/t treatment of disease

Readiness for enhanced **Knowledge** of treatment of disease

See CHF (Congestive Heart Failure), if appropriate

Myringotomy

Acute **Pain** r/t surgical procedure

Disturbed **Sensory** perception r/t possible hearing impairment

Fear r/t hospitalization, surgical procedure

Ineffective **Health** maintenance r/t deficient knowledge regarding care after surgery

Risk for **Infection**: Risk factor: invasive procedure

Myxedema

See Hypothyroidism

N

Narcissistic Personality Disorder

Decisional **Conflict** r/t lack of realistic problem-solving skills

Defensive **Coping** r/t grandiose sense of self

Disturbed **Personal** identity r/t psychological impairment

Impaired **Social** interaction r/t self-concept disturbance

Interrupted **Family** processes r/t taking advantage of others to achieve own goals

Risk for **Loneliness** r/t inability to interact appropriately with others

Risk-prone health **Behavior**: Risk factor: low self-efficacy

Risk for **Self-mutilation**: Risk factor: inadequate coping

Narcolepsy

Anxiety r/t fear of lack of control over falling asleep

Insomnia r/t uncontrollable desire to sleep

Readiness for enhanced **Sleep**: expression of willingness to enhance sleep

Risk for **Trauma**: Risk factor: falling

asleep during potentially dangerous activity

Narcotic Use

Risk for **Constipation**: Risk factor: effects of opioids on peristalsis

See Substance Abuse (if relevant)

Nasogastric Suction

Impaired **Oral** mucous membrane r/t presence of nasogastric tube

Risk for deficient **Fluid** volume: Risk factor: loss of gastrointestinal fluids without adequate replacement

Nausea

Nausea: biophysical, situational, treatment related (See **Nausea,** Section II)

N

Near-Drowning

Aspiration r/t aspiration of fluid into the lungs

Fear: parental r/t possible death of child, possible permanent and debilitating sequelae

Grieving/Risk for Complicated **Grieving** r/t potential death of child, unknown sequelae, guilt about accident

Hypothermia r/t central nervous system injury, prolonged submersion in cold water

Impaired **Gas** exchange r/t laryngospasm, holding breath, aspiration

Ineffective **Airway** clearance r/t aspiration, impaired gas exchange

Ineffective **Health** maintenance r/t parental deficient knowledge regarding safety measures appropriate for age

Readiness for enhanced **Spiritual** well-being: struggle with survival of life-threatening situation

Risk for delayed **Development** and disproportionate growth: Risk factors: hypoxemia, cerebral anoxia

Risk for **Infection**: Risk factors: aspiration, invasive monitoring

See Child with Chronic Condition; Hospitalized Child; Safety, Childhood; Terminally Ill Child/Death of Child, Parent

Nearsightedness

Effective **Therapeutic** regimen management: early diagnosis and appropriate referral for eyeglasses or contact lenses when nearsightedness is suspected; signs that may indicate a vision problem, including sitting close to television, holding books very close when reading, or having difficulty reading the blackboard in school or signs on a wall

Nearsightedness; Corneal Surgery

See LASIK Eye Surgery (Laser-Assisted in Situ Keratomileusis)

Neck Vein Distention

Decreased **Cardiac** output r/t decreased contractility of heart resulting increased preload

Excess **Fluid** volume r/t excess fluid intake, compromised regulatory mechanisms

See CHF (Congestive Heart Failure)

Necrosis, Renal Tubular; ATN (Acute Tubular Necrosis); Necrosis, Acute Tubular

See Renal Failure

Necrotizing Enterocolitis (NEC)

Deficient **Fluid** volume r/t vomiting, gastrointestinal bleeding

Disturbed **Energy** field r/t illness

Imbalanced **Nutrition**: less than body requirements r/t decreased ability to absorb nutrients, decreased perfusion to gastrointestinal tract

Ineffective **Breathing** pattern r/t abdominal distention, hypoxia

Ineffective **Tissue** perfusion: gastrointestinal r/t shunting of blood away from mesenteric circulation and toward vital organs as a result of perinatal stress, hypoxia

Risk for **Infection**: Risk factors: bacterial invasion of gastrointestinal tract, invasive procedures

See Hospitalized Child; Premature Infant (Child)

Necrotizing Fasciitis (Flesh-Eating Bacteria)

Acute **Pain** r/t toxins interfering with blood flow

Decreased **Cardiac** output r/t tachycardia and hypotension

Fear r/t possible fatal outcome of disease

Grieving r/t poor prognosis associated with disease

Hyperthermia r/t presence of infection

Ineffective **Protection** r/t cellulites resistant to treatment

Ineffective **Tissue** perfusion: peripheral r/t thrombosis of the subcutaneous blood vessels, leading to necrosis of nerve fibers

See Renal Failure; Septicemia; Shock

Negative Feelings About Self

Chronic low **Self-esteem** r/t longstanding negative self-evaluation

Readiness for enhanced **Self-concept** r/t expresses willingness to enhance self-concept

Self-esteem disturbance r/t inappropriate learned negative feelings about self

Neglect, Unilateral

See Neglect, Unilateral Section III

Neglectful Care of Family Member

Caregiver role strain r/t care demands of family member, lack of social or financial support

Deficient **Knowledge** r/t care needs

Disabled family **Coping** r/t highly ambivalent family relationships, lack of respite care

Ineffective community **Therapeutic** regimen management r/t deficits in community for support of caregivers, detection of client neglect

Interrupted **Family** processes r/t situational transition or crisis

Risk for compromised human **Dignity**: Risk factor: inadequate participation in decision making

Neonate

See Newborn, Normal; Newborn, Postmature; Newborn, Small for Gestational Age (SGA)

Neoplasm

Fear r/t possible malignancy

See Cancer

Nephrectomy

Acute **Pain** r/t incisional discomfort

Anxiety r/t surgical recovery, prognosis

Constipation r/t lack of return of peristalsis

Impaired **Urinary** elimination r/t loss of kidney

Ineffective **Breathing** pattern r/t location of surgical incision

Risk for deficient **Fluid** volume: Risk factors: vascular losses, decreased intake

Risk for **Infection** Risk factors: invasive procedure, lack of deep breathing because of location of surgical incision

Spiritual distress r/t chronic illness

Nephrostomy, Percutaneous

Acute **Pain** r/t invasive procedure

Impaired **Urinary** elimination r/t nephrostomy tube

Risk for **Infection**: Risk factor: invasive procedure

N

Nephrotic Syndrome

Activity intolerance r/t generalized edema

Disturbed **Body** image r/t edematous appearance and side effects of steroid therapy

Excess **Fluid** volume r/t edema resulting from oncotic fluid shift caused by serum protein loss and renal retention of salt and water

Imbalanced **Nutrition**: less than body requirements r/t anorexia, protein loss

Imbalanced **Nutrition**: more than body requirements r/t increased appetite attributable to steroid therapy

Risk for impaired **Skin** integrity: Risk factor: edema

Risk for **Infection**: Risk factor: altered immune mechanisms caused by disease and effects of steroids

Risk for **Noncompliance**: Risk factor: side effects of home steroid therapy

Social isolation r/t edematous appearance

See Child with Chronic Condition; Hospitalized Child

Nerve Entrapment

See Carpal Tunnel Syndrome

Neural Tube Defects (Meningocele, Myelomeningocele, Spina Bifida, Anencephaly)

Chronic low **Self-esteem** r/t perceived differences, decreased ability to participate in physical and social activities at school

Constipation r/t immobility or less than adequate mobility

Delayed **Growth** and development r/t physical impairments, possible cognitive impairment

Disturbed **Sensory** perception: visual r/t altered reception caused by strabismus

Grieving r/t loss of perfect child, birth of child with congenital defect

Impaired **Mobility** r/t neuromuscular impairment

Impaired **Skin** integrity r/t incontinence

Readiness for enhanced family **Coping**: effective adaptive response by family members

Readiness for enhanced **Family** processes: family supports each other

Reflex **Incontinence** r/t neurogenic impairment

Risk for imbalanced **Nutrition**: more than body requirements: Risk factors: diminished, limited, or impaired physical activity

Risk for impaired **Skin** integrity: lower extremities: Risk factor: decreased sensory perception

Risk for latex **Allergy** response: Risk factor: multiple exposures to latex products

Risk for **Powerlessness**: Risk factor: debilitating disease

Total urinary **Incontinence** r/t neurogenic impairment

Urge urinary **Incontinence** r/t neurogenic impairment

See Child with Chronic Condition; Premature Infant (Child)

Neuritis

Activity intolerance r/t pain with movement

Acute **Pain** r/t stimulation of affected nerve endings, inflammation of sensory nerves

Ineffective **Health** maintenance r/t deficient knowledge regarding self-care with neuritis

Neurofibromatosis

Compromised **Family** coping r/t cost and emotional needs of disease

Disturbed **Energy** field r/t disease

Disturbed **Sensory** perception r/t optic nerve gliomas associated with disease

Effective **Therapeutic** regimen management: evaluate visual disturbances associated with NF1 optic pathway tumors: dimness of vision, headache, visual field defects, nystagmus and distortion of binocular fixation, decreased visual acuity, proptosis or a droopy eyelid

Impaired **Skin** integrity r/t café-au-lait spots

Readiness for enhanced **Decision** making: expresses desire to enhance understanding of choices and meaning of choices, genetic counseling

Readiness for enhanced **Therapeutic** regimen management: seeks cancer screening, education and genetic counseling

Risk for delayed **Development**: learning disorders including attention deficit–hyperactivity disorder, low intelligent quotient scores, and developmental delay: Risk factor: genetic disorder

Risk for decreased **Cardiac** output: Risk factor: hypertension associated with condition

Risk for **Constipation**: Risk factor: intestinal neurofibromas

Risk for disproportionate **Growth**: short stature, precocious puberty, delayed maturation, thyroid disorders: Risk factor: genetic disorder

Risk for **Injury**: Risk factor: possible problems with balance

Risk for **Spiritual** distress: Risk factor: possible severity of disease

See Abdominal Distension; Surgery, Perioperative; Surgery, Postoperative; Surgery, Preoperative

Neurogenic Bladder

Overflow urinary **Incontinence** r/t detrusor external sphincter dyssynergia

Reflex **Incontinence** r/t neurological impairment

Risk for latex **Allergy** response: Risk factors: repeated exposures to latex associated with possible repeated catheterizations

Urinary retention r/t interruption in the lateral spinal tracts

Neurological Disorders

Acute **Confusion** r/t dementia, alcohol abuse, drug abuse, delirium

Disturbed **Energy** field r/t illness

Grieving r/t loss of usual body functioning

Imbalanced **Nutrition**: less than body requirements r/t impaired swallowing, depression, difficulty feeding self

Impaired **Home** maintenance r/t client's or family member's disease

Impaired **Memory** r/t neurological disturbance

Impaired physical **Mobility** r/t neuromuscular impairment

Impaired **Swallowing** r/t neuromuscular dysfunction

Ineffective **Airway** clearance r/t perceptual or cognitive impairment, decreased energy, fatigue

Ineffective **Coping** r/t disability requiring change in lifestyle

Interrupted **Family** processes r/t situational crisis, illness, or disability of family member

Powerlessness r/t progressive nature of disease

Risk for **Disuse** syndrome: Risk factors: physical immobility, neuromuscular dysfunction

Risk for impaired **Religiosity**: Risk factor: life transition

Risk for impaired **Skin** integrity: Risk factors: altered sensation, altered mental status, paralysis

Risk for **Injury**: Risk factors: altered mobility, sensory dysfunction, cognitive impairment

Self-care deficit: specify r/t neuromuscular dysfunction

Sexual dysfunction r/t biopsychosocial alteration of sexuality

Social isolation r/t altered state of wellness

Wandering r/t cognitive impairment

Neuropathy, Peripheral

Chronic **Pain** r/t damage to nerves in the peripheral nervous system as a result of medication side effects, vitamin deficiency, or diabetes

Ineffective **Thermoregulation** r/t decreased ability to regulate body temperature

Risk for **Injury**: Risk factors: lack of muscle control, decreased sensation

Risk for **Peripheral** neurovascular dysfunction: Risk factors: compression, entrapment

See Peripheral Vascular Disease

Neurosurgery

See Craniectomy/Craniotomy

Newborn, Normal

Effective **Breastfeeding** r/t normal oral structure and gestational age greater than 34 weeks

Ineffective **Protection** r/t immature immune system

Ineffective **Thermoregulation** r/t immaturity of neuroendocrine system

Readiness for enhanced organized **Infant** behavior r/t pain

Readiness for enhanced **Parenting**: providing emotional and physical needs of infant

Risk for **Infection**: Risk factor: open umbilical stump

Risk for **Injury**: Risk factors: immaturity, need for caretaking

Risk for sudden infant **Death** syndrome: Risk factors: lack of knowledge regarding infant sleeping in prone or side-lying position, prenatal or postnatal infant smoke exposure, infant overheating or overwrapping, loose articles in the sleep environment

Newborn, Postmature

Hypothermia r/t depleted stores of subcutaneous fat

Impaired **Skin** integrity r/t cracked and peeling skin as a result of decreased vernix

Risk for ineffective **Airway** clearance: Risk factor: meconium aspiration

Risk for unstable **Glucose** level: Risk factor: depleted glycogen stores

Risk for **Injury**: Risk factor: hypoglycemia caused by depleted glycogen stores

Newborn, Small for Gestational Age (SGA)

Imbalanced **Nutrition**: less than body requirements r/t history of placental insufficiency

Ineffective **Thermoregulation** r/t decreased brown fat, subcutaneous fat

Risk for delayed **Development**: Risk factor: history of placental insufficiency

Risk for disproportionate **Growth**: Risk factor: history of placental insufficiency

Risk for **Injury**: Risk factors: hypoglycemia, perinatal asphyxia, meconium aspiration

Risk for sudden infant **Death** syndrome: Risk factor: low birth weight

Nicotine Addiction

Ineffective **Health** maintenance r/t lack of ability to make a judgment about smoking cessation

Powerlessness r/t perceived lack of control over ability to give up nicotine

Readiness for enhanced **Decision** making: expresses desire to enhance understanding and meaning of choices

Readiness for enhanced **Therapeutic** regimen management: expresses desire to learn measures to stop smoking

NIDDM (Non-Insulin-Dependent Diabetes Mellitus)

Health-seeking behaviors r/t desiring information on exercise and diet to manage diabetes

See Diabetes Mellitus

Nightmares

Disturbed **Energy** field r/t disharmony of body and mind

Post-trauma syndrome r/t disaster, war, epidemic, rape, assault, torture, catastrophic illness, or accident

Rape-trauma syndrome: compound reaction or silent reaction r/t forced violent sexual penetration against the victim's will and consent

Nipple Soreness

Acute **Pain** r/t injury to nipples

See Painful Breasts, Sore Nipples

Nocturia

Impaired **Urinary** elimination r/t sensory motor impairment, urinary tract infection

Risk for **Powerlessness**: Risk factor: inability to control nighttime voiding

Total **Urinary** incontinence r/t neuropathy preventing transmission of reflex indicating bladder fullness; neurological dysfunction causing triggering of micturition at unpredictable times; independent contraction of detrusor reflex as result of surgery, trauma, or disease affecting spinal cord nerves; anatomical fistula

Urge urinary **Incontinence** r/t decreased bladder capacity, irritation of bladder stretch receptors causing spasm, alcohol, caffeine, increased fluids, increased urine concentration, overdistention of bladder

Nocturnal Myoclonus

See Restless Leg Syndrome; Stress

Nocturnal Paroxysmal Dyspnea

See PND (Paroxysmal Nocturnal Dyspnea)

Noncompliance

Noncompliance (See **Noncompliance,** Section II)

Non-Insulin-Dependent Diabetes Mellitus (NIDDM)

See Diabetes Mellitus

Normal Pressure Hydrocephalus (NPH)

Acute **Confusion** r/t dementia caused by obstruction to flow of cerebrospinal fluid

Impaired **Memory** r/t neurological disturbance

Impaired verbal **Communication** r/t obstruction of flow of cerebrospinal fluid

Ineffective **Tissue** perfusion: cerebral r/t obstruction to flow of cerebrospinal fluid as a result of closed-head injury, craniotomy, meningitis, or subarachnoid hemorrhage

Risk for **Falls**: Risk factor: unsteady gait as a result of obstruction of cerebrospinal fluid

Norwalk Virus

See Viral Gastroenteritis

NSTEMI (non-ST-elevation myocardial infarction)

See MI (Myocardial Infarction)

Nursing

See Breastfeeding, Effective; Breastfeeding, Ineffective; Breastfeeding, Interrupted

Nutrition

Readiness for enhanced **Nutrition** (See **Nutrition,** readiness for enhanced, Section II)

Nutrition, Imbalanced

Imbalanced **Nutrition**: less than body requirements (See **Nutrition,** imbalanced: less than body requirements, Section II)

Imbalanced **Nutrition**: more than body requirements (See **Nutrition,** imbalanced: more than body requirements, Section II)

Risk for imbalanced **Nutrition**: more than body requirements (See **Nutrition,** risk for imbalanced: more than body requirements, Section II)

Obesity

Chronic low **Self-esteem** r/t ineffective coping, overeating

Disturbed **Body** image r/t eating disorder, excess weight

Imbalanced **Nutrition**: more than body requirements r/t caloric intake exceeding energy expenditure

Readiness for enhanced **Nutrition**: expresses willingness to enhance nutrition

OBS (Organic Brain Syndrome)

See Organic Mental Disorders

Obsessive-Compulsive Disorder

Anxiety r/t threat to self-concept, unmet needs

Decisional **Conflict** r/t inability to make a decision for fear of reprisal

Disabled family **Coping** r/t family process being disrupted by client's ritualistic activities

Disturbed **Thought** processes r/t persistent thoughts, ideas, impulses that seem irrelevant and will not relent

Ineffective **Coping** r/t expression of feelings in an unacceptable way, ritualistic behavior

Powerlessness r/t unrelenting repetitive thoughts to perform irrational activities

Risk for situational low **Self-esteem**: Risk factor: inability to control repetitive thoughts and actions

Risk-prone health **Behavior** r/t inadequate comprehension associated with repetitive thoughts

Obstruction, Bowel

See Bowel Obstruction

Obstructive Sleep Apnea

Health-seeking behaviors r/t seeking nutritional information to control weight that may be contributing to sleep apnea

Imbalanced **Nutrition**: more than body requirements r/t excessive intake related to metabolic need

Insomnia r/t blocked airway

See PND (Paroxysmal Nocturnal Dyspnea)

ODD

See Oppositional Defiant Disorder (ODD)

Older Adult

See Aging

Oligohydramnios

Anxiety: maternal r/t fear of unknown, threat to fetus

Risk for **Injury**: fetal: Risk factor: decreased umbilical cord blood flow as a result of compression

Oliguria

Deficient **Fluid** volume r/t active fluid loss, failure of regulatory mechanism

See Cardiac Output Decrease; Renal Failure; Shock

Omphalocele

See Gastroschisis/Omphalocele

Onychomycosis

See Ringworm of Nails

Oophorectomy

Risk for ineffective **Sexuality** pattern: Risk factor: altered body function

See Surgery, Perioperative; Surgery, Postoperative; Surgery, Preoperative

OPCAB (Off-Pump Coronary Artery Bypass)

Acute **Confusion** r/t possible decreased cerebral tissue perfusion

Acute **Pain** r/t possible gastrointestinal dysfunction

Decreased **Cardiac** output r/t increased vasodilation

Impaired **Gas** exchange r/t alveolar-capillary membrane changes

Impaired **Memory** r/t possible decreased cerebral tissue perfusion

Readiness for enhanced **Therapeutic** regimen management r/t preoperative and postoperative care associated with surgery

Risk for deficient **Fluid** volume: Risk factor: bleeding associated with anticoagulant therapy

See Angioplasty, Coronary; Coronary Artery Bypass Grafting

Open Heart Surgery

Decreased **Cardiac** output r/t altered preload or afterload

Impaired **Gas** exchange r/t cardiac surgery

See Coronary Artery Bypass Grafting; Dysrhythmia

Open Reduction of Fracture with Internal Fixation (Femur)

Anxiety r/t outcome of corrective procedure

Impaired physical **Mobility** r/t postoperative position, abduction of leg, avoidance of acute flexion

Powerlessness r/t loss of control, unanticipated change in lifestyle

Risk for perioperative positioning **Injury**: Risk factor: immobilization

Risk for **Peripheral** neurovascular dysfunction: Risk factors: mechanical compression, orthopedic surgery, immobilization

See Surgery, Postoperative Care

Opiate Use

Risk for **Constipation**: Risk factor: effects of opiates on peristalsis

See Drug Abuse; Drug Withdrawal

Opportunistic Infection

Delayed **Surgical** recovery r/t abnormal blood profiles, impaired healing

Risk for **Infection**: Risk factor: abnormal blood profiles

See AIDS (Acquired Immune Deficiency Syndrome); HIV (Human Immunodeficiency Virus)

Oppositional Defiant Disorder (ODD)

Anxiety r/t feelings of anger and hostility toward authority figures

Chronic or situational low **Self-esteem** r/t poor self-control and disruptive behaviors

Disabled **Family** coping r/t feelings of anger, hostility; defiant behavior toward authority figures

Disturbed **Thought** processes r/t difficulty thinking, making appropriate decisions

Impaired **Social** interaction r/t being touchy or easily annoyed, blaming others for own mistakes, constant trouble in school

Ineffective **Coping** r/t lack of self-control or perceived lack of self-control

Ineffective family **Therapeutic** regimen

management r/t difficulty in limit setting and managing oppositional behaviors

Risk for impaired **Parenting**: Risk factors: children's difficult behaviors and inability to set limits

Risk for other-directed **Violence**: Risk factors: history of violence, threats of violence against others; history of antisocial behavior; history of indirect violence

Risk for **Powerlessness**: Risk factor: inability to deal with difficulty behaviors

Risk for **Spiritual** distress: Risk factors: anxiety and stress in dealing with difficulty behaviors

Risk prone Health **Behavior** r/t multiple stressors associated with condition

Social isolation r/t unaccepted social behavior

O

Oral Mucous Membrane, Impaired

Impaired **Oral** mucous membrane (See **Oral,** mucous membrane, impaired, Section II)

Oral Thrush

See Candidiasis, Oral

Orchitis

Readiness for enhanced **Therapeutic** regimen management r/t follows recommendations for mumps vaccination

See Epididymitis

Organic Mental Disorders

Adult **Failure** to thrive r/t undetected organic mental disorder

Impaired **Social** interaction r/t disturbed thought processes

Risk for **Injury**: Risk factors: disorientation to time, place, person

See Dementia

Orthopedic Traction

Impaired **Social** interaction r/t limited physical mobility

Impaired **Transfer** ability r/t limited physical mobility

Ineffective **Role** performance r/t limited physical mobility

Risk for impaired **Religiosity**: Risk factor: immobility

See Traction and Casts

Orthopnea

Decreased **Cardiac** output r/t inability of heart to meet demands of body

Ineffective **Breathing** pattern r/t inability to breathe with head of bed flat

Orthostatic Hypotension

See Dizziness

Osteoarthritis

Activity intolerance r/t pain after exercise or use of joint

Acute **Pain** r/t movement

Impaired **Transfer** ability r/t pain

See Arthritis

Osteomyelitis

Acute **Pain** r/t inflammation in affected extremity

Deficient **Diversional** activity r/t prolonged immobilization, hospitalization

Fear: parental r/t concern regarding possible growth plate damage caused by infection, concern that infection may become chronic

Hyperthermia r/t infectious process

Impaired physical **Mobility** r/t imposed immobility as a result of infected area

Ineffective **Health** maintenance r/t continued immobility at home, possible extensive casts, continued antibiotics

Risk for **Constipation**: Risk factor: immobility

Risk for impaired **Skin** integrity: Risk factor: irritation from splint or cast

Risk for **Infection**: Risk factor: inadequate primary and secondary defenses

See Hospitalized Child

Osteoporosis

Acute **Pain** r/t fracture, muscle spasms

Deficient **Knowledge** r/t diet, exercise, need to abstain from alcohol and nicotine

Effective **Therapeutic** regimen management: individual: appropriate choices for diet and exercise to prevent and manage condition

Imbalanced **Nutrition**: less than body requirements r/t inadequate intake of calcium and vitamin D

Impaired physical **Mobility** r/t pain, skeletal changes

Readiness for enhanced **Therapeutic** regimen management: expresses desire to manage the treatment of illness and prevent complications

Risk for **Injury**: fracture: Risk factors: lack of activity, risk of falling resulting from environmental hazards, neuromuscular disorders, diminished senses, cardiovascular responses, responses to drugs

Risk for **Powerlessness**: Risk factor: debilitating disease

Ostomy

See Child with Chronic Condition; Colostomy; Ileal Conduit; Ileostomy

Otitis Media

Acute **Pain** r/t inflammation, infectious process

Disturbed **Sensory** perception: auditory r/t incomplete resolution of otitis media, presence of excess drainage in middle ear

Readiness for enhanced **Knowledge** of information: information on treatment and prevention of disease

Risk for delayed speech and language **Development**: Risk factor: frequent otitis media

Risk for **Infection**: Risk factors: eustachian tube obstruction, traumatic eardrum perforation, infectious disease process

Ovarian Carcinoma

Death **Anxiety** r/t unknown outcome, possible poor prognosis

Fear r/t unknown outcome, possible poor prognosis

Ineffective **Health** maintenance r/t deficient knowledge regarding self-care, treatment of condition

See Chemotherapy; Hysterectomy; Radiation Therapy

Oxyuriasis

See Pinworms

P

Pacemaker

Acute **Pain** r/t surgical procedure

Anxiety r/t change in health status, presence of pacemaker

Death **Anxiety** r/t worry over possible malfunction of pacemaker

Deficient **Knowledge** r/t self-care program, when to seek medical attention

Readiness for enhanced **Therapeutic** regimen management appropriate health care management of pacemaker

Risk for decreased **Cardiac** output: Risk factor: malfunction of pacemaker

Risk for **Infection**: Risk factors: invasive procedure, presence of foreign body (catheter and generator)

Risk for **Powerlessness**: Risk factor: presence of electronic device to stimulate heart

Paget's Disease

Chronic **Sorrow** r/t chronic condition with altered body image

Deficient **Knowledge** r/t appropriate diet high in protein and calcium, mild exercise

Disturbed **Body** image r/t possible enlarged head, bowed tibias, kyphosis

Risk for **Trauma**: fracture r/t excessive bone destruction

Pain, Acute

Acute **Pain** (See **Pain**, acute, Section II)

Disturbed **Energy** field r/t unbalanced energy field

Pain, Chronic

Chronic **Pain** (See **Pain**, chronic, Section II)

Disturbed **Energy** field r/t unbalanced energy field

Painful Breasts, Engorgement

Acute **Pain** r/t distention of breast tissue

Impaired **Tissue** integrity r/t excessive fluid in breast tissues

Ineffective **Role** performance r/t change in physical capacity to assume role of breastfeeding mother

Risk for ineffective **Breastfeeding**: Risk factors: pain, infant's inability to latch on to engorged breast

Risk for **Infection**: Risk factor: milk stasis

Painful Breasts, Sore Nipples

Acute **Pain** r/t cracked nipples

Impaired **Skin** integrity r/t mechanical factors involved in suckling, breastfeeding management

Ineffective **Breastfeeding** r/t pain

Ineffective **Role** performance r/t change in physical capacity to assume role of breastfeeding mother

Risk for **Infection**: Risk factor: break in skin

Pallor of Extremities

Ineffective **Tissue** perfusion: peripheral r/t interruption of vascular flow

Palpitations (Heart Palpitations)

See Dysrhythmia

Pancreatic Cancer

Death **Anxiety** r/t possible poor prognosis of disease process

Deficient **Knowledge** r/t disease-induced diabetes, home management

Fear r/t poor prognosis of the disease

Grieving r/t shortened life span

Ineffective family **Coping** r/t poor prognosis

Spiritual distress r/t poor prognosis

See Cancer; Chemotherapy; Radiation Therapy; Surgery, Perioperative; Surgery, Postoperative; Surgery, Preoperative

Pancreatitis

Acute **Pain** r/t irritation and edema of the inflamed pancreas

Adult **Failure** to thrive r/t pain

Chronic **Sorrow** r/t chronic illness

Diarrhea r/t decrease in pancreatic secretions resulting in steatorrhea

Deficient **Fluid** volume r/t vomiting, decreased fluid intake, fever, diaphoresis, fluid shifts

Imbalanced **Nutrition**: less than body requirements r/t inadequate dietary intake, increased nutritional needs as a result of acute illness, increased metabolic needs caused by increased body temperature

Ineffective **Breathing** pattern r/t splinting from severe pain

Ineffective **Denial** r/t ineffective coping, alcohol use

Ineffective **Health** maintenance r/t deficient knowledge concerning diet, alcohol use, medication

Nausea r/t irritation of gastrointestinal system

Readiness for enhanced **Comfort** r/t expresses desire to enhance comfort

Panic Disorder

Anxiety r/t situational crisis

Ineffective **Coping** r/t personal vulnerability

Post-trauma syndrome r/t previous catastrophic event

Readiness for enhanced **Coping**: seeks problem-oriented and emotion-oriented strategies to manage condition

Risk for **Loneliness**: Risk factor: inability to socially interact because of fear of losing control

Risk for **Post-trauma** syndrome: Risk factors: perception of the event, diminished ego strength

Risk for **Powerlessness**: Risk factor: ineffective coping skills

Social isolation r/t fear of lack of control

See Anxiety; Anxiety Disorder

Paralysis

Acute **Pain** r/t prolonged immobility

Chronic **Sorrow** r/t loss of physical mobility

Constipation r/t effects of spinal cord disruption, inadequate fiber in diet

Disturbed **Body** image r/t biophysical changes, loss of movement, immobility

Impaired **Home** maintenance r/t physical disability

Impaired physical **Mobility** r/t neuromuscular impairment

Impaired **Transfer** ability r/t paralysis

Impaired wheelchair **Mobility** r/t neuromuscular impairment

Ineffective **Health** maintenance r/t deficient knowledge regarding self-care with paralysis

Powerlessness r/t illness-related regimen

Readiness for enhanced **Self-care**: expresses desire to enhance knowledge and responsibility for strategies for self-care

Reflex **Incontinence** r/t neurological impairment

Risk for **Disuse** syndrome: Risk factor: paralysis

Risk for **Falls**: Risk factor: paralysis

Risk for impaired **Religiosity**: Risk factors: immobility, possible lack of transportation

Risk for impaired **Skin** integrity: Risk factors: altered circulation, altered sensation, immobility

Risk for **Injury**: Risk factors: altered mobility, sensory dysfunction

Risk for latex **Allergy** response: Risk factor: possible repeated urinary catheterizations

Risk for **Post-trauma** syndrome: Risk factor: event causing paralysis

Risk for situational low **Self-esteem**: Risk factor: change in body image and function

Self-care deficit: specify r/t neuromuscular impairment

Sexual dysfunction r/t loss of sensation, biopsychosocial alteration

See Child with Chronic Condition; Hemiplegia; Hospitalized Child; Neural Tube Defects; Spinal Cord Injury

Paralytic Ileus

Acute **Pain** r/t pressure, abdominal distention

Constipation r/t decreased gastric motility

Deficient **Fluid** volume r/t loss of fluids from vomiting, retention of fluid in bowel

Impaired **Oral** mucous membrane r/t presence of nasogastric tube

Nausea r/t gastrointestinal irritation

Paranoid Personality Disorder

Anxiety r/t uncontrollable intrusive, suspicious thoughts

Chronic low **Self-esteem** r/t inability to trust others

Disturbed personal **Identity** r/t difficulty with reality testing

Disturbed **Sensory** perception: specify r/t psychological dysfunction, suspicious thoughts

Disturbed **Thought** processes r/t psychological conflicts

Risk-prone health **Behavior** r/t intense emotional state

Risk for **Loneliness**: Risk factor: social isolation

Risk for other-directed **Violence**: Risk factor: being suspicious of others and others' actions

Risk for **Post-trauma** syndrome: Risk factor: exaggerated sense of responsibility

Risk for **Suicide**: Risk factor: psychiatric illness

P

Social isolation r/t inappropriate social skills

Paraplegia

See Spinal Cord Injury

Parathyroidectomy

Anxiety r/t surgery

Risk for impaired verbal **Communication**: Risk factors: possible laryngeal damage, edema

Risk for ineffective **Airway** clearance: Risk factors: edema or hematoma formation, airway obstruction

Risk for **Infection**: Risk factor: surgical procedure

See Hypocalcemia

Parent Attachment

Chronic **Sorrow** r/t difficult parent-child relationship

Risk for impaired parent/child **Attachment** (See **Attachment,** impaired parent/child, risk for, Section II)

Risk for **Spiritual** distress: Risk factor: altered relationships

Parental Role Conflict

Chronic **Sorrow** r/t difficult parent-child relationship

Parental role **Conflict** r/t (See **Conflict,** parental role, Section II)

Readiness for enhanced **Parenting**: willingness to enhance parenting

Risk for **Spiritual** distress: Risk factor: altered relationships

Parenting

Readiness for enhanced **Parenting** (See **Parenting,** readiness for enhanced, Section II)

Parenting, Impaired

Chronic **Sorrow** r/t difficult parent-child relationship

Impaired **Parenting** (See **Parenting,** impaired, Section II)

Risk for **Spiritual** distress: Risk factor: altered relationships

Parenting, Risk for Impaired

Chronic **Sorrow** r/t difficult parent-child relationship

Risk for impaired **Parenting** (See **Parenting,** impaired, risk for, Section II)

Risk for **Spiritual** distress: Risk factors: altered relationships

Paresthesia

Disturbed **Sensory** perception: tactile r/t altered sensory reception, transmission, integration

Risk for **Injury** r/t inability to feel temperature changes, pain

Parkinson's Disease

Chronic **Sorrow** r/t loss of physical capacity

Constipation r/t weakness of defecation

muscles, lack of exercise, inadequate fluid intake, decreased autonomic nervous system activity

Imbalanced **Nutrition**: less than body requirements r/t tremor, slowness in eating, difficulty in chewing and swallowing

Impaired verbal **Communication** r/t decreased speech volume, slowness of speech, impaired facial muscles

Risk for **Injury**: Risk factors: tremors, slow reactions, altered gait

See Neurological Disorders

Paroxysmal Nocturnal Dyspnea

See PND (Paroxysmal Nocturnal Dyspnea)

Patent Ductus Arteriosus (PDA)

See Congenital Heart Disease/Cardiac Anomalies

Patient-Controlled Analgesia

See PCA (Patient-Controlled Analgesia)

Patient Education

Deficient **Knowledge** r/t lack of exposure to information, information misinterpretation, unfamiliarity with information resources

Effective **Therapeutic** regimen management: verbalizes desire to manage illness

Health-seeking behaviors: expresses desire to seek control of health practices

Readiness for enhanced **Decision** making: expresses desire to enhance understanding of choices for decision making

Readiness for enhanced **Knowledge** (specify): interest in learning

Readiness for enhanced **Spiritual** well-being: desires to reach harmony with self, others, higher power/God

Readiness for enhanced **Therapeutic** regimen management: expresses desire for information to manage the illness

PCA (Patient-Controlled Analgesia)

Deficient **Knowledge** r/t self-care of pain control

Effective **Therapeutic** regimen management: ability to manage pain with appropriate use of PCA

Pruritus r/t side effects of medication

Nausea r/t side effects of medication

Readiness for enhanced **Knowledge**: appropriate management of PCA

Risk for **Injury**: Risk factors: possible complications associated with PCA

Pediculosis

See Lice

Pelvic Inflammatory Disease

See PID (Pelvic Inflammatory Disease)

Penile Prosthesis

Health-seeking behaviors r/t information regarding use and care of prosthesis

Ineffective **Sexuality** pattern r/t use of penile prosthesis

Risk for **Infection**: Risk factor: invasive surgical procedure

Risk for situational low **Self-esteem**: Risk factors: ineffective sexuality pattern

See Impotence; Erectile Dysfunction (ED)

Peptic Ulcer

See Ulcer, Peptic (Duodenal or Gastric)

Percutaneous Transluminal Coronary Angioplasty (PTCA)

See Angioplasty, Coronary

Pericardial Friction Rub

Acute **Pain** r/t inflammation, effusion

Decreased **Cardiac** output r/t inflammation in pericardial sac, fluid accumulation compressing heart

Delayed **Surgical** recovery r/t complications associated with cardiac problems

Pericarditis

Activity intolerance r/t reduced cardiac reserve, prescribed bed rest

Acute **Pain** r/t biological injury, inflammation

Decreased **Cardiac** output r/t inflammation in pericardial sac, fluid accumulation compressing heart function

Delayed **Surgical** recovery r/t complications associated with cardiac problems

Deficient **Knowledge** r/t unfamiliarity with information sources

Ineffective **Tissue** perfusion: cardiopulmonary/peripheral r/t risk for development of emboli

Risk for imbalanced **Nutrition**: less than body requirements r/t fever, hypermetabolic state associated with fever

Perioperative Positioning

Risk for perioperative positioning **Injury**: Risk factors: (See **Injury**, perioperative, risk for, Section II)

Peripheral Neuropathy

See Neuropathy, Peripheral

Peripheral Neurovascular Dysfunction

Risk for **Peripheral** neurovascular dysfunction: Risk factors: (See **Peripheral** neurovascular dysfunction, risk for, Section II)

See Neuropathy, Peripheral; Peripheral Vascular Disease

Peripheral Vascular Disease

Activity intolerance r/t imbalance between peripheral oxygen supply and demand

Chronic **Pain**: intermittent claudication r/t ischemia

Ineffective **Health** maintenance r/t deficient knowledge regarding self-care and treatment of disease

Ineffective **Tissue** perfusion: peripheral r/t interruption of vascular flow

Readiness for enhanced **Therapeutic** regimen management; self-care and treatment of disease

Risk for **Falls**: Risk factor: altered mobility

Risk for impaired **Skin** integrity: Risk factor: altered circulation or sensation

Risk for **Injury**: Risk factors: tissue hypoxia, altered mobility, altered sensation

Risk for **Peripheral** neurovascular dysfunction: Risk factor: possible vascular obstruction

See Neuropathy, Peripheral; Peripheral Neurovascular Dysfunction

Peritoneal Dialysis

Acute **Pain** r/t instillation of dialysate, temperature of dialysate

Chronic **Sorrow** r/t chronic disability

Deficient **Knowledge** r/t treatment procedure, self-care with peritoneal dialysis

Impaired **Home** maintenance r/t complex home treatment of client

Risk for **Fluid** volume excess: Risk factor: retention of dialysate

Risk for ineffective **Breathing** pattern: Risk factor: pressure from dialysate

Risk for ineffective **Coping**: Risk factor: disability requiring change in lifestyle

Risk for **Infection**: peritoneal: Risk factor: invasive procedure, presence of catheter, dialysate

Risk for **Powerlessness**: Risk factor: chronic condition and care involved

See Child with Chronic Condition; Hospitalized Child; Renal Failure; Renal Failure, Acute/Chronic, Child

Peritonitis

Acute **Pain** r/t inflammation, stimulation of somatic nerves

Constipation r/t decreased oral intake, decrease of peristalsis

Deficient **Fluid** volume r/t retention of fluid in bowel with loss of circulating blood volume

Imbalanced **Nutrition**: less than body requirements r/t nausea, vomiting

Ineffective **Breathing** pattern r/t pain, increased abdominal pressure

Nausea r/t gastrointestinal irritation

Pernicious Anemia

Diarrhea r/t malabsorption of nutrients

Effective **Therapeutic** regimen management r/t follows treatment plan; lifelong replacement of vitamin B_{12}

Fatigue r/t imbalanced nutrition: less than body requirements

Imbalanced **Nutrition**: less than body requirements r/t lack of appetite associated with nausea and altered oral mucous membrane

Impaired **Memory** r/t anemia; lack of adequate red blood cells

Impaired **Oral** mucous membranes r/t vitamin deficiency; inability to absorb vitamin B_{12} associated with lack of intrinsic factor

Nausea r/t altered oral mucous membrane; sore tongue, bleeding gums

Risk for **Peripheral** neurovascular dysfunction: Risk factor: anemia

Risk for **Falls**: Risk factor: dizziness, lightheadedness

Persistent Fetal Circulation

See Congenital Heart Disease/Cardiac Anomalies

Personal Identity Problems

Disturbed personal **Identity** r/t situational crisis, psychological impairment, chronic illness, pain

Personality Disorder

Chronic low **Self-esteem** r/t inability to set and achieve goals

Compromised family **Coping** r/t inability of client to provide positive feedback to family, chronicity exhausting family

Decisional **Conflict** r/t low self-esteem, feelings that choices will always be wrong

Disturbed personal **Identity** r/t lack of consistent positive self-image

Impaired **Social** interaction r/t knowledge or skill deficit regarding ways to interact effectively with others, self-concept disturbances

Readiness for enhanced **Self-concept**: expresses willingness to enhance self-concept

Risk for **Loneliness**: Risk factor: inability to interact appropriately with others

Risk for **Self-mutilation**: Risk factors: disturbed interpersonal relationships, borderline personality disorders

Risk for situational low **Self-esteem**: Risk factor: history of learned helplessness

Risk-prone health **Behavior** r/t ambivalent behavior toward others, testing of others' loyalty

Spiritual distress r/t lack of identifiable values, lack of meaning to life

See Antisocial Personality Disorder; Borderline Personality Disorder; Obsessive-Compulsive Disorder; Paranoid Personality Disorder

Pertussis (Whooping Cough)

See Respiratory Infections, Acute Childhood

Pesticide Contamination

Contamination r/t use of environmental contaminants; pesticides

Effective **Therapeutic** regimen management: verbalizes intent to reduce risk factors associated with environmental toxins; meticulous hand hygiene

Health-seeking behaviors r/t expression of concern about environmental conditions

Risk for disproportionate **Growth**: Risk factor: environmental contamination

Petechiae

See Clotting Disorder; Anticoagulant Therapy; DIC (Disseminated Intravascular Coagulation); Hemophilia

Petit Mal Seizure

Effective **Therapeutic** regimen management r/t follows prescribed medication regimen

Readiness for enhanced **Therapeutic** regimen management: wears medical alert bracelet; limits hazardous activities such as driving, swimming, working at heights, operating equipment

See Epilepsy

Pharyngitis

See Sore Throat

Phenylketonuria

See PKU (Phenylketonuria)

Pheochromocytoma

Anxiety r/t symptoms from increased catecholamines—headache, palpitations, sweating, nervousness, nausea, vomiting, syncope

Ineffective **Health** maintenance r/t deficient knowledge regarding treatment and self-care

Insomnia r/t high levels of catecholamines

Nausea r/t increased catecholamines

Risk for ineffective **Tissue** perfusion: cardiopulmonary and renal: Risk factor: episodes of hypertension

See Surgery, Perioperative; Surgery, Postoperative; Surgery, Preoperative

Phlebitis

See Thrombophlebitis

Phobia (Specific)

Anxiety r/t inability to control emotions when dreaded object or situation is encountered

Fear r/t presence or anticipation of specific object or situation

Ineffective **Coping** r/t transfer of fears from self to dreaded object situation

Powerlessness r/t anxiety about encountering unknown or known entity

Readiness for enhanced **Communication**: willingness to discuss situation

Readiness for enhanced **Power**: expresses readiness to enhance identification of choices that can be made for change

Risk for **Post-trauma** syndrome: Risk factor: exposure to dreaded object or situation

Risk for **Powerlessness**: Risk factor: inadequate coping patterns

Risk for situational low **Self-esteem**: Risk factor: decreased power/control over fears

See Anxiety; Anxiety Disorder; Panic Disorder

Photosensitivity

Ineffective **Health** maintenance r/t deficient knowledge regarding medications inducing photosensitivity

Risk for impaired **Skin** integrity: Risk factor: exposure to sun

Physical Abuse

See Abuse, Child; Abuse, Spouse, Parent, or Significant Other

Pica

Anxiety r/t stress from urge to eat nonnutritive substances

Imbalanced **Nutrition**: less than body requirements r/t eating nonnutritive substances

Impaired **Parenting** r/t lack of supervision, food deprivation

Risk for **Constipation**: Risk factor: presence of undigestible materials in gastrointestinal tract

Risk for **Infection**: Risk factor: ingestion of infectious agents via contaminated substances

Risk for **Poisoning**: Risk factor: ingestion of substances containing lead

PID (Pelvic Inflammatory Disease)

Acute **Pain** r/t biological injury; inflammation, edema, congestion of pelvic tissues

Ineffective **Health** maintenance r/t deficient knowledge regarding self-care, treatment of disease

Ineffective **Sexuality** pattern r/t medically imposed abstinence from sexual activities until acute infection subsides, change in reproductive potential

Risk for **Infection**: Risk factors: insufficient knowledge to avoid exposure to pathogens; proper hygiene, nutrition, other health habits

Risk for urge urinary **Incontinence**: Risk factors: inflammation, edema, congestion of pelvic tissues

See Maturational Issues, Adolescent

PIH (Pregnancy-Induced Hypertension/Preeclampsia)

Anxiety r/t fear of the unknown, threat to self and infant, change in role functioning

Death **Anxiety** r/t threat of preeclampsia

Deficient **Diversional** activity r/t bed rest

Deficient **Knowledge** r/t lack of experience with situation

Excess **Fluid** volume r/t decreased renal function

Impaired **Home** maintenance r/t bed rest

Impaired **Parenting** r/t bed rest

Impaired physical **Mobility** r/t medically prescribed limitations

Impaired **Social** interaction r/t imposed bed rest

Ineffective **Role** performance r/t change in physical capacity to assume role of pregnant woman or resume other roles

Interrupted **Family** processes r/t situational crisis

Powerlessness r/t complication threatening pregnancy, medically prescribed limitations

Readiness for enhanced **Knowledge**: desire for information on managing condition

Risk for imbalanced **Fluid** volume: Risk factors: hypertension, altered renal function

Risk for **Injury**: fetal: Risk factors: decreased uteroplacental perfusion, seizures

Risk for **Injury**: maternal: Risk factors: vasospasm, high blood pressure

Situational low **Self-esteem** r/t loss of idealized pregnancy

See Malignant Hypertension

Piloerection

Hypothermia r/t exposure to cold environment

Pimples

See Acne

Pinworms

Effective **Therapeutic** regimen management: adheres to guidelines for infected person and appropriate care

Impaired **Home** maintenance r/t inadequate cleaning of bed linen and toilet seats

Insomnia r/t discomfort

Pruritus r/t inflammation of skin

Readiness for enhanced **Therapeutic**

regimen: proper hand washing; short clean fingernails; avoiding hand, mouth, nose contact with unwashed hands; appropriate cleaning of bed linen and toilet seats

Pituitary Cushing's

See Cushing's Syndrome

PKU (Phenylketonuria)

Effective management of **Therapeutic** regimen: testing of newborn for PKU and following prescribed dietary regimen if test is positive

Risk for delayed **Development**: Risk factors: not following strict dietary program; eating foods extremely low in phenylalanine; avoiding eggs, milk, any foods containing aspartame (Nutrasweet)

P

Placenta Abruptio

Acute **Pain**: abdominal/back r/t premature separation of placenta before delivery

Death **Anxiety** r/t threat of mortality associated with bleeding

Fear r/t threat to self and fetus

Ineffective **Health** maintenance r/t deficient knowledge regarding treatment and control of hypertension associated with placenta abruptio

Risk for deficient **Fluid** volume r/t maternal blood loss

Risk for **Powerlessness**: Risk factors: complications of pregnancy and unknown outcome

Risk for **Spiritual** distress: Risk factor: fear from unknown outcome of pregnancy

Placenta Previa

Death **Anxiety** r/t threat of mortality associated with bleeding

Deficient **Diversional** activity r/t long-term hospitalization

Disturbed **Body** image r/t negative feelings about body and reproductive ability, feelings of helplessness

Fear r/t threat to self and fetus, unknown future

Impaired **Home** maintenance r/t maternal bed rest, hospitalization

Impaired physical **Mobility** r/t medical protocol, maternal bed rest

Ineffective **Coping** r/t threat to self and fetus

Ineffective **Role** performance r/t maternal bed rest, hospitalization

Ineffective **Tissue** perfusion: placental r/t dilation of cervix, loss of placental implantation site

Interrupted **Family** processes r/t maternal bed rest, hospitalization

Risk for **Constipation**: Risk factor: bed rest, pregnancy

Risk for deficient **Fluid** volume: Risk factor: maternal blood loss

Risk for imbalanced **Fluid** volume: Risk factor: maternal blood loss

Risk for impaired **Parenting**: Risk factors: maternal bed rest, hospitalization

Risk for **Injury**: fetal and maternal: Risk factors: threat to uteroplacental perfusion, hemorrhage

Risk for **Powerlessness**: Risk factors: complications of pregnancy and unknown outcome

Situational low **Self-esteem** r/t situational crisis

Spiritual distress r/t inability to participate in usual religious rituals, situational crisis

Pleural Effusion

Acute **Pain** r/t inflammation, fluid accumulation

Excess **Fluid** volume r/t compromised regulatory mechanisms; heart, liver, or kidney failure

Hyperthermia r/t increased metabolic rate secondary to infection

Ineffective **Breathing** pattern r/t pain

Pleural Friction Rub

Acute **Pain** r/t inflammation, fluid accumulation

Ineffective **Breathing** pattern r/t pain

See cause of Pleural Friction Rub

Pleural Tap

See Pleural Effusion

Pleurisy

Acute **Pain** r/t pressure on pleural nerve endings associated with fluid accumulation or inflammation

Impaired **Gas** exchange r/t ventilation perfusion imbalance

Ineffective **Breathing** pattern r/t pain

Risk for impaired physical **Mobility**: Risk factors: activity intolerance, inability to "catch breath"

Risk for ineffective **Airway** clearance: Risk factors: increased secretions, ineffective cough because of pain

PMS (Premenstrual Tension Syndrome)

Acute **Pain** r/t hormonal stimulation of gastrointestinal structures

Deficient **Knowledge** r/t methods to deal with and prevent syndrome

Excess **Fluid** volume r/t alterations of hormonal levels inducing fluid retention

Fatigue r/t hormonal changes

Readiness for enhanced **Communication**: willingness to express thoughts and feelings about PMS

Readiness for enhanced **Therapeutic** regimen management: desire for information to manage and prevent symptoms

Risk for **Powerlessness**: Risk factors: lack of knowledge and ability to deal with symptoms

PND (Paroxysmal Nocturnal Dyspnea)

Anxiety r/t inability to breathe during sleep

Decreased **Cardiac** output r/t failure of the left ventricle

Ineffective **Breathing** pattern r/t increase in carbon dioxide levels, decrease in oxygen levels

Insomnia r/t suffocating feeling from fluid in lungs on awakening from sleep

Readiness for enhanced **Sleep**: expresses willingness to learn measures to enhance sleep

Risk for **Powerlessness**: Risk factor: inability to control nocturnal dyspnea

Sleep deprivation r/t inability to breathe during sleep

Pneumonia

Activity intolerance r/t imbalance between oxygen supply and demand

Deficient **Knowledge** r/t Risk factors predisposing person to pneumonia, treatment

Hyperthermia r/t dehydration, increased metabolic rate, illness

Imbalanced **Nutrition**: less than body requirements r/t loss of appetite

Impaired **Gas** exchange r/t decreased functional lung tissue

Impaired **Oral** mucous membrane r/t dry mouth from mouth breathing, decreased fluid intake

Ineffective **Airway** clearance r/t inflammation and presence of secretions

Ineffective **Health** maintenance r/t deficient knowledge regarding self-care and treatment of disease

Risk for deficient **Fluid** volume: Risk factor: inadequate intake of fluids

See Respiratory Infections, Acute Childhood

Pneumothorax

Acute **Pain** r/t recent injury, coughing, deep breathing

Fear r/t threat to own well-being, difficulty breathing

Impaired **Gas** exchange r/t ventilation-perfusion imbalance

Risk for **Injury**: Risk factor: possible complications associated with closed chest drainage system

Poisoning, Risk for

External/Internal

Risk for **Poisoning**: Risk factors: (See **Poisoning,** risk for, Section II)

Polydipsia

Readiness for enhanced **Fluid** balance: no excessive thirst when diabetes is controlled

P

See Diabetes Mellitus

Polyphagia

Readiness for enhanced **Nutrition**: knowledge of appropriate diet for diabetes

See Diabetes Mellitus

Polyuria

Readiness for enhanced **Urinary** elimination: willingness to learn measures to enhance urinary elimination

See Diabetes Mellitus

Postoperative Care

See Surgery, Postoperative

Postpartum Blues

Anxiety r/t new responsibilities of parenting

Chronic **Sorrow** r/t loss of ideal postpartum experience or ideal parent-infant relationship

Deficient **Knowledge** r/t lifestyle changes

Disturbed **Body** image r/t normal postpartum recovery

Fatigue r/t childbirth, postpartum state

Impaired **Home** maintenance r/t fatigue, care of newborn

Impaired **Parenting** r/t hormone-induced depression

Impaired **Social** interaction r/t change in role functioning

Ineffective **Coping** r/t hormonal changes, maturational crisis

Ineffective **Role** performance r/t new responsibilities of parenting

Readiness for enhanced **Hope**: Expresses desire to enhance hope and interconnectedness with others

Risk for **Post-trauma** syndrome: Risk factors: trauma or violence associated with labor and birth process, medical/surgical interventions, history of sexual abuse

Risk for situational low **Self-esteem**: Risk factor: decreased power over feelings of sadness

Risk for **Spiritual** distress: Risk factors: altered relationships, social isolation

Risk-prone health **Behavior** r/t lack of support systems

Sexual dysfunction r/t fear of another pregnancy, postpartum pain, lochia flow

Sleep deprivation r/t environmental stimulation of newborn

Postpartum Hemorrhage

Activity intolerance r/t anemia from loss of blood

Acute **Pain** r/t nursing and medical interventions to control bleeding

Death **Anxiety** r/t threat of mortality associated with bleeding

Decreased **Cardiac** output r/t hypovolemia

Deficient **Fluid** volume r/t uterine atony, loss of blood

Deficient **Knowledge** r/t lack of exposure to situation

Disturbed **Body** image r/t loss of ideal childbirth

Fear r/t threat to self, unknown future

Impaired **Home** maintenance r/t lack of stamina

Ineffective **Tissue** perfusion r/t hypovolemia

Interrupted **Breastfeeding** r/t separation from infant for medical treatment

Risk for imbalanced **Fluid** volume: Risk factor: maternal blood loss

Risk for **Infection**: Risk factors: loss of blood, depressed immunity

Risk for impaired **Parenting**: Risk factor: weakened maternal condition

Risk for **Powerlessness**: Risk factor: acute illness

Postpartum, Normal Care

Acute **Pain** r/t episiotomy, lacerations, bruising, breast engorgement, headache, sore nipples, epidural or intravenous (IV) site, hemorrhoids

Anxiety r/t change in role functioning, parenting

Constipation r/t hormonal effects on smooth muscles, fear of straining with defecation, effects of anesthesia

Deficient **Knowledge**: infant care r/t lack of preparation for parenting

Effective **Breastfeeding** r/t basic breastfeeding knowledge, support of partner and health care provider

Fatigue r/t childbirth, new responsibilities of parenting, body changes

Health-seeking behaviors r/t postpartum recovery and adaptation

Impaired **Skin** integrity r/t episiotomy, lacerations

Impaired **Urinary** elimination r/t effects of anesthesia, tissue trauma

Ineffective **Breastfeeding** r/t lack of knowledge, lack of support, lack of motivation

Ineffective **Role** performance r/t new responsibilities of parenting

Readiness for enhanced family **Coping**: adaptation to new family member

Readiness for enhanced **Parenting**: expressing willingness to enhance parenting skills

Risk for **Constipation**: Risk factors: hormonal effects on smooth muscles, fear of straining with defecation, effects of anesthesia

Risk for imbalanced **Fluid** volume: Risk factors: shift in blood volume, edema

Risk for impaired **Parenting**: Risk factors: lack of role models, deficient knowledge

Risk for **Infection**: Risk factors: tissue trauma, blood loss

Risk for **Post-trauma** syndrome: Risk factors: trauma or violence associated with labor and birth process, medical/surgical interventions, history of sexual abuse

Risk for urge urinary **Incontinence**: Risk factors: effects of anesthesia or tissue trauma

Sexual dysfunction r/t fear of pain or pregnancy

Sleep deprivation r/t care of infant

Post-Trauma Syndrome

Post-trauma syndrome r/t (See **Post-trauma** syndrome, Section II)

Post-Trauma Syndrome, Risk for

Risk for **Post-trauma** syndrome: Risk factors: (See **Post-trauma** syndrome, risk for, Section II)

Post-Traumatic Stress Disorder

Anxiety r/t exposure to internal or external cues that symbolize or resemble an aspect of the traumatic event

Death **Anxiety** r/t psychological stress associated with traumatic event

Disturbed **Energy** field r/t disharmony of mind, body, spirit

Disturbed **Sensory** perception r/t psychological stress

P

Disturbed **Thought** processes r/t sense of reliving the experience (flashbacks)

Ineffective **Breathing** pattern r/t hyperventilation associated with anxiety

Ineffective **Coping** r/t extreme anxiety

Insomnia r/t recurring nightmares

Post-trauma syndrome r/t exposure to a traumatic event

Readiness for enhanced **Comfort**: expresses desire to enhance relaxation

Readiness for enhanced **Communication**: willingness to express feelings and thoughts

Readiness for enhanced **Spiritual** well-being: desire for harmony after stressful event

Risk for **Powerlessness**: Risk factors: flashbacks, reliving event

Risk for self- or other-directed **Violence**: Risk factors: fear of self or others

P

Sleep deprivation r/t nightmares associated with traumatic event

Spiritual distress r/t feelings of detachment or estrangement from others

Potassium, Increase/Decrease

See Hyperkalemia; Hypokalemia

Power/Powerlessness

Powerlessness r/t (See **Powerlessness,** Section II)

Readiness for enhanced **Power** (See **Power,** readiness for enhanced, Section II)

Risk for **Powerlessness** Risk factors: (See **Powerlessness,** risk for, Section II)

Preeclampsia

See PIH (Pregnancy-Induced Hypertension/Preeclampsia)

Pregnancy, Cardiac Disorders

See Cardiac Disorders in Pregnancy

Pregnancy-Induced Hypertension/ Preeclampsia

See PIH (Pregnancy-Induced Hypertension/Preeclampsia)

Pregnancy Loss

Acute **Pain** r/t surgical intervention

Anxiety r/t threat to role functioning, health status, situational crisis

Chronic **Sorrow** r/t loss of a fetus or child

Complicated **Grieving** r/t sudden loss of pregnancy, fetus, or child

Compromised family **Coping** r/t lack of support by significant other because of personal suffering

Ineffective **Coping** r/t situational crisis

Grieving r/t loss of pregnancy, fetus, or child

Complicated **Grieving** r/t sudden loss of pregnancy, fetus, or child

Ineffective **Role** performance r/t inability to assume parenting role

Ineffective **Sexuality** pattern r/t self-esteem disturbance resulting from pregnancy loss and anxiety about future pregnancies

Readiness for enhanced **Communication**: willingness to express feelings and thoughts about loss

Readiness for enhanced **Hope**: expresses desire to enhance hope

Readiness for enhanced **Spiritual** well-being: desire for acceptance of loss

Risk for deficient **Fluid** volume: blood loss

Risk for complicated **Grieving**: Risk factor: loss of pregnancy

Risk for **Infection**: Risk factor: retained products of conception

Risk for **Powerlessness**: Risk factor: situational crisis

Risk for **Spiritual** distress: Risk factor: intense suffering

Spiritual distress r/t intense suffering

Pregnancy, Normal

Deficient **Knowledge** r/t primiparity

Disturbed **Body** image r/t altered body function and appearance

Fear r/t labor and delivery

Health-seeking behaviors r/t desire to promote optimal fetal and maternal health

Imbalanced **Nutrition**: less than body requirements r/t growing fetus, nausea

Imbalanced **Nutrition**: more than body requirements r/t deficient knowledge regarding nutritional needs of pregnancy

Ineffective **Coping** r/t personal vulnerability, situational crisis

Interrupted **Family** processes r/t developmental transition of pregnancy

Nausea r/t hormonal changes of pregnancy

Readiness for enhanced family **Coping**: satisfying partner relationship, attention to gratification of needs, effective adaptation to developmental tasks of pregnancy

Readiness for enhanced **Parenting**: expresses willingness to enhance parenting skills

Sexual dysfunction r/t altered body function, self-concept, body image with pregnancy

Sleep deprivation r/t sleep deprivation secondary to uncomfortable pregnancy state

See Discomforts of Pregnancy

Premature Dilation of the Cervix (Incompetent Cervix)

Deficient **Diversional** activity r/t bed rest

Deficient **Knowledge** r/t treatment regimen, prognosis for pregnancy

Fear r/t potential loss of infant

Grieving r/t potential loss of infant

Ineffective **Coping** r/t bed rest, threat to fetus

Ineffective **Role** performance r/t inability to continue usual patterns of responsibility

Impaired physical **Mobility** r/t imposed bed rest to prevent preterm birth

Impaired **Social** interaction r/t bed rest

Powerlessness r/t inability to control outcome of pregnancy

Risk for **Infection**: Risk factors: invasive procedures to prevent preterm birth

Risk for **Injury**: fetal: Risk factors: preterm birth, use of anesthetics

Risk for **Injury**: maternal: Risk factors: surgical procedures to prevent preterm birth (e.g., cerclage)

Risk for **Spiritual** distress: Risk factors; physical/psychological stress

Sexual dysfunction r/t fear of harm to fetus

Situational low **Self-esteem** r/t inability to complete normal pregnancy

Premature Infant (Child)

Delayed **Growth** and development: developmental lag r/t prematurity, environmental and stimulation deficiencies, multiple caretakers

Disorganized **Infant** behavior r/t prematurity

Disturbed **Sensory** perception r/t noxious stimuli, noisy environment

Insomnia r/t noisy and noxious intensive care environment

Imbalanced **Nutrition**: less than body requirements r/t delayed or understimulated rooting reflex, easy fatigue during feeding, diminished endurance

Impaired **Gas** exchange r/t effects of cardiopulmonary insufficiency

Impaired **Swallowing** r/t decreased or absent gag reflex, fatigue

Ineffective **Thermoregulation** r/t large

body surface/weight ratio, immaturity of thermal regulation, state of prematurity

Readiness for enhanced organized **Infant** behavior: prematurity

Risk for delayed **Development**: Risk factor: prematurity

Risk for disproportionate **Growth**: Risk factor: prematurity

Risk for **Infection**: Risk factors: inadequate, immature, or undeveloped acquired immune response

Risk for **Injury**: Risk factor: prolonged mechanical ventilation, retinopathy of prematurely (ROP) secondary to 100% oxygen environment

Premature Infant (Parent)

Chronic **Sorrow** r/t threat of loss of a child, prolonged hospitalization

Complicated **Grieving** (prolonged) r/t unresolved conflicts

Compromised family **Coping** r/t disrupted family roles and disorganization, prolonged condition exhausting supportive capacity of significant persons

Decisional **Conflict** r/t support system deficit, multiple sources of information

Grieving r/t loss of perfect child possibly leading to complicated grieving

Ineffective **Breastfeeding** r/t disrupted establishment of effective pattern secondary to prematurity or insufficient opportunities

Parental role **Conflict** r/t expressed concerns, expressed inability to care for child's physical, emotional, or developmental needs

Readiness for enhanced **Family** process: adaptation to change associated with premature infant

Risk for impaired parent/child **Attachment**: Risk factors: separation, physical barriers, lack of privacy

Risk for **Powerlessness**: Risk factor: inability to control situation

Risk for **Spiritual** distress: Risk factors: challenged belief or value systems regarding moral or ethical implications of treatment plans

Spiritual distress r/t challenged belief or value systems regarding moral or ethical implications of treatment plans

See Child with Chronic Condition; Hospitalized Child

Premature Rupture of Membranes

Anxiety r/t threat to infant's health status

Disturbed **Body** image r/t inability to carry pregnancy to term

Grieving r/t potential loss of infant

Ineffective **Coping** r/t situational crisis

Risk for **Infection**: Risk factor: rupture of membranes

Risk for **Injury**: fetal r/t risk of premature birth

Situational low **Self-esteem** r/t inability to carry pregnancy to term

Premenstrual Tension Syndrome

See PMS (Premenstrual Tension Syndrome)

Prenatal Care, Normal

Anxiety r/t unknown future, threat to self secondary to pain of labor

Constipation r/t decreased gastrointestinal motility secondary to hormonal stimulation

Deficient **Knowledge** r/t lack of experience with pregnancy and care

Fatigue r/t increased energy demands

Health-seeking behaviors r/t consistent prenatal care and education

Imbalanced **Nutrition**: less than body requirements r/t nausea from normal hormonal changes

Impaired **Urinary** elimination r/t frequency caused by increased pelvic pressure and hormonal stimulation

Ineffective **Breathing** pattern r/t increased intrathoracic pressure and decreased energy secondary to enlarged uterus

Insomnia r/t discomforts of pregnancy and fetal activity

Interrupted **Family** processes r/t developmental transition

Readiness for enhanced **Knowledge**: appropriate prenatal care

Readiness for enhanced **Nutrition**: desire for knowledge of appropriate nutrition during pregnancy

Readiness for enhanced **Parenting**: realistic expectations of new role as parent

Readiness for enhanced **Spiritual** well-being: new role as parent

Risk for **Activity** intolerance: Risk factors: enlarged abdomen, increased cardiac workload

Risk for **Constipation**: Risk factors: decreased gastrointestinal motility secondary to hormonal stimulation

Risk for **Injury**: maternal: Risk factors: change in balance and center of gravity secondary to enlarged abdomen

Risk for **Sexual** dysfunction: Risk factors: enlarged abdomen, fear of harm to infant

Prenatal Testing

Acute **Pain** r/t invasive procedures

Anxiety r/t unknown outcome, delayed test results

Health-seeking behaviors r/t desire to have information regarding prenatal testing

Risk for **Infection** r/t invasive procedures during amniocentesis or chorionic villi sampling

Risk for **Injury**: fetal r/t invasive procedures

Preoperative Teaching

Health-seeking behaviors: preoperative regimens, postoperative precautions, expectations of role of client during preoperative or postoperative time

See Surgery, Preoperative Care

Pressure Ulcer

Acute **Pain** r/t tissue destruction, exposure of nerves

Imbalanced **Nutrition**: less than body requirements r/t limited access to food, inability to absorb nutrients because of biological factors, anorexia

Impaired bed **Mobility** r/t intolerance to activity, pain, cognitive impairment, depression, severe anxiety

Impaired **Skin** integrity: stage I or II pressure ulcer r/t physical immobility, mechanical factors, altered circulation, skin irritants

Impaired **Tissue** integrity: stage III or IV pressure ulcer r/t altered circulation, impaired physical mobility

Risk for **Infection**: Risk factors: physical immobility, mechanical factors (shearing forces, pressure, restraint, altered circulation, skin irritants)

Total urinary **Incontinence** r/t neurological dysfunction

Preterm Labor

Anxiety r/t threat to fetus, change in role functioning, change in environment and interaction patterns, use of tocolytic drugs

Deficient **Diversional** activity r/t long-term hospitalization

Grieving r/t loss of idealized pregnancy, potential loss of fetus

Impaired **Home** maintenance r/t medical restrictions

Impaired physical **Mobility** r/t medically imposed restrictions

Impaired **Social** interaction r/t prolonged bed rest or hospitalization

Ineffective **Coping** r/t situational crisis, preterm labor

Ineffective **Role** performance r/t inability to carry out normal roles secondary to bed rest or hospitalization, change in expected course of pregnancy

Readiness for enhanced **Comfort**: expresses desire to enhance relation

Readiness for enhanced **Communication**: willingness to discuss thoughts and feelings about situation

Risk for **Injury**: Risk factors: fetal: premature birth, immature body systems

Risk for **Injury**: Risk factor: maternal: use of tocolytic drugs

Risk for **Powerlessness**: Risk factor: lack of control over pre-term labor

Sexual dysfunction r/t actual or perceived limitation imposed by preterm labor and/or prescribed treatment, separation from partner because of hospitalization

Situational low **Self-esteem** r/t threatened ability to carry pregnancy to term

Sleep deprivation r/t change in usual pattern secondary to contractions, hospitalization, treatment regimen

Problem-Solving Ability

Defensive **Coping** r/t situational crisis

Ineffective **Coping** r/t situational crisis

Readiness for enhanced **Communication** r/t willingness to share ideas with others

Readiness for enhanced **Spiritual** well-being: desires to draw on inner strength and find meaning and purpose to life

Risk-prone health **Behavior** r/t altered locus of control

Projection

Anxiety r/t threat to self-concept

Chronic low **Self-esteem** r/t failure

Defensive **Coping** r/t inability to acknowledge that own behavior may be a problem, blaming others

Impaired **Social** interaction r/t self-concept disturbance, confrontational communication style

Risk for **Loneliness**: Risk factor: blaming others for problems

Risk for **Post-trauma** syndrome: Risk factor: diminished ego strength

Prolapsed Umbilical Cord

Fear r/t threat to fetus, impending surgery

Ineffective **Tissue** perfusion: fetal r/t interruption in umbilical blood flow

Risk for **Injury**: fetal: Risk factors: cord compression, ineffective tissue perfusion

Risk for **Injury**: maternal: Risk factor: emergency surgery

Prolonged Gestation

Anxiety r/t potential change in birthing plans, need for increased medical intervention, unknown outcome for fetus

Defensive **Coping** r/t underlying feeling of inadequacy regarding ability to give birth normally

Imbalanced **Nutrition**: less than body requirements (fetal) r/t aging of placenta

Powerlessness r/t perceived lack of control over outcome of pregnancy

Situational low **Self-esteem** r/t perceived inadequacy of body functioning

Prostatectomy

See TURP (Transurethral Resection of the Prostate)

Prostatic Hypertrophy

Ineffective **Health** maintenance r/t deficient knowledge regarding self-care and prevention of complications

Insomnia r/t nocturia

Risk for **Infection**: Risk factors: urinary residual after voiding, bacterial invasion of bladder

Risk for urge urinary **Incontinence**: Risk factor: small bladder capacity

Urinary retention r/t obstruction

See BPH (Benign Prostatic Hypertrophy)

Prostatitis

Ineffective **Health** maintenance r/t deficient knowledge regarding treatment

Ineffective **Protection** r/t depressed immune system

Risk for urge **Incontinence** r/t irritation of bladder

Protection, Altered

Ineffective **Protection** r/t (See **Protection,** ineffective, Section II)

Pruritus

Deficient **Knowledge** r/t methods to treat and prevent itching

Pruritus r/t (See **Pruritus,** Section II)

Risk for impaired **Skin** integrity: Risk factor: scratching from pruritus

Psoriasis

Disturbed **Body** image r/t lesions on body

Impaired **Skin** integrity r/t lesions on body

Ineffective **Health** maintenance r/t deficient knowledge regarding treatment modalities

Powerlessness r/t lack of control over condition with frequent exacerbations and remissions

Psychosis

Anxiety r/t unconscious conflict with reality

Chronic **Sorrow** r/t chronic mental illness

Disturbed **Thought** processes r/t inaccurate interpretations of environment

Fear r/t altered contact with reality

Imbalanced **Nutrition**: less than body requirements r/t lack of awareness of hunger, disinterest toward food

Impaired **Home** maintenance r/t impaired cognitive or emotional functioning, inadequate support systems

Impaired **Social** interaction r/t impaired communication patterns, self-concept disturbance, disturbed thought processes

Impaired verbal **Communication** r/t psychosis, inaccurate perceptions, hallucinations, delusions

Ineffective **Coping** r/t inadequate support systems, unrealistic perceptions, disturbed thought processes, impaired communication

Ineffective **Health** maintenance r/t cognitive impairment, ineffective individual and family coping

Insomnia r/t sensory alterations contributing to fear and anxiety

Interrupted **Family** processes r/t inability to express feelings, impaired communication

Readiness for enhanced **Hope**: expresses desire to enhance problem-solving to meet goals

Risk for **Post-trauma** syndrome: Risk factor: diminished ego strength

Risk for self- or other-directed **Violence**: Risk factors: lack of trust, panic, hallucinations, delusional thinking

Risk for **Suicide**: Risk factors: psychiatric illness/disorder

Self-care deficit r/t loss of contact with reality, impairment of perception

Self-esteem disturbance r/t excessive use of defense mechanisms (e.g., projection, denial, rationalization)

Social isolation r/t lack of trust, regression, delusional thinking, repressed fears

See Schizophrenia

PTCA (Percutaneous Transluminal Coronary Angioplasty)

See Angioplasty, Coronary

Pulmonary Edema

Anxiety r/t fear of suffocation

Impaired **Gas** exchange r/t extravasation of extravascular fluid in lung tissues and alveoli

P

Ineffective **Breathing** pattern r/t presence of tracheo-bronchial secretions

Ineffective **Health** maintenance r/t deficient knowledge regarding treatment regimen

Sleep deprivation r/t inability to breathe

See CHF (Congestive Heart Failure)

Pulmonary Embolism

Acute **Pain** r/t biological injury, lack of oxygen to cells

Decreased **Cardiac** output r/t right ventricular failure secondary to obstructed pulmonary artery

Deficient **Knowledge** r/t activities to prevent embolism, self-care after diagnosis of embolism

Delayed **Surgical** recovery r/t complications associated with respiratory difficulty

Fear r/t severe pain, possible death

Impaired **Gas** exchange r/t altered blood flow to alveoli secondary to lodged embolus

Ineffective **Tissue** perfusion: pulmonary r/t interruption of pulmonary blood flow secondary to lodged embolus

See Anticoagulant Therapy

Pulmonary Stenosis

See Congenital Heart Disease/Cardiac Anomalies

Pulse Deficit

Decreased **Cardiac** output r/t dysrhythmia

See Dysrhythmia

Pulse Oximetry

Readiness for enhanced **Knowledge**: information associated with treatment regimen

See Hypoxia

Pulse Pressure, Increased

See Intracranial Pressure, Increased

Pulse Pressure, Narrowed

See Shock

Pulses, Absent or Diminished Peripheral

Ineffective **Tissue** perfusion: peripheral r/t interruption of arterial flow

Risk for **Peripheral** neurovascular dysfunction: Risk factors: fractures, mechanical compression, orthopedic surgery trauma, immobilization, burns, vascular obstruction

See cause of Absent or Diminished Peripheral Pulses

Purpura

See Clotting Disorder

Pyelonephritis

Acute **Pain** r/t inflammation and irritation of urinary tract

Impaired **Urinary** elimination r/t irritation of urinary tract

Ineffective **Health** maintenance r/t deficient knowledge regarding self-care, treatment of disease, prevention of further urinary tract infections

Insomnia r/t urinary frequency

Risk for urge urinary **Incontinence**: Risk factor: irritation of urinary tract

Pyloric Stenosis

Acute **Pain** r/t surgical incision

Deficient **Fluid** volume r/t vomiting, dehydration

Imbalanced **Nutrition**: less than body requirements r/t vomiting secondary to pyloric sphincter obstruction

Ineffective **Health** maintenance r/t parental deficient knowledge regarding home care feeding regimen, wound care

See Hospitalized Child

Q

Quadriplegia

Disturbed **Energy** field r/t illness, grieving for loss of normal function

Grieving r/t loss of normal lifestyle, severity of disability

Impaired **Transfer** ability r/t quadriplegia

Impaired wheelchair **Mobility** r/t quadriplegia

Ineffective **Breathing** pattern r/t inability to use intercostal muscles

Readiness for enhanced **Spiritual** well being: r/t heightened coping associated with disability

Risk for **Autonomic** dysreflexia: Risk factors: bladder distention, bowel distention, skin irritation, lack of client and caregiver knowledge

Risk for impaired **Religiosity**: Risk factors: immobility, possible lack of transportation

See Spinal Cord Injury

R

RA (Rheumatoid Arthritis)

See Rheumatoid Arthritis

Rabies

Acute **Pain** r/t multiple immunization injections

Health-seeking behaviors r/t prophylactic immunization of domestic animals, avoidance of contact with wild animals

Hopelessness r/t poor prognosis

Ineffective **Health** maintenance r/t deficient knowledge regarding care of wound, isolation, and observation of infected animal

Radial Nerve Dysfunction

Acute **Pain** r/t trauma to hand or arm

See Neuropathy, Peripheral

Radiation Therapy

Activity intolerance r/t fatigue from possible anemia

Deficient **Knowledge** r/t what to expect with radiation therapy

Diarrhea r/t irradiation effects

Disturbed **Body** image r/t change in appearance, hair loss

Imbalanced **Nutrition**: less than body requirements r/t anorexia, nausea, vomiting, irradiation of areas of pharynx and esophagus

Impaired **Oral** mucous membrane r/t irradiation effects

Ineffective **Protection** r/t suppression of bone marrow

Nausea r/t side effects of radiation

Risk for impaired **Skin** integrity: Risk factor: irradiation effects

Risk for **Powerlessness**: Risk factors: medical treatment and possible side effects

Risk for **Spiritual** distress: Risk factors: radiation treatment, prognosis

Radical Neck Dissection

See Laryngectomy

Rage

Risk for other-directed **Violence**: Risk factors: panic state, manic excitement, organic brain syndrome

Risk for **Self-mutilation**: Risk factor: command hallucinations

Risk for **Suicide**: Risk factor: desire to kill oneself

Risk-prone health **Behavior** r/t multiple stressors

Stress overload r/t multiple coexisting stressors

Rape-Trauma Syndrome

Chronic **Sorrow** r/t forced loss of virginity

Rape-trauma syndrome (See **Rape-trauma** syndrome, Section II)

Rape-trauma syndrome: compound reaction (See **Rape-trauma** syndrome, compound reaction, Section II)

Rape-trauma syndrome: silent reaction (See **Rape-trauma** syndrome, silent reaction, Section II)

Risk for **Post-trauma** syndrome: Risk factors: trauma or violence associated with rape

Risk for **Powerlessness**: Risk factor: inability to control thoughts about incident

Risk for **Spiritual** distress: Risk factor: forced loss of virginity

Rash

Impaired **Skin** integrity r/t mechanical trauma

Pruritus r/t inflammation of skin

Risk for **Infection**: Risk factors: traumatized tissue, broken skin

Risk for latex **Allergy**: Risk factor: allergy to products associated with latex

Rationalization

Defensive **Coping** r/t situational crisis, inability to accept blame for consequences of own behavior

Ineffective **Denial** r/t fear of consequences, actual or perceived loss

Readiness for enhanced **Communication**: expressing desire to share thoughts and feelings

Readiness for enhanced **Spiritual** well-being: possibility of seeking harmony with self, others, higher power, God

Risk for **Post-trauma** syndrome: Risk factor: survivor's role in event

Rats, Rodents in the Home

Impaired **Home** maintenance r/t lack of knowledge, insufficient finances

See Filthy Home Environment

Raynaud's Disease

Deficient **Knowledge** r/t lack of information about disease process, possible complications, self-care needs regarding disease process and medication

Ineffective **Tissue** perfusion: peripheral r/t transient reduction of blood flow

RDS (Respiratory Distress Syndrome)

See Respiratory Conditions of the Neonate

Rectal Fullness

Constipation r/t decreased activity level, decreased fluid intake, inadequate fiber in diet, decreased peristalsis, side effects from antidepressant or antipsychotic therapy

Risk for **Constipation**: Risk factor: habitual denial or ignoring of urge to defecate

Rectal Lump

See Hemorrhoids

Rectal Pain/Bleeding

Acute **Pain** r/t pressure of defecation

Constipation r/t pain on defecation

Deficient **Knowledge** r/t possible causes of rectal bleeding, pain, treatment modalities

Risk for deficient **Fluid** volume: bleeding: Risk factor: untreated rectal bleeding

Rectal Surgery

See Hemorrhoidectomy

Rectocele Repair

Acute **Pain** r/t surgical procedure

Constipation r/t painful defecation

Ineffective **Health** maintenance r/t deficient knowledge of postoperative care of surgical site, dietary measures, exercise to prevent constipation

Risk for **Infection**: Risk factors: surgical

procedure, possible contamination of site with feces

Risk for urge urinary **Incontinence**: Risk factor: edema from surgery

Urinary retention r/t edema from surgery

Reflex Incontinence

Reflex **Incontinence** r/t neurological impairment

Regression

Anxiety r/t threat to or change in health status

Defensive **Coping** r/t denial of obvious problems, weaknesses

Ineffective **Role** performance r/t powerlessness over health status

Powerlessness r/t health care environment

See Hospitalized Child; Separation Anxiety

Regretful

Anxiety r/t situational or maturational crises

Death **Anxiety** r/t feelings of not having accomplished goals in life

Risk for **Spiritual** distress: Risk factor: inability to forgive

Rehabilitation

Impaired physical **Mobility** r/t injury, surgery, psychosocial condition warranting rehabilitation

Ineffective **Coping** r/t loss of normal function

Readiness for enhanced **Comfort**: expresses desire to enhance feeling of comfort

Readiness for enhanced **Self-concept**: accepts strengths and limitations

Readiness for enhanced **Therapeutic** regimen management: expression of desire to manage rehabilitation

Self-care deficit r/t impaired physical mobility

Relaxation Techniques

Anxiety r/t disturbed energy field

Health-seeking behaviors r/t requesting information about ways to relieve stress

Readiness for enhanced **Comfort**: expresses desire to enhance relaxation

Readiness for enhanced **Religiosity**: requests religious materials or experiences

Readiness for enhanced **Self-concept**: willingness to enhance self-concept

Readiness for enhanced **Spiritual** well-being: seeking comfort from higher power

Religiosity

Impaired **Religiosity** (See **Religiosity**, impaired, Section II)

Readiness for enhanced **Religiosity** (See **Religiosity**, readiness for enhanced, Section II)

Risk for impaired **Religiosity** (See **Religiosity**, risk for impaired, Section II)

R

Religious Concerns

Readiness for enhanced **Spiritual** well-being: desire for increased spirituality

Risk for impaired **Religiosity**: Risk factors: ineffective support, coping, caregiving

Risk for **Spiritual** distress: Risk factors: physical or psychological stress

Spiritual distress r/t separation from religious or cultural ties

Relocation Stress Syndrome

Relocation stress syndrome (See **Relocation** stress syndrome, Section II)

Risk for **Relocation** stress syndrome (See **Relocation** stress syndrome, risk for, Section II)

Renal Failure

Activity intolerance r/t effects of anemia, congestive heart failure

Chronic **Sorrow** r/t chronic illness

Death **Anxiety** r/t unknown outcome of disease

Decreased **Cardiac** output r/t effects of congestive heart failure, elevated potassium levels interfering with conduction system

Excess **Fluid** volume r/t decreased urine output, sodium retention, inappropriate fluid intake

Fatigue r/t effects of chronic uremia and anemia

Imbalanced **Nutrition**: less than body requirements r/t anorexia, nausea, vomiting, altered taste sensation, dietary restrictions

Impaired **Oral** mucous membranes r/t irritation from nitrogenous waste products

Impaired **Urinary** elimination r/t effects of disease, need for dialysis

Ineffective **Coping** r/t depression resulting from chronic disease

Pruritus r/t effects of uremia

Risk for impaired **Oral** mucous membranes: Risk factors: dehydration, effects of uremia

Risk for **Infection**: Risk factor: altered immune functioning

Risk for **Injury**: Risk factors: bone changes, neuropathy, muscle weakness

Risk for **Noncompliance**: Risk factor: complex medical therapy

Risk for **Powerlessness**: Risk factor: chronic illness

Spiritual distress r/t dealing with chronic illness

Renal Failure, Acute/Chronic, Child

Deficient **Diversional** activity r/t immobility during dialysis

Disturbed **Body** image r/t growth retardation, bone changes, visibility of dialysis access devices (shunt, fistula), edema

See Child with Chronic Condition; Hospitalized Child; Renal Failure

Renal Failure, Nonoliguric

Anxiety r/t change in health status

Risk for deficient **Fluid** volume: Risk factor: loss of large volumes of urine

See Renal Failure

Renal Transplantation, Donor

Decisional **Conflict** r/t harvesting of kidney from traumatized donor

Moral Distress r/t conflict among decision makers, end-of-life decisions, time constraints for decision making

Readiness for enhanced **Communication**: r/t expressing thoughts and feelings about situation

Readiness for enhanced family **Coping**: decision to allow organ donation

Readiness for enhanced **Decision making**: expresses desire to enhance understanding and meaning of choices

Readiness for enhanced **Spirituality**: inner peace resulting from allowance of organ donation

Spiritual distress r/t grieving from loss of significant person

See Nephrectomy

Renal Transplantation, Recipient

Anxiety r/t possible rejection, procedure

Deficient **Knowledge** r/t specific nutritional needs, possible paralytic ileus, fluid or sodium restrictions

Impaired **Health** maintenance r/t long-term home treatment after transplantation, diet, signs of rejection, use of medications

Impaired **Urinary** elimination r/t possible impaired renal function

Ineffective **Protection** r/t immunosuppression therapy

Readiness for enhanced **Spiritual** well-being: acceptance of situation

Risk for **Infection**: Risk factor: use of immunosuppressive therapy to control rejection

Rhabdomyolysis

Impaired physical **Mobility** r/t myalgia and muscle weakness

Impaired **Urinary** elimination r/t presence of myoglobin in the kidneys

Ineffective **Coping** r/t seriousness of condition

Readiness for enhanced **Therapeutic** regimen management: r/t seeks information to avoid condition

Risk for deficient **Fluid** volume: Risk factor: reduced blood flow to kidneys

See Renal Failure

Rheumatic Fever

See Endocarditis

Rheumatoid Arthritis

Chronic **Pain** r/t swollen or inflamed joints, restricted movement, physical therapy

Effective **Therapeutic** regimen management: following prescribed medication and adhering to exercise program; physical therapy

Fatigue r/t chronic inflammatory disease

Impaired physical **Mobility** r/t pain, limited range of motion

Imbalanced **Nutrition**: less than body requirements r/t loss of appetite

Risk for impaired **Skin** integrity: Risk factors: splints, adaptive devices

Risk for **Injury**: Risk factors: impaired physical mobility, splints, adaptive devices, increased bleeding potential as a result of antiinflammatory medications

Risk for situational low **Self-esteem**: Risk factor: disturbed body image

Self-care deficits: feeding, bathing, hygiene, dressing, grooming, toileting r/t restricted joint movement, pain

See Arthritis; JRA (Juvenile Rheumatoid Arthritis)

Rib Fracture

Acute **Pain** r/t movement, deep breathing

Ineffective **Breathing** pattern r/t fractured ribs

See Ventilator Client (if relevant)

Ridicule of Others

Defensive **Coping** r/t situational crisis, psychological impairment, substance abuse

Risk for **Post-trauma** syndrome: Risk factor: perception of the event

Ringworm of Body

Impaired **Skin** integrity r/t presence of macules associated with fungus

Ineffective **Therapeutic** regimen management r/t deficient knowledge of prevention, treatment

See Itching; Pruritus

Ringworm of Nails

Disturbed **Body** image r/t appearance of nails, removed nails

Ineffective **Therapeutic** regimen management r/t deficient knowledge of prevention, treatment

Ringworm of Scalp

Disturbed **Body** image r/t possible hair loss (alopecia)

Ineffective **Therapeutic** regimen management r/t deficient knowledge of prevention, treatment

See Itching; Pruritus

Risk for Relocation Stress Syndrome

See Relocation Stress Syndrome, Section I

Roaches, Invasion of Home with

Impaired **Home** maintenance r/t lack of knowledge, insufficient finances

See Filthy Home Environment

Role Performance, Altered

Ineffective **Role** performance (See **Role** performance, ineffective, Section II)

ROP

See Retinopathy of Prematurity (ROP)

RSV (Respiratory Syncytial Virus)

See Respiratory Infection, Acute Childhood

Rubella

See Communicable Diseases, Childhood

Rubor of Extremities

Ineffective **Tissue** perfusion: peripheral r/t interruption of arterial flow

See Peripheral Vascular Disease

Ruptured Disk

See Low Back Pain

S

SAD (Seasonal Affective Disorder)

Effective **Therapeutic** regimen management: uses SAD lights during winter months

See Depression (Major Depressive Disorder)

Sadness

Adult **Failure** to thrive r/t depression, apathy

Complicated **Grieving** r/t actual or perceived loss

Readiness for enhanced **Communication**: willingness to share feelings and thoughts

Readiness for enhanced **Spiritual** well-being: desire for harmony after actual or perceived loss

Risk for **Powerlessness**: Risk factor: actual or perceived loss

Risk for **Spiritual** distress: Risk factor: loss of loved one

Spiritual distress r/t intense suffering

See Depression (Major Depressive Disorder); Major Depressive Disorder

Safe Sex

Effective **Therapeutic** regimen management: taking appropriate precautions during sexual activity to keep from contacting a sexually transmitted disease

See Sexuality, Adolescent; STD (Sexually Transmitted Disease)

Safety, Childhood

Deficient **Knowledge**: potential for enhanced health maintenance r/t parental knowledge and skill acquisition regarding appropriate safety measures

Health-seeking behaviors r/t enhanced parenting r/t adequate support systems, appropriate requests for help, desire and request for safety information

Readiness for enhanced **Immunization** status: expresses desire to enhance immunization status

Risk for altered **Health** maintenance: Risk factors: parental deficient knowledge regarding appropriate safety needs per developmental stage, child-proofing house

Risk for **Aspiration** (See **Aspiration,** risk for, Section II)

Risk for impaired **Parenting**: Risk factors: lack of available and effective role model, lack of knowledge, misinformation from other family members (old wives' tales)

Risk for **Injury/Trauma**: Risk factors: developmental age, altered home maintenance

Risk for **Poisoning**: Risk factors: use of lead-based paint; presence of asbestos or radon gas; drugs not locked in cabinet; household products left in accessible area (bleach, detergent, drain cleaners, household cleaners); alcohol and perfume within reach of child; presence of poisonous plants; atmospheric pollutants

Salmonella

Readiness for enhanced **Therapeutic** regimen management: avoiding improperly prepared or stored food, wearing gloves when handling pet reptiles or their feces

Impaired **Home** maintenance r/t improper preparation or storage of food, lack of safety measures when caring for pet reptile

See Gastroenteritis; Gastroenteritis, Child

Salpingectomy

Decisional **Conflict** r/t sterilization procedure

Grieving r/t possible loss from tubal pregnancy

Risk for impaired **Urinary** elimination: Risk factor: trauma to ureter during surgery

See Hysterectomy; Surgery, Perioperative Care; Surgery, Postoperative Care; Surgery, Preoperative Care

Sarcoidosis

Acute **Pain** r/t possible disease affecting joints

Anxiety r/t change in health status

Decreased **Cardiac** output r/t dysrhythmias

Impaired **Gas** exchange r/t ventilation-perfusion imbalance

Ineffective **Health** maintenance r/t deficient knowledge regarding home care and medication regimen

SARS (Severe Acute Respiratory Syndrome)

Risk for **Infection**: Risk factor: increased environmental exposure (travelers in close proximity to infected persons, traveling when a fever is present)

Readiness for enhanced **Knowledge** r/t information regarding travel and precautions to avoid exposure to SARS

Effective **Therapeutic** regimen management r/t uses appropriate hand hygiene

See Pneumonia

SBE (Self Breast Examination)

Effective **Therapeutic** regimen management r/t practices SBE per recommended protocol

Health-seeking behaviors r/t desires to have information about SBE

Readiness for enhanced **Knowledge**: self-breast examination

Scabies

See Communicable Diseases, Childhood

Scared

Anxiety r/t threat of death, threat to or change in health status

Death **Anxiety** r/t unresolved issues surrounding end-of-life decisions

Fear r/t hospitalization, real or imagined threat to own well-being

Readiness for enhanced **Communication**: willingness to share thoughts and feelings

Schizophrenia

Anxiety r/t unconscious conflict with reality

Chronic **Sorrow** r/t chronic mental illness

Deficient **Diversional** activity r/t social isolation, possible regression

Disturbed **Sensory** perception r/t biochemical imbalances for sensory distortion (illusions, hallucinations)

Disturbed **Thought** processes r/t inaccurate interpretations of environment

Fear r/t altered contact with reality

Imbalanced **Nutrition**: less than body requirements r/t fear of eating, lack of awareness of hunger, disinterest toward food

Impaired **Home** maintenance r/t impaired cognitive or emotional functioning, insufficient finances, inadequate support systems

Impaired **Social** interaction r/t impaired communication patterns, self-concept disturbance, disturbed thought processes

Impaired verbal **Communication** r/t psychosis, disorientation, inaccurate perception, hallucinations, delusions

S

Ineffective **Coping** r/t inadequate support systems, unrealistic perceptions, inadequate coping skills, disturbed thought processes, impaired communication

Ineffective **Health** maintenance r/t cognitive impairment, ineffective individual and family coping, lack of material resources

Ineffective family **Therapeutic** regimen management r/t chronicity and unpredictability of condition

Insomnia r/t sensory alterations contributing to fear and anxiety

Interrupted **Family** processes r/t inability to express feelings, impaired communication

Readiness for enhanced **Hope**: expresses desire to enhance interconnectedness with others and problem-solve to meet goals

Readiness for enhanced **Power**: expresses willingness to enhance participation in choices for daily living and health and enhance knowledge for participation in change

Risk for **Caregiver** role strain: Risk factors: bizarre behavior of client, chronicity of condition

Risk for compromised human **Dignity**: Risk factor: stigmatizing label

Risk for impaired **Religiosity**: Risk factors: ineffective coping, lack of security

Risk for **Loneliness**: Risk factor: inability to interact socially

Risk for **Post-trauma** syndrome: Risk factor: diminished ego strength

Risk for **Powerlessness**: Risk factor: intrusive, distorted thinking

Risk for self- and other-directed **Violence**: Risk factors: lack of trust, panic, hallucinations, delusional thinking

Risk for **Suicide**: Risk factor: psychiatric illness

Self-care deficit r/t loss of contact with reality, impairment of perception

Sleep deprivation r/t intrusive thoughts, nightmares

Social isolation r/t lack of trust, regression, delusional thinking, repressed fears

Spiritual distress r/t loneliness, social alienation

Sciatica

See Neuropathy, Peripheral

Scoliosis

Acute **Pain** r/t musculoskeletal restrictions, surgery, reambulation with cast or spinal rod

Chronic **Sorrow** r/t chronic disability

Disturbed **Body** image r/t use of therapeutic braces, postsurgery scars, restricted physical activity

Impaired **Gas** exchange r/t restricted lung expansion as a result of severe presurgery curvature of spine, immobilization

Impaired physical **Mobility** r/t restricted movement, dyspnea caused by severe curvature of spine

Impaired **Skin** integrity r/t braces, casts, surgical correction

Ineffective **Breathing** pattern r/t restricted lung expansion caused by severe curvature of spine

Ineffective **Health** maintenance r/t deficient knowledge regarding treatment modalities, restrictions, home care, postoperative activities

Readiness for enhanced **Therapeutic** regimen management r/t desire for knowledge regarding treatment for condition

Risk for **Infection**: Risk factor: surgical incision

Risk for perioperative positioning **Injury**: Risk factor: prone position

Risk-prone health **Behavior** r/t lack of developmental maturity to comprehend long-term consequences of noncompliance with treatment procedures

See Hospitalized Child; Maturational Issues, Adolescent

Sedentary Lifestyle

Activity intolerance r/t sedentary lifestyle

Readiness for enhanced **Coping** r/t seeking knowledge of new strategies to adjust to sedentary lifestyle

Sedentary **Lifestyle** (See **Lifestyle,** sedentary, Section II)

Seizure Disorders, Adult

Acute **Confusion** r/t postseizure state

Impaired **Memory** r/t seizure activity

Ineffective **Health** maintenance r/t lack of knowledge regarding anticonvulsive therapy

Readiness for enhanced **Knowledge** r/t anticonvulsive therapy

Readiness for enhanced **Self-care:** expresses desire to enhance knowledge and responsibility for self-care

Risk for disturbed **Thought** processes: Risk factor: effects of anticonvulsant medications

Risk for **Falls**: Risk factor: uncontrolled seizure activity

Risk for ineffective **Airway** clearance: Risk factor: accumulation of secretions during seizure

Risk for **Injury**: Risk factors: uncontrolled movements during seizure, falls, drowsiness caused by anticonvulsants

Risk for **Powerlessness**: Risk factor: possible seizure

Social isolation r/t unpredictability of seizures, community-imposed stigma

See Epilepsy

Seizure Disorders, Childhood (Epilepsy, Febrile Seizures, Infantile Spasms)

Ineffective **Health** maintenance r/t lack of knowledge regarding anticonvulsive therapy, fever reduction (febrile seizures)

Risk for delayed **Development** and disproportionate growth: Risk factors: effects of seizure disorder, parental overprotection

Risk for disturbed **Thought** processes: Risk factor: effects of anticonvulsant medications

Risk for **Falls**: Risk factor: possible seizure

Risk for ineffective **Airway** clearance: Risk factor: accumulation of secretions during seizure

Risk for **Injury**: Risk factors: uncontrolled movements during seizure, falls, drowsiness caused by anticonvulsants

Social isolation r/t unpredictability of seizures, community-imposed stigma

See Epilepsy

S

Self Breast Examination

See SBE (Self Breast Examination)

Self-Care

Readiness for enhanced **Self-Care** (See **Self-care,** readiness for enhanced, Section II)

Self-Care Deficit, Bathing/ Hygiene

Bathing/hygiene **Self-care** deficit (See **Self-care** deficit, bathing, hygiene, Section II)

Self-Care Deficit, Dressing/ Grooming

Dressing/grooming **Self-care** deficit (See **Self-care** deficit, dressing/grooming, Section II)

Self-Care Deficit, Feeding

Feeding **Self-care** deficit (See **Self-care** deficit, feeding, Section II)

S

Self-Care Deficit, Toileting

Toileting **Self-care** deficit (See **Self-care** deficit, toileting, Section II)

Self-Concept

Readiness for enhanced **Self-concept** (See **Self-concept,** readiness for, Section II)

Self-Destructive Behavior

Post-trauma response r/t unresolved feelings from traumatic event

Risk for self-directed **Violence**: Risk factors: panic state, history of child abuse, toxic reaction to medication

Risk for **Self-mutilation**: Risk factors: feelings of depression, rejection, self-hatred, depersonalization; command hallucinations

Risk for **Suicide**: Risk factor: history of self-destructive behavior

Self-Esteem, Chronic Low

Chronic low **Self-esteem** (See **Self-esteem,** chronic low, Section II)

Self-Esteem, Situational Low

Risk for situational low **Self-esteem** (See **Self-esteem,** situational low, risk for, Section II)

Self-esteem disturbance r/t inappropriate and learned negative feelings about self

Situational low **Self-esteem** (See **Self-esteem,** situational low, Section II)

Self-Mutilation, Risk for

Risk for **Self-mutilation** (See **Self-mutilation,** risk for, Section II)

Self-mutilation (See **Self-mutilation,** Section II)

Senile Dementia

Sedentary **lifestyle** r/t lack of interest

See Dementia

Sensory/Perceptual Alterations

Disturbed **Sensory** perception: visual, auditory, kinesthetic, gustatory, tactile, olfactory (See **Sensory perception,** disturbed, Section II)

Separation Anxiety

Ineffective **Coping** r/t maturational and situational crises, vulnerability related to developmental age, hospitalization, separation from family and familiar surroundings, multiple caregivers

Insomnia r/t separation for significant others

Risk for impaired parent/child **Attachment**: Risk factor: separation

See Hospitalized Child

Sepsis, Child

Delayed **Surgical** recovery r/t presence of infection

Imbalanced **Nutrition**: less than body requirements r/t anorexia, generalized weakness, poor sucking reflex

Ineffective **Thermoregulation** r/t infectious process, septic shock

Ineffective **Tissue** perfusion: cardiopulmonary, peripheral r/t arterial or venous blood flow exchange problems, septic shock

Risk for impaired **Skin** integrity: Risk factors: desquamation caused by disseminated intravascular coagulation

See Hospitalized Child; Premature Infant, Child

Septicemia

Deficient **Fluid** volume r/t vasodilation of peripheral vessels, leaking of capillaries

Imbalanced **Nutrition**: less than body requirements r/t anorexia, generalized weakness

Ineffective **Tissue** perfusion r/t decreased systemic vascular resistance

See Sepsis, Child; Shock; Shock, Septic

Severe Acute Respiratory Syndrome

See SARS (Severe Acute Respiratory Syndrome); Pneumonia

Sexual Dysfunction

Chronic **Sorrow** r/t loss of ideal sexual experience, altered relationships

Sexual dysfunction (See **Sexual** dysfunction, Section II)

See Erectile Dysfunction

Sexuality, Adolescent

Decisional **Conflict**: sexual activity r/t undefined personal values or beliefs, multiple or divergent sources of information, lack of relevant information

Deficient **Knowledge**: potential for enhanced health maintenance r/t multiple or divergent sources of information or lack of relevant information regarding sexual transmission of disease, contraception, prevention of toxic shock syndrome

Disturbed **Body** image r/t anxiety caused by unachieved developmental milestone (puberty) or deficient knowledge regarding reproductive maturation as manifested by amenorrhea or expressed concerns regarding lack of growth of secondary sex characteristics

Risk for **Rape-trauma** syndrome: Risk factors: date rape, campus rape, insufficient knowledge regarding self-protection mechanisms

See Maturational Issues, Adolescent

Sexuality Pattern, Ineffective

Ineffective **Sexuality** pattern (See **Sexuality**, ineffective pattern, Section II)

Sexually Transmitted Disease

See STD (Sexually Transmitted Disease)

Shaken Baby Syndrome

Decreased **Intracranial** adaptive capacity r/t brain injury

Impaired **Parenting** r/t stress, history of being abusive

Risk for other-directed **Violence**: Risk factors: history of violence against others, perinatal complications

Stress overload r/t intense repeated family stressors, family violence

See Child Abuse; Suspected Child Abuse and Neglect (SCAN), Child; Suspected Child Abuse and Neglect (SCAN), Parent

Shakiness

Anxiety r/t situational or maturational crisis, threat of death

Shame

Self-esteem disturbance r/t inability to deal with past traumatic events, blaming of self for events not under one's control

Shingles

Acute **Pain** r/t vesicular eruption along the nerves

Ineffective **Protection** r/t abnormal blood profiles

Pruritus r/t inflammation

Risk for **Infection**: Risk factor: tissue destruction

Social isolation r/t altered state of wellness, contagiousness of disease

See Itching

Shivering

Hypothermia r/t exposure to cool environment

Shock

Fear r/t serious threat to health status

Ineffective **Tissue** perfusion: cardiopulmonary; peripheral r/t arterial/venous blood flow exchange problems

Risk for **Injury**: Risk factor: prolonged shock resulting in multiple organ failure or death

S

See Shock, Cardiogenic; Shock, Hypovolemic; Shock, Septic

Shock, Cardiogenic

Decreased **Cardiac** output r/t decreased myocardial contractility, dysrhythmia

See Shock

Shock, Hypovolemic

Deficient **Fluid** volume r/t abnormal loss of fluid

See Shock

Shock, Septic

Deficient **Fluid** volume r/t abnormal loss of fluid through capillaries, pooling of blood in peripheral circulation

Ineffective **Protection** r/t inadequately functioning immune system

See Sepsis, Child; Septicemia; Shock

Shoulder Repair

Risk for perioperative positioning **Injury**: Risk factor: immobility

Self-care deficit: bathing, hygiene, dressing, grooming, feeding r/t immobilization of affected shoulder

See Surgery, Preoperative; Surgery, Perioperative; Surgery, Postoperative; Total Joint Replacement

Sickle Cell Anemia/Crisis

Activity intolerance r/t fatigue, effects of chronic anemia

Acute **Pain** r/t viscous blood, tissue hypoxia

Deficient **Fluid** volume r/t decreased intake, increased fluid requirements during sickle cell crisis, decreased ability of kidneys to concentrate urine

Impaired physical **Mobility** r/t pain, fatigue

Risk for ineffective **Tissue** perfusion: renal, cerebral, cardiac, gastrointestinal, peripheral: Risk factors: effects of red cell sickling, infarction of tissues

Risk for **Infection**: Risk factor: alterations in splenic function

See Child with Chronic Condition; Hospitalized Child

SIDS (Sudden Infant Death Syndrome)

Anxiety/Fear: parental r/t life-threatening event

Deficient **Knowledge**: potential for enhanced health maintenance r/t knowledge or skill acquisition of cardiopulmonary resuscitation and home apnea monitoring

Grieving r/t potential loss of infant

Insomnia: parental/infant r/t home apnea monitoring

Interrupted **Family** processes r/t stress as a result of special care needs of infant with apnea

Risk for **Powerlessness**: Risk factor: unanticipated life-threatening event

Risk for sudden infant **Death** syndrome (See **Death** syndrome, sudden infant, risk for, Section II)

See Terminally Ill Child/Death of Child, Parent

Situational Crisis

Ineffective **Coping** r/t situational crisis

Interrupted **Family** processes r/t situational crisis

Readiness for enhanced **Communication**: willingness to share feelings and thoughts

Readiness for enhanced **Religiosity**: requests religious material and/or experiences

Readiness for enhanced **Spiritual** well-being: desire for harmony following crisis

SJS (Stevens-Johnson Syndrome)

See Stevens-Johnson Syndrome

Skin Cancer

Impaired **Skin** integrity r/t abnormal cell growth in skin, treatment of skin cancer

Ineffective **Health** maintenance r/t deficient knowledge regarding self-care with skin cancer

Readiness for enhanced **Knowledge** r/t self-care to prevent and treat skin cancer

Skin Disorders

Internal/External

Impaired **Skin** integrity (See **Skin** integrity, impaired, Section II)

Skin Integrity, Risk for Impaired

Internal/External

Risk for impaired **Skin** integrity (See **Skin** integrity, impaired, risk for, Section II)

Skin Turgor, Change in Elasticity

Deficient **Fluid** volume r/t active fluid loss (decreased skin turgor can be a normal finding in the elderly)

Sleep

Readiness for enhanced **Sleep** (See **Sleep,** readiness for enhanced, Section II)

Sleep Apnea

See PND (Paroxysmal Nocturnal Dyspnea)

Sleep Deprivation

Disturbed **Sensory** perception r/t lack of sleep

Fatigue r/t lack of sleep

Sleep deprivation (See **Sleep** deprivation, Section II)

Sleep Pattern Disorders

Insomnia (See **Insomnia,** Section II)

Sleep Pattern, Disturbed, Parent/Child

Insomnia: child r/t anxiety or fear

Insomnia: parent r/t parental responsibilities, stress

See Suspected Child Abuse and Neglect

Slurring of Speech

Impaired verbal **Communication** r/t decrease in circulation to brain, brain tumor, anatomical defect, cleft palate

Situational low **Self-esteem** r/t speech impairment

See Communication Problems

Small Bowel Resection

See Abdominal Surgery

Smell, Loss of Ability to

Risk for **Injury**: Risk factors: inability to detect gas fumes, smoke smells

See Anosmia

Smoke Inhalation

Impaired **Gas** exchange r/t ventilation perfusion imbalance

Ineffective **Airway** clearance r/t smoke inhalation

Readiness for effective **Therapeutic** regimen management: functioning smoke detectors and carbon monoxide detectors in home and work, plan for escape route worked out and reviewed

Risk for acute **Confusion**: Risk factor: decreased oxygen supply

Risk for **Poisoning**: Risk factor: exposure to carbon monoxide

See Atelectasis; Burns; Pneumonia

Smoking Behavior

Altered **Health** maintenance r/t denial of effects of smoking, lack of effective support for smoking withdrawal

Readiness for enhanced **Knowledge** r/t smoking cessation

Social Interaction, Impaired

Impaired **Social** interaction (See **Social** interaction, impaired, Section II)

Social Isolation

Social isolation (See **Social** isolation, Section II)

Sociopathic Personality

See Antisocial Personality Disorder

Sodium, Decrease/Increase

See Hyponatremia/Hypernatremia

Somatization Disorder

Anxiety r/t unresolved conflicts channeled into physical complaints or conditions

Chronic **Pain** r/t unexpressed anger, multiple physical disorders, depression

Ineffective **Coping** r/t lack of insight into underlying conflicts

Ineffective **Denial** r/t displaces psychological stress to physical symptoms

Sore Nipples, Breastfeeding

Ineffective **Breastfeeding** r/t deficient knowledge regarding correct feeding procedure

See Painful Breasts, Sore Nipples

Sore Throat

Acute **Pain** r/t inflammation, irritation, dryness

Deficient **Knowledge** r/t treatment, relief of discomfort

Impaired **Oral** mucous membrane r/t inflammation or infection of oral cavity

Impaired **Swallowing** r/t irritation of oropharyngeal cavity

Sorrow

Chronic **Sorrow** (See **Sorrow**, chronic, Section II)

Grieving r/t loss of significant person, object, or role

Readiness for enhanced **Communication**: expresses thoughts and feelings

Readiness for enhanced **Spiritual** well-being: desire to find purpose and meaning of loss

Spastic Colon

See IBS (Irritable Bowel Syndrome)

Speech Disorders

Anxiety r/t difficulty with communication

Delayed **Growth** and development r/t effects of physical or mental disability

Disturbed **Sensory** perception (auditory) r/t altered sensory reception, transmission, and/or integration

Impaired verbal **Communication** r/t anatomical defect, cleft palate, psychological barriers, decrease in circulation to brain

Spina Bifida

See Neural Tube Defects

Spinal Cord Injury

Chronic **Sorrow** r/t immobility, change in body function

Complicated **Grieving** r/t loss of usual body function

Constipation r/t immobility, loss of sensation

Deficient **Diversional** activity r/t long-term hospitalization, frequent lengthy treatments

Disturbed **Body** image r/t change in body function

Fear r/t powerlessness over loss of body function

Impaired **Home** maintenance r/t change in health status, insufficient family planning or finances, deficient knowledge, inadequate support systems

Impaired physical **Mobility** r/t neuromuscular impairment

Impaired wheelchair **Mobility** r/t neuromuscular impairment

Ineffective **Health** maintenance r/t deficient knowledge regarding self-care with spinal cord injury

Readiness for enhanced **Self-care**: expresses desire to enhance independence in maintaining well-being

Reflex **Incontinence** r/t spinal cord lesion interfering with conduction of cerebral messages

Risk for **Autonomic** dysreflexia: Risk factors: bladder or bowel distention, skin irritation, deficient knowledge of patient and caregiver

Risk for **Disuse** syndrome: Risk factor: paralysis

Risk for impaired **Religiosity**: Risk factor: lack of transportation

Risk for impaired **Skin** integrity: Risk factors: immobility, paralysis

Risk for ineffective **Breathing** pattern: Risk factor: neuromuscular impairment

Risk for **Infection**: Risk factors: chronic disease, stasis of body fluids

Risk for latex **Allergy** response: Risk factor: continuous or intermittent catheterization

Risk for **Loneliness**: Risk factor: physical immobility

Risk for **Powerlessness**: Risk factor: loss of function

Self-care deficit r/t neuromuscular impairment

Sedentary **lifestyle** r/t lack of resources or interest

Sexual dysfunction r/t altered body function

Urinary retention r/t inhibition of reflex arc

See Child with Chronic Condition; Hospitalized Child; Neural Tube Defects

S

Spinal Fusion

Impaired bed **Mobility** r/t impaired ability to turn side to side while keeping spine in proper alignment

Impaired physical **Mobility** r/t musculoskeletal impairment associated with surgery, possible back brace

Readiness for enhanced **Knowledge** r/t expresses interest in information associated with surgery

See Acute Back; Back Pain; Scoliosis; Surgery, Preoperative Care; Surgery, Perioperative Care; Surgery, Postoperative Care

Spiritual Distress

Risk for **Spiritual** distress (See **Spiritual** distress, risk for, Section II)

Spiritual distress (See **Spiritual** distress, Section II)

Spiritual Well-Being

Readiness for enhanced **Spiritual** well-being (See **Spiritual** well-being, readiness for enhanced, Section II)

Splenectomy

See Abdominal Surgery

Sprains

Acute **Pain** r/t physical injury

Effective **Therapeutic** regimen management: not exercising when tired or in pain; maintaining healthy weight; wearing properly fitting shoes; using appropriate warm-up, stretching, and cool down exercises; wearing protective equipment; running on even surfaces; staying physically fit

Impaired physical **Mobility** r/t injury

Stapedectomy

Acute **Pain** r/t headache

Disturbed **Sensory** perception: auditory r/t hearing loss caused by edema from surgery

Risk for **Falls**: Risk factor: dizziness

Risk for **Infection**: Risk factor: invasive procedure

Stasis Ulcer

Impaired **Tissue** integrity r/t chronic venous congestion

See CHF (Congestive Heart Failure); Varicose Veins

STD (Sexually Transmitted Disease)

Acute **Pain** r/t biological or psychological injury

Fear r/t altered body function, risk for social isolation, fear of incurable illness

Ineffective **Health** maintenance r/t deficient knowledge regarding transmission, symptoms, treatment of STD

Ineffective **Sexuality** pattern r/t illness, altered body function

Readiness for enhanced **Knowledge** r/t prevention and treatment of STDs

Risk for **Infection**/spread of infection: Risk factor: lack of knowledge concerning transmission of disease

Social isolation r/t fear of contracting or spreading disease

See Maturational Issues, Adolescent

STEMI (ST-Elevation Myocardial Infarction)

See MI (Myocardial Infarction)

Stent (Coronary Artery Stent)

Decrease **Cardiac** output r/t possible restenosis

Readiness for enhanced **Decision** making: expresses desire to enhance risk benefit analysis, understanding and meaning of choices, and decisions regarding treatment

Risk for **Injury**: Risk factor: complications associated with stent placement

See Angioplasty Coronary, Cardiac Catheterization

Sterilization Surgery

Decisional **Conflict** r/t multiple or divergent sources of information, unclear personal values or beliefs

See Surgery, Preoperative Care; Surgery, Perioperative Care; Surgery, Postoperative Care; Tubal Ligation; Vasectomy

Stertorous Respirations

Ineffective **Airway** clearance r/t pharyngeal obstruction

Stevens-Johnson Syndrome (SJS)

Acute **Pain** r/t painful skin lesions and painful oral mucosa lesions

Impaired **Oral** mucous membrane r/t immunocompromised condition associated with allergic medication reaction

Impaired **Skin** integrity r/t allergic medication reaction

Risk for acute **Confusion**: Risk factors: dehydration, electrolyte disturbances

Risk for deficient **Fluid** volume: Risk factors: factors affecting fluid needs (hypermetabolic state, hyperthermia), excessive losses through normal routes (vomiting and diarrhea)

Stillbirth

See Pregnancy Loss

Stoma

See Colostomy; Ileostomy

Stomatitis

Impaired **Oral** mucous membrane r/t pathological conditions of oral cavity

Stone, Kidney

See Kidney Stone

Stool, Hard/Dry

Constipation r/t inadequate fluid intake, inadequate fiber intake, decreased activity level, decreased gastric motility

Straining with Defecation

Constipation r/t less than adequate fluid intake, less than adequate dietary intake

Risk for decreased **Cardiac** output r/t vagal stimulation with dysrhythmia resulting from Valsalva maneuver

Stress

Anxiety r/t feelings of helplessness, feelings of being threatened

Disturbed **Energy** field r/t low energy level, feelings of hopelessness

Fear r/t powerlessness over feelings

Ineffective **Coping** r/t ineffective use of problem-solving process, feelings of apprehension or helplessness

Readiness for enhanced **Communication** r/t willingness to share thoughts and feelings

Readiness for enhanced **Spiritual** well-being r/t desire for harmony and peace in stressful situation

Risk for **Post-trauma** syndrome: Risk factors: perception of event, survivor's role in event

Self-esteem disturbance r/t inability to deal with life events

Stress overload r/t intense or multiple stressors

Stress Overload

Stress overload (See **Stress** overload, Section II)

Stress Urinary Incontinence

Risk for urge urinary **Incontinence** r/t involuntary sphincter relaxation

Stress urinary **Incontinence** r/t degenerative change in pelvic muscles

See Incontinence of Urine

Stridor

Ineffective **Airway** clearance r/t obstruction, tracheobronchial infection, trauma

Stroke

See CVA (Cerebrovascular Accident)

Stuttering

Anxiety r/t impaired verbal communication

Impaired verbal **Communication** r/t anxiety, psychological problems

Subarachnoid Hemorrhage

Acute **Pain**: headache r/t irritation of meninges from blood, increased intracranial pressure

Ineffective **Tissue** perfusion: cerebral r/t bleeding from cerebral vessel

See Intracranial Pressure, Increased

Substance Abuse

Anxiety r/t loss of control

Compromised/disabled family **Coping** r/t codependency issues

Defensive **Coping** r/t substance abuse

Dysfunctional **Family** processes: alcohol r/t inadequate coping skills

Imbalanced **Nutrition**: less than body requirements r/t anorexia

Ineffective **Coping** r/t use of substances to cope with life events

Ineffective **Denial** r/t refusal to acknowledge substance abuse problem

Ineffective **Protection** r/t malnutrition, sleep deprivation

Insomnia r/t irritability, nightmares, tremors

Powerlessness r/t substance addiction

Readiness for enhanced **Coping**: seeking social support and knowledge of new strategies

Readiness for enhanced **Self-concept**: accepting strengths and limitations

Risk for impaired parent/child **Attachment**: Risk factor: substance abuse

Risk for **Injury**: Risk factor: alteration in sensory perception

Risk for self- or other-directed **Violence**: Risk factors: reactions to substances used, impulsive behavior, disorientation, impaired judgment

Risk for **Suicide**: Risk factor: substance abuse

Self-esteem disturbance r/t failure at life events

Social isolation r/t unacceptable social behavior or values

See Maturational Issues, Adolescent

Substance Abuse, Adolescent

See Alcohol Withdrawal; Maturational Issues, Adolescent; Substance Abuse

Substance Abuse in Pregnancy

Defensive **Coping** r/t denial of situation, differing value system

Deficient **Knowledge** r/t lack of exposure to information regarding effects of substance abuse in pregnancy

Health-seeking behaviors (substance abuse counseling) r/t desire to provide child with substance-free perinatal period

Ineffective **Health** maintenance r/t addiction

Noncompliance r/t differing value system, cultural influences, addiction

Risk for fetal **Injury** r/t effects of drugs on fetal growth and development

Risk for impaired parent/child **Attachment**: Risk factors: substance abuse, inability of parent to meet infant's or own personal needs

Risk for impaired **Parenting**: Risk factor: lack of ability to meet infant's needs

Risk for **Infection**: Risk factors: intravenous drug use, lifestyle

Risk for maternal **Injury**: Risk factor: drug use

See Substance Abuse

Sucking Reflex

Effective **Breastfeeding** r/t regular and sustained sucking and swallowing at breast

Sudden Infant Death Syndrome (SIDS)

See SIDS (Sudden Infant Death Syndrome)

Suffocation, Risk for

Internal/External

Risk for **Suffocation** (See **Suffocation, risk for**, Section II)

Suicide Attempt

Hopelessness r/t perceived or actual loss, substance abuse, low self-concept, inadequate support systems

Ineffective **Coping** r/t anger, complicated grieving

Post-trauma response r/t history of traumatic events, abuse, rape, incest, war, torture

Readiness for enhanced **Communication**: willingness to share thoughts and feelings

Readiness for enhanced **Spiritual** well-being: desire for harmony and inner strength to help redefine purpose for life

Risk for **Post-trauma** syndrome: Risk factor: survivor's role in suicide attempt

Risk for **Suicide** (See **Suicide,** risk for, Section II)

Self-esteem disturbance r/t guilt, inability to trust, feelings of worthlessness or rejection

Social isolation r/t inability to engage in satisfying personal relationships

Spiritual distress r/t hopelessness, despair

See Violent Behavior

Support System

Readiness for enhanced family **Coping**: ability to adapt to tasks associated with care, support of significant other during health crisis

Readiness for enhanced **Family** processes: activities support the growth of family members

Readiness for enhanced **Parenting**: children or other dependent person(s) expressing satisfaction with home environment

Suppression of Labor

See Preterm Labor; Tocolytic Therapy

Surgery, Perioperative Care

Risk for imbalanced **Fluid** volume: Risk factor: surgery

Risk for perioperative positioning **Injury**: Risk factors: predisposing condition, prolonged surgery

Surgery, Postoperative Care

Activity intolerance r/t pain, surgical procedure

Acute **Pain** r/t inflammation or injury in surgical area

Anxiety r/t change in health status, hospital environment

Deficient **Knowledge** r/t postoperative expectations, lifestyle changes

Delayed **Surgical** recovery r/t extensive surgical procedure, postoperative surgical infection

Imbalanced **Nutrition**: less than body requirements r/t anorexia, nausea, vomiting, decreased peristalsis

Nausea r/t manipulation of gastrointestinal tract, postsurgical anesthesia

Risk for **Constipation**: Risk factors: decreased activity, decreased food or fluid intake, anesthesia, pain medication

Risk for deficient **Fluid** volume: Risk factors: hypermetabolic state, fluid loss during surgery, presence of indwelling tubes

Risk for ineffective **Breathing** pattern: Risk factors: pain, location of incision, effects of anesthesia or narcotics

Risk for ineffective **Tissue** perfusion: peripheral: Risk factors: hypovolemia, circulatory stasis, obesity, prolonged immobility, decreased coughing, decreased deep breathing

Risk for **Infection**: Risk factors: invasive procedure, pain, anesthesia, location of incision, weakened cough as a result of aging

Urinary retention r/t anesthesia, pain, fear, unfamiliar surroundings, client's position

Surgery, Preoperative Care

Anxiety r/t threat to or change in health status, situational crisis, fear of the unknown

Deficient **Knowledge** r/t preoperative procedures, postoperative expectations

Insomnia r/t anxiety about upcoming surgery

Readiness for enhanced **Knowledge** of r/t preoperative and postoperative expectations for self-care

Surgical Recovery, Delayed

Delayed **Surgical** recovery (See **Surgical** recovery, delayed, Section II)

Suspected Child Abuse and Neglect (SCAN), Child

Acute **Pain** r/t physical injuries

Anxiety/Fear: child r/t threat of punishment for perceived wrongdoing

Chronic low **Self-esteem** r/t lack of positive feedback, excessive negative feedback

S

Deficient **Diversional** activity r/t diminished or absent environmental or personal stimuli

Delayed **Growth** and development: regression versus delayed r/t diminished or absent environmental stimuli, inadequate caretaking, inconsistent responsiveness by caretaker

Imbalanced **Nutrition**: less than body requirements r/t inadequate caretaking

Impaired **Skin** integrity r/t altered nutritional state, physical abuse

Insomnia r/t hypervigilance, anxiety

Post-trauma response r/t physical abuse, incest, rape, molestation

Rape-trauma syndrome: compound/silent reaction r/t altered lifestyle because of abuse, changes in residence

Readiness for enhanced community **Coping**: obtaining resources to prevent child abuse, neglect

Risk for **Poisoning**: Risk factors: inadequate safeguards, lack of proper safety precautions

Risk for **Suffocation**: secondary to aspiration: Risk factors: propped bottle, unattended child

Risk for **Trauma**: Risk factors: inadequate precautions, cognitive or emotional difficulties

Social isolation: family-imposed r/t fear of disclosure of family dysfunction and abuse

See Hospitalized Child; Maturational Issues, Adolescent

Suspected Child Abuse and Neglect (SCAN), Parent

Chronic low **Self-esteem** r/t lack of successful parenting experiences

Disabled family **Coping** r/t dysfunctional family, underdeveloped nurturing parental role, lack of parental support systems or role models

Dysfunctional **Family** processes: alcoholism r/t inadequate coping skills

Impaired **Home** maintenance r/t disorganization, parental dysfunction, neglect of safe and nurturing environment

Impaired **Parenting** r/t unrealistic expectations of child; lack of effective role model; unmet social, emotional, or maturational needs of parents; interruption in bonding process

Ineffective **Health** maintenance r/t deficient knowledge of parenting skills as a result of unachieved developmental tasks

Powerlessness r/t inability to perform parental role responsibilities

Risk for **Violence** toward child r/t inadequate coping mechanisms, unresolved stressors, unachieved maturational level by parent

Suspicion

Impaired **Social** interaction r/t disturbed thought processes, paranoid delusions, hallucinations

Powerlessness r/t repetitive paranoid thinking

Risk for self- or other-directed **Violence**: Risk factor: inability to trust

Swallowing Difficulties

Impaired **Swallowing** (See **Swallowing**, impaired, Section II)

Syncope

Anxiety r/t fear of falling

Decreased **Cardiac** output r/t dysrhythmia

Impaired physical **Mobility** r/t fear of falling

Ineffective **Tissue** perfusion: cerebral r/t interruption of blood flow

Risk for **Falls**: Risk factor: syncope

Risk for **Injury**: Risk factors: altered sensory perception, transient loss of consciousness, risk for falls

Social isolation r/t fear of falling

Syphilis

See STD (Sexually Transmitted Disease)

Systemic Lupus Erythematosus

See Lupus Erythematosus

T

T & A (Tonsillectomy and Adenoidectomy)

Acute **Pain** r/t surgical incision

Deficient **Knowledge**: potential for enhanced health maintenance r/t insufficient knowledge regarding postoperative nutritional and rest requirements, signs and symptoms of complications, positioning

Ineffective **Airway** clearance r/t hesitation or reluctance to cough because of pain

Nausea r/t gastric irritation, pharmaceuticals, anesthesia

Risk for **Aspiration/Suffocation**: Risk factors: postoperative drainage and impaired swallowing

Risk for deficient **Fluid** volume: Risk factors: decreased intake because of painful swallowing, effects of anesthesia (nausea, vomiting), hemorrhage

Risk for imbalanced **Nutrition**: less than body requirements: Risk factors: hesitation or reluctance to swallow

Tachycardia

See Dysrhythmia

Tachypnea

Ineffective **Breathing** pattern r/t pain, anxiety

See cause of Tachypnea

Tardive Dyskinesia

Deficient **Knowledge** r/t cognitive limitation in assimilating information relating to side effects associated with neuroleptic medications

Disturbed sensory **Perception** r/t tardive dyskinesia

Ineffective management of **Therapeutic** regimen r/t complexity of therapeutic regimen or medications

Risk for **Injury** r/t drug-induced abnormal body movements

Taste Abnormality

Adult **Failure** to thrive r/t imbalanced nutrition: less than body requirements associated with taste abnormality

Disturbed **Sensory** perception: gustatory r/t medication side effects; altered sensory reception, transmission, integration; aging changes

TB (Pulmonary Tuberculosis)

Fatigue r/t disease state

Hyperthermia r/t infection

Impaired **Gas** exchange r/t disease process

Impaired **Home** maintenance management r/t client or family member with disease

Ineffective **Airway** clearance r/t increased secretions, excessive mucus

Ineffective **Breathing** pattern r/t decreased energy, fatigue

Ineffective **Therapeutic** regimen management r/t deficient knowledge of prevention and treatment regimen

Readiness for enhanced **Therapeutic** regimen management r/t taking medications according to prescribed protocol for prevention and treatment

Risk for **Infection**: Risk factors: insufficient knowledge regarding avoidance of exposure to pathogens

TBI (Traumatic Brain Injury)

Acute **Confusion** r/t brain injury

Chronic **Sorrow** r/t change in health status and functional ability

Decreased **Intracranial** adaptive capacity r/t brain injury

Disturbed **Sensory** perception: specify r/t pressure damage to sensory centers in brain

Disturbed **Thought** processes r/t pressure damage to brain

Impaired **Memory** r/t neurological disturbances

Ineffective **Tissue** perfusion: cerebral r/t effects of increased intracranial pressure

Ineffective **Breathing** pattern r/t pressure damage to breathing center in brainstem

Interrupted **Family** processes r/t traumatic injury to family member

Risk for impaired **Religiosity**: Risk factor: impaired physical mobility

Risk for **Post-trauma** syndrome: Risk factor: perception of event causing TBI

TD (Traveler's Diarrhea)

Risk for deficient **Fluid** volume r/t excessive loss of fluids, diarrhea

Risk for **Infection**: Risk factors: insufficient knowledge regarding avoidance of exposure to pathogens (water supply, iced drinks, local cheeses, ice cream, undercooked meat, fish and shellfish, uncooked vegetables, unclean eating utensils, improper handwashing)

Temperature, Decreased

Hypothermia r/t exposure to cold environment

Temperature, Increased

Hyperthermia r/t dehydration, illness, trauma

Temperature Regulation, Impaired

Ineffective **Thermoregulation** r/t trauma, illness

TEN (Toxic Epidermal Necrolysis)

See Toxic Epidermal Necrolysis

Tension

Anxiety r/t threat to or change in health status, situational crisis

Disturbed **Energy** field r/t change in health status, discouragement, pain

Readiness for enhanced **Communication**: r/t willingness to share feelings and thoughts

See Stress

Terminally Ill Adult

Compromised family **Coping** r/t inability to discuss impending death

Death **Anxiety** r/t unresolved issues relating to death and dying

Decisional **Conflict** r/t planning for advance directives

Disturbed **Energy** field r/t impending disharmony of mind, body, spirit

Grieving r/t loss of self or significant other

Readiness for enhanced **Religiosity**: requests religious material and/or experiences

Readiness for enhanced **Spiritual** well-being: desire to achieve harmony of mind, body, spirit

Risk for **Spiritual** distress: Risk factor: impending death

Spiritual distress r/t suffering before death

Terminally Ill Child, Adolescent

Disturbed **Body** image r/t effects of terminal disease, already critical feelings of group identity and self-image

Impaired **Social** interaction/social isolation r/t forced separation from peers

Ineffective **Coping** r/t inability to establish personal and peer identity because of the threat of being different or not being healthy, inability to achieve maturational tasks

See Child with Chronic Condition; Hospitalized Child

Terminally Ill Child, Infant/Toddler

Ineffective **Coping** r/t separation from parents and familiar environment attributable to inability to understand dying process

See Child with Chronic Condition

Terminally Ill Child, Preschool Child

Fear r/t perceived punishment, bodily harm, feelings of guilt caused by magical thinking (i.e., believing that thoughts cause events)

See Child with Chronic Condition

Terminally Ill Child, School-Age Child/Preadolescent

Fear r/t perceived punishment, body mutilation, feelings of guilt

See Child with Chronic Condition

Terminally Ill Child/Death of Child, Parent

Compromised family **Coping** r/t inability or unwillingness to discuss impending death and feelings with child or support child through terminal stages of illness

Decisional **Conflict** r/t continuation or discontinuation of treatment, do-not-resuscitate decision, ethical issues regarding organ donation

Grieving r/t death of child

Hopelessness r/t overwhelming stresses caused by terminal illness

Impaired **Parenting** r/t risk for overprotection of surviving siblings

Impaired **Social** interaction r/t complicated grieving

Ineffective **Denial** r/t complicated grieving

Insomnia r/t grieving process

Interrupted **Family** processes r/t situational crisis

Powerlessness r/t inability to alter course of events

Readiness for enhanced family **Coping**: r/t impact of crisis on family values, priorities, goals, or relationships; expressed interest or desire to attach meaning to child's life and death

Risk for complicated **Grieving**: Risk factors: prolonged, unresolved, obstructed progression through stages of grief and mourning

Social isolation: imposed by others r/t feelings of inadequacy in providing support to grieving parents

Social isolation: self-imposed r/t unresolved grief, perceived inadequate parenting skills

Spiritual distress r/t sudden and unexpected death, prolonged suffering before death, questioning the death of youth, questioning the meaning of one's own existence

Tetralogy of Fallot

See Congenital Heart Disease/Cardiac Anomalies

Therapeutic Regimen Management, Effective

Effective **Therapeutic** regimen management (See **Therapeutic** regimen management, effective, Section II)

Therapeutic Regimen Management, Ineffective

Ineffective **Therapeutic** regimen management (See **Therapeutic** regimen management, ineffective, Section II)

Therapeutic Regimen Management, Ineffective: Community

Ineffective community **Therapeutic** regimen management (See **Therapeutic** regimen management, ineffective community, Section II)

Therapeutic Regimen Management, Ineffective: Family

Ineffective family **Therapeutic** regimen management (See **Therapeutic** regimen management, ineffective family, Section II)

Therapeutic Regimen Management, Readiness for Enhanced

Readiness for enhanced **Therapeutic** regimen management (See **Therapeutic** regimen management, readiness for enhanced, Section II)

Therapeutic Touch

Disturbed **Energy** field r/t low energy levels, disturbance in energy fields, pain, depression, fatigue

Thermoregulation, Ineffective

Ineffective **Thermoregulation** (See **Thermoregulation**, ineffective, Section II)

Thoracentesis

See Pleural Effusion

Thoracotomy

Activity intolerance r/t pain, imbalance between oxygen supply and demand, presence of chest tubes

Acute **Pain** r/t surgical procedure, coughing, deep breathing

Deficient **Knowledge** r/t self-care, effective breathing exercises, pain relief

Ineffective **Airway** clearance r/t drowsiness, pain with breathing and coughing

Ineffective **Breathing** pattern r/t decreased energy, fatigue, pain

Risk for **Infection**: Risk factor: invasive procedure

Risk for **Injury**: Risk factor: disruption of closed-chest drainage system

Risk for perioperative positioning **Injury**: Risk factor: lateral positioning, immobility

Thought Disorders

Disturbed **Thought** processes r/t disruption in cognitive thinking, processing

See Schizophrenia

Thought Processes, Disturbed

Disturbed **Thought** processes (See **Thought** processes, disturbed, Section II)

Thrombocytopenic Purpura

See ITP (Idiopathic Thrombocytopenic Purpura)

Thrombophlebitis

Acute **Pain** r/t vascular inflammation, edema

Constipation r/t inactivity, bed rest

Deficient **Diversional** activity r/t bed rest

Deficient **Knowledge** r/t pathophysiology of condition, self-care needs, treatment regimen and outcome

Delayed **Surgical** recovery r/t complication associated with inactivity

Impaired physical **Mobility** r/t pain in extremity, forced bed rest

Ineffective **Tissue** perfusion: peripheral r/t interruption of venous blood flow

Risk for **Injury**: Risk factor: possible embolus

Sedentary **Lifestyle** r/t deficient knowledge of benefits of physical exercise

See Anticoagulant Therapy

Thyroidectomy

Risk for altered verbal **Communication**: Risk factors: edema, pain, vocal cord of laryngeal nerve damage

Risk for ineffective **Airway** clearance: Risk factors: edema or hematoma formation, airway obstruction

Risk for **Injury**: Risk factor: possible parathyroid damage or removal

See Surgery, Preoperative Care; Surgery, Perioperative Care; Surgery, Postoperative Care

TIA (Transient Ischemic Attack)

Acute **Confusion** r/t hypoxia

Decreased **Cardiac** output r/t dysrhythmia contributing to inadequate oxygen supply to brain

Health-seeking behaviors r/t obtaining knowledge regarding treatment, prevention of inadequate oxygenation

Ineffective **Tissue** perfusion: cerebral r/t lack of adequate oxygen supply to brain

Risk for **Falls**: Risk factor: hypoxia

Risk for **Injury**: Risk factor: possible syncope

See Syncope

Tic Disorder

See Tourette Syndrome (TS)

Tinea Capitis

Pruritus r/t inflammation

See Ringworm of Scalp

Tinea Corporis

See Ringworm of Body

Tinea Cruris

See Jock Itch; Itching; Pruritus

Tinea Pedis

See Athlete's Foot; Itching; Pruritus

Tinea Unguium (Onychomycosis)

See Ringworm of Nails

Tinnitus

Disturbed **Sensory** perception: auditory r/t altered sensory reception, transmission, integration

Ineffective **Health** maintenance r/t deficient knowledge regarding self-care with tinnitus

Tissue Damage, Corneal, Integumentary, or Subcutaneous

Impaired **Tissue** integrity (See **Tissue** integrity, impaired, Section II)

Tissue Perfusion, Decreased

Ineffective **Tissue** perfusion (See **Tissue** perfusion, ineffective, Section II)

Tocolytic Therapy

Ineffective **Health** maintenance r/t deficient knowledge regarding management of preterm labor, treatment regimen

Risk for **Fluid** volume excess: Risk factor: effects of tocolytic drugs

See Preterm Labor

Toilet Training

Health-seeking behaviors: bladder/bowel training r/t achievement of developmental milestone as a result of enhanced parenting skills

Deficient **Knowledge**: parent r/t signs of readiness for training

Risk for **Constipation**: Risk factor: withholding stool

Risk for **Incontinence**: Risk factor: difficulty in maintaining bladder/bowel control

Risk for **Infection**: Risk factor: withholding urination

T

Toileting Problems

Impaired **Transfer** ability r/t neuromuscular deficits

Self-care deficit: toileting r/t impaired transfer ability, impaired mobility status, intolerance of activity, neuromuscular impairment, cognitive impairment

Tonsillectomy and Adenoidectomy

See T & A (Tonsillectomy and Adenoidectomy)

Toothache

Acute **Pain** r/t inflammation, infection

Impaired **Dentition** r/t ineffective oral hygiene, barriers to self-care, economic barriers to professional care, nutritional deficits, lack of knowledge regarding dental health

Total Anomalous Pulmonary Venous Return

See Congenital Heart Disease/Cardiac Anomalies

Total Joint Replacement (Total Hip/Total Knee/Shoulder)

Acute **Pain** r/t possible edema, physical injury, surgery

Deficient **Knowledge** r/t self-care, treatment regimen, outcomes

Disturbed **Body** image r/t large scar, presence of prosthesis

Impaired physical **Mobility** r/t musculoskeletal impairment, surgery, prosthesis

Risk for **Infection**: Risk factors: invasive procedure, anesthesia, immobility

Risk for **Injury**: neurovascular: Risk factors: altered peripheral tissue perfusion, altered mobility, prosthesis

See Surgery, Preoperative Care; Surgery, Perioperative Care; Surgery, Postoperative Care

Total Parenteral Nutrition

See TPN (Total Parenteral Nutrition)

Total Urinary Incontinence

Total urinary **Incontinence** (See **Incontinence**, total urinary, Section II)

Tourette Syndrome (TS)

Hopelessness r/t inability to control behavior

Risk for situational low **Self-esteem** r/t uncontrollable behavior, motor and phonic tics

See Attention Deficit Disorder

Toxemia

See PIH (Pregnancy-Induced Hypertension/Preeclampsia)

Toxic Epidermal Necrolysis

Death **Anxiety** r/t uncertainty of prognosis

Disturbed **Sensory** perception (visual) r/t altered sensory reception associated with visual changes from conjunctival inflammation and scarring

See Stevens-Johnson syndrome

TPN (Total Parenteral Nutrition)

Imbalanced **Nutrition**: less than body requirements r/t inability to ingest or digest food or absorb nutrients as a result of biological or psychological factors

Risk for **Fluid** volume excess: Risk factor; rapid administration of TPN

Risk for **Infection**: Risk factors: concentrated glucose solution, invasive administration of fluids

Tracheoesophageal Fistula

Imbalanced **Nutrition**: less than body requirements r/t difficulties in swallowing

Ineffective **Airway** clearance r/t aspiration of feeding because of inability to swallow

Risk for **Aspiration**: Risk factors: common passage of air and food

See Respiratory Conditions of the Neonate; Hospitalized Child

Tracheostomy

Acute **Pain** r/t edema, surgical procedure

Anxiety r/t impaired verbal communication, ineffective airway clearance

Deficient **Knowledge** r/t self-care, home maintenance management

Disturbed **Body** image r/t abnormal opening in neck

Impaired verbal **Communication** r/t presence of mechanical airway

Risk for **Aspiration** r/t presence of tracheostomy

Risk for ineffective **Airway** clearance: Risk factors: increased secretions, mucous plugs

Risk for **Infection**: Risk factors: invasive procedure, pooling of secretions

Traction and Casts

Acute **Pain** r/t immobility, injury, or disease

Constipation r/t immobility

Deficient **Diversional** activity r/t immobility

Impaired physical **Mobility** r/t imposed restrictions on activity because of bone or joint disease injury

Impaired **Transfer** ability r/t presence of traction, casts

Risk for **Disuse** syndrome: Risk factor: mechanical immobilization

Risk for impaired **Skin** integrity: Risk factor: contact of traction or cast with skin

Risk for **Peripheral** neurovascular dysfunction: Risk factor: mechanical compression

Self-care deficit: feeding, dressing, grooming, bathing, hygiene, toileting r/t degree of impaired physical mobility, body area affected by traction or cast

Transfer Ability

Impaired **Transfer** ability (See **Transfer** ability, impaired, Section II)

Transient Ischemic Attack

See TIA (Transient Ischemic Attack)

Transposition of Great Vessels

See Congenital Heart Disease/Cardiac Anomalies

Transurethral Resection of the Prostate

See TURP (Transurethral Resection of the Prostate)

Trauma in Pregnancy

Acute **Pain** r/t trauma

Anxiety r/t threat to self or fetus, unknown outcome

Deficient **Knowledge** r/t lack of exposure to situation

Impaired **Skin** integrity r/t trauma

Risk for deficient **Fluid** volume: Risk factor: blood loss

Risk for fetal **Injury**: Risk factor: premature separation of placenta

Risk for **Infection**: Risk factor: traumatized tissue

Trauma, Risk for

Internal/External

Risk for **Trauma** (See **Trauma,** risk for, Section II)

Traumatic Brain Injury (TBI)

T

See TBI (Traumatic Brain Injury); Intracranial Pressure, Increased

Traumatic Event

Post-trauma syndrome r/t previously experienced trauma

Traveler's Diarrhea (TD)

See TD (Traveler's Diarrhea)

Trembling of Hands

Anxiety/Fear r/t threat to or change in health status, threat of death, situational crisis

Tricuspid Atresia

See Congenital Heart Disease/Cardiac Anomalies

Trigeminal Neuralgia

Acute **Pain** r/t irritation of trigeminal nerve

Imbalanced **Nutrition**: less than body requirements r/t pain when chewing

Ineffective **Therapeutic** regimen management r/t deficient knowledge regarding prevention of stimuli that trigger pain

Risk for **Injury** (eye): Risk factor: possible decreased corneal sensation

Truncus Arteriosus

See Congenital Heart Disease/Cardiac Anomalies

TS (Tourette's Syndrome)

See Tourette's Syndrome (TS)

TSE (Testicular Self-Examination)

Health-seeking behaviors: testicular self-examinations

Tubal Ligation

Decisional **Conflict** r/t tubal sterilization

See Laparoscopy

Tube Feeding

Risk for **Aspiration**: Risk factors: improperly administered feeding, improper placement of tube, improper positioning of client during and after feeding, excessive residual feeding or lack of digestion, altered gag reflex

Risk for deficient **Fluid** volume: Risk factor: inadequate water administration with concentrated feeding

Risk for imbalanced **Nutrition**: less than body requirements: Risk factors: intolerance to tube feeding, inadequate calorie replacement to meet metabolic needs

Tuberculosis

See TB (Pulmonary Tuberculosis)

TURP (Transurethral Resection of the Prostate)

Acute **Pain** r/t incision, irritation from catheter, bladder spasms, kidney infection

Deficient **Knowledge** r/t postoperative self-care, home maintenance management

Risk for deficient **Fluid** volume: Risk factors: fluid loss, possible bleeding

Risk for **Infection**: Risk factors: invasive procedure, route for bacteria entry

Risk for urge urinary **Incontinence**: Risk factor: edema from surgical procedure

Risk for **Urinary** retention: Risk factor: obstruction of urethra or catheter with clots

Ulcer, Peptic (Duodenal or Gastric)

Acute **Pain** r/t irritated mucosa from acid secretion

Fatigue r/t loss of blood, chronic illness

Ineffective **Health** maintenance r/t lack of knowledge regarding health practices to prevent ulcer formation

Nausea r/t gastrointestinal irritation

See GI Bleed (Gastrointestinal Bleeding)

Ulcerative Colitis

See Inflammatory Bowel Disease (Child and Adult)

Ulcers, Stasis

See Stasis Ulcer

Unilateral Neglect of One Side of Body

Unilateral **Neglect** (See **Neglect,** unilateral, Section II)

Unsanitary Living Conditions

Impaired **Home** maintenance r/t impaired cognitive or emotional functioning, lack of knowledge, insufficient finances

Urgency to Urinate

Risk for urge urinary **Incontinence** (See **Incontinence,** urge urinary, risk for, Section II)

Urge urinary **Incontinence** (See **Incontinence,** urge urinary, Section II)

Urinary Diversion

See Ileal Conduit

Urinary Elimination, Impaired

Impaired **Urinary** elimination (See **Urinary** elimination, impaired, Section II)

Urinary Incontinence

See Incontinence of Urine

Urinary Readiness

Readiness for enhanced **Urinary** elimination (See **Urinary** elimination, readiness for enhanced, Section II)

Urinary Retention

Urinary retention (See **Urinary** retention, Section II)

Urinary Tract Infection (UTI)

See UTI (Urinary Tract Infection)

Urolithiasis

See Kidney Stone

Uterine Atony in Labor

See Dystocia

Uterine Atony in Postpartum

See Postpartum Hemorrhage

Uterine Bleeding

See Hemorrhage; Postpartum Hemorrhage; Shock

UTI (Urinary Tract Infection)

Acute **Pain**: dysuria r/t inflammatory process in bladder

Impaired **Urinary** elimination: frequency r/t urinary tract infection

Ineffective **Health** maintenance r/t deficient knowledge regarding methods to treat and prevent UTIs

Risk for urge urinary **Incontinence**: Risk factor: hyperreflexia from cystitis

V

VAD

See Ventricular Assist Device (VAD)

Vaginal Hysterectomy

Risk for **Infection** r/t surgical site

Risk for **Perioperative** positioning injury: Risk factor: lithotomy position

Risk for urge urinary **Incontinence**: Risk factors: edema, congestion of pelvic tissues

Urinary retention r/t edema at surgical site

See Postpartum Hemorrhage

Vaginitis

Acute **Pain**: pruritus r/t inflamed tissues, edema

Ineffective **Health** maintenance r/t deficient knowledge regarding self-care with vaginitis

Ineffective **Sexuality** pattern r/t abstinence during acute stage, pain

Pruritus r/t inflammation

Vagotomy

See Abdominal Surgery

Value System Conflict

Decisional **Conflict** r/t unclear personal values or beliefs

Readiness for enhanced **Spiritual** well-being: desire for harmony with self, others, higher power, God

Spiritual distress r/t challenged value system

Varicose Veins

Chronic **Pain** r/t impaired circulation

Ineffective **Health** maintenance r/t deficient knowledge regarding health care practices, prevention, treatment regimen

Ineffective **Tissue** perfusion: peripheral r/t venous stasis

Risk for impaired **Skin** integrity: Risk factor: altered peripheral tissue perfusion

Vascular Dementia (Formerly Called Multiinfarct Dementia)

See Dementia

Vascular Obstruction, Peripheral

Acute **Pain** r/t vascular obstruction

Anxiety r/t lack of circulation to body part

Ineffective **Tissue** perfusion: peripheral r/t interruption of circulatory flow

Risk for **Peripheral** neurovascular dysfunction: Risk factor: vascular obstruction

Vasectomy

Decisional **Conflict** r/t surgery as method of permanent sterilization

Effective **Therapeutic** regimen management: r/t verbalizes desire to manage prevention of sequelae

Vasocognopathy

See Alzheimer's Type Dementia

Venereal Disease

See STD (Sexually Transmitted Disease)

Ventilation, Impaired Spontaneous

Impaired spontaneous **Ventilation** (See **Ventilation,** impaired spontaneous, Section II)

Ventilator Client

Dysfunctional **Ventilatory** weaning response r/t psychological, situational, physiological factors

Fear r/t inability to breathe on own, difficulty communicating

Impaired **Gas** exchange r/t ventilation-perfusion imbalance

Impaired spontaneous **Ventilation** r/t metabolic factors, respiratory muscle fatigue

Impaired verbal **Communication** r/t presence of endotracheal tube, decreased mentation

Ineffective **Airway** clearance r/t increased secretions, decreased cough and gag reflex

Ineffective **Breathing** pattern r/t decreased energy and fatigue as a result of possible altered nutrition: less than body requirements

Powerlessness r/t health treatment regimen

Risk for **Infection**: Risk factors: presence of endotracheal tube, pooled secretions

Risk for latex **Allergy** response: Risk factors: repeated exposure to latex products

Social isolation r/t impaired mobility, ventilator dependence

See Child with Chronic Condition; Hospitalized Child; Respiratory Conditions of the Neonate

Ventilatory, Dysfunctional Weaning Response (DVWR)

Dysfunctional **Ventilatory** weaning response (See **Ventilatory** weaning response, dysfunctional, Section II)

Ventricular Assist Device (VAD)

Readiness for enhanced **Decision** making: r/t Expresses desire to enhance the understanding of the meaning of choices regarding implanting a ventricular assist device

See Open Heart Surgery

Ventricular Fibrillation

See Dysrhythmia

Vertigo

Disturbed **Sensory** perception: kinesthetic r/t altered sensory reception, transmission, integration; medications

Ineffective **Tissue** perfusion: cerebral r/t decreased blood supply to brain

Risk for **Falls**: Risk factor: vertigo

Risk for **Injury**: Risk factor: disturbed sensory perception

Violent Behavior

Risk for other-directed **Violence** (See **Violence,** other directed, risk for, Section II)

Risk for self-directed **Violence**: Risk factors: (See **Violence,** self-directed, risk for, Section II)

Viral Gastroenteritis

Diarrhea r/t infectious process, rotavirus, Norwalk virus

Ineffective **Therapeutic** regimen management r/t inadequate handwashing

Ineffective community **Therapeutic** regimen management r/t contaminated food and/or water

See Gastroenteritis, Child

Vision Impairment

Disturbed **Sensory** perception r/t altered sensory reception associated with impaired vision

Fear r/t loss of sight

Risk for **Injury**: Risk factor: disturbed sensory perception

Self-care deficit: specify r/t perceptual impairment

Social isolation r/t altered state of wellness, inability to see

See Blindness

Vomiting

Nausea r/t chemotherapy, postsurgical anesthesia, irritation to the gastrointestinal system, stimulation of neuropharmacological mechanisms

Risk for deficient **Fluid** volume: Risk factor: decreased intake, loss of fluids with vomiting

Risk for imbalanced **Nutrition**: less than body requirements: Risk factor: inability to ingest food

von Recklinghausen's Disease

See Neurofibromatosis

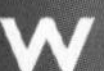

W

Walking Impairment

Impaired **Walking** (See **Walking**, impaired, Section II)

Wandering

Wandering (See **Wandering,** Section II)

Weakness

Fatigue r/t decreased or increased metabolic energy production

Risk for **Falls**: Risk factor: weakness

Weight Gain

Imbalanced **Nutrition**: more than body requirements r/t excessive intake in relation to metabolic need

Weight Loss

Imbalanced **Nutrition**: less than body requirements r/t inability to ingest food because of biological, psychological, economic factors

Wellness-Seeking Behavior

Health-seeking behaviors r/t expressed desire for increased control of health practice

Wernicke Korsakoff Syndrome

See Korsakoff's Syndrome

West Nile Virus

Effective **Therapeutic** regimen management: avoid mosquito bites, use mosquito-repellant products containing DEET, wear long sleeves and pants, mosquito-proof the home, community spray for mosquitos

See Meningitis/Encephalitis

Wheelchair Use Problems

Impaired wheelchair **Mobility** (See **Mobility,** impaired wheelchair, Section II)

Wheezing

Ineffective **Airway** clearance r/t tracheobronchial obstructions, secretions

Wilms' Tumor

Acute **Pain** r/t pressure from tumor

Constipation r/t obstruction associated with presence of tumor

See Chemotherapy; Hospitalized Child; Radiation Therapy; Surgery, Preoperative Care; Surgery, Perioperative Care; Surgery, Postoperative Care

Withdrawal from Alcohol

See Alcohol Withdrawal

Withdrawal from Drugs

See Drug Withdrawal

Wound Debridement

Acute **Pain** r/t debridement of wound

Impaired **Tissue** integrity r/t debridement, open wound

Risk for **Infection**: Risk factors: open wound, presence of bacteria

Wound Dehiscence, Evisceration

Fear r/t client fear of body parts "falling out," surgical procedure not going as planned

Imbalanced **Nutrition**: less than body requirements r/t inability to digest nutrients, need for increased protein for healing

Risk for deficient **Fluid** volume: Risk factors: inability to ingest nutrients, obstruction, fluid loss

Risk for delayed **Surgical** recovery: Risk factors: separation of wound, exposure of abdominal contents

Risk for **Injury**: Risk factor: exposed abdominal contents

Wound Infection

Disturbed **Body** image r/t dysfunctional open wound

Hyperthermia r/t increased metabolic rate, illness, infection

Imbalanced **Nutrition**: less than body requirements r/t biological factors, infection, hyperthermia

Impaired **Tissue** integrity r/t wound, presence of infection

Risk for deficient **Fluid** volume: Risk factor: increased metabolic rate

Risk for delayed **Surgical** recovery: Risk factor: presence of infection

Risk for **Infection**: spread of: Risk factor: imbalanced nutrition: less than body requirements

SECTION

II

Guide to Planning Care

Section II is a listing of nursing diagnosis care plans according to NANDA-I. The care plans are arranged alphabetically by diagnostic concept.

MAKING AN ACCURATE NURSING DIAGNOSIS

Verify the accuracy of the previously suggested nursing diagnoses (from Section I) for the client. To do this:

- Read the definition for the suggested nursing diagnosis and determine if it sounds appropriate
- Compare the Defining Characteristics with the symptoms that were identified from the client data collected or
- Compare the Risk Factors with the symptoms that were identified from the client data collected (if it is a "Risk for" Nursing Diagnosis, they do not have defining characteristics)

WRITING OUTCOMES, STATEMENTS, AND NURSING INTERVENTIONS

After selecting the appropriate nursing diagnosis, use this section to write outcomes and interventions by using the Client Outcomes/Nursing Interventions as written.

Following these steps, you will be able to write a nursing care plan:

- Follow this care plan to administer nursing care to the client.
- Document all steps and evaluate and update the care plan as needed.

Activity intolerance

NANDA Definition

Insufficient physiological or psychological energy to endure or complete required or desired daily activities

Defining Characteristics

Abnormal blood pressure response to activity; abnormal heart rate response to activity; electrocardiographic changes reflecting arrhythmias; electrocardiographic changes reflecting ischemia; exertional discomfort; exertional dyspnea; verbal report of fatigue; verbal report of weakness

Related Factors (r/t)

Bed rest; generalized weakness; imbalance between oxygen supply/demand; immobility, sedentary lifestyle

Client Outcomes

Client Will (Specify Time Frame):

- Participate in prescribed physical activity with appropriate changes in heart rate, blood pressure, and breathing rate; maintains monitor patterns (rhythm and ST segment) within normal limits
- State symptoms of adverse effects of exercise and report onset of symptoms immediately
- Maintain normal skin color and skin is warm and dry with activity
- Verbalize an understanding of the need to gradually increase activity based on testing, tolerance, and symptoms
- Demonstrate increased tolerance to activity

Nursing Interventions

- Determine cause of activity intolerance (see Related Factors) and determine whether cause is physical, psychological, or motivational.
- If mainly on bed rest, minimize cardiovascular deconditioning by positioning the client in an upright position several times daily.
- Assess the client daily for appropriateness of activity and bed rest orders.

- • If client is mostly immobile, consider use of a transfer chair, or a chair that becomes a stretcher.
- • When appropriate, gradually increase activity, allowing the client to assist with positioning, transferring, and self-care as possible. Progress from sitting in bed to dangling, to standing, to ambulation.
- • When getting a client up, observe for symptoms of intolerance such as nausea, pallor, dizziness, visual dimming, and impaired consciousness, as well as changes in vital signs.
- ▲ If a client experiences syncope with activity, refer for evaluation by a physician.
- • Perform range-of-motion (ROM) exercises if the client is unable to tolerate activity or is mostly immobile. See care plan for **risk for Disuse syndrome.**
- • Monitor and record the client's ability to tolerate activity: note pulse rate, blood pressure, monitor pattern, dyspnea, use of accessory muscles, and skin color before and after activity. If the following signs and symptoms of cardiac decompensation develop, activity should be stopped immediately:
  - ■ Onset of chest discomfort
  - ■ Dyspnea
  - ■ Palpitations
  - ■ Excessive fatigue
  - ■ Lightheadedness, confusion, ataxia, pallor, cyanosis, nausea, or any peripheral circulatory insufficiency
  - ■ Dysrhythmia (symptomatic supraventricular tachycardia, ventricular tachycardia, exercise-induced intraventricular conduction defect, second- or third-degree atrioventricular block, frequent premature ventricular contractions)
  - ■ Exercise hypotension (drop in systolic blood pressure of 10 mm Hg from baseline blood pressure despite an increase in workload)
  - ■ Excessive rise in blood pressure (systolic >180 mm Hg or diastolic >110 mm Hg) NOTE: These are upper limits; activity may be stopped before reaching these values
  - ■ Inappropriate bradycardia (drop in heart rate >10 beats/min or <50 beats/min)
  - ■ Increased heart rate above 100 beats/min
- ▲ Instruct the client to stop the activity immediately and report to the physician if the client is experiencing the following symp-

toms: new or worsened intensity or increased frequency of discomfort; tightness or pressure in chest, back, neck, jaw, shoulders, and/or arms; palpitations; dizziness; weakness; unusual and extreme fatigue; excessive air hunger.

- • Assess for constipation. If present, refer to care plan for **Constipation.**
- ▲ Refer the client to physical therapy to help increase activity levels and strength.
- ▲ Consider dietitian referral to assess nutritional needs related to activity intolerance. Recognize that undernutrition causes significant morbidity due to the loss of lean body mass.
- • Identify the factors that contribute to malnutrition in hospital clients, especially in older clients.
- • Provide emotional support and encouragement to the client to gradually increase activity.
- • Observe for pain before activity. If possible, treat pain before activity and ensure that the client is not heavily sedated.
- ▲ Obtain any necessary assistive devices or equipment needed before ambulating the client (e.g., walkers, canes, crutches, portable oxygen).
- • Use a gait walking belt when ambulating the client.
- • Work with the client to set mutual goals that increase activity levels.
- ▲ If the client is scheduled for a surgical intervention that will result in bed rest in intensive care, consider referring to physical therapy for a program including warm-up, aerobic conditioning, strength building, and flexibility enhancement to increase strength and endurance before surgery.

Activity Intolerance Due to Respiratory Disease

- • If the client is able to walk and has chronic obstructive pulmonary disease (COPD), consider the use of an accelerometer to assess walking ability or use the traditional 6-minute walk distance.
- ▲ Ensure that the chronic pulmonary client has oxygen saturation testing with exercise. Use supplemental oxygen to keep oxygen saturation 90% or above or as prescribed with activity.
- • Monitor a COPD client's response to activity by observing for

symptoms of respiratory intolerance such as increased dyspnea, loss of ability to control breathing rhythmically, use of accessory muscles, and skin tone changes such as pallor and cyanosis.

- Instruct and assist a COPD client in using conscious, controlled breathing techniques, including pursed-lip breathing, and inspiratory muscle training.

▲ Refer the COPD client to a pulmonary rehabilitation program.

Activity Intolerance Due to Cardiovascular Disease

- If the client is able to walk and has heart failure, consider use of the 6-minute walk test to determine physical ability.
- Allow for periods of rest before and after planned exertion periods such as meals, baths, treatments, and physical activity.

▲ Refer to heart failure program or cardiac rehabilitation program for education, evaluation, and guided support to increase activity and rebuild life.

- See care plan for **Decreased Cardiac output** for further interventions.

Geriatric

- Slow the pace of care. Allow the client extra time to carry out activities.
- Encourage families to help/allow an elderly client to be independent in whatever activities possible.

▲ Evaluate medications the client is taking to see if they could be causing activity intolerance. Medications such as beta-blockers, lipid-lowering agents, which can damage muscle, and some antihypertensives such as Clonidine, and lowering the blood pressure to normal in the elderly can result in decreased functioning.

▲ If the client has heart disease causing activity intolerance, refer for cardiac rehabilitation.

▲ Refer the client to physical therapy for resistance exercise training as able, including abdominal crunch, leg press, leg extension, leg curl, calf press, and more.

- When mobilizing the elderly client, watch for orthostatic hypotension accompanied by dizziness and fainting.
- Once the client is able to walk independently and needs an exercise program, suggest the client enter an exercise program with a friend.

A

Home Care

- ▲ Begin discharge planning as soon as possible with case manager or social worker to assess need for home support systems and the need for community or home health services.
- ▲ Assess the home environment for factors that contribute to decreased activity tolerance such as stairs or distance to the bathroom. Refer to occupational therapy if needed to assist the client in restructuring the home and ADL patterns.
- ▲ Refer to physical therapy for strength training and possible weight training, to regain strength, increase endurance, and improve balance. If the client is homebound, the physical therapist can also initiate cardiac rehabilitation.
- ▲ Support strength training program prescribed by physical therapist.
- • Normalize the client's activity intolerance; encourage progress with positive feedback.
- • Teach the client/family the importance of and methods for setting priorities for activities, especially those having a high energy demand (e.g., home/family events). Instruct in realistic expectations.
- • Provide the client/family with resources such as senior centers, exercise classes, educational and recreational programs, and volunteer opportunities that can aid in promoting socialization and appropriate activity.
- • Discuss the importance of sexual activity as part of daily living. Instruct the client in adaptive techniques to conserve energy during sexual interactions.
- • Instruct the client and family in the importance of maintaining proper nutrition. Instruct in use of dietary supplements as indicated.
- ▲ Refer to medical social services as necessary to assist the family in adjusting to major changes in patterns of living.
- ▲ Assess the need for long-term supports for optimal activity tolerance of priority activities (e.g., assistive devices, oxygen, medication, catheters, massage), especially for a hospice client. Evaluate intermittently.
- ▲ Refer to home health aide services to support the client and family through changing levels of activity tolerance. Introduce aide support early. Instruct the aide to promote independence in activity as tolerated.

- • Allow terminally ill clients and their families to guide care.
- • Provide increased attention to comfort and dignity of the terminally ill client in care planning.
- ▲ Institute case management of frail elderly to support continued independent living.

Client/Family Teaching

- • Instruct the client on rationale and techniques for avoiding activity intolerance.
- • Teach the client to use controlled breathing techniques with activity.
- • Teach the client the importance and method of coughing, clearing secretions.
- • Instruct the client in the use of relaxation techniques during activity.
- • Help the client with energy conservation and work simplification techniques in ADLs.
- ▲ Describe to the client the symptoms of activity intolerance, including which symptoms to report to the physician.
- ▲ Explain to the client how to use assistive devices, oxygen, or medications before or during activity.
- • Help client set up an activity log to record exercise and exercise tolerance.

Risk for Activity intolerance

NANDA Definition

At risk for experiencing insufficient physiological or psychological energy to endure or complete required or desired daily activities

Risk Factors

Deconditioned status; history of previous intolerance; inexperience with activity; presence of circulatory problems; presence of respiratory problems

Client Outcomes, Nursing Interventions, and Client/Family Teaching

See care plan for **Activity intolerance.**

Ineffective Airway clearance

NANDA Definition

Inability to clear secretions or obstructions from the respiratory tract to maintain a clear airway

Defining Characteristics

Absent or ineffective cough; adventitious breath sounds; changes in respiratory rate; changes in respiratory rhythm; cyanosis; difficulty vocalizing diminished breath sounds; dyspnea; excessive sputum; orthopnea; restlessness; wide-eyed

Related Factors (r/t)

Environmental

Second-hand smoke; smoking; smoke inhalation

Obstructed Airway

Airway spasm; excessive mucus; exudates in the alveoli; foreign body in airway; presence of artificial airway; retained secretions; secretions in the bronchi

Physiological

Allergic airways; asthma; chronic obstructive pulmonary disease; hyperplasia of the bronchial walls; infection; neuromuscular dysfunction

Client Outcomes

Client Will (Specify Time Frame):

- Demonstrate effective coughing and clear breath sounds
- Cyanotic free skin
- Maintain a patent airway at all times
- Relate methods to enhance secretion removal
- Relate the significance of changes in sputum to include color, character, amount, and odor
- Identify and avoid specific factors that inhibit effective airway clearance

Nursing Interventions

- • Auscultate breath sounds q1 to 4 hours. Breath sounds are normally clear or scattered fine crackles at bases, which clear with deep breathing.
- • Monitor respiratory patterns, including rate, depth, and effort.
- • Monitor blood gas values and pulse oxygen saturation levels as available.
- • Position the client to optimize respiration (e.g., head of bed elevated 45 degrees and repositioned at least every 2 hours).
- • If the client has unilateral lung disease, alternate a semi-Fowler's position with a lateral position (with a 10- to 15-degree elevation and "good lung down") for 60 to 90 minutes. This method is contraindicated for a client with a pulmonary abscess or hemorrhage or with interstitial emphysema.
- • Help the client deep breathe and perform controlled coughing. Have the client inhale deeply, hold breath for several seconds, and cough two or three times with mouth open while tightening the upper abdominal muscles.
- • If the client has COPD, cystic fibrosis, or bronchiectasis, consider helping the client use the forced expiratory technique, the "huff cough." The client does a series of coughs while saying the word "huff."
- • Encourage the client to use an incentive spirometer.
- • Assist with clearing secretions from pharynx by offering tissues and gentle suction of the oral pharynx if necessary.
- • Observe sputum, noting color, odor, and volume.
- • When suctioning an endotracheal tube or tracheostomy tube for a client on a ventilator, do the following:
  - ■ Explain the process of suctioning before and ensure the client is not in pain or overly anxious.
  - ■ Hyperoxygenate before and between endotracheal suction sessions.
  - ■ Use a closed, in-line suction system.
  - ■ Avoid saline instillation during suctioning.
  - ■ Document results of coughing and suctioning, particularly client tolerance and secretion characteristics such as color, odor, and volume.

A

- • Encourage activity and ambulation as tolerated. If unable to ambulate the client, turn the client from side to side at least every 2 hours. See interventions for **Impaired Gas exchange** for further information on positioning a respiratory client.
- ▲ If client is intubated, consider use of kinetic therapy, using a kinetic bed that slowly moves the client with 40-degree turns.
- • Encourage fluid intake of up to 2500 mL/day within cardiac or renal reserve.
- ▲ Administer oxygen as ordered.
- ▲ Administer medications such as bronchodilators or inhaled steroids as ordered. Watch for side effects such as tachycardia or anxiety with bronchodilators, or inflamed pharynx with inhaled steroids.
- ▲ Provide postural drainage, percussion, and vibration only as ordered.
- ▲ Refer for physical therapy or respiratory therapy for further treatment.

Geriatric

- • Encourage ambulation as tolerated without causing exhaustion.
- • Actively encourage the elderly to deep breathe and cough.
- • Ensure adequate hydration within cardiac and renal reserves.

Home Care

- • Some of the above interventions may be adapted for home care use.
- ▲ Begin discharge planning as soon as possible with case manager or social worker to assess need for home support systems, assistive devices, and community or home health services.
- • Assess home environment for factors that exacerbate airway clearance problems (e.g., presence of allergens, lack of adequate humidity in air, poor air flow, stressful family relationships).
- • Assess affective climate within family and family support system. Refer to care plan for **Caregiver role strain.**
- ▲ Refer to GOLD and ACP-ASIM/ACCP guidelines for management of home care and indications of hospital admission criteria.
- • Provide the client with emotional support in dealing with symptoms of respiratory distress.

- When respiratory procedures are being implemented, explain equipment and procedures to family members, and provide needed emotional support.
- When electrically based equipment for respiratory support is being implemented, evaluate home environment for electrical safety, proper grounding, and so on. Ensure that notification is sent to the local utility company, the emergency medical team, and police and fire departments.
- Support clients' efforts at self-care. Ensure they have all the information they need to participate in care.
- Provide family with support for care of a client with chronic or terminal illness. Refer to care plan for **Powerlessness.**

▲ Instruct the client to avoid exposure to persons with upper respiratory infections.

▲ Provide/teach percussion and postural drainage per physician orders. Teach adaptive breathing techniques.

- Determine client adherence to medical regimen. Instruct the client and family in importance of reporting effectiveness of current medications to physician.
- Teach the client when and how to use inhalant or nebulizer treatments at home.

▲ Teach the client/family importance of maintaining regimen and having PRN drugs easily accessible at all times.

- Teach the client/family the importance of and methods for setting priorities for activities, especially those having a high energy demand (e.g., home/family events). Instruct in realistic expectations.
- Instruct the client and family in the importance of maintaining proper nutrition, adequate fluids, rest, and behavioral pacing for energy conservation and rehabilitation.
- Instruct in use of dietary supplements as indicated.
- Identify an emergency plan, including criteria for use.

▲ Refer for home health aide services for assistance with ADLs.

▲ Assess family for role changes and coping skills. Refer to medical social services as necessary.

Client/Family Teaching

▲ Teach importance of not smoking. Be aggressive in approach, ask to set a date for smoking cessation, and recommend nicotine

replacement therapy (nicotine patch or gum). Refer to smoking cessation programs, and encourage clients who relapse to keep trying to quit.

- ▲ Teach the client how to use a flutter clearance device if ordered, which vibrates to loosen mucus and gives positive pressure to keep airways open.
- ▲ Teach the client how to use peak expiratory flow rate (PEFR) meter if ordered and when to seek medical attention if PEFR reading drops. Also teach how to use metered dose inhalers and self-administer inhaled corticosteroids as ordered following precautions to decrease side effects.
- • Teach the client how to deep breathe and cough effectively.
- • Teach the client/family to identify and avoid specific factors that exacerbate ineffective airway clearance, including known allergens and especially smoking (if relevant) or exposure to second-hand smoke.
- • Educate the client and family about the significance of changes in sputum characteristics, including color, character, amount, and odor.
- • Teach the client/family the need to take ordered antibiotics until the prescription has run out.

Latex Allergy response

NANDA Definition

A hypersensitive reaction to natural latex rubber products

Defining Characteristics

Life-threatening reactions occurring <1 hour after exposure to latex protein: Bronchospasm; cardiac arrest; contact urticaria progressing to generalized symptoms; dyspnea; edema of the lips; edema of the throat; edema of the tongue; edema of the uvula; hypotension; respiratory arrest; syncope; tightness in chest; wheezing

Orofacial characteristics: Edema of eyelids; edema of sclera; erythema of the eyes; facial erythema; facial itching; itching of the eyes; oral itching; nasal congestion; nasal erythema; nasal itching; rhinorrhea; tearing of the eyes

Gastrointestinal characteristics: Flushing; generalized discomfort; generalized edema; increasing complaint of total body warmth; restlessness

Generalized characteristics: Flushing; generalized discomfort; generalized edema; increasing complaint of total body warmth; restlessness

Type 1V reactions occurring >1 hour after exposure to latex protein: Discomfort reaction to additives such as thiurams and carbamates; eczema; irritation; redness

Related Factors (r/t)

Hypersensitivity to natural latex rubber protein

Client Outcomes

Client Will (Specify Time Frame):

- Identify presence of NRL allergy
- List history of risk factors
- Identify type of reaction
- State reasons not to use or to have anyone use latex products
- Experience a latex-safe environment for all healthcare procedures
- Avoid areas where there is powder from NRL gloves
- State the importance of wearing a Medic-Alert bracelet and wear one
- State the importance of carrying an emergency kit with a supply of nonlatex gloves, antihistamines, and an autoinjectable epinephrine syringe (Epi-pen), and carry one

Nursing Interventions

- Identify clients at risk: those persons who are most likely to exhibit a sensitivity to NRL that may result in varying degrees of reactivity. Consider the following client groups:
  - ■ Persons with neural tube defects including spina bifida, myelomeningocele/meningocele.
  - ■ Children who have experienced three or more surgeries, particularly as a neonate.
  - ■ Children with chronic renal failure.
  - ■ Atopic individuals (persons with a tendency to have multiple allergic conditions) including allergies to food products. Particular allergies to fruits and vegetables including bananas,

avocado, celery, fig, chestnut, papaya, potato, tomato, melon, and passion fruit are significant.

- ■ Persons who possess a known or suspected NRL allergy by having exhibited an allergic or anaphylactic reaction, positive skin testing, or positive IgE antibodies against latex.
- ■ Persons who have had an ongoing occupational exposure to NRL, including healthcare workers, rubber industry workers, bakers, laboratory personnel, food handlers, hairdressers, janitors, policemen, and firefighters.

- • Take a thorough history of the client at risk.
- • Question the client about associated symptoms of itching, swelling, and redness after contact with rubber products such as rubber gloves, balloons, and barrier contraceptives, or swelling of the tongue and lips after dental examinations.
- • Consider a skin prick test with NRL extracts to identify IgE-mediated immunity.
- • All latex-sensitive clients are treated as if they have NRL allergy.
- • Clients with spina bifida and others with a positive history of NRL sensitivity or NRL allergy should have all medical/surgical/dental procedures performed in a latex-controlled environment.
- • The most effective approach to preventing NRL anaphylaxis is complete latex avoidance. Medications may reduce certain symptoms.
- • Materials and items that contain NRL must be identified, and latex-free alternatives must be found.
- • In healthcare settings, general use of latex gloves having negligible allergen content, powder-free latex gloves, and nonlatex gloves and medical articles should be considered in an effort to minimize exposure to latex allergen.
- ▲ If latex gloves are chosen for protection from blood or body fluids, a reduced-protein, powder-free glove should be selected.

Home Care

- • Assess the home environment for presence of NRL products (e.g., balloons, condoms, gloves, and products of related allergies, such as bananas, avocados, and poinsettia plants).

A

- At onset of care, assess client history and current status of NRL allergy response.
- ▲ Seek medical care as necessary.
- Do not use NRL products in caregiving.
- Assist the client in identifying and obtaining alternatives to NRL products.

Client/Family Teaching

- Provide written information about NRL allergy and sensitivity.
- ▲ Instruct the client to inform healthcare professionals if he or she has an NRL allergy, particularly if he or she is scheduled for surgery.
- Teach the client what products contain NRL and to avoid direct contact with all latex products and foods that trigger allergic reactions.
- Teach the client to avoid areas where powdered latex gloves are used, as well as where latex balloons are inflated or deflated.
- Instruct the client with NRL allergy to wear a medical identification bracelet and/or carry a medical identification card.
- Instruct the client to carry an emergency kit with a supply of nonlatex gloves, antihistamines, and an autoinjectable epinephrine syringe (Epi-Pen).

Risk for latex Allergy response

NANDA Definition

At risk for allergic response to natural rubber latex (NRL) products

Risk Factors

Children with three or more surgeries, especially as a neonate; neural tube defects (e.g., spina bifida); children with chronic renal failure; allergies to bananas, avocados, tropical fruits, kiwis, chestnuts, apples, carrots, celery, potatoes, tomatoes; professions with daily exposure to latex (e.g., healthcare workers, rubber industry workers, food handlers, hairdressers, janitors, police, firefighters); conditions needing continuous or intermittent catheterization; history of reactions to latex (e.g., balloons, condoms, gloves); atopic individuals (persons with a tendency to have multiple allergic conditions)

Client Outcomes

Client Will (Specify Time Frame):

- State risk factors for NRL allergy
- Request latex-free environment
- Demonstrate knowledge of plan to treat NRL allergic reaction

Nursing Interventions

- Clients at high risk need to be identified, such as those with frequent bladder catheterizations, occupational exposure to latex, past history of atopy (hay fever, asthma, dermatitis, or food allergy to fruits such as bananas, avocados, papaya, chestnut, or kiwi); those with a history of anaphylaxis of uncertain etiology, especially if associated with surgery; healthcare workers; and females exposed to barrier contraceptives and routine examinations during gynecological and obstetric procedures.
- Clients with spina bifida are a high-risk group for NRL allergy and should remain latex free from the first day of life.
- Children who are on home ventilation should be assessed for NRL allergy.
- Children with chronic renal failure should be assessed for NRL allergy.
- Assess for NRL allergy in clients who are exposed to "hidden" latex.
- See care plan for **Latex Allergy response.**

Home Care

▲ Ensure that the client has a medical plan if a response develops.
- See care plan for **Latex Allergy response.** Note client history and environmental assessment.

Client/Family Teaching

▲ A client who has had symptoms of NRL allergy or who suspects he or she is allergic to latex should tell his or her employer and contact his or her institution's occupational health services.
- Provide written information about latex allergy and sensitivity.
- Healthcare workers should avoid the use of latex gloves and seek alternatives such as gloves made from nitrile.
- Healthcare institutions should develop prevention programs for

the use of latex-free gloves and the absence of powdered gloves; they should also establish latex-safe areas in their facilities.

Anxiety

NANDA Definition

A vague uneasy feeling of discomfort or dread accompanied by an autonomic response (the source often nonspecific or unknown to the individual); a feeling of apprehension caused by anticipation of danger. It is an alerting signal that warns of impending danger and enables the individual to take measures to deal with threat

Defining Characteristics

Behavioral

Diminished productivity; expressed concerns due to change in life events; extraneous movement; fidgeting; glancing about; insomnia; poor eye contact; restlessness; scanning; vigilance

Affective

Apprehensive; anguish; distressed; fearful; feelings of inadequacy; focus on self; increased wariness; irritability; jittery; overexcited; painful increased helplessness; persistent increased helplessness; rattled; regretful; scared; uncertainty; worried

Physiological

Facial tension; hand tremors; increased perspiration; increased tension; shakiness; trembling; voice quivering

Sympathetic

Anorexia; cardiovascular excitation; diarrhea; dry mouth; facial flushing; heart pounding; increased blood pressure; increased pulse; increased reflexes; increased respiration; pupil dilation; respiratory difficulties; superficial vasoconstriction; twitching; weakness

Parasympathetic

Abdominal pain; decreased blood pressure; decreased pulse; diarrhea; faintness; fatigue; nausea; sleep disturbance; tingling in extremities; urinary frequency; urinary hesitancy; urinary urgency

Cognitive

Awareness of physiologic symptoms; blocking of thought; confusion; decreased perceptual field; difficulty concentrating; diminished ability to learn; diminished ability to problem solve; fear of unspecified consequences; forgetfulness; impaired attention; preoccupation; rumination; tendency to blame others

Related Factors (r/t)

Change in: economic status, environment, health status, interaction patterns, role function, role status; exposure to toxins; familial association; heredity; interpersonal contagion; interpersonal transmission; maturational crises; situational crises; stress; substance abuse; threat of death; threat to: economic status, environment, health status, interaction patterns, role function, role status; threat to self-concept; unconscious conflict about essential goals of life; unconscious conflict about essential values; unmet needs

Client Outcomes

Client Will (Specify Time Frame):

- Identify and verbalize symptoms of anxiety
- Identify, verbalize, and demonstrate techniques to control anxiety
- Verbalize absence of or decrease in subjective distress
- Have vital signs that reflect baseline or decreased sympathetic stimulation
- Have posture, facial expressions, gestures, and activity levels that reflect decreased distress
- Demonstrate improved concentration and accuracy of thoughts
- Identify and verbalize anxiety precipitants, conflicts, and threats
- Demonstrate return of basic problem-solving skills
- Demonstrate increased external focus
- Demonstrate some ability to reassure self

Nursing Interventions

- Assess the client's level of anxiety and physical reactions to anxiety (e.g., tachycardia, tachypnea, nonverbal expressions of anxiety). Consider using The Face Anxiety Scale.
- Rule out withdrawal from alcohol, sedatives, or smoking as the cause of anxiety.

A

- Identify and limit, discontinue, or be aware of the use of any stimulants such as caffeine, nicotine, theophylline, terbutaline sulfate, amphetamines, and cocaine.
- If the situational response is rational, use empathy to encourage the client to interpret the anxiety symptoms as normal.
- If irrational thoughts or fears are present, offer the client accurate information and encourage him or her to talk about the meaning of the events contributing to the anxiety.
- Encourage the client to use positive self-talk such as, "Anxiety won't kill me," "I can do this one step at a time," "Right now I need to breathe and stretch," "I don't have to be perfect."
- Intervene when possible to remove sources of anxiety.
- Explain all activities, procedures, and issues that involve the client; use nonmedical terms and calm, slow speech. Do this in advance of procedures when possible, and validate the client's understanding
- Ascertain client preferences about the desire to be distracted before and during noxious medical procedures.
- Provide backrubs/massage for the client to decrease anxiety.
- Use therapeutic touch and healing touch techniques.
- Guided imagery can be used to decrease anxiety.
- Provide clients with a means to listen to music of their choice or audiotapes. Provide a quiet place and encourage clients to listen for 20 minutes.

Geriatric

▲ Monitor the client for depression. Use appropriate interventions and referrals.
- Observe for adverse changes if anti-anxiety drugs are taken.
- Provide alternative interventions such as massage therapy, guided imagery, and aromatherapy to complement traditional medical regimens.

Multicultural

- Assess for the presence of culture-bound anxiety states.
- Identify how anxiety is manifested in the culturally diverse client.
- Acknowledge that value conflicts from acculturation stresses may contribute to increased anxiety.

- For the diverse client experiencing preoperative anxiety, provide music of their choice.

Home Care

- Above interventions may be adapted for home care use.
- ▲ Assess for suicidal ideation. Implement emergency plan as indicated. Refer to care plan for **Risk for Suicide.**
- Assess for influence of anxiety on medical regimen.
- Assess for presence of depression.
- Assist family to be supportive of the client in the face of anxiety symptoms.
- ▲ Consider referral for the prescription of anti-anxiety or antidepressant medications for clients who have panic disorder (PD) or other anxiety-related psychiatric disorders.
- ▲ Assist the client/family to institute medication regimen appropriately. Instruct in side effects, importance of taking medications as ordered, and effects to report immediately to nurse or physician.
- ▲ Refer for psychiatric home healthcare services for client reassurance and implementation of a therapeutic regimen.

Client/Family Teaching

- ▲ Teach use of appropriate community resources in emergency situations (e.g., suicidal thoughts), such as hotlines, emergency departments, law enforcement, and judicial systems.
- Teach the client/family the symptoms of anxiety.
- Help client to define anxiety levels (from "easily tolerated" to "intolerable") and select appropriate interventions.
- Teach the client techniques to self-manage anxiety.
- Teach progressive muscle relaxation techniques.
- Teach relaxation breathing for occasional use: client should breathe in through nose, fill slowly from abdomen upward while thinking "re," and then breathe out through mouth, from chest downward, and think "lax."
- Teach the client to visualize or fantasize about the absence of anxiety or pain, successful experience of the situation, resolution of conflict, or outcome of procedure.
- Teach relationship between a healthy physical and emotional lifestyle and a realistic mental attitude.
- ▲ Provide family members with information to help them to dis-

tinguish between a panic attack and serious physical illness symptoms. Instruct family members to consult a healthcare professional if they have questions.

Death Anxiety

NANDA Definition

Vague uneasy feeling of discomfort or dread generated by perceptions of a real or imagined threat to one's existence

Defining Characteristics

Reports concerns of overworking the caregiver; reports deep sadness; reports fear of developing terminal illness; reports fear of loss of mental abilities when dying; reports fear of pain related to dying; reports fear of premature death; reports fear of the process of dying; reports fear of prolonged dying; reports fear of suffering related to dying; reports feeling powerless over dying; reports negative thoughts related to death and dying; reports worry about the impact on one's own death on significant others

Related Factors (r/t)

Anticipating adverse consequences of general anesthesia; anticipating impact of death on others; anticipating pain; anticipating suffering; confronting reality of terminal disease; discussions on topic of death; experiencing dying process; near death experience; nonacceptance of own mortality; observations related to death; perceived proximity of death; uncertainty about an encounter with a higher power; uncertainty about the existence of a higher power; uncertainty about life after death; uncertainty of prognosis

Client Outcomes

Client Will (Specify Time Frame):

- State concerns about impact of death on others
- Express feelings associated with dying
- Seek help in dealing with feelings
- Discuss concerns about God or higher being
- Discuss realistic goals
- Use prayer or other religious practice for comfort

Nursing Interventions

- Assess the psychosocial maturity of the individual.
- Assess clients for pain and provide pain relief measures.
- Assess client for fears related to death.
- Assist clients with life planning: consider and redefine main life goals, focus on areas of strength and/or goals that will provide satisfaction, adopt realistic goals and recognize those that are impossible to achieve.
- Assist clients with life review and reminiscence.
- Provide music of a client's choosing.
- Provide social support for families, understanding what is most important to families who are caring for clients at the end of life.
- Encourage clients to pray.

Geriatric

- Carefully assess older adults for issues regarding death anxiety.
- Provide back massage for clients who have anxiety regarding issues such as death.
- Refer to care plan for **Grieving.**

Multicultural

- Assist clients to identify with their culture and its values.
- Refer to care plans for **Anxiety** and **Grieving.**

Home Care

- Above interventions may be adapted for home care.
- Identify times and places when anxiety is greatest. Provide for psychological support at those times, using such strategies as personal contact, telephone contact, diversionary activities, or therapeutic self.
- Support religious beliefs; encourage client to participate in services and activities of choice.
- ▲ Refer to medical social services or mental health services, including support groups as appropriate (e.g., anticipatory grieving groups from hospice, visiting volunteers of hospice).
- Encourage the client to verbalize feelings to family/caregivers, counselors, and self.
- Identify client's preferences for end-of-life care; provide assistance in honoring preferences as much as practicable.

A

- ▲ Assist the client in making contact with death-related planning organizations, if appropriate, such as the Cremation Society and funeral homes.
- • With client, create a memento book reflecting life achievements. Leave in the home for regular review by client. If family will be the recipient, a memento book serves as both an opportunity for life review and a means of proactively leaving something behind for survivors.
- ▲ Refer for psychiatric home healthcare services for client reassurance and implementation of a therapeutic regimen. Psychiatric home care nurses can address issues relating to client's death anxiety, including family relationships.
- • Refer to care plan for **Powerlessness.**

Client/Family Teaching

- • Promote more effective communication to family members engaged in the care giving role. Encourage them to talk to their loved one about areas of concern.
- • Allow family members to be physically close to their dying loved one, giving them permission, instruction, and opportunities to touch. Keep family members informed.
- • To increase clients' knowledge about end-of-life issues, teach them and their family members about options for care, such as advance directives.

Risk for Aspiration

NANDA Definition

At risk for entry of gastrointestinal secretions, oropharyngeal secretions, solids, or fluids into the tracheobronchial passages

Risk Factors

Decreased gastrointestinal motility; delayed gastric emptying; depressed cough; depressed gag reflex; facial surgery; facial trauma; gastrointestinal tubes; incompetent lower esophageal sphincter; increased gastric residual; increased intragastric pressure; impaired swallowing; medication administration; neck trauma; neck surgery; oral surgery; oral trauma; presence of endotracheal tube; presence of

tracheostomy tube; reduced level of consciousness; situations hindering elevation of upper boy; tube feedings; wired jaws

Client Outcomes

Client Will (Specify Time Frame):

- Swallow and digest oral, nasogastric, or gastric feeding without aspiration
- Maintain patent airway and clear lung sounds

Nursing Interventions

- • Monitor respiratory rate, depth, and effort. Note any signs of aspiration such as dyspnea, cough, cyanosis, wheezing, or fever.
- • Auscultate lung sounds frequently and before and after feedings; note any new onset of crackles or wheezing.
- • Take vital signs frequently, noting onset of a temperature.
- • Before initiating oral feeding, check client's gag reflex and ability to swallow by feeling the laryngeal prominence as the client attempts to swallow.
- • When feeding client, watch for signs of impaired swallowing or aspiration, including coughing, choking, spitting food, or excessive drooling. If client is having problems swallowing, see Nursing Interventions for **Impaired Swallowing.**
- • Have suction machine available when feeding high-risk clients. If aspiration does occur, suction immediately.
- • Keep head of bed elevated when feeding and for at least an hour afterward.
- ▲ Note presence of any nausea, vomiting, or diarrhea. Treat nausea promptly with antiemetics.
- • Listen to bowel sounds frequently, noting if they are decreased, absent, or hyperactive.
- • Note new onset of abdominal distention or increased rigidity of abdomen.
- ▲ If client has a tracheostomy, ask for referral to speech pathologist for swallowing studies before attempting to feed. After evaluation, decision should be made to have cuff either inflated or deflated when client eats.
- • If client shows symptoms of nausea and vomiting, position on side.

- If client needs to be fed, feed slowly and allow adequate time for chewing and swallowing. Position upright during and after feedings.

Enteral Feedings

- Insert nasogastric feeding tube using the internal nares to distal-lower esophageal-sphincter distance, an updated version of the Hanson method.
- ▲ Check to make sure initial nasogastric feeding tube placement was confirmed by x-ray, with the openings of the tube in the stomach, not the esophagus. This is especially important if a small-bore feeding tube is used, although larger tubes used for feedings or medication administration should be verified by x-ray also. If unable to use x-ray for verification, check the pH of the aspirate. If pH reading is 4 or less, the tube is probably in the stomach.
- Keep nasogastric tube securely taped.
- Measure and record the length of the tube that is outside of the body at defined intervals to help ensure correct placement.
- Note the placement of the tube on any x-rays that are done on the client.
- Determine placement of feeding tube before each feeding or every 4 hours if client is on continuous feeding. Note length of tube outside of body, any recent x-ray results, and characteristic appearance of aspirate; do not rely on air insufflation method.
- ▲ Check for gastric residual volume during continuous feedings or before feedings; if residual is greater than 200 mL, hold feedings following institutional protocol.
- ▲ Test for the presence of glucose in tracheobronchial secretions or the presence of pepsin to detect aspiration of enteral feedings.
- ▲ Do not use blue dye to tint enteral feedings.
- During enteral feedings, position client with head of bed elevated 30 to 45 degrees; maintain for 30 to 45 minutes after feeding.
- Use a closed versus an open enteral delivery system of tube feeding if possible.
- Stop continual feeding temporarily when turning or moving client.

A

Geriatric

- Carefully check elderly client's gag reflex and ability to swallow before feeding.
- Watch for signs of aspiration pneumonia in the elderly with cerebrovascular accidents, even if there are no apparent signs of difficulty swallowing or of aspiration.
- ▲ Use central nervous system depressants cautiously; elderly clients may have an increased incidence of aspiration with altered levels of consciousness.
- Keep the elderly, mostly bedridden client sitting upright for 2 hours following meals.
- ▲ Recommend to families that tube feedings not be used for clients with dementia; instead use increased feeding assistance, modified food consistency as needed, or environmental alterations.

Home Care

- Above interventions may be adapted for home care use.
- ▲ For clients at high risk for aspiration, obtain complete information from the discharging institution regarding institutional management.
- Assess the client and family for willingness and cognitive ability to learn and cope with swallowing, feeding, and related disorders.
- Assess caregiver understanding and reinforce teaching regarding positioning and assessment of the client for possible aspiration.
- Provide the client with emotional support in dealing with fears of aspiration. Refer to care plan for **Anxiety.**
- Establish emergency and contingency plans for care of client.
- ▲ Have a speech and occupational therapist assess client's swallowing ability and other physiological factors and recommend strategies for working with client in the home (e.g., pureeing foods served to client; providing adaptive equipment for independence in eating).
- Obtain suction equipment for the home as necessary.
- Teach caregivers safe, effective use of suctioning devices. Inform client and family that only individuals instructed in suctioning should perform the procedure.
- ▲ Institute case management of frail elderly to support continued independent living.

Client/Family Teaching

- Teach the client and family signs of aspiration and precautions to prevent aspiration.
- Teach the client and family how to safely administer tube feeding.

Risk for impaired parent/child Attachment

NANDA Definition

Disruption of the interactive process between parent/significant other and infant/child that fosters the development of a protective and nurturing reciprocal relationship

Risk Factors

Anxiety associated with the parent role; ill infant/child who is unable to effectively initiate parental contact due to altered behavioral organization; inability of parents to meet personal needs; lack of privacy; parental conflict due to altered behavioral organization; physical barriers; premature infant who is unable to effectively initiate parental contact due to altered behavioral organization; separation; substance abuse

Client Outcomes

Parent(s)/Caregiver(s) Will (Specify Time Frame):

- Be willing to consider pumping breast milk (and storing appropriately) or breastfeeding, if feasible
- Demonstrate behaviors that indicate secure attachment to infant/child
- Provide a safe environment, free of physical hazards
- Provide nurturing environment sensitive to infant/child's need for nutrition/feeding, sleeping, comfort, and social play
- Read and respond contingently to infant/child's behavior cues that signal approach/engagement or avoidance/disengagement
- Be able to calm and relieve infant/child's distress
- Support infant's self-regulation capabilities, intervening when needed
- Engage in mutually satisfying interactions that provide opportunities for attachment

A

- Give infant nurturing sensory experiences (e.g., holding, cuddling, stroking, rocking)
- Demonstrate an awareness of developmentally appropriate activities that are pleasurable, emotionally supportive, and growth fostering
- Avoid physical and emotional abuse and/or neglect as retribution for parent's perception of infant/child's misbehavior
- Be knowledgeable of appropriate community resources and support services

Nursing Interventions

- • Establish a trusting relationship with parent/caregiver.
- • Encourage mothers to breastfeed their infants, and provide support.
- ▲ Identify factors related to postpartum depression (PPD) and major depression and offer appropriate interventions and referrals.
- • Nurture parents so that they in turn can nurture their infant/child.
- • Offer a safe, nonjudgmental environment in which parents can express their feelings.
- • Offer parents opportunities to verbalize their childhood fears.
- • Suggest journaling as a way for parents of hospitalized infants to cope with their stress and emotional reactions.
- • Offer parent-to-parent support to parents of NICU hospitalized infants.
- • Support parents' behaviors that will result in "secure" rather than "avoidant" or "ambivalent" attachment.
- • Encourage parents of hospitalized infants to "personalize the baby" by bringing in clothing, pictures of themselves, toys, and tapes of their voices.
- • Encourage physical closeness using skin-to-skin experiences for parents and infants as appropriate.
- • Assist parents in developing new caregiving competencies and/or revising and extending old ones.
- • Plan ways for parents to interact/assist with caregiving for their hospitalized/institutionalized infant/child.
- • Educate parents about reading and responding sensitively to their infant's unique "body language" (behavior cues) that communicate approach ("I'm ready to play"), avoidance/stress ("I'm

unhappy. I need a change."), and self-calming ("I'm helping myself").

- Educate and support parent's ability to relieve infant/child's stress/distress.
- Guide parents in adapting their behaviors and activities with infant/child cues and changing needs.
- Attend to both the parent and infant/child in an effort to strengthen high-quality parent-infant interactions.
- Assist parents with providing pleasurable sensory learning experiences (i.e. sight, sound, movement, touch, and body awareness).
- Encourage parents and caregivers to massage their infants and children.

Infant

- Recognize and support infant/child's capacity for self-regulation and intervene when appropriate.
- Provide lyrical, soothing music in the nursery and home that is appropriate for age (i.e., corrected, in the case of premature infants) and contingent with state and behavioral cues.
- Recognize and support infant/child's attention capabilities.
- Encourage opportunities for mutually satisfying interactions between infant and parent.
- Encourage opportunities for physical closeness.

Multicultural

- Discuss cultural norms with families to provide care that is appropriate for enhancing attachment with the infant/child.
- Promote the attachment process in women who have abused substances by providing a treatment environment that is culturally based and women-centered.
- Empower family members to draw on personal strengths in which multiple worldviews and values of individual members are recognized, incorporated, and negotiated.
- Encourage positive involvement and relationship development between children and noncustodial fathers to enhance health and development.

Home Care

- Above interventions may be adapted for home care use.
- Assess quality of interaction between parent and infant/child.

• Use "interaction coaching" (i.e., teaching mother to let the infant lead) so that the mother will match her style of interaction to the baby's cues.

▲ Provide home visitation for infants with depressed mothers and for highly stressed parents of preterm infants.

▲ Identify community resources and supportive network systems for mothers showing depressive symptoms.

Autonomic dysreflexia

NANDA Definition

Life-threatening, uninhibited sympathetic response of the nervous system to a noxious stimulus after a spinal cord injury at T7 or above

Defining Characteristics

Blurred vision; bradycardia; chest pain, chilling; conjunctival congestion; diaphoresis (above the injury); headache (a diffuse pain in different portions of the head and not confined to any nerve distribution area); Horner's syndrome; metallic taste in mouth; nasal congestion; pallor (below the injury); paroxysmal hypertension; pilomotor reflex; red splotches on skin (above the injury); tachycardia

Related Factors (r/t)

Bladder distention; bowel distention; deficient caregiver knowledge; deficient patient knowledge; skin irritation

Client Outcomes/Goals

Client Will (Specify Time Frame):

- Maintain normal vital signs
- Remain free of dysreflexia symptoms
- Explain symptoms, prevention, and treatment of dysreflexia

Nursing Interventions

• Monitor the client for symptoms of dysreflexia, particularly those with high-level and more extensive spinal cord injuries. See Defining Characteristics.

▲ Collaborate with healthcare practitioners to identify the cause of dysreflexia (e.g., distended bladder, impaction, pressure ulcer, urinary calculi, bladder infection, acute condition in the abdomen, penile pressure, ingrown toenail, or other source of noxious stimuli).

▲ If symptoms of dysreflexia are present, place client in high Fowler's position, remove all support hoses or binders, and immediately determine the noxious stimuli causing the response. If blood pressure cannot be decreased within 1 minute, notify the physician STAT.

▲ To determine the stimulus for dysreflexia:
  - First, assess bladder function. Check for distention, and if present, catheterize using an anesthetic jelly as a lubricant. Do not use Valsalva maneuver or Crede's method to empty the bladder. Ensure existing catheter patency. Also note signs of urinary tract infection.
  - Second, assess bowel function. Numb the bowel area with a topical anesthetic as ordered, and once agent is effective (5 minutes), check for impaction.
  - Third, assess the skin, looking for any points of pressure.

▲ Initiate antihypertensive therapy as soon as ordered.

▲ Be careful not to increase noxious sensory stimuli. If numbing agent is ordered, use it on anus and 1 inch of rectum before attempting to remove a fecal impaction. Also spray pressure ulcer with it. If necessary to replace an obstructed catheter, use an anesthetic jelly as ordered.

• Monitor vital signs every 3 to 5 minutes during acute event; continue to monitor vital signs after event is resolved.

▲ Watch for complications of dysreflexia, including signs of cerebral hemorrhage, seizures, MI, or intraocular hemorrhage.

• Accurately and completely record any incidences of dysreflexia; especially note the precipitating stimuli.

• Use the following interventions to prevent dysreflexia:
  - Ensure that drainage from Foley catheter is good and that bladder is not distended.
  - Ensure a regular pattern of defecation to prevent fecal impaction.
  - Frequently change position of client to relieve pressure and prevent the formation of pressure ulcers.

▲ If ordered, apply an anesthetic agent to any wound below level of injury before performing wound care.

A

- ▲ Because episodes can reoccur, notify all healthcare team members of the possibility of a dysreflexia episode.
- ▲ For female clients with spinal cord injury who become pregnant, collaborate with obstetrical healthcare practitioners to monitor for signs and symptoms of dysreflexia.

Home Care

- • Above interventions may be adapted for home care use.
- • Instruct the client with any known proclivity toward dysreflexia to wear a medical alert bracelet and carry a medical alert wallet card when not in a safe environment (i.e., not with someone who knows client has the condition and can respond appropriately).
- ▲ Establish an emergency plan: obtain physician orders for medications to be used in situations in which first aid does not work and plans to identify potential stimuli.
- ▲ If orders have not been obtained or client does not have medications, use emergency medical services.
- • When episode of dysreflexia is resolved, monitor blood pressure every 30 to 60 minutes for next 5 hours or admit to institution for observation.

Client/Family Teaching

- • Teach recognition of the earliest symptoms of dysreflexia, the actions that should be taken when they occur, and the need to summon help immediately. Give client a written card that contains this information.
- • Teach steps to prevent dysreflexia episodes: care of bladder, bowel, and skin and prevention of other forms of noxious stimuli (i.e., not wearing clothing that is too tight).
- • Discuss the potential impact of sexual intercourse and pregnancy on autonomic dysreflexia.

Risk for Autonomic dysreflexia

NANDA Definition

At risk for life-threatening, uninhibited response of the sympathetic nervous system; post-spinal shock; in an individual with spinal cord injury or lesion at T6 or above (has been demonstrated in clients with injuries at T7 and T8)

Defining Characteristics (Risk Factors)

An injury/lesion at T6 or above and at least one of the following noxious stimuli:

- **Cardiac/pulmonary problems:** pulmonary emboli; deep vein thrombosis
- **Gastrointestinal stimuli:** bowel distention; constipation; difficult passage of stool; digital stimuli; enemas; esophageal reflux; fecal impaction; gallstones; gastric ulcers; GI system pathology; hemorrhoids; suppositories
- **Musculoskeletal**-integumentary stimuli: cutaneous stimulations (e.g., pressure ulcer, ingrown toenail, dressings, burns, rash); fractures, heterotrophic bone; pressure over bony prominences or genitalia; range-of-motion exercises; spasm; sunburns; wounds
- **Neurological stimuli:** painful/irritating stimuli below the level of injury
- **Regulatory stimuli:** extreme environmental temperatures; temperature fluctuations
- **Reproductive stimuli:** ejaculation; labor and delivery; menstruation; ovarian cyst; pregnancy; sexual intercourse
- **Situational stimuli:** constrictive clothing (e.g., straps, stockings, shoes); drug reactions (e.g., decongestants, sympathomimetics, vasoconstrictors); positioning; surgical procedures
- **Urological stimuli:** bladder distention; bladder spasms; calculi; catheterization; cystitis; detrusor sphincter dyssynergia; epididymitis; instrumentation; surgery; urethritis; urinary tract infection

Client Outcomes and Nursing Interventions

Refer to care plan for **Autonomic dysreflexia**

Risk-prone health Behavior

NANDA Definition

Inability to modify lifestyle/behavior in a manner consistent with a change in health status

Defining Characteristics

B

Demonstrates nonacceptance of health status change; failure to achieve optimal sense of control; failure to take action that prevents health problems; minimizes health status change

Related Factors (r/t)

Inadequate comprehension; inadequate social support; low self-efficacy; low socioeconomic status; multiple stressors; negative attitude toward health status change

Client Outcomes

Client Will (Specify Time Frame):

- State acceptance of change in health status
- Request assistance in altering behaviors to adapt to change
- State personal goals for dealing with change in health status and means to prevent further health problems
- State experience of a period of grief that is proportional to the actual or perceived effect of the loss
- Report and/or demonstrate behavior changes mutually agreed upon with nurse as evidence of positive adaptation

Nursing Interventions

- Assess the client's perception about the illness/event. Ask the client to state feelings related to the change in health status.
- Assess for negative affect and internalization of problems.
- Allow the client adequate time to express feelings about the change in health status.
- Use open-ended questions to allow the client free expression (e.g., "Tell me about your last hospitalization" or "How does this time compare?").
- Help the client work through the stages of grief. Denial is usually the initial response and may be an adaptive coping mechanism. Acknowledge that grief takes time, and give the client permission to grieve; accept crying.
- Discuss resources (e.g., the client's support system) that have worked previously when dealing with changes in lifestyle or health status.
- Discuss the client's current goals. If appropriate, have the client list goals so that they can be referred to and steps can be taken

to accomplish them. Support hope that the goals will be accomplished.

- • Allow the client choices in daily care, particularly choices that result from the change in health status.
- • List the client activities that may require assistance and those that can be performed independently.
- • Give the client positive feedback for accomplishments, no matter how small.
- • Manipulate the environment to decrease stress; allow the client to display personal items that have meaning.
- • Maintain consistency and continuity in daily schedule. When possible, provide the same caregiver.
- • Foster communication between the client/family and medical staff.
- • Promote use of positive spiritual influences.
- ▲ Refer to community resources. Provide general and contact information for ease of use.

Geriatric

- ▲ Assess for signs of depression resulting from illness-associated changes and make appropriate referral.
- • Monitor the client for agitation associated with health problems. Support family caring for elders with agitation.

Multicultural

- • Assess for the influence of cultural beliefs, norms, and values on the client's ability to modify health behavior.
- • Assess the role of fatalism on the client's ability to modify health behavior.
- ▲ Assess for signs of depression and level of social support and make appropriate referrals.
- • Identify which family members the client can rely on for support.
- • Encourage spirituality as a source of support for coping.
- • Negotiate with the client regarding the aspects of health behavior that will need to be modified.

Home Care

- • Above interventions may be adapted for home care use.
- • Take the client's perspective into consideration, and use a holis-

tic approach in assessing and responding to client planning for the future.

- Assist client to recognize and exercise power in using self-care management to adjust to health change.
- ▲ Refer the client to counselor or therapist for follow-up care. Initiate community referrals as needed (e.g., grief counseling, self-help groups).
- Refer to care plan for **Powerlessness.**

Client/Family Teaching

- Assess family/caregivers for coping and teaching/learning styles.
- Educate and prepare families regarding the appearance of the client and the environment before initial exposure.
- Teach the client to maintain a positive outlook by listing current strengths.
- Teach a client and his or her family relaxation techniques (controlled breathing, guided imagery) and help them practice.
- Allow the client to proceed at own pace in learning; provide time for return demonstrations (e.g., self-injection of insulin).
- Involve significant others in planning and teaching.
- If long-term deficits are expected, inform the family as soon as possible.
- Teach families intervention techniques for family members such as setting limits, communicating acceptable behavior, and having time-outs.
- Provide clients with information on how to access and evaluate available health information via the internet.

Disturbed Body image

NANDA Definition

Confusion in mental picture of one's physical self

Defining Characteristics

Behaviors of acknowledgment of one's body; behaviors of avoidance on one's body; behaviors of monitoring one's body; nonverbal response to actual change in body (e.g., appearance, structure, or function); nonverbal response to perceived change in body (e.g., appearance, structure, or function); verbalization of feelings that reflect an altered view of one's body (e.g. appearance, structure, function); verbalization of perceptions that reflect an altered view of one's body appearance

Objective

Actual change in function; actual change in structure; behaviors of acknowledging one's body; behaviors of monitoring one's body; change in ability to estimate spatial relationship of body to environment; change in social involvement; extension of body boundary to incorporate environmental objects; intentional hiding of body part; intentional overexposure of body part; missing body part; not looking at body part; not touching body part; trauma to nonfunctioning part; unintentional hiding of body part; unintentional overexposing of body part

Subjective

Depersonalization of loss by impersonal pronouns; depersonalization of part by impersonal pronouns; emphasis of remaining strengths; fear of reaction by others; fear of rejection by others; focus on past appearance; focus on past function; focus on past strength; heightened achievement; negative feelings about body (e.g., feeling of helplessness, hopelessness, or powerlessness); personalization of loss; personalization of part by name; preoccupation with change; preoccupation with loss; refusal to verify actual change; verbalization of change in lifestyle

Related Factors (r/t)

Biophysical; cognitive; cultural; developmental changes; illness; illness treatment; injury; perceptual; psychosocial; spiritual; surgery; trauma

Client Outcomes

Client Will (Specify Time Frame):

- Demonstrate adaptation to changes in physical appearance or body function as evidenced by adjustment to lifestyle change
- Identify and change irrational beliefs and expectations regarding body size or function
- Verbalize congruence between body reality and body perception
- Describe, touch, or observe affected body part

B

- Demonstrate social involvement rather than avoidance and utilize adaptive coping and/or social skills
- Utilize cognitive strategies or other coping skills to improve perception of body image and enhance functioning
- Utilize strategies to enhance appearance (e.g., wig, clothing)

Nursing Interventions

- • Incorporate psychosocial questions related to body image as part of nursing assessment to identify clients at risk for body image disturbance (e.g., body builders, cancer survivors, clients with eating disorders, burns, skin disorders, polycystic ovary disease, or those with stomas/ostomies/colostomies or other disfiguring conditions).
- • If client is at risk for body image disturbance, consider using a tool such as the Body Image Quality of Life Inventory (BIQLI), which quantifies both the positive and negative effects of body image on one's psychosocial quality of life.
- ▲ Assess for body dysmorphic disorder (BDD) and refer to psychiatry or other appropriate provider.
- ▲ Assess for the possibility of muscle dysmorphia (pathological preoccupation with muscularity and leanness; occurs more often in males than in females) and make appropriate referrals.
- • Assess client and family response to surgery that results in a change in body and offer support.
- • If nursing assessment reveals body image concerns related to a disfiguring condition, assist client in voicing his/her concerns and if appropriate, coaching the client in how to respond to questions from others in social situations. If within the nurse's level of expertise, may assist client in graded practice in social situations (e.g., going to hairdresser, swimming pool).
- ▲ Refer clients with body image disturbance for CBT and/or social skills training if indicated.
- • Acknowledge denial, anger, or depression as normal feelings when adjusting to changes in body and lifestyle. However, allow client to share emotions when ready, rather than rushing them.
- • Encourage the client to discuss interpersonal and social conflicts that may arise.
- • Explore opportunities to assist the client to develop a realistic perception of his or her body image.

- Help client describe self-ideal, and identify self-criticisms, to foster acceptance of self.
- Encourage clients to verbalize treatment preferences and play a role in treatment decisions.
- Encourage the clients to write a narrative description of their changes.
- Take cues from clients regarding readiness to look at wound (may ask if client has seen wound yet) and utilize client's questions or comments as way to teach about wound care and healing.
- Encourage the client to continue same personal care routine that was followed before the change in body image. It is preferable that this care be completed in the bathroom and not in bed.
- Encourage the client to purchase clothes that are attractive and that deemphasize their disability.
- Encourage client to participate in regular aerobic exercise when feasible.

▲ Provide client with a list of appropriate community resources (e.g., Reach to Recovery, Ostomy Association).

Geriatric

- Focus on remaining abilities. Have client make a list of strengths.
- Encourage regular exercise for the elderly.

Multicultural

- Assess for the influence of cultural beliefs, norms, and values on the client's body image.
- Assess for the presence of conflicting cultural demands.
- Assess for the presence of depressive symptoms.
- Acknowledge that body image disturbances can affect all individuals regardless of culture, race, or ethnicity.

Home Care

- Above interventions may be adapted for home care use.
- Assess client's level of social support as it is one of the determinants of client's recovery and emotional health.
- Assess family/caregiver level of acceptance of client's body changes.
- Recognize that older women may continue their younger preoccupation with weight and recurrent dieting, despite being at

normal weight. Assess source of low weight or weight loss with this in mind.

- • Encourage client to discuss concerns related to sexuality and provide support or information as indicated. Many conditions that affect body image also affect sexuality.
- • Teach all aspects of care. Involve client and caregivers in self-care as soon as possible. Do this in stages if client still has difficulty looking at or touching changed body part.
- ▲ Refer for prosthetic device if appropriate.

Client/Family Teaching

- • Teach appropriate care of surgical site (e.g., mastectomy site, amputation site, ostomy site).
- • Inform client of available community support groups; offer to make initial phone call.
- ▲ Refer the client to counseling for help adjusting to body change.
- • Provide printed material and didactic information for significant others.
- • Encourage significant others to offer support.
- • Direct social support as follows: instruct regarding practical care (bandaging); encourage appraisal support (listening); encourage self-esteem support (favorable comparisons between client's and others' appearance); and encourage sense of belonging (assist with socializing).
- ▲ Refer clients who are having difficulty with personal acceptance, personal and social body image disruption, sexual concerns, reduced self-care skills, and the management of surgical complications to an interdisciplinary team or specialist (e.g. ostomy nurse) if available.

Risk for imbalanced Body temperature

NANDA Definition

At risk for failure to maintain body temperature within a normal range

Risk Factors

Altered metabolic rate; dehydration; exposure to cold/cool environments; exposure to warm/hot environments; extremes of age or weight; illness affecting temperature regulation; inactivity; inappropriate clothing for environmental temperature; medications causing vasoconstriction; medications causing vasodilation; sedation; trauma affecting temperature regulation; vigorous activity

Client Outcomes

Client Will (Specify Time Frame):

- Maintain temperature within normal range
- Explain measures needed to maintain normal temperature
- Identify symptoms of hypothermia or hyperthermia

Nursing Interventions

Refer to the interventions for **Ineffective Thermoregulation**

Bowel incontinence

NANDA Definition

Change in normal bowel elimination habits characterized by involuntary passage of stool

Defining Characteristics

Constant dribbling of soft stool, fecal odor; inability to delay defecation; rectal urgency; self-report of inability to feel rectal fullness or presence of stool in bowel; fecal staining of underclothing; recognition of rectal fullness but reported inability to expel formed stool; inattention to urge to defecate; inability to recognize urge to defecate; irritation of perianal skin

Related Factors (r/t)

Change in stool consistency (diarrhea, constipation, fecal impaction); abnormal motility (metabolic disorders, inflammatory bowel disease, infectious disease, drug-induced motility disorders, food intolerance); defects in rectal vault function (low rectal compliance from ischemia, fibrosis, radiation, infectious proctitis, Hirschprung's disease, local or infiltrating neoplasm, severe rectocele); sphincter dysfunction (obstetric- or traumatic-induced incompetence, fistula or abscess, prolapse, third-degree hemorrhoids, high-tone pelvic floor muscle dysfunction); neurological disorders impacting gastrointestinal

B

motility, rectal vault function, and sphincter function (cerebrovascular accident, spinal injury, traumatic brain injury, central nervous system tumor, advanced stage dementia, encephalopathy, profound mental retardation, multiple sclerosis, myelodysplasia and related neural tube defects, gastroparesis of diabetes mellitus, heavy metal poisoning, chronic alcoholism, infectious or autoimmune neurological disorders, myasthenia gravis)

Client Outcomes

Client Will (Specify Time Frame):

- Have regular, complete evacuation of fecal contents from the rectal vault (pattern may vary from every day to every 3 to 5 days) (Roig et al, 1993)
- Have regulation of stool consistency (soft, formed stools)
- Reduce or eliminate frequency of incontinent episodes
- Demonstrate intact skin in the perianal/perineal area
- Demonstrate the ability to isolate, contract, and relax pelvic muscles (when incontinence related to sphincter incompetence or high-tone pelvic floor dysfunction)
- Increase pelvic muscle strength (when incontinence related to sphincter incompetence)

Nursing Interventions

• In a private setting, directly question any client at risk about the presence of fecal incontinence. If the client reports altered bowel elimination patterns, problems with bowel control, or "uncontrollable diarrhea," complete a focused nursing history including previous and present bowel elimination routines, dietary history, frequency and volume of uncontrolled stool loss, and aggravating and alleviating factors.

• Women who have been pregnant and have delivered one or more children vaginally should be routinely screened for fecal incontinence.

▲ In close consultation with a physician or advanced practice nurse, consider routine use of a validated tool that focuses on bowel elimination patterns.

• Complete a focused physical assessment including inspection of perineal skin, pelvic muscle strength assessment, digital examination of the rectum for presence of impaction and anal sphinc-

B

ter strength, and evaluation of functional status (mobility, dexterity, visual acuity).

- Complete an assessment of cognitive function.
- Document patterns of stool elimination and incontinent episodes through a bowel record, including frequency of bowel movements, stool consistency, frequency and severity of incontinent episodes, precipitating factors, and dietary and fluid intake.
- Assess stool consistency and its influence on risk for stool loss.
- Identify conditions contributing to or causing fecal incontinence.
- Improve access to toileting:
  - Identify usual toileting patterns among persons in the acute care or long-term care facility and plan opportunities for toileting accordingly.
  - Provide assistance with toileting for clients with limited access or impaired functional status (mobility, dexterity, access).
  - Institute a prompted toileting program for persons with impaired cognitive status (retardation, dementia).
  - Provide adequate privacy for toileting.
  - Respond promptly to requests for assistance with toileting.
- Counsel clients with fecal incontinence associated with liquid stools (diarrhea) about methods to normalize stool consistency via dietary fiber or fiber supplements.
- For the client with intermittent episodes of fecal incontinence related to acute changes in stool consistency, begin a bowel reeducation program consisting of:
  - Cleansing the bowel of impacted stool if indicated
  - Normalizing stool consistency by adequate intake of fluids (30 mL/kg of body weight/day) and dietary or supplemental fiber
  - Establishing a regular routine of fecal elimination based on established patterns of bowel elimination (patterns established prior to onset of incontinence)
- Begin a prompted defecation program for the adult with dementia, mental retardation, or related learning disabilities.
- Begin a scheduled stimulation defecation program for persons

B

with neurological conditions causing fecal incontinence including the following steps:

- Cleanse the bowel of impacted fecal material before beginning the program.
- Implement strategies to normalize stool consistency including adequate intake of fluid and fiber and avoidance of foods associated with diarrhea.
- Determine a regular schedule for bowel elimination (typically every day or every other day) based on prior patterns of bowel elimination whenever feasible.
- Provide a stimulus before assisting the client to a position on the toilet; digital stimulation, a stimulating suppository, "mini-enema," or pulsed evacuation enema may be used for stimulation.

▲ Begin a reeducation or pelvic floor muscle exercise program for the person with sphincter incompetence or high-tone pelvic floor muscle dysfunction of the pelvic muscles, or refer persons with fecal incontinence related to sphincter dysfunction to a nurse specialist or other therapist with clinical expertise in these techniques of care.

• Begin a pelvic muscle biofeedback program among clients with urgency to defecate and fecal incontinence related to recurrent diarrhea.

• Institute a structured skin care regimen that incorporates three essential steps: cleanse, moisturize, and protect. Select a cleanser with a pH range comparable to that of normal skin (usually labeled "pH balanced"), moisturize with an emollient to replace lipids removed with cleansing, and protect with a skin protectant containing a petrolatum, dimethicone, or zinc oxide base, or a no-sting skin barrier. Skin that is exposed to urine and/or stool should be cleansed daily and following major incontinence episodes. When feasible, select a product that combined two or all three of these processes into a single step. Ensure that products are available at the bedside when caring for a client with total incontinence in an inpatient facility.

• Cleanse the perineal and perianal skin following each episode of fecal incontinence.

• Apply a moisture barrier containing dimethicone or zinc oxide to clients with severe urinary incontinence or those with double urinary and fecal incontinence.

- ▲ Consult the physician or advanced practice nurse concerning use of a moisture barrier with active healing ingredients when perineal dermatitis exists. Apply and teach care providers to use the product sparingly when applying to affected areas.
- • Assist the client to select and apply a containment device for occasional episodes of fecal incontinence.
- • Teach the caregiver of the client with frequent episodes of fecal incontinence and limited mobility to regularly monitor the sacrum and perineal area for pressure ulcerations.
- ▲ Teach the client with more frequent stool loss to apply an anal continence plug in consultation with the physician.
- • Apply a fecal pouch to the critically ill client with frequent stool loss, particularly when fecal incontinence produces altered perianal skin integrity.
- ▲ Consult a physician or advanced practice nurse about insertion of a bowel management system in the critically ill client with frequent stool loss, particularly when fecal incontinence produces altered perianal skin integrity.

Geriatric

- • Evaluate all elderly clients for established or acute fecal incontinence when the elderly client enters the acute or long-term care facility and intervene as indicated.
- • Evaluate cognitive status in the elderly person with a NEECHAM confusion scale for acute cognitive changes, a Folstein Mini-Mental Status Examination, or other tool as indicated.

Home Care

- • Above interventions may be adapted for home care use.
- • Assess and teach a bowel management program to support continence. Address timing, diet, fluids, and actions taken independently to deal with bowel incontinence.
- • Instruct caregiver to provide clothing that is nonrestrictive, can be manipulated easily for toileting, and can be changed with ease.
- • Evaluate self-care strategies of community-dwelling elders; strengthen adaptive behaviors and counsel elders about altering strategies that compromise general health.

B

- Assist the family in arranging care in a way that allows the client to participate in family or favorite activities without embarrassment.
- ▲ If the client is limited to bed (or bed and chair), provide a commode or bedpan that can be easily accessed. If necessary, refer the client to physical therapy services to learn side transfers and to build strength for transfers.
- ▲ If the client is frequently incontinent, refer for home health aide services to assist with hygiene and skin care.
- Teach the client and family to perform a bowel reeducation program; scheduled, stimulated program; or other strategies to manage fecal incontinence.
- Teach the client and family about common dietary sources for fiber, as well as supplemental fiber or bulking agents as indicated.
- ▲ Refer the family to support services to assist with in-home management of fecal incontinence as indicated.
- Teach nursing colleagues and nonprofessional care providers the importance of providing toileting opportunities and adequate privacy for the client in an acute or long-term care facility.

NOTE: Refer to nursing diagnoses **Diarrhea** and **Constipation** for detailed management of these related conditions.

Effective Breastfeeding

NANDA Definition

Mother-infant dyad/family exhibits adequate proficiency and satisfaction with the breastfeeding process

Defining Characteristics

Adequate infant elimination patterns for age; appropriate infant weight pattern for age; eagerness of infant to nurse; effective mother/infant communication patterns; infant content after feeding; maternal verbalization of satisfaction with the breastfeeding process; mother able to position infant at breast to promote a successful latching-on response; regular and sustained suckling at the breast; regular and sustained swallowing at the breast; signs of oxytocin release; symptoms of oxytocin release

Related Factors (r/t)

Basic breastfeeding knowledge; infant gestational age >34 weeks; maternal confidence; normal breast structure; normal infant oral structure; support

Client Outcomes

Client Will (Specify Time Frame):

- Maintain effective breastfeeding
- Maintain normal growth patterns (infant)
- Verbalize satisfaction with breastfeeding process (mother)

Nursing Interventions

- • Encourage and facilitate early skin-to-skin contact (SSC) (position includes contact of the naked baby with the mother's bare chest within 2 hours after birth).
- • Encourage rooming-in and breastfeeding on demand.
- • Monitor the breastfeeding process.
- • Identify opportunities to enhance knowledge and experience regarding breastfeeding. Support and teaching must be individualized to the client's level of understanding.
- • Give encouragement/positive feedback related to breastfeeding mother-infant interactions.
- • Monitor for signs and symptoms of nipple pain and/or trauma.
- • Discuss prevention and treatment of common breastfeeding problems.
- • Monitor infant responses to breastfeeding.
- • Identify current support person network and opportunities for continued breastfeeding support.
- • Avoid supplemental bottle feedings and do not provide samples of formula on discharge.
- ▲ Provide follow-up contact; as available provide home visits and/or peer counseling.

Multicultural

- • Assess for the influence of cultural beliefs, norms, and values on current breastfeeding practices.
- • Assess mothers' timing preference to begin breastfeeding.
- • Validate the client's concerns about the amount of milk taken.

Home Care

B

- Above interventions may be adapted for home care use.

Client/Family Teaching

- Include the father and other family members in education about breastfeeding.
- Teach the client the importance of maternal nutrition.
- Reinforce the infant's subtle hunger cues (e.g., quiet-alert state, rooting, sucking, hand-to-mouth activity) and encourage the client to nurse whenever signs are apparent.
- Review guidelines for frequency (every 2 to 3 hours, or 8 to 12 feedings per 24 hours) and duration (until suckling and swallowing slow down and satiety is reached) of feeding times.
- Provide anticipatory guidance about common infant behaviors.
- Provide information about additional breastfeeding resources.

Ineffective Breastfeeding

NANDA Definition

Dissatisfaction or difficulty a mother, infant, or child experiences with the breastfeeding process

Defining Characteristics

Inadequate milk supply; infant arching at the breast; infant crying at the breast; infant inability to latch on to maternal breast correctly; infant exhibiting crying within the first hour after breastfeeding; infant exhibiting fussiness within the first hour after breastfeeding; insufficient emptying of each breast per feeding; insufficient opportunity for suckling at the breast; no observable signs of oxytocin release; nonsustained suckling at the breast; observable signs of inadequate infant intake; perceived inadequate milk supply, persistence of sore nipples beyond first week of breastfeeding; resisting latching on; unresponsive to other comfort measures; unsatisfactory breastfeeding process

Related Factors (r/t)

Infant anomaly; infant receiving supplemental feedings with artificial nipple; interruption in breastfeeding; knowledge deficit; maternal ambivalence; maternal anxiety; maternal breast anomaly; nonsupportive family; nonsupportive partner; poor infant reflex; prematurity; previous breast surgery; previous history of breastfeeding failure

Client Outcomes

Client Will (Specify Time Frame):

- Achieve effective breastfeeding (dyad)
- Verbalize/demonstrate techniques to manage breastfeeding problems (mother)
- Manifest signs of adequate intake at the breast (infant)
- Manifest positive self-esteem in relation to the infant feeding process (mother)
- Explain alternative method of infant feeding if unable to continue exclusive breastfeeding (mother)

Nursing Interventions

- • Identify women with risk factors for lower breastfeeding initiation and continuation rates (age <20 years, low socioeconomic status) as well as factors contributing to ineffective breastfeeding as early as possible in the perinatal experience.
- • Provide time for clients to express expectations and concerns and give emotional support.
- • Use valid and reliable tools to measure breastfeeding performance and to predict early discontinuance of breastfeeding whenever possible/feasible.
- • Observe a full breastfeeding session (every 8 hours in the early postpartum and once per visit on follow-up).
- • Provide teaching and breastfeeding assistance appropriate to the client's individualized needs (see Client/Family Teaching).
- • Promote comfort and relaxation to reduce pain and anxiety.
- • Avoid supplemental feedings.
- • Monitor infant behavioral cues and responses to breastfeeding.
- • Provide necessary equipment/instruction/assistance for milk expression as needed.
- ▲ Provide referrals and resources: lactation consultants, nurse and peer support programs, community organizations, and written and electronic sources of information.
- • If unsuccessful in achieving effective breastfeeding, help client accept and learn an alternate method of infant feeding.
- • See care plan for **Effective Breastfeeding.**

Multicultural

- Assess whether the client's concerns about the amount of milk taken during breastfeeding is contributing to dissatisfaction with the breastfeeding process.
- Assess the influence of family support on the decision to continue or discontinue breastfeeding.
- Assess for the influence of mother's weight on attempts to initiate and sustain breastfeeding.
- See care plan for **Effective Breastfeeding.**

Home Care

- Above interventions may be adapted for home care use.
- Provide anticipatory guidance in relation to home management of breastfeeding.
- Investigate availability/refer to public health department, hospital home follow-up breastfeeding program, or other postdischarge support.
- Monitor for specific difficulties contributing to bonding difficulties between mother and infant. Refer to care plan for **Risk for impaired parent/child Attachment.**

Client/Family Teaching

- Review maternal and infant benefits of breastfeeding.
- Instruct the client on maternal breastfeeding behaviors/techniques (preparation for, positioning, initiation of/promoting latch-on, burping, completion of session, and frequency of feeding). Consider use of a video.
- Teach the client self-care measures for the breastfeeding woman (e.g., breast care, management of breast/nipple discomfort, nutrition/fluid, rest/activity).
- Provide information regarding infant cues and behaviors related to breastfeeding and appropriate maternal responses (e.g., cues that infant is ready to feed, behaviors during feeding that contribute to effective breastfeeding, measures of infant feeding adequacy).
- Provide education to father/family/significant others as needed.

B

Interrupted Breastfeeding

NANDA Definition

Break in the continuity of the breastfeeding process as a result of inability or inadvisability to put baby to breast for feeding

Defining Characteristics

Infant receives no nourishment at the breast for some or all feedings; lack of knowledge regarding expression of breast milk; lack of knowledge regarding storage of breast milk; maternal desire to eventually provide breast milk for infant/child's nutritional needs; maternal desire to maintain breastfeeding for infant/child's nutritional needs; maternal desire to provide breast milk for infant/child's nutritional needs; separation of mother and infant

Related Factors (r/t)

Contraindications to breastfeeding; infant illness; maternal employment; maternal illness; need to abruptly wean infant; prematurity

Client Outcomes

Client Will (Specify Time Frame):
Infant

- Receive mother's breast milk if not contraindicated by maternal conditions (e.g., certain drugs, infections) or infant conditions (e.g., true breast milk jaundice)

Maternal

- Maintain lactation
- Achieve effective breastfeeding or satisfaction with the breastfeeding experience
- Demonstrate effective methods of breast milk collection and storage

Nursing Interventions

- • Discuss mother's desire/intention to begin or resume breastfeeding.
- • Provide anticipatory guidance to the mother/family regarding potential duration of the interruption when possible/feasible.

B

- • Reassure mother/family that early measures to sustain lactation and promote parent-infant attachment can make it possible to resume breastfeeding when the condition/situation requiring interruption is resolved.
- • Reassure the mother/family that the infant will benefit from any amount of breast milk provided.
- ▲ Collaborate with the mother/family/healthcare providers/employers (as needed) to develop a plan for expression of breast milk/infant feeding/kangaroo care/SSC.
- • Monitor for signs indicating infants' ability to and interest in breastfeeding.
- • Observe mother performing psychomotor skill (expression, storage, alternative feeding, kangaroo care, and/or breastfeeding) and assist as needed.
- ▲ Provide and/or assist with arrangements and/or necessary equipment.
- ▲ Use supplementation only as medically indicated.
- • Provide anticipatory guidance for common problems associated with interrupted breastfeeding (e.g., incomplete emptying of milk glands, diminishing milk supply, infant difficulty with resuming breastfeeding, or infant refusal of alternative feeding method).
- ▲ Initiate follow-up and make appropriate referrals.
- • Assist the client to accept and learn an alternative method of infant feeding if effective breastfeeding is not achieved.
- • See care plans for **Effective Breastfeeding** and **Ineffective Breastfeeding**.

Multicultural

- • Assess for the influence of cultural beliefs, norms, and values on current decision to stop breastfeeding.
- • Teach culturally appropriate techniques for maintaining lactation.
- • Validate the client's feelings with regard to the difficulty of or her dissatisfaction with breastfeeding.
- • See care plans for **Effective Breastfeeding** and **Ineffective Breastfeeding**.

Home Care

- • Above interventions may be adapted for home care use.

Client/Family Teaching

- Teach mother effective methods to express breast milk.
- Teach mother/parents about kangaroo care.
- Instruct mother on safe breast milk handling techniques.
- See care plans for **Effective Breastfeeding** and **Ineffective Breastfeeding.**

Ineffective Breathing pattern

NANDA Definition

Inspiration and/or expiration that does not provide adequate ventilation

Defining Characteristics

Alterations in depth of breathing; altered chest excursion; assumption of a 3-point position; bradypnea; decreased expiratory pressure; decreased inspiratory pressure; decreased minute ventilation; decreased vital capacity; dyspnea; increased anterior-posterior diameter; nasal flaring; orthopnea; prolonged expiration phase; pursed-lip breathing; tachypnea; timing ratio; use of accessory muscles to breathe

Related Factors (r/t)

Anxiety; body position; bony deformity; chest wall deformity; cognitive impairment; fatigue hyperventilation; hypoventilation syndrome; musculoskeletal impairment; neurological immaturity; neuromuscular dysfunction; obesity; pain; perception impairment; respiratory muscle fatigue; spinal cord injury

Client Outcomes

Client Will (Specify Time Frame):

- Demonstrate a breathing pattern that supports blood gas results within the client's normal parameters
- Report ability to breathe comfortably
- Demonstrate ability to perform pursed-lip breathing and controlled breathing and use relaxation techniques effectively
- Identify and avoid specific factors that exacerbate episodes of ineffective breathing patterns

Nursing Interventions

B

- • Monitor respiratory rate, depth, and ease of respiration. See Defining Characteristics for guidelines for children.
- • Note pattern of respiration. If client is dyspneic, note what seems to cause the dyspnea, the way in which the client deals with the condition, and how the dyspnea resolves or gets worse. Note amount of anxiety associated with the dyspnea.
- • Attempt to determine if client's dyspnea is physiological or psychological in cause.

Psychological Dyspnea—Hyperventilation

- • Assess cause of hyperventilation by asking client about current emotions and psychological state.
- • Ask the client to breathe with you to slow down respiratory rate. Maintain eye contact and give reassurance.
- ▲ If pain is the cause of hyperventilation, provide medication routinely as ordered to prevent severe pain. Use distraction techniques to help client deal with pain. See interventions for **Acute Pain.**
- ▲ If client has chronic problems with hyperventilation, numbness and tingling in extremities, dizziness, and other signs of panic attacks, refer for counseling.

Physiological Dyspnea

- • Ensure that client in acute dyspneic state has received medications, oxygen, and any other treatment needed.
- • Determine severity of dyspnea using a rating scale such as the modified Borg scale, rating dyspnea 0 (best) to 10 (worst) in severity. Alternative scales are the Visual Analogue Scale (VAS) with dyspnea rated as 0 (best) to 100 (worst), or the Medical Research Council Dyspnea Scale.
- • Note abdominal breathing, use of accessory muscles, nasal flaring, retractions, irritability, confusion, or lethargy.
- • Observe color of tongue, oral mucosa, and skin.
- • Auscultate breath sounds, noting decreased or absent sounds, crackles, or wheezes.
- ▲ Monitor client's oxygen saturation and blood gases.
- ▲ Monitor for presence of pain and provide pain medication for comfort as needed.
- • Using touch on the shoulder, coach the client to slow respiratory

B

rate, demonstrating slower respirations; making eye contact with the client; and communicating in a calm, supportive fashion.

- • Support the client in using pursed-lip and controlled breathing techniques.
- • Position the client in an upright or semi-Fowler's position. See Nursing Interventions for **Impaired Gas exchange** for further information on positioning.
- ▲ Administer oxygen as ordered.
- • Increase client's activity to walking three times per day as tolerated. Assist the client to use oxygen during activity as needed. See Nursing Interventions for **Activity intolerance.**
- • Schedule rest periods before and after activity.
- ▲ Evaluate the client's nutritional status. Refer to a dietitian if needed. Use nutritional supplements to increase nutritional level if needed.
- • Provide small, frequent feedings.
- • Offer a fan to move the air in the environment.
- • Encourage the client to take deep breaths at prescribed intervals and do controlled coughing.
- • Help the client with chronic respiratory disease to evaluate dyspnea experience to determine if similar to previous incidences of dyspnea and to recognize that he or she made it through those incidences. Encourage the client to be self-reliant if possible, use problem-solving skills, and maximize use of social support.
- • See **Ineffective Airway clearance** if client has a problem with increased respiratory secretions.
- ▲ Refer COPD client for pulmonary rehabilitation.

Geriatric

- • Encourage ambulation as tolerated.
- • Encourage elderly clients to sit upright or stand and to avoid lying down for prolonged periods during the day.

Home Care

- • Above interventions may be adapted for home care use.
- • Assist the client and family with identifying other factors that precipitate or exacerbate episodes of ineffective breathing patterns (i.e., stress, allergens, stairs, activities that have high energy requirements).

- • Assess client knowledge of and compliance with medication regimen.
- • Teach the client and family the importance of maintaining regimen and having PRN drugs easily accessible at all times.
- • Provide the client with emotional support in dealing with symptoms of respiratory difficulty. Provide family with support for care of a client with chronic or terminal illness. Refer to care plan for **Anxiety.**
- • When respiratory procedures (e.g., apneic monitoring for an infant) are being implemented, explain equipment and procedures to family members, and provide needed emotional support.
- ▲ When electrically based equipment for respiratory support is being implemented, evaluate home environment for electrical safety, proper grounding, etc. Ensure that notification is sent to the local utility company, the emergency medical team, and police and fire departments.
- • Refer to GOLD and ACP-ASIM/ACCP guidelines for management of home care and indications of hospital admission criteria.
- • Support clients' efforts at self-care. Ensure they have all the information they need to participate in care.
- • Identify an emergency plan including when to call the physician or 911.
- ▲ Refer the client to an outpatient pulmonary rehabilitation program or a home-based training program for COPD.
- ▲ Refer to occupational therapy for evaluation and teaching of energy conservation techniques.
- ▲ Refer to home health aide services as needed to support energy conservation.
- ▲ Institute case management of frail elderly to support continued independent living.

Client/Family Teaching

- • Teach pursed-lip and controlled breathing techniques.
- • Using a prerecorded tape, teach client progressive muscle relaxation techniques.
- • Teach about dosage, actions, and side effects of medications.
- • Teach the client to identify and avoid specific factors that exacerbate ineffective breathing patterns, such as exposure to other sources of air pollution, especially smoking.

Decreased Cardiac output

NANDA Definition

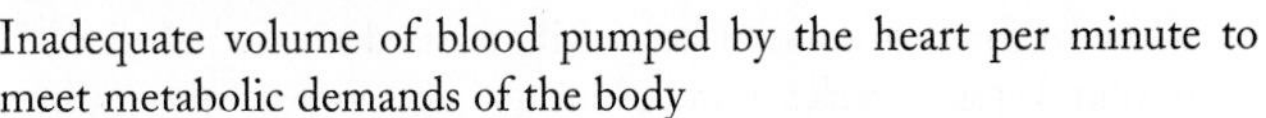

Inadequate volume of blood pumped by the heart per minute to meet metabolic demands of the body

Defining Characteristics

Altered heart rate/rhythm: Arrhythmias; bradycardia; electrocardiographic changes; palpitations; tachycardia

Altered preload: Edema; decreased central venous pressure (CVP); decreased pulmonary artery wedge pressure (PAWP); fatigue; increased central venous pressure (CVP); increased pulmonary artery wedge pressure (PAWP); jugular vein distention; murmurs; weight gain

Altered afterload: Clammy skin; dyspnea; decreased peripheral pulses; decreased pulmonary vascular resistance (PVR); decreased systemic vascular resistance (SVR); increased pulmonary vascular resistance (PVR); increased systemic vascular resistance (SVR); oliguria, prolonged capillary refill; skin color changes; variations in blood pressure readings

Altered contractility: Crackles; cough; decreased ejection fraction; decreased left ventricular stroke work index (LVSWI); decreased stroke volume index (SVI); decreased cardiac index; decreased cardiac output; orthopnea; paroxysmal nocturnal dyspnea; S3 sounds; S4 sounds

Behavioral/emotional: Anxiety; restlessness

Related Factors (r/t)

Altered heart rate; altered heart rhythm; altered stroke volume: altered preload, altered afterload, altered contractility

Client Outcomes

Client Will (Specify Time Frame):

- Demonstrate adequate cardiac output as evidenced by blood pressure and pulse rate and rhythm within normal parameters for client; strong peripheral pulses; and an ability to tolerate activity without symptoms of dyspnea, syncope, or chest pain
- Remain free of side effects from the medications used to achieve adequate cardiac output

- Explain actions and precautions to take for primary or secondary prevention of cardiac disease

C

Nursing Interventions

- • Monitor for symptoms of heart failure and decreased cardiac output; listen to heart sounds, lung sounds; note symptoms, including dyspnea, orthopnea, paroxysmal nocturnal dyspnea, Cheyne-Stokes respirations, fatigue, weakness, third and fourth heart sounds, crackles in lungs, increased venous pressure greater than 16 cm H_2O, and positive hepatojugular reflex.
- ▲ Recognize the importance of cardiac index estimated by thermodilution in the intensive care unit (ICU) client.
- ▲ When using pulmonary arterial catheter technology, be sure to appropriately level and zero the equipment, use minimal tubing, maintain system patency, perform square wave testing, position the client appropriately, and consider correlation to respiratory and cardiac cycles when assessing waveforms and integrating data into client assessment.
- ▲ Hemodynamic pressure and parameters can be obtained either before or after cardiac output measurement.
- ▲ Be aware of the utilization of impedance cardiography in noninvasive hemodynamic monitoring of heart failure.
- ▲ Be aware of the utilization of other cardiac output techniques including the Fick Method and esophageal Doppler imaging.
- • Recognize the effect of sleep disordered breathing in heart failure.
- • Observe for chest pain or discomfort; note location, radiation, severity, quality, duration, associated manifestations such as nausea, indigestion, and diaphoresis; also note precipitating and relieving factors.
- ▲ If chest pain is present, have client lie down, monitor cardiac rhythm, give oxygen, check vital signs, run a monitor strip, medicate for pain, and notify the physician.
- • Monitor intake and output. If client is acutely ill, measure hourly urine output and note decreases in output.
- ▲ Note results of electrocardiography and chest radiography.
- ▲ Note results of diagnostic imaging studies such as echocardiogram, radionuclide imaging, or dobutamine stress echocardiography.
- ▲ Watch laboratory data closely, especially arterial blood gases, electrolytes including potassium, and B-type natriuretic peptide (BNP assay).

▲ Monitor laboratory work such as complete blood count (CBC), sodium level, and serum creatinine.
▲ Administer oxygen as needed per physician's order.
• Place client in semi-Fowler's or high Fowler's position with legs down or position of comfort.
▲ Check blood pressure, pulse, and condition before administering cardiac medications such as angiotensin-converting enzyme (ACE) inhibitors, digoxin, calcium channel blockers, and beta-blockers such as Carvedilol. Notify physician if heart rate or blood pressure is low before holding medications.
• During acute events, ensure client remains on short-term bed rest or maintains activity level that does not compromise cardiac output.
• Gradually increase activity when client's condition is stabilized by encouraging slower paced activities or shorter periods of activity with frequent rest periods following exercise prescription; observe for symptoms of intolerance. Take blood pressure and pulse before and after activity and note changes. See **Activity intolerance.**
• Serve small sodium-restricted, low-cholesterol meals.
• Serve only small amounts of coffee or caffeine-containing beverages if requested (no more than four cups per 24 hours) if no resulting dysrhythmia.
▲ Monitor bowel function. Provide stool softeners as ordered. Caution client not to strain when defecating.
• Have clients use a commode or urinal for toileting and avoid use of a bedpan.
• Provide a restful environment by minimizing controllable stressors and unnecessary disturbances. Schedule rest periods after meals and activities.
• Weigh client at same time daily (after voiding).
▲ Apply graduated compression stockings as ordered. Ensure proper fit by measuring accurately. Remove the stocking at least once a day, then reapply. Assess the condition of the extremity frequently.
• Assess for presence of anxiety. Consider using music to decrease anxiety and improve cardiac function. See Nursing Interventions for **Anxiety** to facilitate reduction of anxiety in clients and family.
▲ Refer for treatment if anxiety is present.

C

- ▲ Closely monitor fluid intake, including intravenous lines. Maintain fluid restriction if ordered.
- ▲ If intravenous fluid is ordered for circulatory failure, administer cautiously and observe for signs of fluid overload. Administering excessive volume is detrimental to cardiac output.
- ▲ Observe for symptoms of cardiogenic shock, including impaired mentation, hypotension with blood pressure lower than 90 mm Hg, decreased peripheral pulses, cold clammy skin, signs of pulmonary congestion, and decreased organ function. If present, notify physician immediately.
- ▲ If shock is present, monitor hemodynamic parameters for an increase in pulmonary wedge pressure, an increase in systemic vascular resistance, or a decrease in cardiac output and index.
- ▲ Titrate inotropic and vasoactive medications within defined parameters to maintain contractility, preload, and afterload per physician's order.
- ▲ Be aware that intraaortic balloon counterpulsation is implemented to treat cardiogenic shock by decreasing the workload of the left ventricle and improving myocardial perfusion.
- ▲ Be aware that mechanical ventilation can decrease cardiac output.
- ▲ Refer to heart failure program or cardiac rehabilitation program for education, evaluation, and guided support to increase activity and rebuild life.
- ▲ Be aware that cardiac resynchronization therapy improves cardiac output and may be ordered for appropriate clients.
- • Be aware that pregnancy increases cardiac output and take into consideration when assessing nutritional needs.

Geriatric

- • Observe for atypical pain; the elderly often have jaw pain instead of chest pain or may have silent myocardial infarctions (MIs) with symptoms of dyspnea or fatigue.
- ▲ If client has heart disease causing activity intolerance, refer for cardiac rehabilitation.
- • Consider the use of graphic feedback with the elderly in exercise adherence.
- • Observe for syncope, dizziness, palpitations, or feelings of weakness associated with an irregular heart rhythm.
- ▲ Observe for side effects from cardiac medications.

Pediatrics/Newborn

- Monitor heart rate continuously in the newborn and report abnormalities immediately.

C

Home Care

- Some of the above interventions may be adapted for home care use.
- ▲ Begin discharge planning as soon as possible with case manager or social worker to assess home support systems and the need for community or home health services. Consider referral for advanced practice nurse (APN) follow-up. Support services may be needed to assist with home care, meal preparations, housekeeping, personal care, transportation to doctor visits, or emotional support.
- ▲ Adopt a clinical pathway to address focused interventions with CHF, coronary artery bypass graft (CABG). National Practice Guidelines for Cardiac Home Care are available to direct intervention for the client post-CABG who is recovering at home.
- ▲ Assess or refer to case manager or social worker to evaluate client ability to pay for prescriptions.
- Continue to monitor client closely for exacerbation of heart failure when discharged home.
- ▲ Monitor women for differential symptoms of MI and institute emergency treatment measures as indicated.
- Instruct women in the differential symptoms of MI in women, and the need to take symptoms seriously and seek help as indicated.
- ▲ Assess client for understanding of and compliance with medical regimen, including medications, activity level, and diet. Client/family may need repetition of instructions received at hospital discharge, and may require reiteration as fear of a recent crisis decreases.
- ▲ Assess and monitor for signs of depression (particularly in adults age 65 years or older) or social isolation. Refer for mental health treatment as indicated.
- Assess for signs/symptoms of cognitive impairment.
- Assess for fatigue and weakness frequently. Assess home environment for safety, as well as resources/obstacles to energy conservation. Instruct client and family members on need for behavioral pacing and energy conservation.
- Instruct family and client about the disease process, complications of disease process, information on medications, need for weighing daily, and when it is appropriate to call doctor.

C

- • Help family adapt daily living patterns to establish life changes that will maintain improved cardiac functioning in the client. Take the client's perspective into consideration, and use a holistic approach in assessing and responding to client planning for the future.
- • Assist client to recognize and exercise power in using self-care management to adjust to health change. Refer to care plan for **Powerlessness.**
- • Support client self-efficacy to increase physical activity by creating a supportive environment, offering encouragement, providing anticipatory guidance, and supplying a realistic assessment of the client's abilities.
- ▲ Explore barriers to medical regimen adherence. Review medications and treatment regularly for needed modifications. Take complaints of side effects seriously and serve as client advocate to address changes as indicated.
- ▲ Refer for cardiac rehabilitation, strengthening exercises if client is not involved in outpatient cardiac rehabilitation.
- ▲ Refer to medical social services as necessary for counseling about the impact of severe or chronic cardiac disease.
- ▲ Institute case management of frail elderly to support continued independent living.
- ▲ As client condition warrants, refer to hospice.
- • Identify emergency plan, including use of cardiopulmonary resuscitation (CPR). Encourage family members to become certified in cardiopulmonary resuscitation.

Client/Family Teaching

- • Teach symptoms of heart failure and appropriate actions to take if client becomes symptomatic.
- • Teach importance of smoking cessation and avoidance of alcohol intake.
- • Teach stress reduction (e.g., imagery, controlled breathing, muscle relaxation techniques).
- • Explain necessary restrictions, including consumption of a sodium-restricted diet, guidelines on fluid intake, and the avoidance of Valsalva maneuver. Teach the importance of pacing activities, work simplification techniques, and the need to rest between activities to prevent becoming overly fatigued.

▲ Teach the client actions, side effects, and importance of consistently taking cardiovascular medications.
• Provide client/family with advance directive information to consider. Allow client to give advance directions about medical care or designate who should make medical decisions if he or she should lose decision-making capacity.
▲ Instruct the client on importance of getting a pneumonia shot (usually one per lifetime) and yearly influenza shots as prescribed by physician.
• Instruct client/family on the need to weigh daily and keep a weight log. Ask if client has a scale at home; if not, assist in getting one. Instruct on establishing baseline weight on own scale when gets home.
• Provide specific written materials and self-care plan for client/caregivers to use for reference.
▲ Consult dietitian or assist client in understanding the need for a sodium-restricted diet. Provide alternatives for salt such as spices, herbs, lemon juice, or vinegar.
• Instruct family regarding cardiopulmonary resuscitation.

C

Caregiver role strain

NANDA Definition

Difficulty in performing family caregiver role

Defining Characteristics

Caregiving Activities

Apprehension about care receiver's care if caregiver unable to provide care; apprehension about the future regarding care receiver's health; apprehension about the future regarding caregiver's ability to provide care; apprehension about possible institutionalization of care receiver; difficulty completing required tasks; difficulty performing required tasks; dysfunctional change in caregiving activities; preoccupation with care routine

Caregiver Health Status—Physical

Cardiovascular disease; diabetes; fatigue; GI upset; headaches; hypertension; rash; weight change

Caregiver Health Status—Emotional

Anger; disturbed sleep; feeling depressed; frustration; impaired individual coping; impatience; increased emotional lability; increased nervousness; lack of time to meet personal needs; somatization; stress

Socioeconomic

Changes in leisure activities; low work productivity; refuses career advancement; withdraws from social life

Caregiver–Care Receiver Relationship

Difficulty watching care receiver go through the illness; grief regarding changed relationship with care receiver; uncertainty regarding changed relationship with care receiver

Family Processes

Concerns about family members; family conflict

Related Factors (r/t)

Care Receiver Health Status

Addiction; codependence; cognitive problems; dependency; illness chronicity; illness severity; increasing care needs; instability of care receiver's health; problem behaviors; psychological problems; unpredictability of illness course

Socioeconomic Factors

Isolation from others; competing role commitments; alienation from family, friends, and coworkers; insufficient recreation

Caregiver Health Status

Addiction; codependency; cognitive problems; inability to fulfill one's own expectations; inability to fulfill other's expectations; marginal coping patterns; physical problems; psychological problems; unrealistic expectations of self

Caregiver–Care Receiver Relationship

History of poor relationship; mental status of elder inhibiting conversation presence of abuse or violence; unrealistic expectations of caregiver by care receiver

Caregiving Activities
24-hour care responsibilities; amount of activities; complexity of activities; discharge of family members to home with significant care needs; ongoing changes in activities; unpredictability of care situation; years of caregiving

Family Processes
History of family dysfunction; history of marginal family coping

Resources
Caregiver is not developmentally ready for caregiver role; deficient knowledge about community resources; difficulty accessing community resources; emotional strength; formal assistance; formal support; inadequate community resources (e.g., respite services, recreational resources); inadequate equipment for providing care; inadequate physical environment for providing care (e.g., housing, temperature, safety); inadequate transportation; inexperience with caregiving; informal assistance; informal support; insufficient finances; insufficient time; lack of caregiver privacy; lack of support; physical energy

Socioeconomic
Alienation from others; competing role commitments; insufficient recreation; isolation from others

Client Outcomes
- Caregiver will feel supported
- Caregiver will report low or no feelings of burden or distress
- Caregiver will maintain own physical and psychological/emotional health
- Caregiver will identify resources available to help in giving care
- Caregiver will verbalize mastery of the care situation, feeling confident and competent to provide care
- Care receiver will obtain quality and safe care

Nursing Interventions
- • Watch for signs of depression and deteriorating physical health in the caregiver, especially if the marital relationship is poor, the care recipient has cognitive or neuropsychiatric symptoms, there is little social support available, the caregiver becomes enmeshed

in the care situation, the caregiver is elderly, female, or has poor preexisting physical or emotional health. Refer to the care plan for **Hopelessness** when appropriate.

- • The impact of providing care on the caregiver's emotional health should be assessed at regular intervals using a reliable and valid instrument such as the Caregiver Strain Index, Caregiver Burden Inventory, Caregiver Reaction Assessment, Screen for Caregiver Burden, and the Subjective and Objective Burden Scale.
- • Identify potential caregiver resources such as mastery, social support, optimism, and positive aspects of care.
- • Screen for caregiver role strain at the onset of the care situation, at regular intervals throughout the care situation, and with changes in care recipient status and care transitions.
- • Watch for caregivers who become enmeshed in the care situation (e.g., becoming overinvolved or unable to disentangle themselves from the caregiver role).
- • Arrange for intervals of respite care for the caregiver; encourage use if available.
- • Help the caregiver to identify and utilize support systems.
- • Encourage the caregiver to grieve over changes in the care receiver's condition and give the caregiver permission to share angry feelings in a safe environment. Refer to nursing interventions for **Grieving.**
- • Help the caregiver find personal time to meet his or her needs, learn stress management techniques, schedule regular health screenings, and schedule regular respite time.
- • Encourage the caregiver to schedule and keep routine healthcare appointments (i.e., annual physicals and screening tests).
- • Encourage the caregiver to talk about feelings, concerns, uncertainties, and fears. Acknowledge the frustration associated with caregiver responsibilities.
- • Observe for any evidence of caregiver or care receiver violence or abuse; if evidence is present, speak with the caregiver and care receiver separately.
- ▲ Involve the family in care transitions; use a multidisciplinary team to provide medical and social services for instruction and planning.
- ▲ Encourage regular communication with the care recipient and with the healthcare team.
- • Help caregiver assess his or her socioeconomic status (services

reimbursed by insurance, available support through community and religious organizations).

- Help the caregiver identify competing occupational demands and potential ways to modify the work role in order to provide care (enact the Family Leave Act, change from full to part time, work from home, take a leave of absence or early retirement).
- When necessary, help the caregiver transition the care recipient to a long-term care facility.
- Help the caregiver problem solve to meet the care recipient's needs.

Geriatric

- Monitor the caregiver for psychological distress and signs of depression, especially if caring for a mentally impaired elder or if there was an unsatisfactory marital relationship before caregiving.
- Assess the health of caregivers at intervals, especially if they have their own chronic illness in addition to caregiving role.
- Assess social support and encourage the use of secondary caregivers with elderly caregivers.
- Provide skills training related to direct care, performing complex monitoring tasks, supervision interpreting client symptoms, assisting with decision making, providing emotional support and comfort, and coordinating care.
- Teach symptom management techniques (assessment, potential causes, aggravating factors, potential alleviating factors, reassessment), particularly for fatigue, constipation, anorexia, and pain.

Multicultural

- Assess for the influence of cultural beliefs, norms, and values on the client's ability to modify health behavior.
- Encourage spirituality as a source of support for coping.
- Negotiate with the client regarding the aspects of health behavior that will need to be modified.
- Assess the role of fatalism on the client's ability to modify health behavior.
- Identify which family members the client can rely on for support.

▲ Assess for signs of depression and level of social support and make appropriate referrals.

- Assess for the presence of conflicting values within the culture.

Home Care

C

- • Identify client and caregiver factors that necessitate the use of formal home care services, that may affect provision of care, or that need to be addressed before the client can be safely discharged from home care.
- • Collaborate with the caregiver and discuss the care needs of the client, disease processes, medications, and what to expect; use a variety of instructional techniques (e.g., explanations, demonstrations, visual aids) until the caregiver is able to express a degree of comfort with care delivery.
- • Assist the caregiver and client in arranging care so that it is compatible with other household patterns.
- • Assess family caregiving skill. The identification of caregiver difficulty with any of a core set of processes highlights areas for intervention.
- • Assess the client and caregiver at every visit for quality of care provided, functional disability of care recipient, caregiver coping, and signs of caregiver stress.
- • Assess the client and caregiver at every visit for quality of relationship, and for the quality of caring that exists.
- • Assess preexisting strengths and weaknesses the caregiver brings to the situation, as well as current responses, depression, and fatigue levels.
- • Identify and support strengths and weaknesses of the caregiver and efforts to gain control of unpredictable situations.
- • Form a trusting and supportive relationship with the caregiver. Allow the caregiver to verbalize frustrations.
- • Explore with the spouse the process of understanding the client's behavior that the spouse has been undergoing; assist with reframing that understanding to be as realistic and positive as possible. Consider use of the Progressively Lowered Stress Threshold psychoeducational nursing intervention to help the spouse understand and handle the behavior changes associated with Alzheimer's disease.
- ▲ Refer the client to home health aide services for assistance with ADLs and light housekeeping. Allow the caregiver to gain confidence in the respite provider.
- ▲ Identify appropriate individual and group interventions for the caregiver; assess for appropriateness of referrals given the caregiver's needs and mobility.

▲ Refer to a caregivers' support group if available or recommend an online support group—see suggested websites listed on the Evolve website.
- Assess the caregiver for over-involvement with the client and client's illness. Encourage the caregiver to address an enmeshed relationship with the client prompted by concerns over the client's illness and altered quality of life by discussing the issue, seeking respite, and attending support groups.

▲ Refer for homemaker or psychiatric home healthcare services for respite, client reassurance, and implementation of a therapeutic regimen.
- As indicated by client status, assist the caregiver in examining the option of adult day care and maintaining realistic expectations of adult day care.

▲ As indicated by deterioration of the client's condition, assist the caregiver in examining options for institutional placement.
- Assess the caregiver's emotional response to placement of the client and provide support, cognitive interventions, and problem solving as needed.
- Be aware that physical and emotional demands on the caregiver tend to increase during the last 3 months of a care recipient's life, which may require more frequent or intense intervention.

Caregiver/Family Teaching

- Assess the caregiver's need for information such as information on symptom management, disease progression, specific skills, and available support.
- Teach the caregiver warning signs for burnout, depression, and anxiety. Help them identify a resource in case they begin to feel overwhelmed.
- Teach the caregiver methods for managing disruptive behavioral symptoms if present. Refer to the care plan for **Chronic Confusion.**
- Teach the caregiver how to provide the care needed and put a plan in place for monitoring the care provided.
- Provide ongoing support and evaluation of care skills as the care situation and care demands change.
- Provide information regarding the care recipient's diagnosis, treatment regimen, and expected course of illness.

▲ Refer to counseling or support groups to assist in adjusting to the caregiver role and periodically evaluate not only the caregiver's emotional response to care but the safety of the care delivered to the care recipient.

C

Risk for Caregiver role strain

NANDA Definition

Caregiver is vulnerable for felt difficulty in performing the family caregiver role

Risk Factors

Addiction; amount of caregiving tasks; care receiver exhibits bizarre behavior; care receiver exhibits deviant behavior; caregiver's competing role commitments; caregiver health impairment; caregiver is female; caregiver is spouse; caregiver isolation; caregiver not developmentally ready for caregiver role; codependency; cognitive problems in care receiver; complexity of caregiving tasks; congenital defect; developmental delay of the care receiver; developmental delay of the caregiver; discharge of family member with significant home care needs; duration of caregiving required; family dysfunction prior to the caregiving situation; family isolation; illness severity of the care receiver; inadequate physical environment for providing care (e.g., housing, transportation, community services, equipment); inexperience with caregiving; instability in the care receiver's health; lack of recreation for caregiver; lack of respite for caregiver; marginal caregiver's coping patterns; marginal family adaptation; past history of poor relationship between caregiver and care receiver; premature birth; presence of abuse; presence of situational stressors that normally affect families (e.g., significant loss, disaster or crisis, economic vulnerability, major life events); presence of violence; psychological problems in care receiver; retardation of the care receiver; retardation of the caregiver; unpredictable illness course

Client Outcomes

Client/Caretaker Will (Specify Time Frame):

- Maintain physical and psychological health
- Identify resources available to help in giving care
- Obtain appropriate care

Nursing Interventions and Client/Family Teaching

Refer to the care plan for **Caregiver role strain**

Readiness for enhanced Comfort

NANDA Definition

A pattern of ease, relief and transcendence in physical, psycho spiritual, environmental, and social dimensions that can be strengthened

Defining Characteristics

Expresses desire to enhance comfort; expresses desire to enhance feelings of contentment; expresses desire to enhance relaxation; expresses desire to enhance resolution of complaints

Client Outcomes

Client Will (Specify Time Frame):

- Assess current level of comfort as acceptable
- Express the need to achieve an enhanced level of comfort
- Identify strategies to enhance comfort
- Perform appropriate interventions as needed for increased comfort
- Evaluate the effectiveness of interventions at regular intervals
- Maintain an enhanced level of comfort when possible

Nursing Interventions

- • Assess client's current level of comfort.
- • Help clients understand that enhanced comfort is a desirable, positive, and achievable goal.
- ▲ Enhance feelings of trust between the client and the healthcare provider.
- • Manipulate the environment as necessary to enhance comfort.
- • Use therapeutic massage for enhancement of comfort.
- • Teach and encourage use of guided imagery.
- • Foster and instill hope in clients whenever possible.
- • See the care plan for **Hopelessness.**
- • Provide opportunities for and enhance spiritual care activities.
- • Enhance social support and family involvement.
- • Encourage mind-body therapies such as meditation as an enhanced comfort activity.

- ▲ Promote participation in creative arts and activity programs.
- ▲ Encourage clients to use Health Information Technology (HIT) as needed.
- • Evaluate the effectiveness of all interventions at regular intervals and adjust therapies as necessary.

Pediatric

- • Assess and evaluate child's level of comfort at frequent intervals.
- • Provide gentle, soothing touch, which may be well-suited for clients who cannot tolerate more stimulating interventions such as simple massage.
- • Skin-to-skin contact (SSC) and selection of most effective method improves the comfort of newborns during routine blood draws.
- • Lower fevers with medication rather than sponging alone or in combination with medication unless there is a clear need to rapidly lower the client's temperature.
- • Adjust the environment as needed to enhance comfort.
- • Encourage parental presence whenever possible. The same basic principles for managing pain in adults and children apply to neonates.
- • Promote use of alternative comforting strategies such as positioning, presence, massage, spiritual care, music therapy, art therapy, and story-telling to enhance comfort when needed. In addition to oral sucrose, other comfort measures should be used to alleviate pain such as swaddling, skin-to-skin contact with mother, nursing, rocking, and holding.

Multicultural

- • Identify cultural beliefs, values, lifestyles, practices, and problem-solving strategies when assessing clients.
- • Enhance cultural knowledge by actively seeking out information regarding different cultural and ethnic groups.
- • Recognize the impact of culture on communication styles and techniques.
- • Provide culturally competent care to clients from different cultural groups.

Home Care

- • The nursing interventions described previously in **Readiness for enhanced Comfort** may be used with clients in the home care setting. When needed, adaptations can be made to meet the needs of specific clients, families, and communities.

▲ Make appropriate referrals to other organizations or providers as needed to enhance comfort.

▲ Promote an interdisciplinary approach to home care.

• Evaluate regularly if enhanced comfort is attainable in the home care setting.

Client/Family Teaching

• Teach client how to regularly assess levels of comfort.

• Instruct client that a variety of interventions may be needed at any given time to enhance comfort.

• Help clients to understand that enhanced comfort is an achievable goal.

• Teach techniques to enhance comfort as needed.

▲ When needed, empower clients to seek out other health professionals as members of the interdisciplinary team to assist with comforting measures and techniques.

• Encourage self-care activities and continued self-evaluation of achieved comfort levels to ensure enhanced comfort will be maintained.

Impaired verbal Communication

NANDA Definition

Decreased, delayed, or absent ability to receive, process, transmit, and use a system of symbols

Defining Characteristics

Absence of eye contact; cannot speak; difficulty in comprehending usual communication pattern; difficulty expressing thoughts verbally (e.g., aphasia, dysphasia, apraxia, dyslexia); difficulty forming sentences; difficulty forming words (e.g., aphonia, dyslalia, dysarthria); difficulty in maintaining usual communication pattern; difficulty in selective attending; difficulty in use of body expressions; difficulty in use of facial expressions; disorientation to person; disorientation to space; disorientation to time; does not speak; dyspnea; inability to speak language of caregiver; inability to use body expressions; inability to use facial expressions; inappropriate verbalization; partial visual deficit; slurring; speaks with difficulty; stuttering; total visual deficit; verbalizes with difficulty; willful refusal to speak

Related Factors (r/t)

Absence of significant others; altered perceptions; alteration in self-concept; alteration in self-esteem; alteration of central nervous system; anatomical defect (e.g., cleft palate, alteration of the neuromuscular visual system, auditory system, phonatory apparatus); brain tumor; cultural differences; decrease in circulation to brain; differences related to development age; emotional conditions; environmental barriers; lack of information; physical barrier (e.g., tracheostomy, intubation); physiological conditions; psychological barriers (e.g., psychosis, lack of stimuli); side effects of medication; stress; weakening of the musculoskeletal system

Client Outcomes

Client Will (Specify Time Frame):

- Use effective communication techniques
- Use alternative methods of communication effectively
- Demonstrate congruency of verbal and nonverbal behavior
- Demonstrate understanding even if not able to speak
- Express desire for social interactions

Nursing Interventions

▲ When the client is having difficulty communicating, assess and refer for consultation for hearing loss. Suspect hearing loss when:

- ■ Client frequently complains that people mumble, speech is not clear, or client hears only parts of conversations when people are talking.
- ■ Client often asks people to repeat what they said.
- ■ Client's friends or relatives tell them that client doesn't seem to hear very well.
- ■ Client does not laugh at jokes because client misses too much of the story.
- ■ Client needs to ask others about the details of a meeting that the client just attended.
- ■ Others say that the client plays the television or radio too loudly.

C

- ■ Client cannot hear the doorbell or the telephone.
- ■ Client finds that looking at people when they talk to them makes it somewhat easier to understand, especially when clients are in a noisy place or where there are competing conversations.

• Involve a familiar person when attempting to communicate with a client who has difficulty with communication, if accepted by the client.

• Avoid making assumptions about the communication choice of those with hearing loss.

▲ Identify the language spoken; obtain a language dictionary or interpreter if possible and accepted by the client.

• Listen carefully. Validate verbal and nonverbal expressions particularly when dealing with pain.

• When communicating with a client with a hearing loss, face toward his or her unaffected side or better ear while allowing client to see speaker's face at a reasonably close distance.

• Provide sufficient light and do not stand in front of window when communicating with a person with a hearing loss.

• Use simple communication; speak in a well-modulated voice, smile, and show concern for the client.

• Maintain eye contact at the client's level.

• When working with clients who have hearing impairments, remove masks or use see-through masks and reduce background noise whenever possible.

• Use touch as appropriate.

• Use presence. Spend time with the client, allow time for responses, and make the call light readily available.

• Explain all healthcare procedures.

• Be persistent in deciphering what the client is saying, and do not pretend to understand when the message is unclear.

▲ Obtain communication equipment such as electronic devices, letter boards, picture boards, and magic slates.

▲ Consider the use of a lipreader translator (LRT) for those who are intubated via a tracheostomy.

• Using an individualized approach, establish an alternative method of communication such as writing or pointing to letters, word phrases, picture cards, or simple drawings of basic needs.

C

- ▲ Consider use of an intelligent keyboard to facilitate communication for clients unable to express themselves verbally.
- ▲ Consultation with a speech pathologist may be helpful. Supplement the work of the speech pathologist with appropriate exercises.
- • Establish an understanding of the client's symbolic speech, especially with clients who have schizophrenia. Ask the client to clarify particular statements.
- • If a comprehension deficit is present, keep the environment quiet when communicating and get the client's attention before attempting to communicate (e.g., touch the client's shoulder, call the client's name).
- • Do not raise your voice or shout at the client.

Pediatric

- • Observe behavioral communication cues in infants.
- • Identify and define variations of communication that may be used by children with significant disabilities. Teach at least two new forms of socially acceptable communication alternatives to teach as repairs when communication breaks down.
- • Teach children with severe disabilities functional communication skills.
- ▲ Refer children with primary speech and language delay/disorder for speech and language therapy interventions.

Geriatric

- • Carefully assess all clients for hearing difficulty using an audiometer.
- • Avoid use of "elderspeak."
- • Initiate communication with the client with dementia.
- • Encourage the client to wear hearing aids, if appropriate.
- • Facilitate communication and reminiscing with remembering boxes that contain objects, photographs, and writings that have meaning for the client.

Multicultural

- • Nurses should become more sensitive to the meaning of a culture's nonverbal communication modes, such as eye contact, facial expression, touching, and body language.
- • Assess for the influence of cultural beliefs, norms, and values on the client's communication process.

- Assess personal space needs, acceptable communication styles, acceptable body language, interpretation of eye contact, perception of touch, and use of paraverbal modes when communicating with the client.
- Assess for how language barriers contribute to health disparities among ethnic and racial minorities.
- Although touch is generally beneficial, there may be certain instances where it may not be advisable due to cultural considerations.
- Modify and tailor the communication approach in keeping with the client's particular culture.
- Use reminiscence therapy as a language intervention.
- Use of the Office of Minority Health (OMH) of the U.S. Department of Health and Human Services (DHHS) standards on culturally and linguistically appropriate services (CLAS) in healthcare should be used as needed.

Home Care

- The interventions described previously may be adapted for home care use.

Client/Family Teaching

- Teach the client and family techniques to increase communication, including the use of communication devices.
- Encourage significant others to use touch, such as holding the client's hand or stroking the arm.
- ▲ Refer the client to a speech-language pathologist (SLP) or audiologist.
- ▲ Refer to a specialist for possible surgical intervention when clients have surgical defects caused by cancer of the maxillary sinus and alveolar ridge.

Readiness for enhanced Communication

NANDA Definition

A pattern of exchanging information and ideas with others that is sufficient for meeting one's needs and life's goals and can be strengthened

Defining Characteristics

C

Able to speak a language; able to write a language; expresses feelings; expresses satisfaction with ability to share ideas with others; expresses satisfaction with ability to share information with others; expresses thoughts; expresses willingness to enhance communication; forms phrases; forms sentences; forms words; interprets nonverbal cues appropriately; uses nonverbal cues appropriately

Client Outcomes

Client Will (Specify Time Frame):

- Express willingness to enhance communication
- Demonstrate ability to speak or write a language
- Form words, phrases, and language
- Express thoughts and feelings
- Use and interpret nonverbal cues appropriately
- Express satisfaction with ability to share information and ideas with others

Nursing Interventions

- • Establish a therapeutic nurse-client relationship: provide appropriate education for the client, demonstrate caring by being present to the client.
- • Carefully assess the client's readiness to communicate, using an individualized approach. Avoid making assumptions regarding the client's preferred communication method.
- • Assess the client's literacy level.
- • Listen attentively and provide a comfortable environment for communicating; use these practical guidelines to assist in communication: Slow down and listen to the client's story; use augmentative and alternative communication methods (such as lip-reading, communication boards, writing, body language, and computer/electronic communication devices) as appropriate; repeat instructions if necessary; limit the amount of information given; have the client "teach back" to confirm understanding; avoid asking, "Do you understand?"; be respectful, caring, and sensitive.
- ▲ Provide communication with specialty nurses who have knowledge about the client's situation.
- ▲ Refer couples in maladjusted relationships for psychosocial intervention and social support to strengthen communication; consider nurse specialists.

- Consider using music to enhance communication between client who is dying and his/her family.
- See care plan for **Impaired verbal Communication.**

Pediatric

▲ All individuals involved in the care and everyday life of children with learning difficulties need to have a collaborate approach to communication.

- See care plan for **Impaired verbal Communication.**

Geriatric

▲ Assess for hearing and vision impairments and make appropriate referrals for hearing aids.

- Use touch if culturally acceptable when communicating with older clients and their families.
- Caregivers may sing when delivering care and instructions for clients with dementia.
- See care plan for **Impaired verbal Communication.**

Multicultural

- See care plan for **Impaired verbal Communication.**

Home Care and Client/Family Teaching

- The interventions described previously may be used in home care.
- See care plan for **Impaired verbal Communication.**

Decisional Conflict (specify)

NANDA Definition

Uncertainty about course of action to be taken when choice among competing actions involves risk, loss, or challenge to values and beliefs

Defining Characteristics

Delayed decision making; physical signs of distress or tension (e.g., increased heart rate, increased muscle tension, restlessness); questioning moral principles while attempting a decision; questioning

C

moral rules while attempting a decision; questioning moral values while attempting a decision; questioning personal beliefs while attempting a decision; questioning personal values while attempting a decision; self-focusing; vacillation among alternative choices; verbalizes feeling of distress while attempting a decision; verbalizes uncertainty about choices; verbalizes undesired consequences of alternative actions being considered

Related Factors (r/t)

Divergent sources of information; interference with decision making; lack of experience with decision making; lack of relevant information; moral obligations require performing action; moral obligations require not performing action; moral principles support courses of action; moral rules support mutually inconsistent courses of action; moral values support mutually inconsistent courses of action; multiple sources of information; perceived threat to value system; support system deficit; unclear personal beliefs; unclear personal values

Client Outcomes

Client Will (Specify Time Frame):

- State the advantages and disadvantages of choices
- Share fears and concerns regarding choices and responses of others
- Seek resources and information necessary for making an informed choice
- Make an informed choice

Nursing Interventions

- • Observe for factors causing or contributing to conflict (e.g., value conflicts, fear of outcome, poor problem-solving skills).
- • Work with and allow the client to make decisions in a way that is comfortable for the client, such as deferring (allowing others to decide), delaying (choosing an alternative that meets basic requirements), or deliberating (looking at all alternatives).
- • Give the client time and permission to express feelings associated with decision making.
- • Demonstrate reassurance with unconditional respect for and acceptance of the client's values, spiritual beliefs, and cultural norms.

C

- ▲ Use decision aids or computer-based decision aid to assist clients in making decisions.
- ▲ Initiate health teaching and referrals when needed.
- • Facilitate communication between the client and family members regarding the final decision; offer support to the person actually making the decision.
- ▲ Provide detailed information on benefits and risks using functional terms and probabilities tailored to clinical risk, plus steps for considering the issues and means for making a decision, including values clarification and decision aids, when clients are faced with difficult treatment choices.
- ▲ Encourage client to communicate values, beliefs, goals, life plans and the ultimate decision with other healthcare providers, as appropriate.

Geriatric

- • Carefully assess clients with dementia regarding ability to make decisions.
- • If end-of-life discussions are being avoided, nurses are in a better position than any other health team member to facilitate discussions of healthcare choices among older adults and their family members.
- ▲ Discuss the purpose of a living will and advance directives.
- ▲ Discuss choices or changes to be made (e.g., moving in with children, into a nursing home, or into an adult foster care home).

Multicultural

- • Assess for the influence of cultural beliefs, norms, and values on the client's decision-making conflict.
- • Identify who will be involved in the decision-making process.
- • Use cross-cultural decision aids whenever possible to enhance an informed decision-making process.
- • Provide support for client's decision making.

Home Care

- • The interventions described previously may be adapted for home care use.
- ▲ Before providing any home care, assess the client plan for advance directives (living will and power of attorney). If a plan

C

exists, place a copy in the client file. If no plan exists, offer information on advance directives according to agency policy. Refer for assistance in completing advance directives as necessary. Do not witness a living will.

- • Assess the client and family for consensus (or lack thereof) regarding the issue in conflict. When the conflict involves end-of-life decisions, work to shift the client's and family's expectations from curative to palliative.
- • Refer to the care plan for **Anxiety** as indicated.

Client/Family Teaching

- ▲ Instruct the client and family members to provide advance directives in the following areas:
  - ■ Person to contact in an emergency
  - ■ Preference (if any) to die at home or in the hospital
  - ■ Desire to sign a living will
  - ■ Desire to donate an organ
  - ■ Funeral arrangements (i.e., burial, cremation)
- ▲ Inform the family of treatment options; encourage and defend self-determination.
- • Identify reasons for family decisions regarding care. Explore ways in which family decisions can be respected.
- • Recognize and allow the client to discuss the selection of complementary therapies available, such as spiritual support, relaxation, imagery, exercise, lifestyle changes, diet (e.g., macrobiotic, vegetarian), and nutritional supplementation.
- ▲ Provide the Physician Orders for Life-Sustaining Treatment (POLST) form for clients and families faced with end-of-life choices across the healthcare continuum.

Parental role Conflict

NANDA Definition

Parent's experience of role confusion and conflict in response to crisis

Defining Characteristics

Anxiety; demonstrated disruption in caretaking routines; expresses concern about perceived loss of control over decisions relating to their child; fear; parent(s) express(es) concern(s) about changes in parental role; parent(s) express(es) concern(s) about family (e.g., functioning, communication, health); parent(s) express(es) concerns(s) of inadequacy to provide for child's needs (e.g., physical, emotional); parent(s) express(es) feeling(s) of inadequacy to provide for child's needs (e.g., physical, emotional); reluctant to participate in usual caretaking activities even with encouragement and support; verbalizes feelings of frustration; verbalizes feelings of guilt

Related Factors (r/t)

Change in marital status; home care of a child with special needs; interruptions of family life due to home care regimen (e.g., treatments, caregivers, lack of respite); intimidation with invasive modalities (e.g., intubation); intimidation with restrictive modalities (e.g., isolation); separation from child due to chronic illness; specialized care center

Client Outcomes

Client Will (Specify Time Frame):

- Express feelings and perceptions regarding impacts of illness, disability, and/or hospitalization on parental role
- Participate in hospital and home care as much as able given the availability of resources and support systems
- Exhibit assertiveness and responsibility in active family decision making regarding care of the child
- Describe and select available resources to support parental management of the child's and family's needs

Nursing Interventions

- • Assess and support parents' previous coping behaviors.
- • Explore parent/family sources of stress, usual methods of coping, and perceptions of illness/condition. Capitalize on the strengths identified.
- • Evaluate the family's perceived strength of its social support system. Encourage the family to use social support to increase its resiliency and to moderate stress.
- • Determine the older-than-average mother's support systems and self-expectations for motherhood.
- • Consider the use of family theory as a framework to help guide interventions (e.g., family stress theory, role theory, social exchange theory).

- • Be available to discuss concerns and be a good listener.
- ▲ Sustain parental involvement in shared decision making with regard to care by using the following steps: Incorporate parents' information concerning the child's typical routines, behaviors, fears, likes, and dislikes; provide clear and direct firsthand information concerning the child's condition and progress; normalize the home/hospital environment as much as possible; collaborate in care by providing choices when possible.
- • Seek and support parental participation in care.
- • Provide support for each parent's primary coping strategies.
- ▲ Offer respite care to assist parents in maintaining sufficient energy and personal resources to continue caregiving responsibilities.
- • Encourage the parent to meet his or her own needs for rest, nutrition, and hygiene. Provide facilities so that the parent may stay with the sick child (e.g., cot, reclining chair).
- • Provide family-centered care. Demonstrate safe places where the parent may touch or stroke the child. Encourage the parent to talk or sing to the child. Adjust equipment so that the parent is able to hold the child, and provide a comfortable chair, preferably a rocking chair. Provide opportunities and offer praise for successful caregiving.
- ▲ Refer parents to available telephone counseling services.
- ▲ Support young grandmothers of teen mothers in areas of mother-daughter conflict such as child-rearing decisions, time with friends, household chores, and teens' choices/priorities with appropriate community referrals.

Multicultural

- • Acknowledge racial/ethnic differences at the onset of care.
- • Assess for the influence of cultural beliefs, norms, and values on the client's perceptions of the parental role.
- • Acknowledge that value conflicts arising from acculturation stresses may contribute to increased anxiety and significant conflict with the parental role.
- • Promote the female parenting role by providing a treatment environment that is culturally based and woman-centered.

Home Care

- • The interventions described previously may be adapted for home care use.

C

- Assess family adjustment prenatally and postpartum; assist new parents to renegotiate behavior around issues such as amount of time spent together, sexual relationship, resolution of disagreements, and provision of sufficient time for leisure/recreational activities. Encourage the father to take an active role in infant care.

▲ Assess interference with family functioning. Refer for family counseling as indicated.

Client/Family Teaching

- Furnish clear explanations and answer questions about condition, disease or disability, associated treatments, and prognosis.
- For parents with medically fragile and developmentally disabled children, support the family's way of coping in addition to "normalization."

▲ Refer parents of children with behavioral problems to parenting programs.

▲ Involve parents in formal and/or informal social support situations, such as internet support groups.

▲ Teach the client about available community resources (e.g., therapists, ministers, counselors, self-help groups).

▲ Encourage parents with human immunodeficiency virus/acquired immune deficiency syndrome (HIV/AIDS) to implement custody plans for their children.

Acute Confusion

NANDA Definition

Abrupt onset of reversible disturbances of consciousness attention, cognition, and perception that develop over a short period of time

Defining Characteristics

Fluctuation in cognition; level of consciousness; psychomotor activity; hallucinations; increased agitation; increased restlessness; lack of motivation to follow through with goal-directed behavior; lack of motivation to follow through with purposeful behavior; lack of motivation to initiate goal-directed behavior; lack of motivation to initiate purposeful behavior; misperceptions

Related Factors (r/t)

Alcohol abuse; delirium; dementia; drug abuse; fluctuation in sleep-wake cycle; over 60 years of age; polypharmacy

C

Client Outcomes

Client Will (Specify Time Frame):

- Demonstrate restoration of cognitive status to baseline
- Obtain adequate amount of sleep
- Demonstrate appropriate motor behavior
- Maintain functional capacity
- Optimize hydration and nutrition

Nursing Interventions

- • Assess the client's behavior and cognition systematically and continually throughout the day and night, as appropriate.
- • Perform an accurate mental status examination that includes the following:
  - ■ Overall appearance, manner, and attitude
  - ■ Behavior characteristics and level of psychomotor behavior
  - ■ Mood and affect (presence of suicidal or homicidal ideation as observed by others and reported by the client)
  - ■ Insight and judgment
  - ■ Cognition as evidenced by level of consciousness, orientation (to time, place, and person), thought process, and content (perceptual disturbances such as illusions and hallucinations, paranoia, delusions, abstract thinking)
  - ■ Level of attention
- ▲ Assess for and report possible physiological alterations (e.g., sepsis, hypoglycemia, hypoxia, hypotension, infection, changes in temperature, fluid and electrolyte imbalance, use of medications with known cognitive and psychotropic side effects).
- ▲ Treat the underlying causes of delirium in collaboration with the healthcare team: Establish/maintain normal fluid and electrolyte balance; establish/maintain normal nutrition, normal body temperature, normal oxygenation (if the client experiences low oxygen saturation, deliver supplemental oxygen), normal blood glucose levels, normal blood pressure.
- ▲ Communicate client status, cognition, and behavioral manifestations to all necessary providers.

- ■ Monitor for any trends occurring in these manifestations of delirium.

▲ Laboratory results should be closely monitored and physiological support given as appropriate.
- Establish or maintain elimination patterns.
- Plan care that allows for an appropriate sleep-wake cycle.

▲ Conduct a medication review.
- Modulate sensory exposure and establish a calm environment.
- Provide reality orientation, including identifying self by name at each contact with the client; calling the client by their preferred name; using orientation techniques; providing familiar objects from home such as an afghan; providing clocks, calendars; and gently correcting misperceptions.
- Avoid use of validation therapy with the confused client, other than to validate the feelings the client may be expressing.
- Use appropriate communication techniques for clients at risk for confusion including communicating clearly and providing simple explanations as needed.
- Provide supportive nursing care including meeting of basic needs such as feeding, toileting, and hydration.

▲ Identify, evaluate, and treat pain quickly (see care plans for **Acute Pain** or **Chronic Pain**).

▲ Facilitate appropriate sensory input by having clients use aids (e.g., glasses, hearing aids) as needed.

▲ Recognize that delirium is frequently treated with an antipsychotic medication. Watch for side effects of the medications.

Geriatric

- Mobilize the client as soon as possible; provide active and passive range of motion.

▲ Evaluate all medications for potential to cause or exacerbate delirium. Review the Beers Criteria for Potentially Inappropriate Medication Use in Elderly.

▲ Provide sufficient medication to relieve pain.
- Explain hospital routines and procedures slowly and in simple terms; repeat information as necessary.
- Provide continuity of care when possible (e.g., provide the same caregivers, avoid room changes).
- If clients know that they are not thinking clearly, acknowledge the concern.

- Keep the client's sleep-wake cycle as normal as possible (e.g., avoid letting the client take daytime naps, avoid waking the client at night, give sedatives but not diuretics at bedtime, provide pain relief and back rubs).
- Maintain normal sleep-wake patterns (treat with bright light for 2 hours in the early evening).

Home Care

- Some of the interventions described previously may be adapted for home care use.
- Assess and monitor for acute changes in cognition and behavior.
- Recognize that delirium is reversible but can become chronic if untreated. The client may be discharged from the hospital to home care in a state of undiagnosed delirium.
- Assess for treatable causes of changes in cognition and behavior. The mnemonic DEMENTIA can be used to remember potential causes of acute or chronic confusion:
  - **D:** Drugs and alcohol—including over-the-counter drugs
  - **E:** Eyes and ears—disorientation due to visual/auditory distortion
  - **M:** Medical disorders—e.g., diabetes, hypothyroidism
  - **E:** Emotional and psychological disturbances—e.g., mood or paranoid disorders
  - **N:** Neurological disorders—e.g., multi-infarct dementia
  - **T:** Tumors and trauma
  - **I:** Infections—e.g., urinary tract or upper respiratory tract
  - **A:** Arteriosclerosis—leading to heart failure, insufficient blood supply to heart and brain, confusion
- Assess fluid intake, dementia status, and occurrence of a fall within the past 30 days in evaluating confusion.
- Avoid preconceptions about the source of acute confusion; assess each occurrence on the basis of available evidence.

▲ Institute case management of frail elderly clients to support continued independent living, if possible, once delirium has resolved.

Client/Family Teaching

▲ Teach the family to recognize signs of early confusion and seek medical help.

- Counsel the client and family regarding the management of delirium and its sequelae.

Chronic Confusion

NANDA Definition

Irreversible, long-standing, and/or progressive deterioration of intellect and personality characterized by decreased ability to interpret environmental stimuli; decreased capacity for intellectual thought processes; and manifested by disturbances of memory, orientation, and behavior

Defining Characteristics

Altered interpretation; altered personality; altered response to stimuli; clinical evidence of organic impairment; impaired long-term memory; impaired short-term memory; impaired socialization; long-standing cognitive impairment; no change in level of consciousness; progressive cognitive impairment

Related Factors (r/t)

Alzheimer's disease; cerebral vascular attack; head injury; Korsakoff's psychosis; multi-infarct dementia

Client Outcomes

Client Will (Specify Time Frame):

- Remain content and free from harm
- Function at maximal cognitive level
- Participate in activities of daily living at the maximum of functional ability
- Have minimal episodes of agitation since agitation occurs in up to 70% of patients with dementia

Nursing Interventions

- Determine the client's cognitive level using a screening tool such as the Mini-Mental State Exam (MMSE). The Mini-Cog is also a useful screening tool to be used in a busy setting.
- Gather information about the client's predementia cognitive functioning.
- Assess the client for signs of depression: insomnia, poor appetite, flat affect, and withdrawn behavior.
- Determine client's normal routines and attempt to maintain them.

- Begin each interaction with the client by identifying yourself and calling the client by name. Approach the client with a caring, loving, and accepting attitude, and speak calmly and slowly.
- Use a calm approach in interactions and use reminiscence therapy and validation (validating what the clients say is real instead of correcting them).
- Provide scheduled activities that are matched to the client's abilities and personality.
- Provide periods of rest along with periods of activities.
- Give one simple direction at a time and repeat it as necessary. Use verbal and physical prompts, and model the desired action if needed and possible.
- Break down self-care tasks into simple steps (e.g., instead of saying, "Take a shower," say to the client, "Please follow me. Sit down on the bed. Take off your shoes. Now take off your socks.").
- Engage the client in communication by individualizing the nurse's interactions to maximize client interaction and response.
- For anxious clients who are having problems relaxing enough to eat, try having them listen to music during meals.
- Assess the cause of and consequences of wandering before attempting to control the wandering.
- For individuals who have wandering behavior, individualize interventions such as those that provide a safe environment with physical barriers to exits, safe walking paths, and a daily schedule of activities. See the care plan for **Wandering.**
- Use symbols rather than words to identify areas such as the bathroom or kitchen. Utilize environmental cues such as clocks and a sign with mealtimes to decrease common mealtime questions and thus decrease agitation around mealtimes.
- Set up scheduled quiet periods in a recliner or room. Use afghans and environmental cues to define rest periods.
- Provide structured social and physical activities that are individualized for the client.
- Provide quiet activities such as listening to music of the client's preference or introduce other cues that promote relaxation in the afternoon or early evening.
- Provide simple activities for the client, such as folding washcloths and sorting or stacking activities or other hobbies the individual enjoyed prior to the onset of dementia.

- • Use cues, such as picture boards denoting day, time, and location, to help client with orientation.
- • Use reminiscence and life review therapeutic interventions; ask questions about the client's work, children, or time spent in military service. Ask questions such as, "What was really important to you as you look back?" to engage the client in storytelling.
- ▲ If the client becomes increasingly confused and agitated, perform the following steps:
  - ■ Assess the client for physiological causes, including acute hypoxia, pain, medication effects, malnutrition, infections such as urinary tract infection, fatigue, electrolyte disturbances, and constipation.
  - ■ Assess for psychological causes, including changes in the environment, caregiver, and routine; demands to perform beyond capacity; or multiple competing stimuli, including discomfort.
  - ■ In clients with agitated behaviors, rather than confronting the client, provide diversional behaviors such as singing, games, and the provision of textured items to handle.
- • Decrease stimuli in the environment (e.g., turn off the television, take the client to a quiet place). Institute activities associated with pleasant emotions, such as playing soft music the client likes, looking through a photo album, providing favorite food, or using simulated presence therapy.
- • If clients with dementia become more agitated, assess for pain.
- • Avoid using restraints if at all possible.
- ▲ Use PRN or low-dose regular dosing of psychotropic or antianxiety drugs only as a last resort. They can be effective in managing symptoms of psychosis and aggressive behavior, but have undesirable side effects. Start with the lowest possible dose.
- ▲ Avoid the use of anticholinergic medications such as Benadryl.
- • For predictable difficult times, such as during bathing and grooming, try the following:
  - ■ Massage the client's hands lovingly or use therapeutic touch to relax the client.
  - ■ When bathing a client with dementia, minimize the client's discomfort by using the Bag Bath (if available).
  - ■ Approach the client in a client-centered framework as this offers a sense of control and promotes self-esteem.
  - ■ Involve family in care of the client.

C

- For care of early dementia clients with primarily symptoms of memory loss, see the care plan for **Impaired Memory.**
- For care of clients with self-care deficits, see the appropriate care plan **(Feeding Self-care deficit; Dressing/grooming Self-care deficit;** and **Toileting Self-care deficit).**

Geriatric

NOTE: All interventions are appropriate with geriatric clients.

Multicultural

- Assess for the influence of cultural beliefs, norms, and values on the family's or caregiver's understanding of chronic confusion or dementia.
- Inform the client's family or caregiver of the meaning of and reasons for common behavior observed in clients with dementia.
- Assist the family or caregiver in identifying barriers that would prevent the use of social services or other supportive services that could help reduce the impact of caregiving.
- Assess the client for the presence of an instrumental activity of daily living (IADL) disability and chronic health conditions.
- ▲ Refer the family to social services or other supportive services to assist in meeting the demands of caregiving for the client with dementia.
- ▲ Encourage the family to make use of support groups or other service programs.
- Validate the family members' feelings with regard to the impact of the client's behavior on family lifestyle.

NOTE: Black and Latino community-dwelling clients with moderate to severe dementia have a higher prevalence of dementia-related behaviors than Caucasian clients. Therefore, as the aging minority population grows, it will be especially important to target caregiver education, in-home support, and resources to minority communities.

Home Care

NOTE: Keeping the client as independent as possible is important. Because community-based care is usually less structured than institutional care; however, in the home setting the goal of maintaining safety for the client takes on primary importance.

- The interventions described previously may be adapted for home care use.

- ▲ Provide information to the family and home care client regarding advanced directives.
- • Assess the client's memory and executive function deficits before assuming the inability to make any medical decisions.
- ▲ Assess the home for safety features and client needs for assistive devices. Refer to the interventions for **Feeding Self-care deficit, Dressing Self-care deficit,** and **Bathing Self-care deficit** as needed.
- • Elements of reality orientation therapy may be applied in the home, incorporating person-centered respect, reminiscence, validation, and sensory-motor stimulation.
- ▲ Provide education and support to the family of the client with a chronic and disabling condition; be prepared to offer support and information to family members who live at a distance as well.
- • Use familiar aspects of the environment (smells, music, foods, pictures) to cue the client, capitalizing on habit to remind the client of activities in which the client can participate (e.g., cooperating with medication administration).
- • Instruct the caregiver to provide a balanced activity schedule that does not stress the client nor deprive him or her of stimulation; avoid sustained low- or high-stimulation activity.
- ▲ If the client will require extensive supervision on an ongoing basis, evaluate the client for day care programs. Refer the family to medical social services to assist with this process if necessary.
- • Encourage the family to include the client in family activities when possible. Reinforce the use of therapeutic communication guidelines (see Client/Family Teaching) and sensitivity to the number of people present.
- • Assess family caregivers for caregiver stress, loneliness, and depression.
- • Refer to the care plan for **Caregiver role strain.**
- ▲ Refer the client to medical social services as necessary to evaluate financial resources and initiate benefits or access to providers.
- ▲ Institute case management for frail elderly clients to support continued independent living.

Client/Family Teaching

- • In the early stages of confusion (e.g., initial period following stroke), provide the caregiver with information on illness processes, needed care, and likely trajectory of progress.

C

- Teach the family how to converse with a memory-impaired person. Individuals with dementia have a variety of communication difficulties.
- Teach the family how to provide physical care for the client (bathing, feeding, and ADLs).
- Instruct the family and care providers that faith, humor, patience, and contact with friends and family have been identified as positive approaches in keeping a client with dementia engaged in their care.
- Discuss with the family what to expect as the dementia progresses.

▲ Counsel the family about resources available regarding end-of-life decisions and legal concerns.

▲ Inform the family that as dementia progresses, hospice care may be available in the home in the terminal stages to help the caregiver.

NOTE: The nursing diagnoses **Impaired Environmental interpretation syndrome** and **Chronic Confusion** are very similar in definition and interventions. **Impaired Environmental interpretation syndrome** must be interpreted as a syndrome when other nursing diagnoses would also apply. **Chronic Confusion** may be interpreted as the human response to a situation or situations that require a level of cognition of which the individual is no longer capable. Further research is underway to make this distinction clear to the practicing nurse.

Risk for acute Confusion

NANDA Definition

At risk for reversible disturbances of consciousness, attention, cognition, and perception that develop over a short period of time

Risk Factors

Alcohol use; decreased mobility; decreased restraints; dementia; fluctuation in sleep-wake cycle; history of stroke; impaired cognition; infection; male gender; medication/drugs: anesthesia, anticholinergics, diphenhydramine, multiple medications, opioids, psychoactive drugs; metabolic abnormalities: azotemia, decreased hemoglobin, dehydration, electrolyte imbalances, increased BUN/creatine; malnutrition; over 60 years of age; pain; sensory deprivation; substance abuse; urinary retention

Client Outcomes

Client Will (Specify Time Frame):

- Demonstrate restoration of cognitive status to baseline
- Obtain adequate amount of sleep
- Demonstrate appropriate motor behavior
- Maintain functional capacity
- Optimize hydration and nutrition

Nursing Interventions

See the nursing interventions for **Acute Confusion.**

Constipation

NANDA Definition

Decrease in normal frequency of defecation, accompanied by difficult or incomplete passage of stool and/or passage of excessively hard, dry stool

Defining Characteristics

Abdominal pain; abdominal tenderness with palpable muscle resistance; abdominal tenderness without palpable muscle resistance; anorexia; atypical presentations in older adults (e.g., change in mental status, urinary incontinence, unexplained falls, elevated body temperature); borborygmi; bright red blood with stool; change in bowel pattern; decreased frequency; decreased volume of stool; distended abdomen; feeling of rectal fullness; feeling of rectal pressure; generalized fatigue; hard; formed stool; headache; hyperactive bowel sounds; hypoactive bowel sounds; increased abdominal pressure; indigestion; nausea; oozing liquid stool; palpable abdominal mass; palpable rectal mass; presence of soft; paste-like stool in rectum; percussed abdominal dullness; pain with defecation; severe flatus; straining with defecation; unable to pass stool; vomiting

Related Factors (r/t)

Functional

Abdominal muscle weakness; habitual denial; habitual ignoring of urge to defecate; inadequate toileting (e.g., timeliness, positioning for defecation, privacy); irregular defecation habits; insufficient physical activity; recent environmental changes

Psychological
Depression; emotional stress; mental confusion

Pharmacological
Aluminum containing antiacids; anticholinergics; anticonvulsants; antidepressants; antilipemic agents; bismuth salts; calcium carbonate; calcium channel blockers; diuretics; iron salts; laxative overuse use; nonsteroidal anti-inflammatory drugs; opiates; phenothiazines; sedatives; sympathomimetics

Mechanical
Electrolyte imbalance; hemorrhoids; Hirschsprung's disease; neurological impairment; obesity; postsurgical obstruction; pregnancy; prostate enlargement; rectal abscess; rectal anal fissures; rectal anal stricture; rectal prolapse; rectal ulcer; rectocele; tumors

Physiological
Change in eating patterns; change in usual foods; decreased motility of gastrointestinal tract; dehydration; inadequate dentition; inadequate oral hygiene; insufficient fiber intake; insufficient fluid intake; poor eating habits

Client Outcomes

Client Will (Specify Time Frame):
- Maintain passage of soft, formed stool every 1 to 3 days without straining
- State relief from discomfort of constipation
- Identify measures that prevent or treat constipation

Nursing Interventions

- Assess usual pattern of defecation, including time of day, amount and frequency of stool, consistency of stool; history of bowel habits or laxative use; diet, including fiber and fluid intake; exercise patterns; personal remedies for constipation; obstetrical/gynecological history; surgeries; diseases that affect bowel motility; alterations in perianal sensation; present bowel regimen.

C

- • Have the client or family keep a diary of bowel habits using a Management of Constipation Assessment Inventory, including information such as time of day; usual stimulus; consistency, amount, and frequency of stool; fluid consumption; and use of any aids to defecation.
- ▲ Review the client's current medications.
- ▲ If the client is receiving temporary opioids (e.g., for acute postoperative pain), request an order for routine stool softeners from the primary care practitioner, monitor bowel movements, and request a laxative if the client develops constipation. If the client is receiving round-the-clock opiates (e.g., for palliative care), request an order for Senokot-S and institute a bowel regimen.
- • If new onset of constipation, determine if the client has recently stopped smoking.
- • Palpate for abdominal distention, percuss for dullness, and auscultate bowel sounds.
- ▲ Check for impaction; if present, perform digital removal per physician's order.
- ▲ If the client is uncomfortable or in pain due to constipation or has acute or chronic constipation that does not respond to increased fiber, fluid, activity, and appropriate toileting, refer the client to the primary care practitioner for an evaluation of bowel function and health status.
- • Encourage fiber intake of 20 g/day (for adults), ensuring that the fiber is palatable to the individual and that fluid intake is adequate. Add fiber gradually to decrease bloating and flatus.
- ▲ Use a mixture of bran cereal, applesauce, and prune juice; begin administration in small amounts and gradually increase amount. Keep refrigerated. Always check with the primary care practitioner before initiating this intervention. It is important that the client also ingest sufficient fluids.
- • Provide prunes or prune juice daily.
- ▲ If client would prefer to increase fiber intake using a pill, recommend that client use a tablet that contains methylcellulose. See fluid intake below.
- • Encourage a fluid intake of 1.5 to 2 L/day (six to eight glasses of liquids per day), unless contraindicated because of renal insufficiency.
- • Encourage clients to resume walking and activities of daily living as soon as possible if their mobility has been restricted.

C

Encourage turning and changing positions in bed, lifting the hips off the bed, performing range-of-motion exercises, alternately lifting each knee to the chest, doing wheelchair lifts, doing waist twists, stretching the arms away from the body, and pulling in the abdomen while taking deep breaths.

• Ask clients when they normally have a bowel movement and assist them to the bathroom at that same time every day to establish regular elimination. An optimal time for many individuals is 30 minutes after breakfast because of the gastrocolic reflex.
• Provide privacy for defecation. If not contraindicated, help the client to the bathroom and close the door.
• Help clients onto a bedside commode or toilet so they can either squat or lean forward while sitting.
• Teach clients to respond promptly to the defecation urge.
▲ Provide laxatives, suppositories, and enemas only as needed if other more natural interventions are not effective, and as ordered only; establish a client goal of eliminating their use.
• When giving large-volume enema solutions (e.g., soapsuds or tap water enemas), measure the amount of fluid given and the amount expelled, especially when giving repeated enemas. Use a low concentration of Castile soap in the soapsuds enema.

Geriatric

• Explain the importance of adequate fiber intake, fluid intake, activity, and established toileting routines to ensure soft, formed stool.
• Determine the client's perception of normal bowel elimination; promote adherence to a regular schedule.
• Explain Valsalva maneuver and the reason it should be avoided.
• Respond quickly to the client's call for help with toileting.
• Avoid regular use of enemas in the elderly.
▲ Use opioids cautiously. If they are ordered, use stool softeners and bran mixtures to prevent constipation.
• Position the client on the toilet or commode and place a small footstool under the feet.

Home Care

• The interventions described previously may be adapted for home care use.
• Take complaints seriously and evaluate claims of constipation in

a matter-of-fact manner. Refer to the care plan for **Perceived Constipation.**

- • Assess the self-care management activities the client is already using.
- ▲ The following treatment recommendations have been offered:
  - ■ Acknowledge the client's lifelong experience of bowel function; respect beliefs, attitudes, and preferences, and avoid patronizing responses.
  - ■ Make available comprehensive, useful written information about constipation and possible solutions.
  - ■ Make available empathetic and accessible professional care to provide treatment and advice; a multidisciplinary approach (including physician, nurse, and pharmacist) should be used.
  - ■ Institute a bowel management program.
  - ■ Consider affordability when suggesting solutions to constipation; discuss cost-saving strategies.
  - ■ Discuss a range of solutions to constipation and allow the client to choose the preferred options.
- ▲ Have orders in place for a suppository and enema as the need may occur.
- • Although the use of a bedside commode may be necessitated by the client's condition, allow the client to use the toilet in the bathroom when possible and provide assistance.
- • In older clients, routinely advise consumption of fluids, fruits, and vegetables as part of the diet, and ambulation if the client is able. Introduce a bowel management program at the first sign of constipation.
- ▲ Refer for consideration of the use of polyethylene glycol 3350 (PEG-3350) for constipation.
- • Advise the client against attempting to remove impacted feces on his or her own.
- • When using a bowel program, establish a pattern that is very regular and allows the client to be part of the family unit.

Client/Family Teaching

- • Instruct the client on normal bowel function and the need for adequate fluid and fiber intake, activity, and a defined toileting pattern in a bowel program.
- • Encourage the client to heed defecation warning signs and

C

develop a regular schedule of defecation by using a stimulus such as a warm drink or prune juice.
- Encourage the client to avoid long-term use of laxatives and enemas and to gradually withdraw from their use if they are used regularly.
- If not contraindicated, teach the client how to do bent-leg sit-ups to increase abdominal tone; also encourage the client to contract the abdominal muscles frequently throughout the day. Help the client develop a daily exercise program to increase peristalsis.

Perceived Constipation

NANDA Definition

Self-diagnosis of constipation and abuse of laxatives, enemas, and suppositories to ensure a daily bowel movement

Defining Characteristics

Expectation of a daily bowel movement; expectation of passage of stool at same time every day; overuse of laxatives; overuse of enemas; overuse of suppositories

Related Factors (r/t)

Cultural health beliefs; family health beliefs; faulty appraisals; impaired thought processes

Client Outcomes

Client Will (Specify Time Frame):

- Regularly defecate soft, formed stool without using any aids
- Explain the need to decrease or eliminate the use of stimulant laxatives, suppositories, and enemas
- Identify alternatives to stimulant laxatives, enemas, and suppositories for ensuring defecation
- Explain that defecation does not have to occur every day

Nursing Interventions

- Have the client keep a diary of bowel habits using a Management of Constipation Assessment Inventory, including information such as time of day; usual stimulus; consistency, amount, and frequency of stool; fluid consumption; and use of any aids to defecation.

- • Determine the client's perception of an appropriate defecation pattern.
- • Monitor the use of laxatives, suppositories, or enemas and suggest replacing them with increased fiber intake along with increased fluids to 2 L/day.
- • Encourage fiber intake of 20 g/day (for adults), ensuring that the fiber is palatable to the individual and that fluid intake is adequate. Add fiber gradually to decrease bloating and flatus.
- ▲ Use a mixture of bran cereal, applesauce, and prune juice; begin administration in small amounts and gradually increase amount. Keep refrigerated. Always check with the primary care practitioner before initiating this intervention. It is important that the client also ingest sufficient fluids.
- • Teach clients to respond promptly to the defecation urge.
- ▲ If the client is uncomfortable or in pain due to constipation or has chronic constipation that does not respond to increased fiber and fluid intake, activity, and appropriate toileting, refer the client to a gastroenterologist for an evaluation of bowel function and health status.
- ▲ Obtain a dietary referral for analysis of the client's diet and input on how to improve the diet to ensure adequate fiber intake and nutrition.
- ▲ Assess for signs of depression, other psychological disorders, and a history of physical or sexual abuse.
- • Encourage the client to increase activity, walking for at least 30 minutes at least 5 days a week as tolerated.
- ▲ Observe for the presence of an eating disorder or the use of laxatives to control or decrease weight; refer for counseling if needed.

Home Care

- • The interventions described previously may be adapted for home care use.
- • Take complaints seriously and evaluate claims of constipation in a matter-of-fact manner.
- • Obtain family and client histories of bowel or other patterned behavior problems.

C

- Observe family cultural patterns related to eating and bowel habits.
- Encourage a mindset and program of self-care management. Elicit from the client the self-talk he or she uses to describe body perceptions; correct fatalistic interpretations.
- Instruct the client in a healthy lifestyle that supports normal bowel function (e.g., activity, fluid intake, diet) and encourage progressive inclusion of these elements into daily activities.
- Discuss the client's self-image. Help the client to reframe the self-concept as capable.
- Instruct the client and family in appropriate expectations for having bowel movements.
- Offer instruction and reassurance regarding explanations for variation from the previous pattern of bowel movements.
- Contract with the client and/or a responsible family member regarding the use of laxatives. Have the client maintain a bowel pattern diary. Observe for diarrhea or frequent evacuation.

▲ Teach the family to carry out the bowel program per the physician's orders.

▲ Refer for home health aide services to assist with personal care, including the bowel program, if appropriate.

- Identify a contingency plan for bowel care if the client is dependent on outside persons for such care.

Client/Family Teaching

- Explain normal bowel function and the necessary ingredients for a regular bowel regimen (e.g., fluid, fiber, activity, and regular schedule for defecation).
- Work with the client and family to develop a diet that fits the client's lifestyle and includes increased fiber.
- Teach the client that it is not necessary to have daily bowel movements and that the passage of anywhere from three stools each day to three stools each week is considered normal.
- Explain to the client the harmful effects of the continual use of defecation aids such as laxatives and enemas.
- Encourage the client to gradually decrease the use of the usual laxatives and/or enemas, and recognize it may take months for the process to do it gradually.
- Determine a method of increasing the client's fluid intake and fit this practice into the client's lifestyle.

- Explain what Valsalva maneuver is and why it should be avoided.
- Work with the client and family to design a bowel-training routine that is based on previous patterns (before laxative or enema abuse) and incorporates the consumption of warm fluids, increased fiber, and increased fluids; privacy; and a predictable routine.

Additional Nursing Interventions and Client/Family Teaching

See care plan for **Constipation.**

Risk for Constipation

NANDA Definition

At risk for a decrease in normal frequency of defecation accompanied by difficult or incomplete passage of stool and/or passage of excessively hard, dry stool

Related Factors (r/t)

Functional

Habitual denial/ignoring urge to defecate; recent environmental changes; inadequate toileting (e.g., timeliness, positioning for defecation, privacy); irregular defecation habits; insufficient physical activity; abdominal muscle weakness

Psychological

Depression; emotional stress; mental confusion

Physiological

Change in usual eating patterns; change in usual foods; decreased motility of gastrointestinal tract; dehydration; inadequate dentition; inadequate oral hygiene; insufficient fiber intake; insufficient fluid intake; poor eating habits

Pharmacological

Aluminum containing antiacids; anticholinergics; anticonvulsants; antidepressants; antilipemic agents; bismuth salts; calcium carbonate;

calcium channel blockers; diuretics; iron salts; laxative overuse use; nonsteroidal anti-inflammatory drugs; opiates; phenothiazines; sedatives; and sympathomimetics

C

Mechanical

Electrolyte imbalance; hemorrhoids; Hirschsprung's disease; neurological impairment; obesity; postsurgical obstruction; pregnancy; prostate enlargement; rectal abscess; rectal anal fissures; rectal anal stricture; rectal prolapse; rectal ulcer; rectocele; tumors

Client Outcomes

Client Will (Specify Time Frame):

- Maintain passage of soft, formed stool every 1 to 3 days without straining
- Identify measures that prevent constipation
- Explain rationale for not using laxatives and enemas

Nursing Interventions and Client/Family Teaching

See care plan for **Constipation.**

Contamination

NANDA Definition

Exposure to environmental contaminants in doses sufficient to cause adverse health effects

Defining Characteristics

Pesticides, Chemicals, Biologicals

Cardiovascular: Cardiac dysrhythmia; hypertension; hypotension

Gastrointestinal: Stomachache; diarrhea; cramping; nausea; vomiting

Neuromuscular: Muscle weaknesses; joint and muscle aches; hallucinations; confusion; seizures; decreased level of consciousness; pupil changes; blurred vision

Respiratory: difficulty breathing; cough; flu symptoms; labored breathing; cyanosis

Skin: skin lesions (rash, pustules, scabs)

C

Radiation

History of exposure to radiation; pregnancies resulting in birth defects; weakness; fatigue; paresthesia; confusion; lethargy; changes to level of consciousness; skin irritation; itching; blistering; burns; erythema; dry or moist desquamation; ulceration; nausea; abdominal pain; diarrhea; visual changes; cataracts; irregular heartbeat; changes in the electrocardiogram; hypertension; labored breathing; cough; presence of skin cancer; thyroid cancer; leukemia; bone marrow suppression

Symptoms of radiation sickness: Weakness; hair loss; changes in blood chemistries; hemorrhage; diminished organ function

Waste

Nausea; abdominal cramps; anorexia; diarrhea; weight loss; jaundice; weakness; fever

Pollution

Difficulty breathing; lung irritation; chest pain; headaches; eye irritation; wheezing; shortness of breath; pulmonary or nasal congestion; developmental delay

Community

Measurement of contaminants exceeding acceptable levels; clusters of patients seeking care for similar signs or symptoms; large numbers of patients with rapidly fatal illnesses; presence of sick, dying, or dead animals or fish; absence of insects; unusual liquids, sprays, or vapors at work or home; anger over loss of security and safety; confusion related to trying to understand highly technical information; community conflict

Related Factors

Presence of bacteria, viruses, toxins, vectors; exposure to heavy metals or chemicals, atmospheric pollutants, radiation; concomitant or previous exposures; nutritional factors or dietary practices; pre-existing disease states; gender, occupation, history of smoking; developmental characteristics; gestational age during exposure; recent vaccinations; insufficient or absent use of decontamination protocol; no use of or inappropriate use of protective clothing; bioterrorism; flooding, earthquakes, or other natural disasters;

sewer line leaks; contamination of aquifers by septic tanks; intentional/accidental contamination of food and water supply; industrial plant emissions; discharge of contaminants by industries or businesses; physical factors: climactic conditions such as temperature, wind, geographic area; social factors: crowding, sanitation, poverty, personal and household hygiene practices, lack of access to health care; use of environmental contaminants in the home; playing in outdoor areas where environmental contaminants are present; community dynamics

Client Outcomes

Client Will (Specify Time Frame):

- Have minimal health effects associated with contamination
- Cooperate with appropriate decontamination protocol
- Participate in appropriate isolation precautions

Community Will (Specify Time Frame):

- Utilize health surveillance data system to monitor for contamination incidents
- Utilize disaster plan to evacuate and triage affected members
- Have minimal health effects associated with contamination

Nursing Interventions

- Help individuals cope with contamination incident by doing the following:
  - Use groups that have survived terrorist attacks as useful resource for victims
  - Provide accurate information on risks involved, preventive measures, use of antibiotics, and vaccines
  - Assist to deal with feelings of fear, vulnerability, and grief
  - Encourage individuals to talk to others about their fears
  - Assist victims to think positively and to move toward the future
- Triage, stabilize, transport, and treat affected community members.
- Utilize approved procedures for decontamination of persons, clothing, and equipment.
- Utilize appropriate isolation precautions: universal, airborne, droplet, and contact isolation.

- Monitor individual for therapeutic effects, side effects, and compliance with postexposure drug therapy.

▲ Collaborate with other agencies (local health department, emergency medical service [EMS], state and federal agencies).

Geriatric

- Help the client identify age-related factors that may affect response to contamination incidents.
- Encourage family members to acknowledge and validate the client's concerns.

Pediatric

- Provide environmental health hazard information.

Home Care

- Assess current environmental stressors and identify community resources.

Client/Family Teaching

- Provide truthful information to the person or family affected
- Discuss signs and symptoms of contamination
- Explain decontamination protocols
- Explain need for isolation procedures

Risk for Contamination

NANDA Definition

Accentuated risk of exposure to environmental contaminants in doses sufficient to cause adverse health effects

Risk Factors

Presence of bacteria, viruses, toxins, vectors; exposure to heavy metals or chemicals, atmospheric pollutants, radiation; concomitant or previous exposures; nutritional factors or dietary practices; pre-existing disease states; gender, occupation, history of smoking; developmental characteristics; gestational age during exposure; recent vaccinations; insufficient or absent use of decontamination protocol; no use of or inappropriate use of protective clothing; bioterrorism; flooding, earthquakes, or other natural disasters; sewer line leaks or contamination of aquifers by septic tanks; intentional/accidental contamination of food and water supply; industrial plant emissions; discharge of contaminants by industries or businesses

Physical factors: Climactic conditions such as temperature, wind; geographic area

Social factors: Crowding, sanitation, poverty, personal and household hygiene practices, lack of access to health care; use of environmental contaminants in the home; playing in outdoor areas where environmental contaminants are present; community dynamics

Client Outcomes

Client Will (Specify Time Frame):

- Remain free of adverse effects of contamination

Community Will (Specify Time Frame):

- Utilize health surveillance data system to monitor for contamination incidents
- Participate in mass casualty and disaster readiness drills
- Remain free of contamination-related health effects
- Minimize exposure to contaminants

Nursing Interventions

▲ Conduct surveillance for environmental contamination. Notify agencies authorized to protect the environment of contaminants in the area.

- Assist individuals to modify the environment to minimize risk or assist in relocating to safer environment.
- Schedule mass casualty and disaster readiness drills.
- Provide accurate information on risks involved, preventive measures, use of antibiotics, and vaccines.
- Assist to deal with feelings of fear and vulnerability.
- Assist with decontamination of persons, clothing, and equipment using approved procedure.
- Utilize appropriate isolation precautions: universal, airborne, droplet, and contact isolation.
- Monitor individual for therapeutic effects, side effects, and compliance with postexposure drug therapy.

▲ Collaborate with other agencies (local health department, emergency medical service [EMS], state and federal agencies.

Geriatric

- Help the client identify age-related factors that may affect response to contamination incidents.
- Encourage family members to acknowledge and validate the client's concerns.

Pediatric

- Provide environmental health hazard information relevant to children.

Home Care

- Assess current environmental stressors and identify community resources.

Client/Family Teaching

- Provide truthful information to the person or family
- Discuss signs and symptoms of contamination
- Explain decontamination protocols
- Explain need for isolation procedures

Compromised family Coping

NANDA Definition

Usually supportive primary person (family member or close friend) provides insufficient, ineffective, or compromised support, comfort, assistance, or encouragement that may be needed by the client to manage or master adaptive tasks related to his/her health challenge

Defining Characteristics

Objective

Significant person attempts assistive behaviors with unsatisfactory results; significant person attempts supportive behaviors with unsatisfactory results; significant person displays protective behavior disproportionate to client's abilities; significant person displays protective behavior disproportionate to client's need for autonomy; significant person enters into limited personal communication with client; significant person withdraws from client.

C

Subjective

Client expresses a complaint about significant other's response to health problem; client expresses a concern about significant other's response to health problem; significant person expresses an inadequate knowledge base, which interferes with effective supportive behaviors; significant person expresses an inadequate understanding, which interferes with supportive behaviors; significant person describes preoccupation with personal reaction (e.g., fear, anticipatory grief, guilt, anxiety) to client's need.

Related Factors (r/t)

Coexisting situations affecting the significant person; developmental crises the significant person may be facing; exhaustion of supportive capacity of significant people; inadequate information by a primary person; inadequate understanding of information by a primary person; incorrect information by a primary person; lack of reciprocal support; little support provided by client, in turn, for primary person; prolonged disease that exhausts supportive capacity of significant people; situational crises the significant person may be facing; temporary family disorganization; temporary family role changes; temporary preoccupation by a significant person

Client Outcomes

Family/Significant Person Will (Specify Time Frame):

- Verbalize internal resources to help deal with the situation
- Verbalize knowledge and understanding of illness, disability, or disease
- Provide support and assistance as needed
- Identify need for and seek outside support

Nursing Interventions

- Assess the strengths and deficiencies of the family system.
- Assess how family members interact with each other; observe verbal and nonverbal communication and individual and group responses to stress.
- Establish rapport with families by providing accurate communication.
- Consider the use of family theory as a framework to help guide interventions (e.g., family stress theory, role theory, social exchange theory, family systems theory).

- Help family members recognize the need for help and teach them how to ask for it.
- Encourage expression of positive thoughts and emotions.
- Encourage family members to verbalize feelings. Spend time with them, sit down and make eye contact, and offer coffee and other nourishment.
- Provide opportunities for families to discuss spirituality.
- Mothers may require additional support in their role of caring for chronically ill children.
- Provide privacy during family visits. If possible, maintain flexible visiting hours to accommodate more frequent family visits. If possible, arrange staff assignments so the same staff members have contact with the family. Familiarize other staff members with the situation in the absence of the usual staff member.
- Determine whether the family is suffering from additional stressors (e.g., child care issues, financial problems).
- ▲ Refer the family with ill family members to appropriate resources for assistance as indicated (e.g., counseling, psychotherapy, financial assistance, or spiritual support).

Pediatric

- Assess the adolescent's perception of support from family and friends during crisis.
- Provide educational interventions and psychosocial interventions such as coping skills training in treatment for families and their adolescents who have type 1 diabetes.
- Encourage the use of family rituals such as connection, spirituality, love, recreation, and celebration, especially in single-parent families.
- Encourage laughing, playing, singing, talking, and praying with seriously injured children.
- Staff should involve the family in decision-making processes, especially during hospital discharge planning.
- ▲ Link trained volunteers with "vulnerable" first-time parents. Provide social support and information related to age-appropriate expectations of infants.

Geriatric

- Perform a holistic assessment of all needs of informal spousal caregivers.

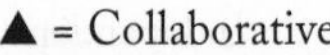

- • Help caregivers establish one's priorities and concentrate on them, believe in themselves and their ability to handle the situation, taking life one day at a time, looking for positive things in each situation, and relying on their own individual expertise and experience.
- ▲ Refer caregivers of clients with Alzheimer's disease to a monthly psychoeducational support group (i.e., the Alzheimer's Association).
- ▲ Consider the use of telephone support for caregivers of family members with dementia.
- • Assist in finding transportation to enable family members to visit or arrange alternate ways of maintaining contact.

Multicultural

- • Assess for the influence of cultural beliefs, norms, and values on the family's perceptions of coping.
- • Understand the importance of cultural beliefs and values the family may hold.
- • Acknowledge racial/ethnic differences at the onset of care.
- • Validate the family's feelings regarding the impact of the client's illness on the family's lifestyle.
- • Approach families of color with respect, warmth, and professional courtesy.
- • Provide rationale when assessing families with regard to sensitive issues.
- • Use a family-centered approach when working with Latino, Asian, African-American, and Native-American clients.

Home Care

- • The interventions described previously may be adapted for home care use.
- • Assess the reason behind the breakdown of family coping. Refer to the care plan for **Caregiver role strain.**
- ▲ Assess the needs of the caregiver in the home. Intervene to meet needs as appropriate, and explore all available resources that may be used to provide adequate home care (e.g., parish nursing as an effective adjunct, home health aide services to relieve the caregiver's fatigue).
- • During the time of compromised coping, increase visits to ensure the safety of the client, support of the family, and assis-

tance with coping strategies. Provide reassurance regarding expectations for prognosis as appropriate.

- • With a cancer client, encourage family discussion of stressors (including the meaning of the illness, fear of recurrence, the client's employment status) and resources (family social support).
- ▲ When a terminal illness is the precipitating factor for ineffective coping, offer hospice services and support groups as possible resources.
- ▲ If compromised family coping interferes with the ability to support the client's treatment plan, refer for psychiatric home healthcare services for family counseling and implementation of a therapeutic regimen.

Client/Family Teaching

- • Provide truthful information and support for the family and significant people regarding the client's specific illness or condition.
- ▲ Refer women with recurrent breast cancer and their family caregivers to a FOCUS Program (family involvement, optimistic attitude, coping effectiveness, uncertainty reduction, and symptom management), a family-based program of care.
- • Promote individual and family relaxation and stress-reduction strategies.
- ▲ Provide a parent support and education group to provide opportunities for parents to access support, learn new parenting skills, and, ultimately, optimize their relationships with their children in families of children in residential care.

Defensive Coping

NANDA Definition

Repeated projection of falsely positive self-evaluation based on a self-protective pattern that defends against underlying perceived threats to positive self-regard

Defining Characteristics

Denial of obvious problems; denial of obvious weaknesses; difficulty establishing relationships; difficulty maintaining relationships; diffi-

C

culty in perception of reality; difficulty in perception of reality testing; grandiosity; hostile laughter; hypersensitivity of criticism; hypersensitivity to slight; lack of follow-through in therapy; lack of follow-through in treatment; lack of participation in therapy; lack of participation in treatment; projection of blame; projection of responsibility; rationalization of failures; ridicule of others; superior attitude toward others

Client Outcomes

Client Will (Specify Time Frame):

- Acknowledge need for change in coping style
- Accept responsibility for own behavior
- Establish realistic goals with validation from caregivers
- Solicit caregiver validation in decision making

Nursing Interventions

- • Assess for the presence of denial as a coping mechanism.
- • Do not confront denial if its consequences are not a significant threat to health.
- • Ask appropriate questions to assess whether denial (defensive coping) is being used in association with alcoholism.
- • Develop a trusting, therapeutic relationship with the client and family.
- • Determine whether the client has a positive or negative overall appraisal of a given event.
- • Determine the client's perception of the problem and then provide reality-based examples of the true situation (e.g., witnesses to an accident, blood alcohol levels, problems caused by alcohol).
- • Help the client identify patterns of response in life that may be maladaptive.
- ▲ Promote the client's feelings of self-worth by using group or individual therapy, role playing, one-to-one interactions, and role modeling.
- • Support strengths and normal observations with "I note that" or "I want you to notice." Tell clients when they do something well.
- • Teach the client to use positive thinking by blocking negative thoughts with the word "Stop!" and inserting positive thoughts (e.g., "I'm a good [person, friend, student]").

- Provide feedback regarding others' perceptions of the client's behavior through group or milieu therapy or one-to-one interactions.
- Encourage the client to use "I" statements and to accept responsibility for and consequences of actions.
- Refer to the care plans for **Readiness for enhanced Coping, Ineffective Denial** and **Dysfunctional Family processes: alcoholism.**

Geriatric

- Assess the client for anger and identify previous outlets for anger.
- Assess the client for dementia or depression.
- ▲ It is essential to identify problems with alcohol in the elderly with the appropriate tools and make appropriate referrals.
- ▲ Encourage exercise for positive coping.
- If a traumatic event has occurred, support positive religious coping behaviors.

Multicultural

- Assess for the influence of cultural beliefs, norms, and values on the client's feelings of defensiveness.
- Acknowledge racial/ethnic differences at the onset of care.
- Use therapeutic communication techniques that emphasize acceptance, offer the self, validate the client's concerns, and convey respect.

Home Care

- The interventions described previously may be adapted for home care use.
- Observe family dynamics for dysfunctional and supportive communication.
- ▲ Refer to a mental health professional for possible psychodrama therapy, especially if the client experiences difficulty in coping with a traumatic event.
- ▲ If medical diagnoses coexist with defensive coping, confirm and validate the client's mental health plan and progress.

Client/Family Teaching

- ▲ Teach the client the actions and side effects of medications and the importance of taking them as prescribed, even when the client is feeling good.

▲ Work with the client's support group to identify harmful behaviors and to seek help for the client if he or she is unable to control behavior.
• Support family efforts using religious coping behaviors.

Disabled family Coping

NANDA Definition

Behavior of significant person (family member or other primary person) that disables his/her capacity and the client's capacity to effectively address tasks essential to either person's adaptation to the health challenge

Defining Characteristics

Abandonment; aggression; agitation; carrying on usual routines without regard for client's needs; client's development of dependence; depression; desertion; disregarding client's needs; distortion of reality regarding client's health problem; family behaviors that are detrimental to well-being; hostility; impaired individualization; impaired restructuring of a meaningful life for self; intolerance; neglectful care of client in regard to basic human needs; neglectful care of client in regard to illness treatment; neglectful relationships with other family members; prolonged overconcern for client; psychosomaticism; rejection; taking on illness signs of client

Related Factors (r/t)

Arbitrary handling of family's resistance to treatment; dissonant coping styles for dealing with adaptive tasks by the significant person and client; dissonant coping styles among significant people; highly ambivalent family relationships; significant person with pressed feelings (e.g., guilt, anxiety, hostility, despair)

Client Outcomes

Family/Significant Person Will (Specify Time Frame):

- Express realistic understanding and expectations of the client
- Participate positively in the client's care within the limits of his or her abilities
- Identify responses that are harmful

- Acknowledge and accept the need for assistance with circumstances
- Express feelings openly, honestly, and appropriately

C

Nursing Interventions

Refer to care plan **Compromised family Coping** for additional interventions

- • Identify current behaviors of family members, such as withdrawal (e.g., not visiting, briefly visiting, ignoring client when visiting), anger and hostility toward the client and others, or expression of guilt.
- • Note other stressors in the family (e.g., financial, job-related).
- ▲ Evaluate the family's perceived strength of its social support system. Encourage the family to use social support to increase its resiliency and to moderate stress.
- ▲ Observe for any symptoms of elder or child abuse or neglect Prompt reporting of abuse according to local and state law is necessary.
- • Encourage family members to spend time with the client and to assist in care when possible. Support thoughts for positive outcome when possible.
- ▲ Encourage family members to participate in appropriate support programs (e.g., chronic obstructive pulmonary disease [COPD] support groups, Arthritis I Can Cope groups, Alzheimer's support groups, Art making groups, telesupport).

Geriatric

- ▲ If actual or potential abuse or neglect is an issue, report it to the appropriate agency.
- ▲ Refer the family to appropriate senior community resources (e.g., senior centers, Medicare assistance, meal programs, parish nursing services, charitable organizations).
- • Work with the family to manage common challenges related to normal aging.
- ▲ Provide support for family caregivers of persons with dementia and related disorders: Encourage pleasant event therapies (i.e., interventions that teach caregivers to identify and pursue experiences that give them pleasure on a regular basis). Provide dietary and physical activity interventions. Screen for signs of depression.

C

Multicultural

- • Work to provide caregivers who understand the importance of cultural beliefs and values the family may hold.
- ▲ Develop programs to prevent injury from abuse and suffocation for the African-American community.

Home Care

- • The interventions described previously may be adapted for home care use.
- ▲ If disabled family coping interferes with the family member's ability to support the client's treatment plan, refer for psychiatric home healthcare services for family and client counseling and implementation of a therapeutic regimen.

Client/Family Teaching

- • Involve the client and family in the planning of care as often as possible; mutual goal setting is now considered part of "client safety."
- • Discuss with the family appropriate ways to demonstrate feelings such as reminiscence.
- ▲ Refer combat service members and their families for mental health treatment before and during deployment.

Ineffective Coping

NANDA Definition

Inability to form a valid appraisal of the stressors, inadequate choices of practiced responses, and/or inability to use available resources

Defining Characteristics

Abuse of chemical agents; change in usual communication patterns; decreased use of social support; destructive behavior toward others; destructive behavior toward self; fatigue; high illness rate; inability to meet basic needs; inability to meet role expectations; inadequate problem solving; lack of goal-directed behavior/resolution of problem, including inability to attend to and difficulty organizing information; poor concentration; risk taking; sleep disturbance; use of forms of coping that impede adaptive behavior;

verbalization of inability to ask for help; verbalization of inability to cope

Related Factors

Disturbance in pattern of appraisal of threat; disturbance in pattern of tension release; gender differences in coping strategies; high degree of threat; inability to conserve adaptive energies; inadequate level of confidence in ability to cope; inadequate level of perception of control; inadequate opportunity to prepare for stressor; inadequate resources available; inadequate social support created by characteristics of relationships; maturational crisis; situational crisis; uncertainty

Client Outcomes

Client Will (Specify Time Frame):

- Use effective coping strategies
- Use behaviors to decrease stress
- Remain free of destructive behavior toward self or others
- Report decrease in physical symptoms of stress
- Report increase in psychological comfort
- Seek help from a healthcare professional as appropriate

Nursing Interventions

- Monitor the client's risk of harming self or others and intervene appropriately. See care plan for **Risk for Suicide.**
- Observe for contributing factors of ineffective coping such as poor self-concept, grief, lack of problem-solving skills, lack of support, recent change in life situation, or gender differences in coping strategies.
- Use verbal and nonverbal therapeutic communication approaches including empathy, active listening, and confrontation to encourage the client and family to express emotions such as sadness, guilt, and anger (within appropriate limits); verbalize fears and concerns; and set goals.
- Collaborate with the client to identify strengths such as the ability to relate the facts and to recognize the source of stressors.
- Encourage the client to describe previous stressors and the coping mechanisms used.
- Be supportive of coping behaviors; allow the client time to relax.
- Provide opportunities for the client to discuss the meaning the situation might have for the client.

C

- • Assist the client to set realistic goals and identify personal skills and knowledge.
- • Provide information regarding care before care is given.
- • Discuss changes with the client before making them.
- • Encourage the client to make choices (as appropriate) and participate in planning care and scheduled activities.
- • Provide mental and physical activities within the client's ability (e.g., reading, television, radio, crafts, outings, movies, dinners out, social gatherings, exercise, sports, games).
- • Encourage moderate aerobic exercise (as appropriate).
- • Discuss the client's and family's power to change a situation or the need to accept a situation.
- • Offer instruction regarding alternative coping strategies.
- • Encourage use of spiritual resources as desired.
- • Encourage use of social support resources.
- ▲ Refer for additional or more intensive therapies as needed.

Geriatric

- ▲ Assess and report possible physiological alterations (e.g., sepsis, hypoglycemia, hypotension, infection, changes in temperature, fluid and electrolyte imbalances, and use of medications with known cognitive and psychotropic side effects).
- • Screen for elder neglect or other forms of elder mistreatment.
- • Target selected coping mechanisms for older persons based on client features, use, and preferences.
- ▲ Increase and mobilize support available to older persons by encouraging a variety of mechanisms involving family, friends, peers, and healthcare providers.
- • Actively listen to complaints and concerns.
- • Engage the client in reminiscence.

Multicultural

- • Assess for the influence of cultural beliefs, norms, and values on the client's perceptions of effective coping.
- • Assess the influence of fatalism on the client's coping behavior.
- • Assess the influence of cultural conflicts that may affect coping abilities.
- • Assess for intergenerational family problems that can overwhelm coping abilities.
- • Encourage spirituality as a source of support for coping.

- Negotiate with the client with regard to the aspects of coping behavior that will need to be modified.
- Identify which family members the client can count on for support.
- Support the inner resources that clients use for coping.
- Use an empowerment framework to redefine coping strategies.

Home Care

- The interventions described previously may be adapted for home care use.
- ▲ Assess for suicidal tendencies. Refer for mental health care immediately if indicated.
- Identify an emergency plan should the client become suicidal. Refer to the care plan for **Risk for Suicide.**
- Observe the family for coping behavior patterns. Obtain family and client history as possible.
- ▲ Assess for effective symptoms after cerebrovascular accident (CVA) in the elderly, particularly emotional lability and depression. Refer for evaluation and treatment as indicated.
- Encourage the client to use self-care management to increase the experience of personal control. Identify with the client all available supports and sense of attachment to others. Refer to the care plan for **Powerlessness.**
- ▲ Refer to medical social services for evaluation and counseling, which will promote adequate coping as part of the medical plan of care. If no primary medical diagnosis has been made, request medical social services to assist with community support contacts.
- ▲ Refer the client and family to support groups.
- ▲ If monitoring medication use, contract with the client or solicit assistance from a responsible caregiver.
- ▲ Institute case management for frail elderly clients to support continued independent living.
- ▲ If the client is homebound, refer for psychiatric home health-care services for client reassurance and implementation of a therapeutic regimen.

Client/Family Teaching

- Teach the client to problem solve. Have the client define the problem and cause, and list the advantages and disadvantages of the options.

- • Provide the seriously ill client and his or her family with needed information regarding the condition and treatment.
- • Teach relaxation techniques.
- • Work closely with the client to develop appropriate educational tools that address individualized needs.
- ▲ Teach the client about available community resources (e.g., therapists, ministers, counselors, self-help groups).

Ineffective community Coping

NANDA Definition

Pattern of community activities for adaptation and problem solving that is unsatisfactory for meeting the demands or needs of the community

Defining Characteristics

Community does not meet its own expectations; deficits in community participation; excessive community conflicts; expressed community powerlessness; expressed vulnerability; high illness rates; increased social problems (e.g., homicides, vandalism, arson, terrorism, robbery, infanticide, abuse, divorce, unemployment, poverty, militancy, mental illness); stressors perceived as excessive

Related Factors (r/t)

Deficits in community social support services; deficits in community social support resources; natural disasters; man-made disasters; inadequate resources for problem solving; ineffective community systems (e.g., lack of emergency medical system, transportation system, or disaster planning systems); nonexistent community systems

Community Outcomes

A Broad Range of Community Members Will (Specify Time Frame):

- • Participate in community actions to improve power resources
- • Develop improved communication among community members
- • Participate in problem solving
- • Demonstrate cohesiveness in problem solving
- • Develop new strategies for problem solving
- • Express power to deal with change and manage problems

Nursing Interventions

NOTE: The diagnosis of **Ineffective Coping** does not apply and should not be used when stress is being imposed by external sources or circumstance. If the community is a victim of circumstances, using the nursing diagnosis **Ineffective Coping** is equivalent to blaming the victim. See the care plans for **Ineffective community Therapeutic regimen management** and **Readiness for enhanced community Coping.**

- • Establish a collaborative partnership with the community (see the care plan for **Ineffective community Therapeutic regimen management**).
- • Assist the community with team building.
- • Participate with community members in the identification of stressors and assessment of distress; for example, observe and participate in faith-based organizations that want to improve community stress management.
- • Identify community strengths with community members.
- • Assist community members to articulate the local perspective based on years of experience with the issue or concern.
- ▲ Identify the health services and information resources that are currently available in the community.
- ▲ Consult with community mediation services, for example, the National Association of Community Mediation.
- • Work with community members to increase awareness of ineffective coping behaviors (e.g., conflicts that prevent community members from working together, anger and hate that paralyze the community, health risk behaviors of adolescents).
- • Provide support to the community and help community members to identify and mobilize additional supports.
- • Use focus group methods to evaluate and strengthen interventions.
- • Use mentoring strategies for community members.
- • Advocate for the community in multiple arenas (e.g., television, newspapers, and governmental agencies).
- • Work with community groups to improve the economic status and reduce unemployment.
- • Write grant proposals to help community members obtain funds for programs that reduce stress or improve coping.
- • Work with members of the community to identify and develop coping strategies that promote a sense of power (e.g., obtaining sources for funding, collaborating with other communities).

C

- Obtain police support for community partnerships aimed at healthy coping.
- Engage emotions during conflict mediation.
- Protect children from exposure to community conflicts.

Multicultural

- Acknowledge the stressors unique to racial/ethnic communities.
- Work with members of the community to prioritize and target health goals specific to the community.
- Approach community leaders and members of color with respect, warmth, and professional courtesy.
- Establish and sustain partnerships with key individuals within communities when developing and implementing programs.
- Use community church settings as a forum for advocacy, teaching, and program implementation.
- Ask political leaders to become part of the partnership process.

Community Teaching

- Teach strategies for stress management.
- Explain the relationship between enhancing power resources and coping.

Readiness for enhanced Coping

NANDA Definition

Pattern of cognitive and behavioral efforts to manage demands that is sufficient for well-being and can be strengthened

Defining Characteristics

Acknowledges power; aware of possible environmental changes; defines stressors as manageable; seeks knowledge of new strategies; seeks social support; uses a broad range of emotion-oriented strategies; uses a broad range of strategies; uses spiritual resources

Client Outcomes

Client Will (Specify Time Frame):

- Verbalize ability to cope and ask for help when needed
- Demonstrate ability to solve problems related to current needs

- Communicate needs and negotiate with others to meet needs
- State that stressors are manageable
- Demonstrate new effective coping strategies
- Seek social support for problems associated with coping
- Seek spiritual support of personal choice

Nursing Interventions

- Observe for strengths such as the ability to relate the facts and to recognize the source of stressors.
- Use empathetic communication and encourage the client and family to verbalize fears, express emotions, and set goals. Be present for clients physically or by telephone.
- Help the client set realistic goals and identify personal skills and knowledge.
- Encourage expression of positive thoughts and emotions.
- Encourage the use of cognitive behavioral relaxation (e.g., music therapy, guided imagery).

▲ Refer for cognitive behavioral therapy.

- Encourage the client to use spiritual coping mechanisms such as faith and prayer.
- Help the client with depression to maintain social support networks or assist in building new ones.

▲ Consider a workplace stress management program to enhance coping skills.

▲ Refer the client with breast cancer to a psychosocial group intervention for coping skills training, stress management, relaxation exercises, and psychosocial support.

- Refer to the care plans for **Readiness for enhanced Communication** and **Readiness for enhanced Spiritual well-being.**

Pediatric

- Encourage exercise for children and adolescents to promote positive self-esteem, to enhance coping, and to prevent behavioral and psychological problems.

Geriatric

- Consider the use of telephone support for caregivers of family members with dementia.

C

- ▲ Refer the client with Alzheimer's disease who is terminally ill to hospice.
- ▲ Refer the widowed older client to self-help support groups.

Multicultural

- • Encourage spirituality as a source of support for coping.
- • Refer to care plans for **Ineffective Coping.**

Home Care

- • The interventions described previously may be adapted for home care use.
- • Observe the family for coping behavior patterns. Obtain family and client history as possible.
- • Encourage the client to use self-care management to increase the experience of personal control. Identify with the client all available supports and sense of attachment to others.
- ▲ Refer the client and family to support groups.
- ▲ Refer the client for a behavioral program that teaches coping skills via "Lifeskills" workshop and/or video.
- ▲ Refer combat veterans and service members directly involved in combat as well as those providing support to combatants, including nurses for mental health services.

Client/Family Teaching

- • Teach relaxation techniques.
- ▲ Teach the client about available community resources (e.g., therapists, ministers, counselors, self-help groups).

Readiness for enhanced community Coping

NANDA Definition

Pattern of community activities for adaptation and problem solving that is satisfactory for meeting the demands or needs of the community but that can be improved for management of current and future problems/stressors

Defining Characteristics

One or more characteristics that indicate effective coping: Active planning by community for predicted stressors; active problem solving by community when faced with issues; agreement that community is responsible for stress management; positive communication among community members; positive communication between community/aggregates and larger community; programs available for recreation; programs available for relaxation; resources sufficient for managing stressors

C

Related Factors (r/t)

Community has sense of power to manage stressors; resources available for problem solving; social supports available

Community Outcomes

Community Will (Specify Time Frame):

- Develop enhanced coping strategies
- Maintain effective coping strategies for management of stress

Nursing Interventions

NOTE: Interventions depend on the specific aspects of community coping that can be enhanced (e.g., planning for stress management, communication, development of community power, community perceptions of stress, community coping strategies). Nursing interventions are conducted in collaboration with key members of the community, community/public health nurses, and members of other disciplines.

- • Describe the roles of community/public health nurses in working with healthy communities.
- • Help the community to obtain funds for additional programs.
- • Encourage positive attitudes toward the community through the media and other sources.
- • Help community members to collaborate with one another for power enhancement and coping skills.
- • Assist community members with cognitive skills and habits of mind for problem solving.
- • Demonstrate optimum use of the power resources.
- • Reduce poverty whenever possible.
- ▲ Collaborate with community members to improve educational levels within the community.

Multicultural

- Refer to care plan **Ineffective community Coping.**

C

Community Teaching

- Review coping skills, power for coping, and the use of power resources.

Readiness for enhanced family Coping

NANDA Definition

Effective management of adaptive tasks by family member involved with client's health challenge, who now exhibits desire and readiness for enhanced health and growth with regard to self and in relation to client

Defining Characteristics

Individual expresses interest in making contact with others who have experienced a similar situation; family member attempts to describe growth impact of crisis; family member moves in direction of enriching lifestyle; family member moves in direction of health promotion; chooses experiences that optimize wellness

Related Factors (r/t)

Adaptive tasks effectively addressed to enable goals of self-actualization to surface; needs sufficiently gratified to enable goals of self-actualization to surface

Client Outcomes

Family Will (Specify Time Frame):

- State a plan for growth
- Perform tasks needed for change
- State positive effects of changes made

Nursing Interventions

Refer to **Compromised family Coping** for additional interventions

- Assess the structure, resources, and coping abilities of families.
- Establish rapport with families through effective and accurate communication.

▲ Encourage family caregivers to become involved with mutual support groups.
▲ Develop and encourage the use of counseling services for family caregivers.
• Provide family-focused education to family caregivers to encourage adherence to medical care plans.
• Acknowledge the importance of cultural influences and ensure assessment tools are culturally appropriate.
• Develop and implement psycho-educational interventions for family members and clients to improve overall functioning, coping, and health outcomes.
• Increase the use of technology in providing supportive and educational services to family members.
▲ Identify and refer to support groups that discuss problems and concerns similar to those faced by the family (e.g., Alzheimer's Association; MUMS – National Parent to Parent Network; OncoChat–Online cancer support for clients, families, and friends).

Pediatric

• Provide expecting parents with educational resources and support to encourage the use of prenatal health services.
• Implement developmentally supportive family-centered services for infants and their caregivers.
• Empower parental caregivers through educational and behavioral enhancement programs.
• Employ family support programs that deliver services in multiple formats to maximize potential efficacy.

Geriatric

• Encourage family caregivers to participate in supportive counseling programs.
• Encourage family caregivers to become involved with mutual support groups.
▲ Provide psychosocial services to family caregivers that focus on skill-building, information, and support.
• Older adults living in residential facilities should be provided with companion animals and plants and frequent visits with children.
• Enhance the coping abilities of family caregivers of relatives living in long-term care settings.

- Provide psycho-educational support for family members providing end-of-life care in the home setting.

Multicultural, Home Care, and Client/Family Teaching

D

Refer to **Compromised family Coping** for additional interventions

Risk for sudden infant Death syndrome

NANDA Definition

Presence of risk factors for sudden death of an infant under 1 year of age

Risk Factors

Modifiable: Delayed prenatal care; infant overheating; infant overwrapping; infants placed to sleep in the prone position; infants placed to sleep in the side-lying position; lack of prenatal care; postnatal infant smoke exposure; prenatal infant smoke exposure; soft underlayment (loose articles in the sleep environment)

Potentially Modifiable: Low birth weight, prematurity, young maternal age

Nonmodifiable: Ethnicity (e.g., African American or Native American), male gender, seasonality of SIDS deaths (e.g., winter and fall months), infant age of 2-4 months, identified genetic component

Client Outcomes

Client Will (Specify Time Frame):

- Explain appropriate measures to prevent SIDS
- Demonstrate correct techniques for positioning the infant, protecting the infant from harm

Nursing Interventions

- Position infant on back to sleep, do not position in the prone position.
- Avoid use of loose bedding, such as blankets and sheets for sleeping. If blankets are used, they should be tucked in around the crib mattress so the infant's face is less likely to become covered by bedding.

- To avoid overbundling and overheating the infant, lightly clothe the child for sleep. The infant should not feel hot to touch.
- Provide the infant a certain amount of time in prone position, or "tummy time," while the infant is awake and observed.
- Consider offering the infant a pacifier during sleep times.

▲ Use electronic respiratory or cardiac monitors to detect cardiorespiratory arrest only if ordered.

Home Care

- Most of the interventions above are relevant to home care.
- Evaluate home for potential safety hazards, such as inappropriate cribs, cradles, or strollers.
- Determine where and how the child sleeps, and provide instructions on safe sleeping positions and environments as needed.

Multicultural

- Discuss cultural norms with families to provide care that is appropriate for promoting safety for the infant in sleeping arrangements and care.
- Encourage American-Indian mothers to avoid drinking alcoholic beverages and to avoid wrapping infants in excessive blankets or clothing.
- Encourage African-American mothers to find alternatives to bed sharing and to avoid placing pillows, soft toys, and soft bedding in the sleep environment.

Client/Family Teaching

- Teach families to position infants to sleep on their back rather than in the prone position.
- Teach the parents to place the infant supine to sleep with the head rotated to one side for a week, and then to the other side for the next week. Parents should also change the orientation of the crib at intervals, so the infant turns the head in alternate directions.
- Recommend the following infant care practices to parents:
  - ■ Infants should not be put to sleep on soft surfaces such as waterbeds, sofas, or soft mattresses.
  - ■ Avoid placing soft materials in the infant's sleeping environment such as pillows, quilts, and comforters. Do not use sheepskins under a sleeping infant.

  - Avoid the use of loose bedding, such as blankets and sheets.
- • Teach parents the need to obtain a crib that conforms to the safety standards of the Consumer Product Safety Commission.

- • Teach parents not to place the infant in an adult bed to sleep, or a sofa or chair. Infants should sleep in a crib.
- • Teach parents not to sleep with an infant, especially if alcohol or medications/illicit drugs are used by the parents.
- • Recommend an alternative to sleeping with an infant; parents might consider placing the infant's crib near their bed to allow for more convenient breastfeeding and parent contact.
- • Teach parents to avoid overbundling and overheating the infant by lightly clothing the child for sleep. The infant should not feel hot to touch. The bedroom temperature should be comfortable for an adult wearing light bedclothing.
- • Question parents regarding following recommendations for the prevention of SIDS at each well-baby visit or visit with health-care practitioner for illness. Strongly encourage compliance with precautions to prevent SIDS.
- • Teach the need to stop smoking during pregnancy and to not smoke around the infant, because smoking is a risk factor for SIDS.
- • Recommend that parents with infants in child care make it very clear to the employees that the infant must always be placed in the supine position to sleep, not prone or in a side-lying position.
- ▲ Suggest speaking with a physician about genetic counseling.
- • Teach child care employees how best to position infants for sleeping and the dangers of a too soft environment.
- • Teach parents living in deprived areas of precautions to prevent SIDS.
- ▲ Involve family members in learning and practicing rescue techniques, including treatment of choking, breathing, and cardiopulmonary resuscitation (CPR). Initiate referral to formal training classes.

Readiness for enhanced Decision-making

NANDA Definition

A pattern of choosing courses of action that is sufficient for meeting short and long term health-related goals and can be strengthened

D

Defining Characteristics

Expresses desire to enhance decision making; expresses desire to congruency of decisions with personal values and goals; expresses desire to congruency of decisions with sociocultural values and goals; expresses desire to risk benefit analysis of decisions; expresses desire to understand choices for decision making; expresses desire to enhance understanding of the meaning of choices; expresses desire to enhance use of reliable evidence for decisions

Client Outcomes

Client Will (Specify Time Frame):

- Review treatment options with providers
- Ask questions about the benefits and risks of treatment options
- Communicate decisions about treatment options to providers in relation to personal preferences, values, and goals

Nursing Interventions

- Support and encourage clients and their representatives to engage in healthcare decisions.
- Respect personal preferences, values, needs, and rights.
- Determine the degree of participation desired by the client.
- Provide access to healthcare services as needed.
- Provide information that is appropriate, relevant, and timely.
- Tailor information to the specific needs of individual clients, according to principles of health literacy.
- Motivate clients to be as independent as possible in decision making.
- Identify the client's level of choice in decision making.
- Focus on the positive aspects of decision making, rather than decisional conflicts.

D

- Use existing decision aids for particular types of decisions, or develop decision aids as indicated.
- Design educational interventions for decision support.
- Provide clients with the benefits of decisions at the same time you help them to identify strategies to reduce the barriers for healthful decisions.
- Acknowledge the complexity of everyday self-care decisions related to self-management of chronic illnesses.
- Determine the health literacy of clients and their representatives before helping with decision making.
- Reframe professional image, role, and values to incorporate a vision of clients as the experts in their own care.

Home Care

- The previously mentioned interventions should be adapted for home care use.
- Develop clinical practice guidelines that include shared decision making.
- Contribute to home care policy making that supports the adequacy of home care services.

Client/Family Teaching

- Before teaching, identify client preferences in involvement with decision making.

Ineffective Denial

NANDA Definition

The conscious or unconscious attempt to disavow the knowledge or meaning of an event to reduce anxiety/fear, but leading to the detriment of health

Defining Characteristics

Delays seeking healthcare attention to the detriment of health; displaces fear of impact of the condition; displaces source of symptoms to other organs; displays inappropriate affect; does not admit fear of death; does not admit fear of invalidism; does not perceive personal relevance of danger; does not perceive personal relevance of symptoms; makes dismissive comments when speaking of distressing events; minimizes symptoms; refuses healthcare attention to the detriment of health; unable to admit impact of disease on life pattern; uses self-treatment

Related Factors (r/t)

Anxiety; fear of death; fear of loss of autonomy; fear of separation; lack of competency in using effective coping mechanisms; lack of control of life situation; lack of emotional support from others; overwhelming stress; threat of inadequacy in dealing with strong emotions; threat of unpleasant reality

Client Outcomes

Client Will (Specify Time Frame):

- Seek out appropriate healthcare attention when needed
- Use home remedies only when appropriate
- Display appropriate affect and verbalize fears
- Remain substance free
- Actively engage in treatment program related to identified "substance" of abuse
- Demonstrate alternate adaptive coping mechanism

Nursing Interventions

- Assess the client's understanding of symptoms and illness.
- Spend time with the client, and allow time for responses.
- Assess whether the use of denial is helping or hindering the client's care. Provide support for clients who are using denial as a way of coping.
- Allow the client to express and use denial as a coping mechanism.
- Assess for subtle signs of denial (e.g., unrealistic display of optimism, downplaying of symptoms, inability to admit one's own fear).
- Avoid confrontation.
- Support the client's spiritual coping measures.
- Develop a trusting, therapeutic relationship with the client/family.
- Encourage individual family members to share their concerns and worries.
- Sit at eye level.

D

- Use touch if appropriate and with permission. Touch the client's hand or arm.
- Explain signs and symptoms of illness; as necessary, reinforce use of the prescribed treatment plan.
- Have the client make choices regarding treatment and actively involve him or her in the decision-making process.
- Help the client recognize existing and additional sources of support; allow time for adjustment.
- Refer to care plans **Defensive Coping** and **Dysfunctional Family processes: alcoholism**

Geriatric

- Identify recent losses of the client, because grieving may prolong denial. Encourage the client to take one day at a time.
- Encourage the client to verbalize feelings.
- Encourage communication among family members.
- Recognize denial.
- Use reality-focusing techniques. Wherever possible, provide realistic feedback, allowing the client to validate his or her perceptions.

Multicultural

- Assess for the influence of cultural beliefs, norms, and values on the client's understanding of and ability to acknowledge health status.
- Discuss with the client those aspects of his or her health behavior/lifestyle that will remain unchanged by health status.
- Negotiate with the client regarding the aspects of health behavior that will need to be modified as a result of health status.
- Assess the role of fatalism on the client's ability to acknowledge health status.
- Validate the client's feelings of anxiety and fear related to health status.

Home Care

- Previously mentioned interventions may be adapted for home care use.
- Observe family interaction and roles. Assess whether denial is being used to meet the needs of another family member.

▲ Refer the client/family for follow-up if prolonged denial is a risk.

- Encourage communication between family members, particularly when dealing with the loss of a significant person.

Client/Family Teaching

- Teach signs and symptoms of illness and appropriate responses (e.g., taking medication, going to the emergency department, calling the physician). Provide a list of names and numbers.
- Teach family members that denial may continue throughout the adjustment to treatment and they should not be confrontational.

▲ If the problem is substance abuse, refer to an appropriate community agency (e.g., Alcoholics Anonymous).

- Teach families of clients with brain injuries that denial has been associated with damage to the right hemisphere.
- Inform family of available community support resources.

Impaired Dentition

NANDA Definition

Disruption in tooth development/eruption patterns or structural integrity of individual teeth

Defining Characteristics

Abraded teeth, absence of teeth; asymmetrical facial expression; crow caries; erosion of enamel; excessive calculus; excessive plaque; halitosis; incomplete eruption for age (may be primary or permanent teeth); loose teeth; malocclusion; missing teeth; premature loss of primary teeth; root caries; tooth enamel discoloration; tooth fracture(s); tooth misalignment; toothache; worn down teeth

Related Factors (r/t)

Barriers to self-care; bruxism; chronic use of coffee; chronic use of tea; chronic use of red wine; chronic use of tobacco; chronic vomiting; deficient knowledge regarding dental health; dietary habits; economic barriers to professional care; excessive use of abrasive cleaning agents; excessive intake of fluorides; genetic predisposition; ineffective oral hygiene; lack of access to professional care; nutritional deficits; selected prescription medications; sensitivity to cold; sensitivity to heat

Client Outcomes

Client Will (Specify Time Frame):

- Have clean teeth, gums healthy pink color, mouth with pleasant odor
- Demonstrate ability to masticate foods without difficulty
- State no pain originating from teeth
- Demonstrate measures can take to improve dental hygiene

Nursing Interventions

▲ Inspect oral cavity/teeth at least once daily and note any discoloration; presence of debris; amount of plaque buildup; presence of lesions, edema, or bleeding; and intactness of teeth. Refer to a dentist or periodontist as appropriate.

- If the client is free of bleeding disorders and is able to swallow, encourage the client to brush teeth with a soft toothbrush, using fluoride-containing toothpaste at least twice daily and to floss teeth daily.
- Use a powered sonic toothbrush for removal of dental plaque and prevention of gingivitis.
- If the client is unable to brush his or her teeth, follow this procedure:
  1. Position the client upright or on side.
  2. Use a soft bristle baby toothbrush.
  3. Use fluoride toothpaste and tap water or saline as a solution.
  4. Brush teeth in an up-and-down manner.
  5. Suction as needed.
- Avoid using foam sticks to clean teeth; use them only to swab out the oral cavity.
- Monitor the client's nutritional and fluid status to determine if adequate. Recommend the client eat a balanced diet and limit between meal snacks.
- Recommend the client decrease or preferably stop intake of soft drinks.
- If client has halitosis, review good oral care with the client, including brushing teeth, using floss, and brushing the tongue.

▲ Assess the client for an underlying medical condition that may be causing halitosis.

- Determine the client's mental status and manual dexterity; if the client is unable to care for self, nursing personnel must provide dental hygiene. The nursing diagnosis **Bathing/hygiene Self-Care deficit** is then applicable.

- • Determine the client's usual method of oral care. Whenever possible, build on the client's existing knowledge and current practices to develop an individualized plan of care.
- • Tell the client to direct the toothbrush vertically toward the tooth surfaces.
- • Instruct the client to clean the tongue when performing oral hygiene. Brush tongue with tongue scraper and follow with a mouth rinse.
- • Use tap water or saline only for a mouth rinse. Avoid the use of hydrogen peroxide, lemon-glycerin swabs, or alcohol-based mouthwashes.
- • If the client does not have a bleeding disorder, encourage the client to floss daily with approximately 18 inches of floss, using a gentle up-and-down rubbing motion.
- ▲ Recommend client see a dentist at prescribed intervals, generally two times per year if teeth are in satisfactory condition.
- ▲ If there are any signs of bleeding when the teeth are brushed, refer the client to a dentist; or if there are obvious signs of inflamed gums, refer the client to a periodontist.
- • If platelet numbers are decreased, or if the client is edentulous, use moistened toothettes or a specially made, very soft toothbrush for oral care.
- • Provide scrupulous dental care to critically ill clients.
- • If teeth are nonfunctional for chewing, modification of oral intake (e.g., edentulous diet, soft diet) may be necessary. The nursing diagnosis **Imbalanced Nutrition: less than body requirements** may apply.
- • If the client is unable to swallow, keep suction nearby when providing oral care.
- • See care plan for **Impaired Oral mucous membrane.**

Pregnant Client

- • Encourage the expectant mother to eat a healthy, balanced diet that is rich in calcium.

Infant Oral Hygiene

- • Gently wipe baby's gums with a washcloth or sterile gauze at least once a day.

- Never allow child to fall asleep with a bottle containing milk, formula, fruit juice, or sweetened liquid, or give child a pacifier dipped in any sweet liquid. Avoid filling a child's bottle with such liquids as sugar water and soft drinks.
- When multiple teeth appear, brush with a small toothbrush with a small (pea-size) amount of fluoride toothpaste. Recommend that the child use either a fluoride gel or fluoride varnish.

Older Children

▲ Encourage the family to talk with the dentist about dental sealants, which can help prevent cavities in permanent teeth.
▲ Recommend the child use dental floss to help prevent gum disease. The dentist will give guidelines on when to start using floss.
• Recommend to parents that they not permit the child to smoke or chew tobacco, and stress the importance of setting a good example by not using products themselves.
• Recommend the child drink fluoridated water when possible.
• If a child has halitosis, consider the presence of parasites in the gastrointestinal system as a cause.

Geriatric

▲ Provide dentists with accurate medication history to avoid drug interaction.
• Carefully observe oral cavity and lips for abnormal lesions when providing dental care.
▲ Consider professional oral health care for older adults in nursing homes.
• Ensure that dentures are removed and cleaned regularly, preferably after every meal and before bedtime; select appropriate adhesives to improve breath.
• Support other care givers providing oral hygiene.
▲ The medication profile should be reviewed to determine if an older adult is taking anticoagulants. If so, the International Normalized Ration (INR) should be reviewed before providing dental care.

Multicultural

• Assess for the influence of cultural beliefs, norms, and values on the client's understanding of dental care.

- Assess for barriers to access to dental care, such as lack of insurance.
- Instruct mothers on the danger of feeding infants bottles filled with soda, juice, or milk when the infant goes to sleep.
- Assess for dental anxiety.

▲ Introduce the dental home concept to improve families' access to dental care.

Home Care

- Assess client patterns for daily and professional dental care and related patterns (e.g., smoking, nail biting). Assess for environmental influences on dental status (e.g., fluoride).
- Assess client facilities and financial resources for providing dental care.
- Request a dietary log from the client, adding columns for type of food (i.e., soft, pureed, regular).
- Observe a typical meal to assess the impact of impaired dentition on nutrition.
- Identify mechanical needs for food preparation and ease of ingestion/digestion to meet the client's dental/nutritional needs.
- Assist the client with accessing financial or other resources to support optimum dental and nutritional status.

Client/Family Teaching

- Teach how to inspect the oral cavity and monitor for problems with the teeth and gums.
- Teach how to implement a personal plan of dental hygiene, including appropriate brushing of teeth and tongue and using dental floss.
- Teach the client the value of having an optimal fluoride concentration in drinking water and of brushing teeth twice daily with fluoride toothpaste.
- Teach clients of all ages the need to decrease intake of sugary foods and to brush teeth regularly.
- Suggest chewing gum with sugar to reduce oral malodor.
- Inform individuals who are considering tongue piercing of the potential complications, such as chipping and cracking of teeth and possible trauma to the gingiva. If piercing is done, teach the client how to care for the wound and prevent complications.

Risk for delayed Development

NANDA Definition

D At risk for delay of 25% or more in one or more of the areas of social or self-regulatory behavior or cognitive, language, gross, or fine motor skills

Risk Factors

Prenatal

Endocrine disorders; genetic disorders; illiteracy; inadequate nutrition; infections; lack of prenatal care; late prenatal care; maternal age <15 years; maternal age >35 years; poor prenatal care; poverty; substance abuse; unplanned pregnancy; unwanted pregnancy

Individual

Adopted child; behavior disorders; brain damage (e.g., hemorrhage in postnatal period, shaken baby, abuse, accident); chemotherapy; chronic illness; congenital disorders; failure to thrive; foster child; frequent otitis media; genetic disorders; hearing impairment; inadequate nutrition; lead poisoning; natural disasters; positive drug screen(s); prematurity; radiation therapy; seizures; substance abuse; technology-dependent; vision impairment

Environmental

Poverty; violence

Caregiver

Abuse; mental illness; mental retardation or severe learning disability

Client Outcomes

Client/Parents/Primary Caregiver Will (Specify Time Frame):

- Describe realistic, age-appropriate patterns of development
- Promote activities and interactions that support age-related developmental tasks

Nursing Interventions

• Refer to care plan for **Delayed Growth and development.**

D

Preconception/Pregnancy

- Males and females should avoid exposure to organic solvents before and during pregnancy.
- Avoid exposure to heavy metals, pesticides, herbicides, sterilants, anesthetic gases, and anticancer drugs used in health care.

Multicultural

Parents

- Assess for the influence of cultural beliefs, norms, and values on the client's perceptions of child development.

Infants

- Carefully assess infants for developmental milestones, and supply appropriate preventive interventions, such as adequate nutrition.

Home Care

- Teach the parents to provide toys and books and read aloud to young children in the home.

Client/Family Teaching

▲ Encourage mothers to abstain from alcohol and cocaine use during pregnancy; refer them to treatment programs for substance abuse.
- Encourage adequate antepartum and postpartum care for both mother and child.
- Counsel parents, siblings, and caregivers about the importance of smoking cessation and the necessity of eliminating all secondhand smoke exposure.
- Teach caregivers of children appropriate developmental interactions; use anticipatory guidance to facilitate preparation for developmental milestones.
- Provide developmental care interventions to preterm infants to improve neurodevelopmental outcomes.

▲ Provide information on support groups and education on human immunodeficiency virus (HIV) and caring for infants with this diagnosis.

Diarrhea

NANDA Definition

D

Passage of loose, unformed stools

Defining Characteristics

Abdominal pain; at least 3 loose liquid stools per day; cramping; hyperactive bowel sounds; urgency

Related Factors (r/t)

Psychological

Anxiety; high stress levels

Situational

Adverse effects of medications; alcohol abuse; contaminants; travel; laxative abuse; radiation; toxins; tube feedings

Physiological

Infectious processes; inflammation; irritation; malabsorption; parasites

Client Outcomes

Client Will (Specify Time Frame):

- Defecate formed, soft stool every day to every third day
- Maintain a rectal area free of irritation
- State relief from cramping and less or no diarrhea
- Explain cause of diarrhea and rationale for treatment
- Maintain good skin turgor and weight at usual level
- Contain stool appropriately (if previously incontinent)

Nursing Interventions

- Assess pattern of defecation, or have the client keep a diary that includes the following: time of day defecation occurs; usual stimulus for defecation; consistency, amount, and frequency of stool; type of, amount of, and time food consumed; fluid intake; history of bowel habits and laxative use; diet; exercise patterns; obstetrical/gynecological, medical, and surgical histories; medications; alterations in perianal sensations; and present bowel regimen.

- • Assess stool consistency and its influence on risk for stool loss. Several classification systems for stool have been promulgated.
- ▲ Identify cause of diarrhea if possible based on history (e.g., rotavirus or norovirus exposure; HIV infection; food poisoning; medication effect; radiation therapy; protein malnutrition; laxative abuse; stress). See Related Factors (r/t).
- ▲ If the client has watery diarrhea, a low-grade fever, abdominal cramps, and a history of antibiotic therapy, consider possibility of *Clostridium difficile* infection.
- ▲ Obtain stool specimens as ordered, to either rule out or diagnose an infectious process (e.g., ova and parasites, *C. difficile* infection, bacterial cultures).
- ▲ Use standard precautions when caring for clients with diarrhea to prevent spread of infectious diarrhea; use gloves and hand washing.
- ▲ If the client has diarrhea associated with antibiotic therapy, consult with the primary care practitioner regarding the use of probiotics, such as yogurt, with active cultures to treat diarrhea, or also use probiotics to prevent diarrhea when first beginning antibiotic therapy.
- • Ask the client to examine intake of high fructose corn syrup and fructose sweeteners in relation to onset of diarrhea symptoms. If diarrhea is associated with fructose ingestion, intake should be limited or eliminated.
- • If the client has infectious diarrhea, avoid using medications that slow peristalsis.
- • Inspect, palpate, percuss, and auscultate abdomen; note whether bowel sounds are frequent.
- • Assess for dehydration by observing skin turgor over sternum and inspecting for longitudinal furrows of the tongue. Watch for excessive thirst, fever, dizziness, lightheadedness, palpitations, excessive cramping, bloody stools, hypotension, and symptoms of shock.
- • Observe for symptoms of sodium and potassium loss (e.g., weakness, abdominal or leg cramping, dysrhythmia). Note results of electrolyte laboratory studies.
- • Monitor and record intake and output; note oliguria and dark, concentrated urine.
- • Measure specific gravity of urine if possible.
- • Weigh the client daily and note decreased weight.

D

- • Give dilute clear fluids as tolerated (e.g., clear soda, gelatin dessert), serving at lukewarm temperature.
- ▲ If the client has chronic diarrhea causing fecal incontinence at intervals, consider suggesting use of dietary fiber from psyllium or gum arabic after consultation with primary practitioner.
- ▲ If diarrhea is chronic and there is evidence of malnutrition, consult with primary care for a dietary consult and possible use of a hydrolyzed formula (a clear liquid supplement containing increased protein) to maintain nutrition while the gastrointestinal system heals.
- • Encourage the client to eat small, frequent meals, to consume foods that are easy to digest (e.g., bananas, crackers, pretzels, rice, potatoes, clear soups, applesauce), and to avoid milk products, foods high in fiber, and caffeine (dark sodas, tea, coffee, chocolate).
- • Provide a readily available bedpan, commode, or bathroom.
- • If the client has diarrhea and incontinence, consider use of a Perineal Assessment Tool to measure the risk for perineal skin injury.
- • Thoroughly cleanse and dry the perianal and perineal skin daily and as needed using a cleanser capable of stool removal. Select a product with a slightly acidic pH designed to preserve the skin's acid mantle, and designed to remove irritants from the skin with minimal physical force. Avoid vigorous scrubbing with water, soap, and a washcloth. Consider selection of a product with a moisturizer.
- ▲ If the client is receiving a tube feeding, note rate of infusion, and prevent contamination of feeding by rinsing container every 8 hours and replacing it every 24 hours.
- ▲ If the client is receiving a tube feeding, suggest formulas that contain a bulking agent, such as Jevity, or add soluble dietary fiber to the feeding per physician's/dietitian's order.

Pediatric

- ▲ Recommend the parents give the child oral rehydration fluids to drink in the amounts specified by the physician, especially during the first 4 to 6 hours to replace lost fluid. Once the child is rehydrated, an orally administered maintenance solution should be used along with food.
- • Recommend the mother resume breastfeeding as soon as possible.

- Recommend parents not give the child decarbonated soda, fruit juices, gelatin dessert, or instant fruit drink.
- Recommend parents give children foods with complex carbohydrates, such as potatoes, rice, bread, cereal, yogurt, fruits, and vegetables. The BRAT diet is often advocated. Avoid fatty foods and foods high in simple sugars.

Geriatric

▲ Evaluate medications the client is taking. Recognize that many medications can result in diarrhea, including digitalis, propranolol, angiotensin-converting enzyme (ACE) inhibitors, histamine-receptor antagonists, nonsteroidal antiinflammatory drugs (NSAIDs), anticholinergic agents, oral hypoglycemia agents, antibiotics, and others.

▲ Monitor the client closely to detect whether an impaction is causing diarrhea; remove impaction as ordered.

▲ Seek medical attention if diarrhea is severe or persists for more than 24 hours, or if the client has history of dehydration or electrolyte disturbances, such as lassitude, weakness, or prostration.

- Provide emotional support for clients who are having trouble controlling unpredictable episodes of diarrhea.

Home Care

- Previously mentioned interventions may be adapted for home care use.
- Assess the home for general sanitation and methods of food preparation. Reinforce principles of sanitation for food handling.

▲ Assess for methods of handling soiled laundry if the client is bed bound or has been incontinent. Instruct or reinforce Universal Precautions with family and blood-borne pathogen precautions with agency caregivers.

▲ When assessing medication history, include over-the-counter (OTC) drugs, both general and those currently being used to treat the diarrhea. Instruct clients not to mix OTC medications when self-treating.

▲ Evaluate current medications for indication that specific interventions are warranted.

▲ Consult with physician regarding need for blood work or stool specimens.

▲ Evaluate need for home health aide or homemaker service referral.
▲ Evaluate need for durable medical equipment in the home.

Client/Family Teaching

D

- Encourage avoidance of coffee, spices, milk products, and foods that irritate or stimulate the gastrointestinal tract.
- ▲ Teach appropriate method of taking ordered antidiarrheal medications; explain side effects.
- Explain how to prevent the spread of infectious diarrhea (e.g., careful hand washing, appropriate handling and storage of food).
- Help the client to determine stressors and set up an appropriate stress reduction plan.
- Teach signs and symptoms of dehydration and electrolyte imbalance.
- Teach perirectal skin care.

Risk for compromised Human Dignity

NANDA Definition

At risk for perceived loss of respect and honor

Risk Factors

Cultural incongruity; disclosure of confidential information; exposure of the body; inadequate participation in decision making; loss of control of body functions; perceived dehumanizing treatment; perceived humiliation; perceived intrusion by clinicians; perceived invasion of privacy; stigmatizing label; use of undefined medical terms

Client Outcomes

Client Will (Specify Time Frame):

- Perceive that dignity is maintained throughout hospitalization
- Consistently be called by name of choice
- Have privacy maintained at all times

Nursing Interventions

- Be authentically present when with the client, try to limit extraneous thoughts of self or others, concentrate on the well-being of the client.

- Accept the client as is, with unconditional positive regard.
- Use loving appropriate touch based on client's culture. When first meeting the client, shake hands with younger clients, touch the arm or shoulder of older clients.
- Determine the client's perspective about their health. Example questions include: "Tell me about your health." "What is it like to be in your situation?" "Tell me how you perceive yourself in this situation?" "What meaning are you giving to this situation?" "Tell me about your health priorities." "Tell me about the harmony you wish to reach."
- Create a loving, healing environment for the client to help meet physical, psychological, and spiritual needs as possible.
- Determine the client's preferences for when and how nursing care is needed and follow the client's guidelines if at all possible.
- Include the client in all decision making. If the client does not chose to be part of the decision, or is no longer capable of making a decision, use the named surrogate decision maker.
- Encourage the client to share his/her feelings, both positive and negative as appropriate and as the client is willing.
- Ask the client what they would like to be called and use that name consistently.
- Maintain privacy at all times.
- Avoid authoritative care where the nurse knows what should be done, and the client is powerless.
- Sit down when talking to clients in the bed, establish appropriate eye contact.
- Actively listen to what the client is saying both verbally and non-verbally.
- Encourage the client to share thoughts about spirituality as desires.
- Utilize interventions to instill increased hope; see the care plan **Readiness for enhanced Hope.**
- For further interventions on spirituality, see the care plan for **Readiness for enhanced Spiritual well-being.**

Geriatrics

- Avoid calling elderly clients "sweetie," "honey," "Gramps," or other terms that can be demeaning unless this is acceptable in the client's culture or requested by the client.

- Treat the elderly client with the utmost respect, even if delirium or dementia is present with confusion.
- Avoid use of restraints.

D

Multicultural

- Assess for the influence of cultural beliefs, norms, and values on the client's way of communicating, and follow the client's lead in communicating in matters of eye contact, amount of personal space, voice tones, and amount of touching.

Home Care

- Most of the interventions described previously may be adapted for home care use.
- Recognize that the client with the caregiver have complete autonomy in the home.

Client/Family Teaching

- Teach family and caregivers the need for the dignity of the client to be maintained at all times.

NOTE: Caring is integral to maintaining dignity. A caring occasion is the moment (focal point in space and time) when the nurse and another person come together in such a way that an occasion for human caring is created. Both the one cared-for and the one caring can be influenced by the caring moment through the choices and actions decided within the relationship, thereby, influencing and becoming part of their own life history.

Moral Distress

NANDA Definition

Response to the inability to carry out one's chosen ethical/moral decision/action

Defining Characteristics

Patient/family expresses anguish (e.g., powerlessness, guilt, frustration, anxiety, self-doubt, fear) over difficulty acting on one's moral choice

Related Factors

End-of-life decisions; treatment decisions; time constraints for decision making; conflicting information guiding moral/ethical decision-making; conflict among decision makers; physical distance of decision maker; loss of autonomy; cultural conflicts

Client Outcomes

Client Will (Specify Time Frame):

- Be able to act in accordance with values, goals, and beliefs
- Regain confidence in the ability to make decision and/or act in accord with values, goals, and beliefs
- Expresses satisfaction with the ability to make decisions consistent with values, goals, and beliefs
- Have choices respected

Nursing Interventions

- • Examine the source of moral distress.
- • Affirm and validate the client's feelings and perceptions of others.
- ▲ Provide adequate information and emotional and psychological support to assist in coping and making collaborative decisions with the healthcare team.
- • Assist client in evaluating the situation.
- • Assess personal source of distress to contemplate ability to act.
- • Implement strategies to initiate changes to resolve moral distress.
- • Confront the barrier.
- ▲ Improve communication and collaboration among client, family, and healthcare team.
- • Advocate for the client.
- • Teach the client how to take action.
- ▲ Consult with other healthcare providers that may include the family.
- ▲ Contact an ethicist or the ethics committee to ensure the client's rights are protected.

Risk for Disuse syndrome

NANDA Definition

D

At risk for a deterioration of body systems as the result of prescribed or unavoidable musculoskeletal inactivity

Risk Factors

Altered level of consciousness; mechanical immobilization; paralysis; prescribed immobilization; severe pain (*Note:* Complications from immobility can include pressure ulcer, constipation, stasis of pulmonary secretions, thrombosis, urinary tract infection and/or retention, decreased strength or endurance, orthostatic hypotension, decreased range of joint motion, disorientation, disturbed body image, and powerlessness.)

Client Outcomes

Client Will (Specify Time Frame):

- Maintain full range of motion in joints
- Maintain intact skin, good peripheral blood flow, and normal pulmonary function
- Maintain normal bowel and bladder function
- Express feelings about imposed immobility
- Explain methods to prevent complications of immobility

Nursing Interventions

• Use a functional assessment instrument to evaluate abilities, including such instruments as the Barthel Index, the Katz Index of Activities of Daily Living, or the FIM instrument.

▲ Have the client do exercises in bed if not contraindicated (e.g., flexing and extending feet and quadriceps, performing gluteal and abdominal sitting exercises, lifting small weights to maintain muscle strength).

▲ If not contraindicated by the client's condition, obtain referral to physical therapy for use of tilt table to provide weight bearing on long bones.

• Perform range of motion exercises for all possible joints at least twice daily; perform passive or active range of motion exercises as appropriate.

▲ Use high-top sneakers or specialized boots from the occupational therapy department to prevent foot drop; remove shoes twice daily to provide foot care.

- Position the client so that joints are in normal anatomical alignment at all times.
- When positioning clients on the side, tilt clients 30° or less while lying on their side.
- If client is immobile, consider use of a transfer chair, which is a chair that becomes a stretcher.
- Assess skin condition at least daily and more frequently if needed. Refer to care plan for **risk for impaired Skin integrity.**
- Turn clients at high risk for pressure/shear/friction frequently.
- Provide the client with a pressure-relieving horizontal support surface. For further interventions on skin care, refer to the care plan for **impaired Skin integrity.**
- Assist the client to walk as soon as medically possible.

▲ Recognize that the client who has been in an intensive care environment may develop a neuromuscular disorder resulting in extreme weakness. The client may need a workup to determine the cause before satisfactory ambulation can begin.

▲ Consider use of a continuous lateral rotation therapy bed.

▲ If at all possible, help the client begin a walking program, using a physical therapist as needed.

- Be very careful when helping the client into a chair and when transferring. Be sure to lock beds and wheelchairs. Recognize that there is a high probability for falls.
- Minimize cardiovascular deconditioning by positioning clients as close to upright as possible, several times daily.
- When getting the client up after bed rest, do so slowly and watch for signs of postural hypotension, tachycardia, nausea, diaphoresis, or syncope. Take the blood pressure lying, sitting, and standing, waiting 2 minutes between each reading.

▲ Obtain assistive devices, such as braces, crutches, or canes, to help the client reach and maintain as much mobility as possible.

▲ Request a physical therapy referral to help the client learn how to move self in bed, including bridging, and also how to transfer out of bed.

▲ Apply graduated compression stockings as ordered. Ensure proper fit by measuring, remove at least twice, in the morning with bath and in the evening to assess condition of extremity, then reapply.

- Monitor peripheral circulation and especially note color, pulse, and calf or thigh swelling; check Homans' sign, but recognize that it is an unreliable sign of DVT.
- Have the client cough and take deep breaths or use incentive spirometry every 2 hours while he or she is awake.
- Monitor respiratory functions, noting breath sounds and respiratory rate. Percuss for new onset of dullness in lungs.
- Note bowel function daily. Provide increased fluids, fiber, and natural laxatives, such as prune juice, as needed.
- Increase fluid intake to 2000 mL/day within the client's cardiac and renal reserve.
- Encourage intake of a balanced diet with adequate amounts of fiber and protein.

Geriatrics

- Help the mostly immobile client achieve mobility as soon as possible, depending on physical condition.
- Use the Outcome Expectation for Exercise Scale to determine client's self-efficacy expectations and outcomes expectations toward exercise.
- If client is frail, ensure good nutrition, appropriate medications, attention to vision and hearing deficits, and increase social support along with exercise.
- If the client is mostly immobile, encourage him or her to attend a low-intensity aerobic chair exercise class that includes stretching and strengthening chair exercises.

▲ Refer the client to physical therapy for resistance exercise training as able, including abdominal crunch, leg press, leg extension, leg curl, calf press, and more.

▲ If the client is elderly and scheduled for an elective surgery that will result in admission into ICU and immobility such as recovering from a knee replacement, initiate a prehabilitation program that includes a warm-up, aerobic strength, flexibility, and functional task work.

- Monitor for signs of depression: flat affect, poor appetite, insomnia, many somatic complaints.
- Keep careful track of bowel function in elderly clients, and do not allow them to become constipated.

Home Care

- • Some of the previously mentioned interventions may be adapted for home care use.
- ▲ Begin discharge planning as soon as possible with case manager or social worker to assess need for home support systems and community or home health services.
- ▲ Become oriented to all programs of care for the client before discharge from institutional care.
- ▲ Confirm the immediate availability of all necessary assistive devices for home.
- • Perform complete physical assessment and recent history at initial visit.
- ▲ Refer to physical and occupational therapies for immediate evaluations of the client's potential for independence and functioning in the home setting and for follow-up care.
- • Allow the client to have as much input and control of the plan of care as possible.
- • Assess knowledge of all care with caregivers. Review as necessary.
- ▲ Support the family of the client in assuming caregiver activities. Refer for home health aide services for assistance and respite as appropriate. Refer to medical social services as appropriate.
- ▲ Institute case management of frail older adults to support continued independent living if possible in the home environment.

Client/Family Teaching

- • Teach how to perform range of motion exercises in bed if not contraindicated.
- • Teach the family how to turn and position the client and provide all care necessary.

NOTE: Nursing diagnoses that are commonly relevant when the client is on bed rest include **Constipation, risk for impaired Skin integrity, disturbed Sensory perception, disturbed Sleep pattern, adult Failure to thrive,** and **Powerlessness.**

Deficient Diversional activity

NANDA Definition

D

Decreased stimulation from (or interest or engagement in) recreational or leisure activities

Defining Characteristics

Patient's statements regarding boredom (e.g., wish there was something to do, to read, etc.); usual hobbies cannot be undertaken in hospital

Related Factor (r/t)

Environmental lack of diversional activity

Client Outcome

Client Will (Specify Time Frame):

- Engage in personally satisfying diversional activities

Nursing Interventions

- Observe for signs of deficient diversional activity: restlessness, unhappy facial expression, and statements of boredom and discontent.
- Observe ability to engage in activities that require good vision and use of hands.
- Discuss activities with clients that are interesting and feasible in the present environment.
- Encourage the client to share feelings about situation of inactivity away from usual life activities.
- Encourage a mix of physical and mental activities if possible (e.g., crafts, videotapes).
- Provide videos and/or DVDs of movies for recreation and distraction.
- Provide magazines and/or books of interest.
- Set up a puzzle in a community space, or provide individual puzzles as desired.
- Provide access to a portable computer so that the client can access e-mail and the Internet. Give client a list of interesting websites, including games and directions on how to use a search engine (e.g., Google) if desired.

- • Help client find a support group for the appropriate condition on the internet if interested, and if support group is available.
- • Use "bread therapy" in long term units—clients/staff bake bread with a bread maker as desired.
- ▲ Arrange animal-assisted therapy if desired, with a dog, cat, or bird for the client to interact with and if possible care for.
- • Encourage the client to schedule visitors so that they are not all present at once or at inconvenient times.
- • Provide reading material, television, radio, and books on tape.
- • If clients are able to write, help them keep journals; if clients are unable to write, have them record thoughts on tape or on videotape.
- ▲ Request recreational or art therapist to assist with providing diversional activities.
- • Provide a change in scenery; get the client out of the room if possible.
- • Help the client experience nature by looking at a nature scene from a window, or walking through a garden if possible.
- • Structure the environment as needed to promote optimal comfort and sensory diversity (e.g., have family bring in posters, banners, or a sound system; change lighting; change direction bed faces).
- • Work with family to provide music that is enjoyable to the client.
- • Structure the client's schedule around personal wishes for time of care, relaxation, and participation in fun activities.
- • Spend time with the client when possible or arrange for a friendly visitor.

Pediatric

- ▲ Request an order for a child life specialist or, if not available, a play therapist for children.
- • Provide activities, such as video projects and access to computer-based support groups for children (e.g., Starbright World: a computer network where children interact virtually, sharing their experiences and escaping hospital routines).
- • Provide computer games and virtual reality experiences for children, which can be used as distraction techniques during venipuncture or other procedures.

Geriatrics

- • If the client is able, arrange attendance with senior citizen group activities.
- • Encourage involvement in senior citizen activities (e.g., AARP, YMCA, church groups). Arrange transportation to activities as needed.
- • Encourage clients to use their ability to help others by volunteering.
- • Provide an environment that promotes activity (e.g., one that has adequate lighting for crafts, large-print books); allow periods of solitude and privacy.
- ▲ Use reminiscence therapy in conjunction with the expression of emotions. Refer to a reminiscence group if available.
- ▲ Use the Eden Alternative with the elderly; bring in appropriate plants for the elderly client to care for; animals, such as birds, fish, dogs, and cats, as appropriate for the client; and children to visit.
- • For clients who love gardening, bring in seeds, soil, and pots for indoor gardening. Use seeds, such as sunflower, pumpkin, and zinnia, that grow rapidly.
- • For clients in assisted living facilities, provide leisure educational programs.
- ▲ Provide recreational therapy exercises in the morning for clients with dementia in the extended care facility.

Multicultural

- • Assess for the influence of cultural beliefs, norms, and values on the client's leisure activity interests.
- • Validate the client's feelings and concerns related to lack of stimulation or interest in leisure activities.

Home Care

NOTE: Many of the previously listed interventions should be administered in the home setting.

- • Explore previous interests with the client; consider related activities that are within the client's capabilities.
- ▲ Assess the client for depression. Refer for mental health services as indicated.
- • Assess the family's ability to respond to the client's psychosocial needs for stimulation. Assist as able.

▲ Refer to occupational therapy to assist the client and family with identifying diversional activities within the capability of the client and family.
▲ Introduce (or continue) friendly volunteer visitors if the client is willing and able to have the company. If transportation is an issue or if the client does not want visitors in the home, consider alternatives (e.g., telephone contacts, computer messaging).
• For clients who are interested and capable, suggest involvement in a community gardening experience through the senior center.
▲ In the presence of a psychiatric disorder, refer for psychiatric home healthcare services for client reassurance and implementation of therapeutic regimen.
• If the client is dying, and is interested, assist in making a videotape, audiotape or memory book for family members with treasured stories, memoirs, pictures, and video clips.

Client/Family Teaching

• Work with the client and family on learning diversional activities that the client is interested in (e.g., knitting, hooking rugs, writing memoirs).
• If the client is in isolation, give the client complete information on why isolation is needed and how it should be accomplished, especially guidelines for visitors.

Disturbed Energy field

NANDA Definition

Disruption of the flow of energy surrounding a person's being results in disharmony of the body, mind, and/or spirit

Defining Characteristics

Perceptions of changes in patterns of energy flow, such as movement (wave, spike, tingling, density, flowing); sounds (tone, words); temperature change (warmth, coolness); visual changes (image, color); disruption of the field (deficit, hole, spike, bulge, obstruction, congestion, diminished flow in energy field)

Related Factors

Slowing or blocking of energy flows secondary to: maturational factors: age-related developmental crisis or difficulties; pathophysiologic factors: illness, injury, pregnancy; situational factors: anxiety, fear, grieving, pain; treatment-related factors: chemotherapy, immobility, labor and delivery, perioperative experience

Client Outcomes

Client Will (Specify Time Frame):

- State sense of well-being
- State feeling of relaxation
- State decreased pain
- State decreased tension
- Demonstrate evidence of physical relaxation (e.g., decreased blood pressure, pulse, respiration rate, muscle tension)

Nursing Interventions

- Refer to care plans for **Anxiety, Acute Pain,** and **Chronic Pain.**
- Consider using Therapeutic Touch (TT) and/or Healing Touch (HT) for clients with anxiety, tension, pain, or other conditions that indicate a disruption in the flow of energy.
- Consider HT treatments for clients with psychological depression.
- Administer TT and/or HT as described in the following discussion (may also include Reiki practice).

Guidelines for Therapeutic Touch and Healing Touch

- TT and HT may be practiced by anyone with the requisite preparation, desire, and commitment.
- Those who are not licensed healthcare professionals may practice TT and HT within their families and religious or spiritual community and on friends.
- NOTE: Nurses who are not trained in TT or HT should consider spending quiet time with clients listening to their concerns.
- TT is conducted according to the standards for its practice developed by Dolores Krieger and Dora Kunz.
- HT is conducted according to the code of ethics and standards of practice developed by Healing Touch International, Inc.
- Administer TT and HT according to the guidelines established by the prospective therapies and programs.

Pediatric

- Consider using TT or HT for pediatric clients with adjunct therapies to decrease stress, anxiety, and pain.
- Teach that when working with the very young, old, or ill, or in the head area, TT should be gentle and used only for short periods.

Geriatric

- Consider TT and HT for agitated clients with Alzheimer's disease.

Multicultural

- Assess for the influence of cultural beliefs, norms, and values on the client's sense of disharmony of mind and spirit.
- Assess for the presence of specific culture-bound syndromes that may manifest as disturbances in energy or spirit.
- Validate the client's feelings and concerns related to sense of disharmony or energy disturbance.

Home Care

- See Guidelines for TT and HT.
- Help the client and family accept TT and HT as healing interventions.
- Assist the family with providing an appropriate space in which TT and or HT can be administered.

▲ Assess clients with bipolar disorder for the occurrence of social rhythm disruption, particularly during periods of stressful life events. Refer for mental health treatment.

▲ In the presence of a psychiatric disorder, refer for psychiatric home healthcare services for client reassurance and implementation of therapeutic regimen.

Client/Family Teaching

- Teach the TT and/or specific HT technique process to clients and family members.
- Teach that when working with the very young, old, or ill, or in the head area, TT should be gentle and used only for short periods.
- Teach the client how to use guided imagery.
- Teach the client to use deep breathing to relax. Ask the client to create an image of the disease, affected organ, or symptom.

After the image has been identified, ask the client to speak with the image to address an unresolved issue.

F

Impaired Environmental interpretation syndrome

NANDA Definition

Consistent lack of orientation to person, place, time, or circumstances for more than 3 to 6 months, necessitating a protective environment

Defining Characteristics

Chronic confusional states; consistent disorientation; inability to concentrate; inability to follow simple directions; inability to reason; loss of occupation; loss of social functioning; slow in responding to questions

Related Factors (r/t)

Dementia; depression; Huntington's disease

Client Outcomes

Client Will (Specify Time Frame):

- Remain content and free from harm
- Function at maximal cognitive level
- Participate in activities of daily living (ADLs) at the maximum of functional ability

Nursing Interventions and Client/Family Teaching

Refer to care plan for **Chronic Confusion.**

Adult Failure to thrive

NANDA Definition

Progressive functional deterioration of a physical and cognitive nature. The individual's ability to live with multisystem diseases, cope with ensuing problems, and manage his or her care are remarkably diminished.

Defining Characteristics

Altered mood state; anorexia; apathy; cognitive decline: problems with responding to environmental stimuli; demonstrated difficulty in concentration; demonstrated difficulty in decision making; demonstrated difficulty in judgment; demonstrated difficulty in memory; demonstrated difficulty in reasoning; decreased perception; consumption of minimal to no food at most meals (i.e., consumes <75% of normal requirements); decreased participation in activities of daily living; decreased social skills; expresses loss of interest in pleasurable outlets; frequent exacerbations of chronic health problems; inadequate nutritional intake; neglect of home environment; neglect of financial responsibilities; physical decline (e.g., fatigue, dehydration, incontinence of bowel and bladder); self-care deficit; social withdrawal; unintentional weight loss (e.g., 5% in 1 month, 10% in 6 months); verbalizes desire for death

Related Factor (r/t)

Depression

Client Outcomes

Client Will (Specify Time Frame):

- Resume highest level of functioning possible
- Express feelings
- Participate in ADLs
- Participate in social interactions
- Consume adequate dietary intake for weight and height
- Maintain usual weight
- Have adequate fluid intake with no signs of dehydration
- Maintain clean personal and home environment

Nursing Interventions

Psychosocial

- Elderly clients who have failure to thrive (FTT) should be evaluated by review of their ADLs, cognitive function, and mood; a targeted history and physical examination; and selected laboratory studies.
- Assess for depression with a geriatric depression scale. Be alert for depression in clients newly admitted to nursing homes.
- Screen for depression in persons with adult macular degeneration and low vision or vision loss.

▲ Carefully assess for elder abuse and refer for treatment.
• Provide reality orientation for clients with mild dementia.
• Instill hope and encourage the expression of positive thoughts.
• Provide music for clients with dementia.
▲ Consider the use of light therapy.
▲ Provide opportunities for visitation from animals.
• Encourage clients to reminiscence and share and compile life histories.
• Encourage clients to pray if they wish.
• Encourage elderly clients to take part in activities and social relationships according to their capacity and wishes.
• Help clients participate in activities by assessing motivation and helping them identify reasons to participate, such as better mobility, more independence, and feelings of well-being.
• Provide physical touch for clients. Touch the client's hand or arm when speaking with him or her; offer hugs with permission.
• Administer TT.

Physiological

▲ Assess possible causes for adult FTT and treat any underlying problems such as malnutrition, diarrhea, renal failure, and illnesses caused by physical and cognitive changes.
▲ Assess for signs of fatigue and sensory changes that may indicate an infection is present that may be related to undetected diabetes mellitus, human immunodeficiency virus (HIV), or *Staphylococcus aureus* bacteremia.
• Monitor weight loss, leaving 25% or more of food uneaten at most meals, psychiatric/mood diagnoses, and deteriorated ability to participate in activities of daily living.
• Assess for signs of dehydration.
• Play soothing music during mealtimes to increase the amount of food eaten and promote decreased agitation.
• Decrease noise and increase lighting in the dining area.
• Serve "family-style" meals.
▲ Refer to a dietician for individualized nutrition therapy.
• Refer to care plan **Readiness for enhanced Nutrition** for additional interventions.
• Assess how often the frail elder living at home goes outdoors. (Ask, "How often do you go outside the house?" Examples

include shopping, taking a walk, working in the garden.) Encourage outside activities.

- Provide opportunities for interaction with the natural environment.
- Assess grip strength.
- Frail elderly clients should also participate in carefully supervised group exercise as well as balance and gait programs accompanied by music.

▲ Refer for possible pharmacological intervention.

- Refer to care plans for **Imbalanced Nutrition: less than body requirements, Hopelessness,** and **Disturbed Energy field.**

F

Multicultural

- Assess for the influence of cultural beliefs, norms, and values on the family's or caregiver's understanding of FTT.
- Actively listen and be sensitive to how communication is shared culturally. Some cultures communication with eye contact and some avoid eye contact.

▲ Refer culturally diverse clients to appropriate social, medical, mental health, and long-term care services.

Home Care

- The above interventions may be adapted for home care use.
- If FTT is attributable to a dementing illness, refer to care plan for **Chronic Confusion.**

▲ Institute case management and refer for care housing of frail elderly to support continued independent living.

▲ Refer for individualized care management for home healthcare services such as homemaker or psychiatric home healthcare services for respite, client reassurance, and implementation of therapeutic regimen.

Client/Family Teaching

▲ Consider use of a nurse-managed telehealth system with clients who have been discharged early from the hospital to monitor symptoms, provide education, and make referrals if necessary.

▲ Refer for medical evaluation when cognitive changes are noticed.

- Encourage family to provide social interaction with the client.
- Instruct the family to monitor the elder person's weight.

▲ Provide referral for evaluation of hearing and appropriate hearing aids.
▲ Refer for psychotherapy and possible medication if the etiology is depression.
▲ Refer for possible medication therapy when the diagnosis is dementia.

Risk for Falls

NANDA Definition

Increased susceptibility to falling that may cause physical harm

Risk Factors (Intrinsic and Extrinsic)

Adults

Age 65 or older; history of falls; lives alone; lower limb prosthesis; use of assistive devices (e.g., walker, cane); wheelchair use

Children

Less than 2 years of age; bed located near window; lack of auto restraints; lack of gate on stairs; lack of window guard; lack of parental supervision; male gender when less than one year of age; unattended infant on elevated surface (e.g., bed/changing table)

Cognitive

Diminished mental status

Environment

Cluttered environment; dimly lit room; no antislip material in bath or shower; restraints; throw rugs; unfamiliar room; weather conditions (e.g., wet floors, ice)

Medications

ACE inhibitors; alcohol use; antianxiety agents; antihypertensive agents; diuretics; hypnotics; narcotics; tranquilizers; tricyclic antidepressants

Physiological

Anemias; arthritis; diarrhea; decreased lower extremity strength; difficult with gait; faintness when extending neck; faintness when turning neck; foot problems; hearing difficulties; impaired balance; impaired physical mobility; incontinence; neoplasms (i.e., fatigue/limited mobility); neuropathy; orthostatic hypotension; postoperative conditions; postprandial blood sugar changes; presence of acute illness; proprioceptive deficits; sleeplessness; urgency; vascular disease; visual difficulties

Client Outcomes

Client Will (Specify Time Frame):

- Remain free of falls
- Change environment to minimize the incidence of falls
- Explain methods to prevent injury

Nursing Interventions

- Determine risk of falling by using an evaluation tool such as the Fall Risk Assessment, The Conley Scale, or the FRAINT Tool for fall risk assessment.
- Complete a fall risk assessment for older adults in acute care using a valid and reliable tool such as The Hendrich II Model.
- Screen all clients for balance and mobility skills (supine to sit, sitting supported and unsupported, sit to stand, standing, walking and turning around, transferring, stooping to floor and recovering, and sitting down). Use tools such as the Balance Scale or the Get Up and Go Scale.
- Recognize that when people attend to another task while walking, such as carrying a cup of water, clothing, or supplies, they are more likely to fall.
- Be careful when getting a mostly immobile client up. Be sure to lock the bed and wheelchair and have sufficient personnel to protect the client from falls. When the client is rising from a lying position, have the client change positions slowly, dangle legs, and stand next to the bed before walking to prevent orthostatic hypotension.
- Identify clients likely to fall by placing a "fall precautions" sign on the doorway and by keying the Kardex and chart. Use a "high-risk fall" armband and room sign to alert staff for increased vigilance and mobility assistance.

▲ Evaluate the client's medications to determine whether they increase the risk of falling; consult physician regarding the client's need for medication if appropriate.

F

- Thoroughly orient the client to the environment. Place the call light within reach and show how to call for assistance; answer call light promptly.
- Use one-quarter- to one-half-length side rails only and maintain bed in a low position. Ensure that wheels are locked on bed and commode. Keep dim light in room at night.
- Routinely assist the client with toileting on his or her own schedule.

▲ Avoid restraints if at all possible. Obtain a physician's order if restraints are necessary, and use the least restrictive device.

- In place of restraints, use the following:
  - Well-staffed and educated nursing personnel with frequent client contact with careful consideration during shift changes
  - Nursing units designed to care for clients with cognitive or functional impairments
  - Nonskid footwear, sneakers preferable
  - Adequate lighting, night light in bathroom
  - Frequent toileting
  - Frequent assessment of the need for invasive devices, tubes, intravenous (IV) lines
  - Tubes hidden with bandages to prevent pulling of tubes
  - Alternative IV placement site to prevent client from pulling it out
  - Alarm systems with ankle, above-the-knee, or wrist sensors
  - Bed or wheelchair alarms
  - Wedge cushions on chairs to prevent slipping
  - Increased observation of the client
  - Locked doors to unit
  - Low or very low height beds
  - Border-defining pillow or mattress to remind the client to stay in bed
- If the client has an acute change in mental status (delirium), recognize that the cause is usually physiological and is a medical emergency. Provide reality orientation when interacting. Have family bring in familiar items, clocks, and watches from home to maintain orientation. See interventions for **Acute Confusion.**
- If the client has chronic confusion with dementia, use validation therapy that reinforces feelings but does not confront reality. See interventions for **Chronic Confusion.**

- Ask family to stay with the client to assist with ADLs and prevent the client from accidentally falling or pulling out tubes.
- ▲ If the client is unsteady on feet, have two nursing staff members alongside when walking the client. Consider referral to physical therapy for gait training and strengthening.
- Place a fall-prone client in a room that is near the nurses' station.
- Help clients sit in a stable chair with arm rests. Avoid use of wheelchairs and "geri-chairs" except for transportation as needed.
- Ensure that the chair or wheelchair fits the build, abilities, and needs of the client to ensure propulsion with legs or arms and ability to reach the floor, eliminating footrests and minimizing problems with shearing.
- Avoid use of wheelchairs as much as possible because they can serve as a restraint device. Most people in wheelchairs do not move.
- ▲ Refer to physical therapy for strengthening exercises, gait training, and help with balance to increase mobility.

Geriatric

- Assess ability to move using the Get Up and Go test. Ask the client to rise from a sitting position, walk 10 feet, turn, and return to the chair to sit.
- Complete a fall risk assessment for older adults in acute care using a valid and reliable tool such as The Hendrich II Model.
- ▲ If new onset of falling, assess for laboratory abnormalities and signs and symptoms of infection and dehydration. Check blood pressure and pulse rate supine, sitting, and standing for orthostatic hypotension.
- Encourage the client to wear glasses and use walking aids when ambulating.
- Help the client obtain and wear a specially designed hip protector when ambulating. Hip protectors are worn in a specially designed stretchy undergarment containing a pocket on each side for placement of the protector.
- If the client experiences dizziness when getting up because of orthostatic hypotension, teach methods to decrease dizziness such as rising slowly, remaining seated several minutes before standing, flexing feet upward several times while sitting, sitting

down immediately if feeling dizzy, and having someone present when standing.

▲ If the client has syncope, determine symptoms that occur before syncope and note medications that the client is taking. Refer for medical care. The circumstances surrounding syncope often suggest the cause.

▲ Observe client for signs of anemia, and refer to primary care practitioner for testing if appropriate.

▲ Evaluate client for chronic alcohol intake as well as mental health and neurologic function.

▲ Refer to physical therapy for strength training with free weights or machines.

▲ If an elderly woman has symptoms of urge incontinence, refer to a urologist for evaluation and ensure the path to the bathroom is well lit and free of obstructions.

Home Care

- Some of the above interventions may be adapted for home care use.
- If the client was identified as a fall risk in the hospital, recognize that there is a high incidence of falls after discharge and use all measures possible to reduce the incidence of falls.
- Assess and monitor for acute changes in cognition and behavior.
- Assess for cause of delirium and/or falls with an interdisciplinary team.
- Assess for additional factors leading to risk for falls.
- Assess home environment for threats to safety including clutter, slippery floors, scatter rugs, and other potential hazards. Additionally, assess external environment (e.g., uneven pavement, unleveled stairs or steps).

▲ Institute a home-based, nurse-delivered exercise program to reduce falls or refer to physical therapy services for client and family education of safe transfers and ambulation and for strengthening exercises for the client.

▲ Instruct the client and family or caregivers on how to correct identified hazards. Refer to physical and occupational therapy services for assistance if needed.

- Use a multifactorial assessment along with interventions targeted to the identified risk factors. Key components of the interventions include evaluating need for all medications, balance, gait and strength training, use of strategies to deal with postural hypotension if present, home safety evaluation with needed modifications, and any needed cardiovascular treatment.

- Encourage the client to eat a balanced diet, with particular inclusion of vitamin D and calcium.
- If the client lives alone or spends a lot of time alone, teach the client what to do if he or she falls and cannot get up, and make sure he or she has a personal emergency response system or a cellular phone that is available from the floor.
- If the client is at risk for falls, use a gait belt and additional persons when ambulating.
- Ensure appropriate nonglare lighting in the home. Ask the client to install indoor strip or "runway" type of lighting to baseboards to help clients balance. Install motion-sensitive lighting that turns on automatically when the client gets out of bed to go to the bathroom.
- Have the client wear supportive low-heeled shoes with good traction when ambulating.
- Avoid use of slip-on footwear (e.g., clogs, slip-on slippers or sneakers).
- Consider the use of external hip protectors for clients at risk of falls.

▲ Refer to physical therapy services for the client and family education of safe transfers and ambulation and for strengthening/balance exercises for the client for ambulation and transfers.

- Provide a signaling device for clients who wander or are at risk for falls.
- Provide a medical identification bracelet for clients at risk for injury from dementia, diabetes, seizures, or other medical disorders.
- Suggest a tai chi class designed for the elderly to selected clients who have sufficient balance to participate.

Client/Family Teaching

- Teach the client how to ambulate safely at home, including using safety measures such as hand rails in bathroom and the need to avoid carrying things or performing other tasks while walking.
- Teach the client the importance of maintaining a regular exercise program such as walking. If the client is afraid of falling

while walking outside during cold or wet weather, suggest walking the length of a local mall.

Dysfunctional Family processes: alcoholism

F

NANDA Definition

Psychosocial, spiritual, and physiological functions of the family unit are chronically disorganized, which leads to conflict, denial of problems, resistance to change, ineffective problem solving, and a series of self-perpetuating crises.

Defining Characteristics

Behavioral

Alcohol abuse; enabling to maintain alcoholic drinking pattern; family special occasions are alcohol centered; inadequate understanding of alcoholism; substance abuse other than alcohol

Feelings

Anger; anxiety; responsibility for alcoholic's behavior

Roles and Relationships

Altered role function; chronic family problems; closed communication systems; deterioration in family relationships/disturbed family dynamics

Related Factors (r/t)

Abuse of alcohol; addictive personality; biochemical influences; family history of alcoholism; family history of resistance to treatment; genetic predisposition; inadequate coping skills; lack of problem-solving skills

Client Outcomes

Family/Client Will (Specify Time Frame):

- Develop relationship with nurse that demonstrates at least minimal level of trust
- Demonstrate an understanding of alcoholism as a family illness and the severity of the threat to emotional and physical health of family members

- Develop and state a belief in feasibility and effectiveness of efforts to address alcoholism
- Demonstrate change from dysfunctional patterns by moving from inappropriate to appropriate role relationships, improving cohesion among family members, decreasing conflict and social isolation, and improving coping behaviors
- Maintain improvements

Nursing Interventions

- • Refer to care plans for **Ineffective Denial** and **Defensive Coping** for additional interventions.
- • When completing a family assessment, assess behaviors of alcohol abuse, loss of control of drinking, denial, nicotine addiction, impaired communication, inappropriate expression of anger, and enabling behaviors.
- • Screen clients for at-risk drinking during routine primary care visits.
- • Instill hope and encourage the expression of positive thoughts.
- • Stress early treatment and brief intervention to resolve the problem.
- • Assist with stabilization and maintenance of positive change in the family. Instruct the alcoholic's family members before the client's discharge to give verbal messages that convey concern about the alcoholic's problem drinking, their observations of the alcoholic's past episodes of drinking, and wishes and support for abstinence.
- • Provide activities that are physical in nature, such as adventure therapy and therapeutic camping, as part of a substance abuse treatment program.
- ▲ Consider alternative therapies such as acupuncture.
- ▲ Refer for possible use of medications such as naltrexone and acamprosate to control problem drinking.

Pediatric

- • Educate family members about available educational and support programs and encourage limited alcohol use in the home.
- • Use closed-ended questions when questioning adolescents about drinking behavior.
- ▲ Provide a brief motivational interviewing and cognitive/

behavioral-based alcohol intervention group program for young people at risk of developing a problem with alcohol.
- • Encourage parent involvement with adolescents for both supervision and emotional support.
- • Work at strengthening adolescents' relationships in and out of the home.

F

- ▲ Provide school-based prevention programs using peer leaders at an early age.
- ▲ Provide a school-based drug-prevention program to junior high students.

Geriatric

- • Include assessment of possible alcohol abuse when assessing elderly family members.
- ▲ Provide alcohol treatment programs for geriatric clients in primary care settings.

Multicultural

- • Acknowledge racial/ethnic differences at the onset of care.
- • Approach families of color with respect, warmth, and professional courtesy.
- • Give rationale when assessing black families about alcohol use and misuse.
- • Use a family-centered approach when working with Latino, Asian-American, African-American, and Native-American clients.
- • When working with Asian-American clients, provide opportunities for the family to save face.
- • Some less-acculturated Latino families may be unwilling to discuss family issues with healthcare providers until they perceive a close personal relationship with the provider.
- • Use family strengthening interventions such as behavioral parent training, family skills training, in-home family support, brief family therapy, and family education when working with culturally diverse families.
- • Work with families in a way that incorporates cultural elements.

Home Care

NOTE: In the community setting, alcoholism as cause of dysfunctional family processes must be considered in two categories

(1) when the client suffers personally from the illness and (2) when a significant other suffers from the illness, that is, the client is not the active alcoholic but may depend on the alcoholic for caregiving. The following considerations apply to both situations with appropriate adaptation for the circumstances.

- • The previous interventions may be adapted for home care use.
- • Identify client and family expectations of the home care nurse and nurse expectations of the client and family by use of a well-defined contract. Be specific and realistic. Adjust the contract only with clear consent and understanding of the client and family.
- • Work with family members to support a sense of valued fit on their part; include them in treatment planning and identify the importance of their roles in the client's care. At the same time, encourage their pursuit of positive outside activities that enhance their sense of belonging.
- ▲ Establish well-defined contingency and emergency plans for the care of the client.
- • Request concrete, measurable tasks of the client and family for caregiving and provide concrete, nonjudgmental instruction to the client and family regarding the interactions of alcohol use with medications and the therapeutic regimen.
- ▲ Observe for abuse of other medications. Notify physician of problems noted.
- ▲ If the client is a recovering alcoholic, extreme care must be taken in the use of psychoactive or pain medications. Notify physician if inappropriate medications have been inadvertently ordered.
- ▲ Refer for medical social work services at the outset of care.
- ▲ Provide information regarding available substance use treatment programs and support groups.
- • Acknowledge without judging when resolution of alcoholism is not a goal of care.
- ▲ Refer for psychiatric home healthcare services for client reassurance and implementation of therapeutic regimen.

Client Family Teaching

- • Suggest the client complete a confidential Internet self-screening test for identification of problems and suggestions for treatment if a problem with alcohol is suspected. Many tools are available.

Interrupted Family processes

NANDA Definition

Change in family relationships and/or functioning

F

Defining Characteristics

Changes in assigned tasks; changes in availability for affective responsiveness; changes in availability for emotional support; changes in communication patterns; changes in effectiveness in completing assigned tasks; changes in expressions of conflict with community resources; changes in expressions of isolation from community resources; changes in expressions of conflict within family; changes in intimacy; changes in mutual support; changes in patterns; changes in participation in problem solving; changes in participation in decision making; changes in power alliances; changes in rituals; changes in satisfaction with family; changes in somatic complaints; changes in stress-reduction behaviors

Related Factors (r/t)

Developmental crises; developmental transition; family roles shift; interaction with community; modification in family finances; modification in family social status; power shift of family members; shift in health status of a family member; situation transition; situational crises

Client Outcomes

Family/Client Will (Specify Time Frame):

- Express feelings (family)
- Identify ways to cope effectively and use appropriate support systems (family)
- Treat impaired family member as normally as possible to avoid overdependence (family)
- Meet physical, psychosocial, and spiritual needs of members or seek appropriate assistance (family)
- Demonstrate knowledge of illness or injury, treatment modalities, and prognosis (family)
- Participate in the development of the plan of care to the best of ability (significant person)

Nursing Interventions

Refer to the care plan **Readiness for enhanced Family processes** for additional interventions.

- • Establish rapport with families by providing accurate communication.
- • Acknowledge the range of emotions and feelings that may be experienced when the health status of a family member changes; counsel family members that it is normal to be angry and afraid.
- • Encourage family members to list their personal strengths.
- • Involve family members in the care, information, and client teaching sessions with the client.
- • Encourage family to visit the client; adjust visiting hours to accommodate family's schedule (e.g., schedule around work, school, babysitting needs). Assist with sleeping arrangements if family is spending the night; provide a place to lie down, pillows, and blankets.
- • Allow and encourage family to assist in the client's care. Allow family presence during invasive procedures and resuscitation.
- ▲ Consider use of video home training as a method of early support in problems of family life control.

Pediatric

- ▲ Carefully assess potential for reunifying children placed in foster care with their birth parents.
- • Allow and encourage family to assist in the client's care.
- ▲ Refer children and mothers exposed to violence in the home to theraplay: an attachment-based intervention that uses the four core elements of nurturing, engagement, structure, and challenge in interactions between mother and her child.

Geriatric

- • Encourage family members to be involved in the care of relatives who are in residential care settings.
- • Support group problem solving among family members and include the older member.
- ▲ Refer family for counseling with a psychotherapist who is knowledgeable about gerontology.
- • Refer to care plan for **Readiness for enhanced Family processes** for additional interventions.

Multicultural

- Refer to the care plan **Readiness for enhanced Family process** for additional interventions.

Home Care

- The nursing interventions described in the care plan for **Compromised family Coping** should be used in the home environment with adaptations as necessary.
- Request help from the family when communicating with clients with advanced stages of cancer who are no longer able to communicate their illness and symptom needs.

Client/Family Teaching

- Refer to Client/Family Teaching in **Compromised family Coping** and **Readiness for enhanced family Coping** for suggestions that may be used with minor adaptations.

Readiness for enhanced Family processes

NANDA Definition

A pattern of family functioning that is sufficient to support the well-being of family members and can be strengthened.

Defining Characteristics

Activities support the growth of family members; activities support the safety of family members; balance exists between autonomy and cohesiveness; boundaries of family members are maintained; communication is adequate; energy level of family supports activities of daily living; expresses willingness to enhance family dynamics; family adapts to change; family functioning meets needs of family members; family resilience is evident; family roles are appropriate for developmental stages; family roles are flexible for developmental stages; family tasks are accomplished; interdependent with community; relationships are generally positive; respect for family members is evident

Client Outcomes

Family/Client Will (Specify Time Frame):

- Identify ways to cope effectively and use appropriate support systems (family)
- Meet physical, psychosocial, and spiritual needs of members or seek appropriate assistance (family)
- Demonstrate knowledge of potential environmental, lifestyle, and genetic risks to health and use appropriate measures to decrease possibility of risk (family)
- Focus on wellness, disease prevention, and maintenance (family and individual)
- Seek balance among exercise, work, leisure, rest, and nutrition (family and individual)

Nursing Interventions

- • Assess the family's stress level and coping abilities during the initial nursing assessment.
- • Consider the use of family theory as a framework to help guide interventions (e.g., family stress theory, role theory, social exchange theory).
- • Use family-centered care and role modeling for holistic care of families.
- • Discuss with family members how they have handled previous crises.
- • Support family empowerment; strength, and resourcefulness.
- • Spend time with family members; allow them to verbalize their feelings.
- • Encourage family members to find meaning in a serious illness such as cancer.
- ▲ Provide family-centered care to explore and use all available resources appropriate for the situation (e.g., counseling, social services, self-help groups, pastoral care).
- ▲ Consider referral for walk-in family therapy.

Pediatric

- • Provide a parenting class series based on individual and couple changes in meaning and identity, roles, and relationships and interaction during the transition to parenthood. Address mother

and father roles, infant communication abilities, and patterns of the first 3 months of life in a mutually enjoyable, possibility focused manner.
- • Encourage families with adolescents to have family meals.
- ▲ Consider the use of adventure therapy for adolescents with cancer.

F

Geriatric

- • Carefully listen to residents and family members in the long-term care facility.
- • Support caregivers' awareness of the positive effects of their contribution to the well-being of parents.
- • Teach family members about the impact of developmental events (e.g., retirement, death, change in health status, and household composition).
- • Encourage social networks; social integration; and social engagement with friends, children, and relatives of the elderly.

Multicultural

- • Assess for the influence of cultural beliefs, norms, and values on the family's perceptions of normal functioning.
- • Identify and acknowledge the stresses unique to racial/ethnic families.
- • Assess and support spiritual needs of families.
- • With the client's consent, facilitate a group meeting for family members to discuss how the family is functioning.
- • Facilitate modeling and role playing for the client and family regarding healthy ways to start a discussion about the client's prognosis.
- • Encourage family mealtimes.

Home Care

- • The previous nursing interventions should be used in the home environment with adaptations as necessary.
- • Provide a videophone network for peer support for frail elderly people living at home.
- • Encourage families to help women caring for husbands with chronic obstructive pulmonary disease by providing respite care so the women may have recreation time.

Client/Family Teaching

- Refer to Client/Family Teaching in **Readiness for enhanced family Coping** for suggestions that may be used with minor adaptations.

F

Fatigue

NANDA Definition

An overwhelming, sustained sense of exhaustion and decreased capacity for physical and mental work at usual level.

Defining Characteristics

Compromised concentration; compromised libido; decreased performance; disinterest in surroundings; drowsy; feelings of guilt for not keeping up with responsibilities; inability to maintain usual level of physical activity; inability to maintain usual routines; inability to restore energy even after sleep; increase in physical complaints; increase in rest requirements; introspection; lack of energy; lethargic; listless; perceived need for additional energy to accomplish routine tasks; tired; verbalization of an unremitting lack of energy; verbalization of an overwhelming lack of energy

Related Factors (r/t)

Psychological

Anxiety; boring lifestyle; depression

Physiological

Anemia; disease states; increased physical exertion; malnutrition; poor physical condition; pregnancy; sleep deprivation

Environmental

Humidity; lights; noise; temperature

Situational

Negative life events; occupation

Client Outcomes

Client Will (Specify Time Frame):

- Identify potential factors that aggravate and relieve fatigue
- Describe ways to assess and track patterns of fatigue
- Describe ways in which fatigue affects the ability to accomplish goals
- Verbalize increased energy and improved well-being
- Explain energy conservation plan to offset fatigue
- Explain energy restoration plan to offset fatigue

Nursing Interventions

- • Assess severity of fatigue on a scale of 0 to 10 (average fatigue, worst and best levels); assess frequency of fatigue (number of days per week and time of day), activities and symptoms associated with increased fatigue (e.g., pain), ability to perform ADLs and instrumental ADLs, interference with social and role function, times of increased energy, ability to concentrate, mood, and usual pattern of activity. Consider use of an instrument such as the Profile of Mood State Short Form Fatigue Subscale, the Multidimensional Assessment of Fatigue, the Lee Fatigue Scale, the Multidimensional Fatigue Inventory, the HIV-Related Fatigue Scale, the Brief Fatigue Inventory, or the Dutch Fatigue Scale to assess fatigue accurately.
- • Evaluate adequacy of nutrition and sleep patterns (napping throughout the day, inability to fall asleep or stay asleep). Encourage the client to get adequate rest, limit naps (particularly in the late afternoon or evening), use a routine sleep/wake schedule, avoid caffeine in the late afternoon or evening, and eat a well-balanced diet with at least eight glasses of water a day. Refer to **Imbalanced Nutrition: less than body requirements** or **Sleep Deprivation** if appropriate.
- ▲ Collaborate with the primary care practitioner to identify physiological and/or psychological causes of fatigue that could be treated, such as anemia, pain, electrolyte imbalance (e.g., altered potassium levels), hypothyroidism, depression, or medication effect.
- ▲ Work with the primary care practitioner to determine if the client has chronic fatigue syndrome.
- • Encourage the client to express feelings about fatigue, including potential causes of fatigue, and possible interventions to alleviate fatigue such as setting small, easily achieved short-term

goals and developing energy management techniques; use active listening techniques and help identify sources of hope.

- • Encourage the client to keep a journal of activities, symptoms of fatigue, and feelings, including how fatigue affects the client's normal activities and roles.
- • Help the client identify sources of support and essential and nonessential tasks to determine which tasks can be delegated to whom. Give the client permission to limit social and role demands if needed (e.g., switch to part-time employment, hire cleaning service).
- ▲ Collaborate with the primary care practitioner regarding the appropriateness of referrals to physical therapy for carefully monitored aerobic exercise program and possible physical aids, such as a walker or cane.
- • Clients may desire multiple strategies to relieve fatigue rather than one single intervention, particularly when there are multiple potential etiologies present.
- ▲ Refer the client to diagnosis-appropriate support groups such as National Chronic Fatigue Syndrome Association, Multiple Sclerosis Association, or cancer fatigue websites such as the Oncology Nurses Association.
- ▲ For a cardiac client, recognize that fatigue is common after a myocardial infarction. Refer to cardiac rehabilitation for carefully prescribed and monitored exercise program.
- • For fatigue associated with multiple sclerosis, encourage energy conservation, "recharging efforts," and excellent self-care; consider use of a cooling suit because fatigue increases in a warm environment.
- ▲ Consider referring for cognitive therapy to help deal with symptoms of fatigue and help change negative thought patterns.
- • If fatigue is associated with cancer or cancer-related treatment, assess for other symptoms that may enhance fatigue (e.g., pain or depression).
- ▲ Collaborate with primary care practitioners to identify attentional fatigue, which may manifest itself as the inability to direct attention necessary to perform usual activities.

Geriatric

- • Review comorbid conditions that may contribute to fatigue, such as congestive heart failure, arthritis, and cancer.

- • Identify recent losses; monitor for depression as a possible contributing factor to fatigue.
- ▲ Review medications for side effects.

Home Care

F

- • The above interventions may be adapted for home care use.
- • Assess the client's history and current patterns of fatigue as they relate to the home environment and environmental and behavioral triggers of increased fatigue.
- ▲ Refer to occupational and/or physical therapy if substantial intervention is needed to assist the client in adapting to home and daily patterns.
- • For clients receiving chemotherapy, intervene to:
  - ■ Relieve symptom distress (negative mood, nausea, difficulty sleeping)
  - ■ Encourage as much physical activity as possible
  - ■ Support a positive attitude for the future
  - ■ Support adequate recovery time between treatments
- ▲ Refer cancer clients to a community-based pain and fatigue management program, such as the I Feel Better program, if available.
- • Teach the client and family the importance of and methods for setting priorities for activities, especially those with high energy demand (e.g., home or family events). Instruct in realistic expectations and behavioral pacing.
- • Assess effect of fatigue on the client's relatedness; recognize that the client's fatigue affects the whole family. Initiate the following interventions:
  - ■ Avoid dismissing reports of fatigue; validate the client's experience and foster hope for eventual treatment, if not resolution, of the fatigue.
  - ■ Identify with the client ways in which he or she continues to be a valued part of his or her social environment.
  - ■ Identify with the client ways in which he or she continues to participate in equitable exchange with others.
  - ■ Encourage the client to maintain regular family routines (e.g., meals, sleep patterns) as much as possible.
  - ■ Initiate cognitive restructuring to refute the client's guilt-producing and negative thought patterns.
  - ■ Assess and intervene with family's and friends' contributions to guilt-inducing self-talk.

- ■ Work with the client to inoculate against the negative thinking of others.
- ■ Explore family life and demands to identify accommodations.
- ■ Support the client's efforts at limit setting on the demands of others.
- ■ Assist the client to move toward a state of parallelism by working to identify and relieve sources of physical or emotional discomfort. Degree of involvement, limited by fatigue, need not be changed.

▲ Refer for family therapy in the event the client's fatigue interferes with normal family functioning.

▲ If fatigue has affected the client's ability to participate in relationships effectively, refer for psychiatric home healthcare services for client reassurance and implementation of therapeutic regimen.

Client/Family Teaching

- Help client to reframe cognitively; share information about fatigue and how to live with it, including need for positive self-talk.
- Teach strategies for energy conservation (e.g., sitting instead of standing during showering, storing items at waist level).
- Teach the client to carry a pocket calendar, make lists of required activities, and post reminders around the house.
- Teach the importance of following a healthy lifestyle with adequate nutrition fluids and rest, pain relief, insomnia correction, and appropriate exercise to decrease fatigue (i.e., energy restoration).
- See **Depression** care plan if appropriate.

Fear

NANDA Definition

Response to perceived threat that is consciously recognized as a danger.

Defining Characteristics

Report of alarm; apprehension; being scared; increased tension; decreased self-assurance; dread; excitement; jitteriness; panic; terror

F

Cognitive
Diminished productivity; learning ability; problem-solving ability; identifies object of fear; stimulus believed to be a threat

Behaviors
Attack or avoidance behaviors; impulsiveness; increased alertness; narrowed focus on the source of fear

Physiological
Anorexia; diarrhea; dry mouth; dyspnea; fatigue; increased perspiration, pulse, respiratory rate, systolic blood pressure; muscle tightness; nausea; pallor; pupil dilation; vomiting

Related Factors (r/t)

Innate origin (e.g., sudden noise, height, pain, loss of physical support); innate releasers (neurotransmitters); language barrier; learned response (e.g., conditioning, modeling from or identification with others); phobic stimulus; sensory impairment; separation from support system in potentially stressful situation (e.g., hospitalization, hospital procedures); unfamiliarity with environmental experience(s)

Client Outcomes

Client Will (Specify Time Frame):
- Verbalize known fears
- State accurate information about the situation
- Identify, verbalize, and demonstrate those coping behaviors that reduce own fear
- Report and demonstrate reduced fear

Nursing Interventions

- • Assess source of fear with the client.
- • Assess for a history of anxiety.
- • Have the client draw the object of his or her fear.
- • Discuss the situation with the client and help distinguish between real and imagined threats to well-being.
- • Encourage the client to explore underlying feelings that may be contributing to the fear.
- • Stay with clients when they express fear; provide verbal and nonverbal (touch and hug with permission and if culturally acceptable) reassurances of safety if safety is within control.

- Explore coping skills previously used by the client to deal with fear; reinforce these skills and explore other outlets.
- Provide backrubs and massage for clients to decrease anxiety.
- Use TT and HT techniques.
- ▲ Refer for cognitive behavior therapy.
- ▲ Animal-assisted therapy can be incorporated into the care of perioperative clients.
- Encourage clients to express their fears in narrative form.
- Refer to care plans for **Anxiety** and **Death Anxiety.**

Pediatric

- Use draw-and-tell conversations with children about fear.
- Explore coping skills previously used by the client to deal with fear.
- Teach parents to use cognitive-behavioral strategies such as positive coping statements ("I am a brave girl [boy]. I can take care of myself in the dark.") and rewards of bravery tokens for appropriate behavior.
- Screen for depression in clients who report social or school fears.
- Teach relaxation techniques to children to induce calmness.

Geriatric

- Establish a trusting relationship so that all fears can be identified.
- Monitor for dementia and use appropriate interventions.
- Provide a protective and safe environment, use consistent caregivers, and maintain the accustomed environmental structure.
- Observe for untoward changes if antianxiety drugs are taken.
- Assess for fear of falls in hospitalized clients with hip fractures to determine risk of poor health outcomes.
- Encourage exercises to improve physical skills and levels of mobility to decrease fear of falling.
- Assist the client in identifying and reducing risk factors of falls, including environmental hazards in and out of the home, the importance of good nutrition and activity, proper footwear, and how to stand up after a fall.

Multicultural

- Assess for the presence of culture-bound anxiety and fear states.
- Assess for the influence of cultural beliefs, norms, and values on the client's perspective of a stressful situation.
- Identify what triggers fear response.

- Identify how the client expresses fear.
- Validate the client's feelings regarding fear.
- Assess for fears of racism in culturally diverse clients.

Home Care

F

- The previous interventions may be adapted for home care use.
- Assess to differentiate the presence of fear versus anxiety.
- Refer to care plan for **Anxiety.**
- During initial assessment, determine whether current or previous episodes of fear relate to the home environment (e.g., perception of danger in the home or neighborhood or of relationships that have a history in the home).
- Identify with the client what steps may be taken to make the home a "safe" place to be.

▲ Encourage the client to seek or continue appropriate counseling to reduce fear associated with stress or resolve alterations in irrational thought processes.

▲ Encourage the client to have a trusted companion, family member, or caregiver present in the home for periods when fear is most prominent. Pending other medical diagnoses, a referral to homemaker or home health aide services may meet this need.

▲ Offer to sit quietly with a terminally ill client as needed by the client or family, or provide hospice volunteers to do the same.

Client/Family Teaching

- Teach the client the difference between warranted and excessive fear.
- Teach clients to use guided imagery when they are fearful; have them use all senses to visualize a place that is "comfortable and safe" for them.

▲ Teach use of appropriate community resources in emergency situations (e.g., hotlines, emergency departments, law enforcement, judicial systems).

▲ Encourage use of appropriate community resources in nonemergency situations (e.g., family, friends, neighbors, self-help and support groups, volunteer agencies, churches, recreation clubs and centers, seniors, youths, others with similar interests).

▲ If fear is associated with bioterrorism, provide accurate information and ensure that healthcare personnel have appropriate training and preparation.

Readiness for enhanced Fluid balance

NANDA Definition

A pattern of equilibrium between fluid volume and chemical composition of body fluids that is sufficient for meeting physical needs and can be strengthened.

Defining Characteristics

Dehydration; expresses willingness to enhance fluid balance; good tissue turgor; intake adequate for daily needs; moist mucous membranes; no evidence of edema; no excessive thirst; specific gravity within normal limits; stable weight; straw-colored urine; urine output appropriate for intake

Client Outcomes

Client Will (Specify Time Frame):

- Maintain light-yellow urine output
- Maintain elastic skin turgor, moist tongue, and mucous membranes
- Explain measures that can be taken to improve fluid intake

Nursing Interventions

- Discuss normal fluid requirements.
- Recommend intake of mainly water, but milk or fruit juice can also be effective in maintaining good fluid balance.
- Recommend the client decrease the use of alcoholic beverages and beverages containing caffeine to provide fluid to the body.
- Recommend the client avoid intake of carbonated beverages; instead suggest the client drink water.

Geriatric

- Encourage the elderly client to develop a pattern of drinking water regularly.

Home Care

- Assess availability of clean drinking water in the home, or assess resources to acquire bottled water.

▲ Assess available and preferred fluids. Refer for social services if resources are needed to purchase adequate fluid.

Client/Family Teaching

- Teach the client to drink water before and while engaging in activities that can quickly result in dehydration, such as distance running or gardening in hot weather.
- Caution the athlete client not to drink excessively during competition or training but to follow the dictates of thirst.
- Teach clients who work in hot environments or exercise in hot environments to increase intake of both water and electrolyte-carbohydrate beverages.
- Ask the client to monitor the color of urine to tell if adequately hydrated.

Deficient Fluid volume

NANDA Definition

Decreased intravascular, interstitial, and/or intracellular fluid. This refers to dehydration, water loss alone without change in sodium level.

Defining Characteristics

Change in mental state; decreased blood pressure; decreased pulse pressure; decreased pulse volume; decreased skin turgor; decreased tongue turgor; decreased urine output; decreased venous filling; dry mucous membranes; dry skin; elevated hematocrit; increased body temperature; increased pulse rate; increased urine concentration; sudden weight loss (except in third spacing); thirst; weakness

Related Factors (r/t)

Active fluid volume loss; failure of regulatory mechanisms

Client Outcomes

Client Will (Specify Time Frame):

- Maintain urine output more than 1300 mL/day (or at least 30 mL/hr)
- Maintain normal blood pressure, pulse, and body temperature
- Maintain elastic skin turgor; moist tongue and mucous membranes; and orientation to person, place, and time

- Explain measures that can be taken to treat or prevent fluid volume loss
- Describe symptoms that indicate the need to consult with healthcare provider

Nursing Interventions

F

- Watch for early signs of hypovolemia, including restlessness, weakness, muscle cramps, headaches, inability to concentrate, and postural hypotension.
- Monitor for the existence of factors causing deficient fluid volume (e.g., vomiting, diarrhea, difficulty maintaining oral intake, fever, uncontrolled type 2 diabetes, diuretic therapy).
- Monitor daily weight for sudden decreases, especially in the presence of decreasing urine output or active fluid loss. Weigh the client on the same scale with the same type of clothing at same time of day, preferably before breakfast.
- Monitor total fluid intake and output every 8 hours (or every hour for the unstable client). Recognize that urine output is not always an accurate indicator of fluid balance.
- Watch trends in output for 3 days; include all routes of intake and output and note color and specific gravity of urine.
- Monitor vital signs of clients with deficient fluid volume every 15 minutes to 1 hour for the unstable client (every 4 hours for the stable client). Observe for tachycardia, tachypnea, decreased pulse pressure first, then hypotension, decreased pulse volume, and increased or decreased body temperature.
- Check orthostatic blood pressures with the client lying, sitting, and standing.
- Monitor for thirst, dry tongue and mucous membranes, longitudinal tongue furrows, speech difficulty, dry skin, sunken eyeballs, weakness (especially of upper body), headache, and confusion.
- Provide frequent oral hygiene, at least twice a day (if mouth is dry and painful, provide hourly while awake).
- Provide fresh water and oral fluids preferred by the client (distribute over a period of 24 hours [e.g., 1200 mL on days, 800 mL on evenings, and 200 mL on nights]); provide prescribed diet; offer snacks (e.g., frequent drinks, fresh fruits, fruit juice); and instruct significant other to assist the client with feedings as appropriate.

- • Provide free water with tube feedings as appropriate: 50 to 100 mL every 4 hours or 30 mL/kg of body weight.
- • Institute measures to rest the bowel when the client is vomiting or has diarrhea (e.g., restrict food or fluid intake when appropriate, decrease intake of milk products).
- ▲ Provide oral replacement therapy as ordered and tolerated with a hypotonic glucose-electrolyte solution when the client has acute diarrhea or nausea and vomiting. Provide small, frequent quantities of slightly chilled solutions.
- ▲ Administer antidiarrheals and antiemetics as appropriate.
- ▲ Hydrate the client with ordered intravenous (IV) solutions if prescribed.
- ▲ If the client requires IV fluid replacement, maintain patent IV access, set an appropriate IV infusion flow rate, and administer at a constant flow rate as ordered.
- • Assist with ambulation if the client has postural hypotension.

Critically Ill

- • If a trauma client, check manual blood pressure until the systolic pressure is 110 mm Hg. Do not rely on automatic blood pressure measurements. Check vital signs frequently.
- • Monitor central venous pressure, right atrial pressure, and pulmonary wedge pressure for decreases.
- • Monitor serum and urine osmolality, serum sodium, BUN/creatinine ratio, and hematocrit for elevations.
- • Use a sublingual capnometry device if available to determine level of tissue hypoxia caused by lack of fluid volume.
- ▲ Insert a Foley catheter if ordered and measure urine output hourly. Notify physician if <30 mL/hour.
- ▲ When ordered, initiate a fluid challenge of crystalloids (0.9% normal saline or Ringer's lactate) for replacement of intravascular volume; monitor the client's response to prescribed fluid therapy and fluid challenge, especially noting central venous pressure and pulmonary capillary wedge pressure readings, vital signs, urine output, blood lactate concentrations, and lung sounds.
- • Position the client flat with legs elevated when hypotensive, if not contraindicated.
- ▲ Monitor trends in serum lactic acid levels and base deficit obtained from blood gases as ordered.

▲ Consult physician if signs and symptoms of deficient fluid volume persist or worsen.

Pediatric

- • Monitor the child for signs of deficient fluid volume, including capillary refill time, skin turgor, and respiratory pattern along with other symptoms.
- ▲ Reinforce the physician's recommendation for the parents to give the child oral rehydration fluids to drink in the amounts specified, especially during the first 4 to 6 hours to replace fluid losses. Once the child is rehydrated, an orally administered maintenance solution should be used along with food.
- • Recommend the mother initiate, continue, or resume breast-feeding as soon as possible.
- • Recommend parents not give the child carbonated soda, fruit juices, gelatin dessert, or instant fruit drink mix.
- • Recommend parents give children foods with complex carbohydrates such as potatoes, rice, bread, cereal, yogurt, fruits, and vegetables.

Geriatric

- • Monitor elderly clients for deficient fluid volume carefully, noting new onset of weakness, dizziness, or dry mouth with longitudinal furrows on the tongue.
- • Evaluate the risk for dehydration using the Dehydration Risk Appraisal Checklist.
- • Check skin turgor of elderly clients on the forehead, sternum, or inner thigh; also look for the presence of longitudinal furrows on the tongue and dry mucous membranes.
- • Encourage fluid intake by offering fluids regularly to cognitively impaired clients.
- • Incorporate regular hydration into daily routines (e.g., extra glass of fluid with medication or social activities). Consider use of a beverage cart and a hydration assistant to routinely offer increased beverages to clients in extended care.
- • If client is identified as having chronic dehydration, flag the food tray to indicate to caregivers they should finish 75% to 100% of their food and fluids.
- • Recognize that lower blood pressures and a higher BUN/

creatinine ratio can be significant signs of dehydration in the elderly.

- Note the color of urine and compare against a urine color chart to monitor adequate fluid intake.
- Monitor elderly clients for excess fluid volume during the treatment of deficient fluid volume: listen to lung sounds, watch for edema, and note vital signs.

Home Care

- Teach family members how to monitor output in the home (e.g., use of commode "hat" in the toilet, urinal, or bedpan or use of catheter and closed drainage). Instruct them to monitor both intake and output.
- When weighing the client, use the same scale each day. Be sure scale is on a flat, not cushioned, surface. Do not weigh the client with scale placed on any kind of rug. Use bed or chair scales for clients who are unable to stand.
- ▲ Teach family about complications of deficient fluid volume and when to call physician.
- ▲ If the client is receiving IV fluids, there must be a responsible caregiver in the home. Teach caregiver about administration of fluids, complications of IV administration (e.g., fluid volume overload, speed of medication reactions), and when to call for assistance. Assist caregiver with administration for as long as necessary to maintain client safety.
- Identify an emergency plan, including when to call 911.
- If the client is terminal, determine if it is appropriate to intervene for deficient fluid volume or allow the client to die comfortably without fluids as desired.

Client/Family Teaching

- Instruct the client to avoid rapid position changes, especially from supine to sitting or standing.
- Teach the client and family about appropriate diet and fluid intake.
- Teach the client and family how to measure and record intake and output accurately.
- Teach the client and family about measures instituted to treat hypovolemia and prevent or treat fluid volume loss.
- Instruct the client and family about signs of deficient fluid

volume that indicate they should contact the healthcare provider.

Excess Fluid volume

F

NANDA Definition

Increased isotonic fluid retention

Defining Characteristics

Adventitious breath sounds; altered electrolytes; anasarca; anxiety; azotemia; blood pressure changes; change in mental status; changes in respiratory pattern; decreased hematocrit; decreased hemoglobin; dyspnea; edema; increased central venous pressure; intake exceeds output; jugular vein distention; oliguria; orthopnea; pleural effusion; positive hepatojugular reflex; pulmonary artery pressure changes; pulmonary congestion; restlessness; specific gravity changes; S_3 heart sound; weight gain over short period of time

Related Factors (r/t)

Compromised regulatory mechanism; excess fluid intake; excess sodium intake

Client Outcomes

Client Will (Specify Time Frame):

- Remain free of edema, effusion, anasarca; weight appropriate for the client
- Maintain clear lung sounds, no evidence of dyspnea or orthopnea
- Remain free of jugular vein distention, positive hepatojugular reflex, and gallop heart rhythm
- Maintain normal central venous pressure, pulmonary capillary wedge pressure, cardiac output, and vital signs
- Maintain urine output within 500 mL of intake with normal urine osmolality and specific gravity
- Explain measures that can be taken to treat or prevent excess fluid volume, especially fluid and dietary restrictions and medications

- Describe symptoms that indicate the need to consult with healthcare provider

Nursing Interventions

F

- • Monitor location and extent of edema; use a millimeter tape in the same area at the same time each day to measure edema in extremities.
- • Monitor daily weight for sudden increases; use same scale and type of clothing at same time each day, preferably before breakfast.
- • Monitor lung sounds for crackles, monitor respirations for effort, and determine the presence and severity of orthopnea.
- • With head of bed elevated 30 to 45 degrees, monitor jugular veins for distention in the upright position; assess for positive hepatojugular reflex.
- ▲ Monitor central venous pressure, mean arterial pressure, pulmonary artery pressure, pulmonary capillary wedge pressure, and cardiac output; note and report trends indicating increasing pressures over time.
- • Monitor vital signs; note decreasing blood pressure, tachycardia, and tachypnea. Monitor for gallop rhythms. If signs of heart failure are present, see the care plan for **Decreased Cardiac output.**
- ▲ Monitor serum osmolality, serum sodium, BUN/creatinine ratio, and hematocrit for decreases.
- • Monitor intake and output; note trends reflecting decreasing urine output in relation to fluid intake.
- • Monitor urine color for lighter colored urine as a sign of fluid overload in the client with functioning kidneys.
- • Monitor the client's behavior for restlessness, anxiety, or confusion; use safety precautions if symptoms are present.
- • Monitor for the development of conditions that increase the client's risk for excess fluid volume.
- ▲ Assist with continuous renal replacement therapy as ordered if the client is critically ill and excessive fluid must be removed.
- ▲ Provide a restricted-sodium diet as appropriate if ordered.
- • Monitor serum albumin level and provide protein intake as appropriate.
- ▲ Administer prescribed diuretics as appropriate; check blood pressure before administration to ensure it is adequate. If ad-

ministering a diuretic IV, note and record urine output after the dose.

- • Monitor for side effects of diuretic therapy: orthostatic hypotension (especially if the client is also receiving ACE inhibitors), hypovolemia and electrolyte imbalances (hypokalemia and hyponatremia). Observe for hyperkalemia in clients receiving a potassium-sparing diuretic, especially with the concurrent administration of an ACE inhibitor.
- ▲ Implement fluid restriction as ordered, especially when serum sodium is low; include all routes of intake. Schedule fluids around the clock and include the type of fluids preferred by the client.
- • Calculate an appropriate daily fluid intake amount and work with client to establish a fluid intake goal.
- • Maintain the rate of all IV infusions carefully with an IV pump.
- • Turn clients with dependent edema frequently (i.e., at least every 2 hours).
- • Provide scheduled rest periods.
- • Promote a positive body image and good self-esteem. Refer to the care plan for **Disturbed Body image.**
- ▲ Consult physician if signs and symptoms of excess fluid volume persist or worsen.

Geriatric

- • Recognize that the presence of risk factors for excess fluid volume is particularly serious in the elderly.

Home Care

- • Assess client and family knowledge of disease process causing excess fluid volume.
- ▲ Teach about disease process and complications of excess fluid volume, including when to contact physician.
- • Assess client and family knowledge and compliance with medical regimen, including medications, diet, rest, and exercise. Assist family with integrating restrictions into daily living.
- ▲ Teach and reinforce knowledge of medications. Instruct the client not to use over-the-counter medications (e.g., diet medications) without first consulting the physician.
- ▲ Instruct the client to make primary physician aware of medications ordered by other physicians.

- • Identify emergency plan for rapidly developing or critical levels of excess fluid volume when diuresing is not safe at home.
- ▲ Teach about signs and symptoms of both excess and deficient fluid volume and when to call physician.

Client/Family Teaching

F

- • Describe signs and symptoms of excess fluid volume and actions to take if they occur.
- ▲ Teach client on diuretics to weigh self daily in the morning and notify the physician of a change in weight of 3 pounds or more.
- ▲ Teach the importance of fluid and sodium restrictions. Help the client and family devise a schedule for intake of fluids throughout the entire day. Refer to dietitian concerning implementation of low-sodium diet.
- ▲ Teach how to take diuretics correctly: take one dose in the morning and second dose (if taken) no later than 4 PM. Adjust potassium intake as appropriate for potassium-losing or potassium-sparing diuretics. Note the appearance of side effects such as weakness, dizziness, muscle cramps, numbness and tingling, confusion, hearing impairment, palpitations or irregular heartbeat, and postural hypotension.
- • Caution the athlete client not to drink excessively during competition or training, but to follow the dictates of thirst.
- • For the client undergoing hemodialysis, spend time with the client to detect any factors that may interfere with the client's compliance with the fluid restriction or restrictive diet.

Risk for deficient Fluid volume

NANDA Definition

At risk for experiencing vascular, cellular, or intracellular dehydration

Risk Factors

Deviations affecting access of fluids; deviations affecting intake of fluids; deviations affecting absorption of fluids; excessive losses through normal routes (e.g., diarrhea); extremes of age; extremes of weight; factors influencing fluid needs (e.g., hypermetabolic state); loss of fluid through abnormal routes (e.g., indwelling tubes); knowledge deficiency; medication (e.g., diuretics)

Client Outcomes

Client Will (Specify Time Frame):

- Maintain urine output of more than 1300 mL/day (or at least 30 mL/hr)
- Maintain normal blood pressure, pulse, and body temperature
- Maintain elastic skin turgor; moist tongue and mucous membranes; and orientation to person, place, and time
- Explain measures that can be taken to treat or prevent fluid volume loss
- Describe symptoms that indicate the need to consult a health-care provider

Nursing Interventions

- Watch for early signs of hypovolemia, including restlessness, weakness, muscle cramps, headaches, inability to concentrate, and postural hypotension.
- Monitor for the existence of factors causing deficient fluid volume (e.g., vomiting, diarrhea, difficulty maintaining oral intake, fever, uncontrolled type 2 diabetes, diuretic therapy).
- Monitor daily weight for sudden decreases, especially in the presence of decreasing urine output or active fluid loss. Weigh the client on the same scale with the same type of clothing at same time of day, preferably before breakfast.
- Monitor total fluid intake and output every 8 hours (or every hour for the unstable client). Recognize that urine output is not always an accurate indicator of fluid balance.
- Check orthostatic blood pressures with the client lying, sitting, and standing.
- Monitor for inelastic skin turgor, thirst, dry tongue and mucous membranes, longitudinal tongue furrows, speech difficulty, dry skin, sunken eyeballs, weakness (especially of upper body), headache, and confusion.
- Use appropriate preoperative fasting guidelines as ordered.
- Refer to care plan for **Deficient Fluid volume.**

Home Care

- • Assess availability of clean drinking water in the home or resources to acquire bottled water.
- ▲ Assess available and preferred fluids. Refer for social services if resources are needed to purchase adequate fluid.

Client/Family Teaching

F

- • Teach clients who work in hot environments or exercise in hot environments to increase intake of both water and electrolyte-carbohydrate beverages.

Risk for imbalanced Fluid volume

NANDA Definition

At risk for a decrease, increase, or rapid shift from one to the other of intravascular, interstitial, and/or intracellular fluid (refers to body fluid loss, gain, or both)

Risk Factor

Scheduled for major invasive procedures

Client Outcomes

- Lung sounds clear, respiratory rate 12 to 20, and free of dyspnea postoperatively
- Urine output greater than 30 mL/hr (Beyea, 2002)
- Blood pressure, pulse rate, temperature, and pulse oximetry within expected range (Beyea, 2002)
- Laboratory values within expected range (Beyea, 2002)
- Nonedematous extremities and dependent areas
- Mental orientation unchanged from preoperative status

Nursing Interventions

- • Monitor vital signs of clients with deficient fluid volume every 15 minutes if unstable or every 4 hours if stable. Observe for tachycardia, tachypnea, and decreased pulse pressure, which will occur first, followed by hypotension, decreased pulse volume, and increased or decreased body temperature.
- • Check the client's orthostatic blood pressure.

- • Monitor for nonelastic skin turgor, thirst, dry tongue and mucous membranes, longitudinal tongue furrows, difficulty speaking, dry skin, sunken eyeballs, weakness (especially upper body), headache, and confusion, which are symptoms of decreased body fluids.
- • Provide frequent oral hygiene—at least twice daily. If the client's mouth is dry and painful, provide oral hygiene hourly while client is awake.
- ▲ Initiate measures to rest the bowel when the client is vomiting or has diarrhea; that is, restrict food or fluid intake when appropriate, and decrease intake of milk products. Hydrate the client with any prescribed (ordered) IV solutions. Refer to care plan for **Diarrhea** or **Nausea.**
- ▲ Provide oral replacement therapy as ordered and tolerated, with a hypotonic glucose-electrolyte solution when the client has acute diarrhea or nausea and vomiting. Provide small, frequent qualities of slightly chilled solutions.
- • Maintain patent IV access if the client requires IV fluid replacement.
- • Monitor for factors causing deficient fluid volume, such as vomiting, diarrhea, difficulty maintaining oral intake, fever, uncontrolled type 2 diabetes, diuretic therapy, and preoperative bowel preparation.
- ▲ When ordered, administer a fluid challenge, giving a specified amount of IV fluid, such as 0.9% normal saline rapidly IV, for replacement of intravascular volume and monitor the client's response by noting vital signs, lung sounds, urine output, and pulmonary capillary wedge pressure or central venous pressures if applicable.
- • Keep all IV fluids on a volumetric pump.
- • Monitor intake and output.
- ▲ Measure urine output hourly. If urine output is less than 30 mL/hr or 0.5 mL/kg/hr, notify the physician.
- • Observe for trends in output for 3 days; include all routes of intake and output and note color and specific gravity of urine.
- • Monitor daily weight for sudden decreases, especially in the presence of decreasing urine output or active fluid loss. Weigh the client on the same scale, in the same type clothing, at the same time of day, preferably before breakfast.
- ▲ Monitor trends in serum lactic acid levels and base deficit, obtained from blood gases as ordered.

Surgical Clients

- ▲ Perform a preoperative assessment to identify clients with increased risk for hemorrhage or hypovolemia (e.g., recent traumatic injury, abnormal bleeding or clotting times; complicated renal or liver disease; diabetes; cardiovascular disease; major organ transplant; history of aspirin or nonsteroidal antiinflammatory drug use or anticoagulant therapy; or history of hemophilia, von Willebrand's disease, or disseminated intravascular coagulation).
- • Monitor for signs of intraoperative hypovolemia (e.g., dry skin, dry mucous membranes, tachycardia, decreased urinary output, decreased central venous pressure, hypotension, increased pulse, and/or deep rapid respirations).
- • Monitor for signs of intraoperative hypervolemia (dyspnea, coarse crackles, increased pulse and respirations, decreased urinary output), all of which could progress to pulmonary edema.
- • Monitor for signs of intraoperative third spacing.
- • In the critically ill surgical client with a pulmonary artery catheter, monitor pressures, especially wedge pressure.
- • Monitor clients undergoing laparoscopic or hysteroscopic procedures for the development of pulmonary edema when Dextran is used as the irrigation fluid.
- • Monitor intraoperative intake and output.
- • Monitor clients undergoing transurethral resection of the prostate (TURP) procedures for TURP syndrome symptoms: headache, visual changes, agitation, lethargy, vomiting, muscle twitching, bradycardia, diminished pupillary reflexes, hypertension, and respiratory distress.
- • If the client is undergoing endometrial ablation under general anesthesia, watch for symptoms of decreased body temperature, decreased oxygen saturation, dilated pupils, and tremulousness.
- • Monitor clients undergoing percutaneous nephrolithotomy procedures for excessive fluid absorption and volume overload.
- • Observe the surgical client for signs of hyperkalemia, that is, cardiac dysrhythmias, heart block, asystole, abdominal distention, and weakness.
- • Observe surgical clients closely for signs of hypokalemia.
- • Recognize that the surgical client may develop hyponatremia related to inappropriate antidiuretic hormone secretion, which can be caused by trauma, thrombosis, abscesses, hemorrhages, or hematomas.

- Clients undergoing abdominal lavage should be monitored for hyperchloremic acidosis.
- Monitor the surgical client for signs and symptoms of hyponatremia: nausea, confusion, disorientation, muscle twitching, seizures, hypovolemia, tachycardia, and/or hypotension.
- Accurately measure blood loss intraoperatively.
- Provide appropriate supplies, instruments, and techniques to control hemorrhage.
- Recognize that evidence-based procedure-specific protocols for administration of fluid postoperatively are unavailable.
- Accurate postoperative assessment and fluid management should include traditional intake and output measurement as well as monitoring of the client's weight, laboratory values, and checks of peripheral pulses.

Geriatric

- Be especially vigilant when monitoring vital signs and fluids in elderly surgical clients.
- Assess preoperatively for symptoms of dehydration: weakness, dizziness, dry mouth, sunken eyes and cheeks, concentrated urine, and decreased skin turgor.
- Ensure that when food intake is reduced or limited it is compensated with an increase in water/fluid intake.
- Check skin turgor of the elderly client on the forehead, sternum, or inner thigh; also look for the presence of longitudinal tongue furrows and dry mucous membranes.
- Encourage fluid intake regularly to cognitively impaired clients.
- Incorporate regular hydration into daily routines, such as providing an extra glass of fluid with medication or during social activities. Consider using a beverage cart and a hydration assistant to routinely offer beverages to clients in extended care facilities.
- Note the color of urine and compare against a urine color chart to monitor adequate fluid intake.
- Monitor elderly clients for excess fluid volume during the treatment of deficient fluid volume: listen to lung sounds, watch for edema, and note vital signs.

Pediatric

- Administer fluids preoperatively until NPO status must be initiated so that fluid deficit is decreased.

Impaired Gas exchange

NANDA Definition

Excess or deficit in oxygenation and/or carbon dioxide elimination at the alveolar-capillary membrane

Defining Characteristics

Abnormal arterial blood gases; abnormal arterial pH; abnormal breathing (e.g., rate, rhythm, depth); abnormal skin color (e.g., pale, dusky); confusion; cyanosis (in neonates only); decreased carbon dioxide; diaphoresis; dyspnea; headache upon awakening; hypercapnia; hypercarbia; hypoxemia; hypoxia; irritability; nasal flaring; restlessness; somnolence; tachycardia; visual disturbances

Related Factors (r/t)

Alveolar-capillary membrane changes; ventilation-perfusion imbalance

Client Outcomes

Client Will (Specify Time Frame):

- Demonstrate improved ventilation and adequate oxygenation as evidenced by blood gas levels within normal parameters for that client.
- Maintain clear lung fields and remain free of signs of respiratory distress.
- Verbalize understanding of oxygen supplementation and other therapeutic interventions.

Nursing Interventions

- Monitor respiratory rate, depth, and effort, including use of accessory muscles, nasal flaring, and abnormal breathing patterns.
- Auscultate breath sounds every 1 to 2 hours. The presence of crackles and wheezes may alert the nurse to airway obstruction, which may lead to or exacerbate existing hypoxia.
- Monitor the client's behavior and mental status for the onset of restlessness, agitation, confusion, and (in the late stages) extreme lethargy.
- Monitor oxygen saturation continuously by pulse oximetry. Note blood gas results as available.

- Observe for cyanosis of the skin; especially note color of the tongue and oral mucous membranes.
- Position clients in semi-Fowler's position, with an upright posture at 45 degrees if possible.
- If the client has unilateral lung disease, alternate semi-Fowler's position in an upright posture with a lateral position (with 10- to 15-degree elevation and "good lung down") for 60 to 90 minutes. This method is contraindicated for clients with pulmonary abscess, hemorrhage, or interstitial emphysema.
- If the client has bilateral lung disease, position the client in either semi-Fowler's or a side-lying position, which increases oxygenation as indicated by pulse oximetry (or, if the client has a pulmonary catheter, venous oxygen saturation).
- Turn the client every 2 hours. Monitor mixed venous oxygen saturation closely after turning. If it drops below 10% or fails to return to baseline promptly, return the client to the supine position and evaluate oxygen status. If the client does not tolerate turning, consider use of a kinetic bed that rotates the client from side to side in a turn of at least 40 degrees.
- If the client is obese or has ascites, consider positioning the client in reverse Trendelenburg position at 45 degrees for periods as tolerated.

▲ If the client has adult respiratory distress syndrome (ARDS) or difficulty maintaining oxygenation, consider positioning the client prone with the upper thorax and pelvis supported, allowing the abdomen to protrude. Monitor oxygen saturation and turn back to supine position if desaturation occurs.

- If the client is acutely dyspneic, consider having the client lean forward over a bedside table if tolerated.
- Help the client deep breathe and perform controlled coughing. Have the client inhale deeply, hold the breath for several seconds, and cough two or three times with the mouth open while tightening the upper abdominal muscles as tolerated. NOTE: If the client has excessive fluid in the respiratory system, see the interventions for **ineffective Airway clearance.**

▲ Monitor the effects of sedation and analgesics on the client's respiratory pattern; use judiciously.

- Schedule nursing care to provide rest and minimize fatigue.

▲ Administer humidified oxygen through an appropriate device (e.g., nasal cannula or Venturi mask per the physician's order);

aim for an oxygen saturation level of 90%. Watch for onset of hypoventilation as evidenced by increased somnolence.
- • Assess nutritional status, including serum albumin level and body mass index (BMI).
- • Help the client eat frequent small meals and use dietary supplements as necessary. For some clients, drinking 30 mL of a supplement such as Ensure or Pulmocare every hour while awake can be helpful.
- • If the client is severely debilitated from chronic respiratory disease, consider the use of a wheeled walker to help in ambulation.
- ▲ Watch for signs of psychological distress, including anxiety, agitation, and insomnia. Refer for counseling as needed.
- ▲ Refer the client with COPD to a pulmonary rehabilitation program. NOTE: If the client becomes ventilator dependent, see the care plan for **Impaired spontaneous Ventilation.**

Geriatric

- ▲ Use central nervous system (CNS) depressants carefully to avoid decreasing respiration rate.
- ▲ Maintain low-flow oxygen therapy.

Home Care

- • Assess the home environment for irritants that impair gas exchange. Help the client adjust the home environment as necessary (e.g., install an air filter to decrease the level of dust).
- ▲ Refer the client to occupational therapy as necessary to help the client adapt the home and environment and conserve energy.
- • Help the client identify and avoid situations that exacerbate impairment of gas exchange (e.g., stress-related situations, exposure to pollution of any kind, proximity to noxious gas fumes such as chlorine bleach).
- • Refer to GOLD and ACP-ASIM/ACCP guidelines for management of home care and indications of hospital admission criteria.
- • Instruct the client to keep the home temperature above 68° F (20° C) and avoid cold weather.
- • Instruct the client to limit exposure to persons with respiratory infections.
- • Instruct the family in the complications of the disease and the

importance of maintaining the medical regimen, including when to call a physician.

- ▲ Refer the client for home health aide services as necessary for assistance with activities of daily living.
- • When respiratory procedures are being implemented, explain equipment and procedures to family members and provide needed emotional support.
- • When electrically based equipment for respiratory support is being implemented, evaluate home environment for electrical safety, proper grounding, and so forth. Ensure that notification is sent to the local utility company, the emergency medical team, and police and fire departments.
- ▲ Assess family role changes and coping ability. Refer the client to medical social services as appropriate for assistance in adjusting to chronic illness.
- • Support the family of the client with chronic illness.

G

Client/Family Teaching

- • Teach the client how to perform pursed-lip breathing, controlled diaphragmatic breathing, and how to use the tripod position. Have the client watch the pulse oximeter to note improvement in oxygenation with these breathing techniques.
- • Teach the client energy conservation techniques and the importance of alternating rest periods with activity. See nursing interventions for **Fatigue.**
- ▲ Teach the importance of not smoking:
  - ■ Be very clear in approach, and ask the client to set a date for smoking cessation.
  - ■ Recommend pharmacological support or else contraindicated (nicotine replacement therapy or antidepressant).
  - ■ Refer the client to smoking-cessation programs.
  - ■ Encourage clients who relapse to keep trying to quit.
- ▲ Instruct the family regarding home oxygen therapy if ordered (e.g., delivery system, liter flow, safety precautions).
- • Teach the client the need to receive a yearly influenza vaccine.
- • Teach the client relaxation techniques to help reduce stress responses and panic attacks resulting from dyspnea.
- • Teach the client to use music along with a rest period to decrease dyspnea and anxiety.

Risk for unstable blood Glucose

NANDA Definition

Risk for variation of blood glucose/sugar levels from the normal range

Risk Factors

G

Deficient knowledge of diabetes management (e.g., action plan); developmental level; dietary intake; inadequate blood glucose monitoring; lack of acceptance of diagnosis; lack of adherence to diabetes management (e.g., action plan); lack of diabetes management (e.g., action plan); medication management; mental health status; physical activity level; physical health status; pregnancy; rapid growth periods; stress; weight gain; weight loss

Client Outcomes

Client Will (Specify Time Frame):

- Maintain preprandial blood glucose level between 90 and 130 mg/dL; consult primary care provider for client-specific goals
- Maintain postprandial glucose level less than 180 mg/dL
- Maintain hemoglobin A1c level <7% (normal, 4%-6%)
- Maintain blood glucose level as close as possible to 110 mg/dL if critically ill
- In gestational diabetes, maintain fasting blood glucose level ≤105 mg/dL, 1-hour after the meal (pc) level ≤155 mg/dL, and 2-hour pc level ≤130 mg/dL
- Demonstrate how to test blood glucose accurately
- Identify self-care actions to take if blood glucose level is too low or too high
- Demonstrate correct administration of prescribed medications

Nursing Interventions

- Monitor blood glucose before meals and at bedtime. Monitor blood glucose every 4 to 6 hours in clients with a nothing-by-mouth order or who are continuously fed. Monitor blood glucose level hourly for clients on continuous insulin drips; may decrease to every 2 hours once stable.
- Evaluate hemoglobin A1c level for glucose control over the previous 2 to 3 months.

- Monitor for signs and symptoms of hypoglycemia. Rapidly falling blood glucose level can cause sympathetic symptoms such as anxiety, dizziness, diaphoresis, tachycardia, headache, tremor, or hunger.
- Be alert to hypoglycemia in clients with heart failure, renal or liver disease, malignancy, infection, sepsis, sudden reduction of corticosteroids, altered ability to self-report symptoms, reduced nutritional intake, emesis, new nothing-by-mouth status, or altered consciousness.
- If a client is experiencing signs and symptoms of hypoglycemia, test glucose. If the result is below 70 mg/dL, administer 15 to 20 g glucose (½ cup fruit juice or regular [not diet] soda, 1 cup milk, 1 small piece of fruit, or 3 to 4 glucose tablets). Repeat test in 60 minutes or if symptoms recur.
- Administer intravenous 50% dextrose or intramuscular glucagon according to agency protocol if client is hypoglycemic and is unable to take oral carbohydrate.
- Monitor for signs and symptoms of hyperglycemia, such as polydipsia, polyuria, and polyphagia.
- Test urine for ketones during acute illness or stress or when blood glucose levels are >300 mg/dL.
- Maintain tight glucose control in critically ill hospitalized clients.
- If client is acutely ill, continue insulin and oral hypoglycemic agents and frequent monitoring. Assure client is receiving adequate fluids and carbohydrates.
- Prime tubing with 20 mL diluted intravenous insulin solution before initiating insulin drip.
- Evaluate the client's medication regimen for medications that can alter blood glucose.
- Evaluate blood glucose level in hospitalized clients before administering oral hypoglycemic agents or insulin.

▲ Refer client to dietitian for carbohydrate counting instruction.

▲ Refer overweight clients to a dietitian for weight loss counseling.

Geriatric

- Assess possible barriers to following nutrition recommendations: food preferences, ability to prepare meals, dentition, swallowing problems, decreased appetite or thirst sensation,

use of taste-altering medications, limited finances, and social isolation.
- Assess for age-related cognitive changes that can impair self-management of diabetes.
- Assess for vision and dexterity impairments that may affect the older client's ability to measure insulin doses accurately.
- Teach client and family caregivers to recognize signs and symptoms of hyperosmolar hyperglycemia.
- Help client set up pill boxes or reminder system for taking medications.

Pediatric

- Ensure that daycare or school personnel are trained in diabetes management and treatment of emergencies.
- Be aware that young children (<6 or 7 years) may not be aware of symptoms of hypoglycemia.

Home Care

▲ Teach family how to use an emergency glucagon kit (if prescribed).

Client Education

- Provide "survival skills" education for hospitalized clients, including information about (1) diabetes and its treatment, (2) medication administration, (3) nutrition therapy, (4) self-monitoring of blood glucose, (5) symptoms and treatment of hypoglycemia, (6) basic foot care, and (7) follow-up appointments for in-depth training.
- Educate clients on self-monitoring of blood glucose.
- Educate clients with type 2 diabetes to monitor blood glucose before meals and bedtime.

▲ Refer client to a diabetes treatment and teaching program for training in flexible intensive insulin therapy and dietary freedom. Most large hospitals or medical centers offer such programs.

▲ Refer client for blood glucose awareness training for instruction in detection, anticipation, avoidance, and treatment of extremes in blood glucose levels.

- Teach client to maintain a blood glucose diary.
- Provide group-based training programs for instruction.

- Educate client about the benefits of smoking cessation.
- Teach client the benefits of regular adherence to prescribed exercise regimen.
- Teach clients who are treated with insulin that they may need to eat extra carbohydrates before exercise, depending on how exercise affects their blood glucose levels.
- Teach client that stopping insulin therapy can lead to hyperglycemic crisis (ketoacidosis or hyperosmolar hyperglycemia). Ensure client has resources to purchase insulin.

Grieving

NANDA Definition

A normal, complex process that includes emotional, physical, spiritual, social, and intellectual responses and behaviors by which individuals, families, and communities incorporate a loss into their daily lives

Defining Characteristics

Alteration in activity level; alterations in immune function; alterations in neuroendocrine function; alteration in sleep patterns; alteration in dream patterns; anger; blame; detachment; despair; disorganization; experiencing relief; maintaining connection to the deceased; making meaning of the loss; pain; panic behavior; personal growth; psychological distress; suffering

Related Factors (r/t)

Anticipatory loss of significant object (e.g., possession, job, status, home, parts & processes of body); anticipatory loss of a significant other; death of a significant other; loss of significant object (e.g., possession, job, status, home, parts & processes of body)

Client/Family Outcomes

Client/Family Will (Specify Time Frame):

- Discuss meaning of the loss to his/her life and the functioning of the family
- Identify ways to support family members and articulate methods of support he or she requires from family and friends

- Utilize effective conflict management strategies
- Accept assistance in meeting the needs of the family from friends/extended family

Nursing Interventions

- • Concentrate on improving communication and providing an environment in which families can physically touch and care for their seriously ill loved one as much as possible. Focus on enhancing coping skills of the person's grieving to alleviate life problems and distressing symptoms such as anxiety and depression. Learning new coping strategies aimed at resuming former roles or assuming new roles is important over time.
- • Understand and support the family's expression of pain in its own way and in its own time. Encourage the family to create quiet and comfortable healing environments.
- • Encourage the family to follow comforting grief rituals such as interacting with nature, lighting votive candles, saying a prayer, or whatever ritual brings spiritual comfort in dealing with the loss.
- ▲ Refer the family members for spiritual counseling if desired.
- • Help the family determine the best way and place to find social support. Encourage family members to continue to use supports for 1 to 2 years.
- ▲ Identify available community resources, including bereavement groups at local hospitals and hospice centers. Volunteers who provide bereavement support can also be effective.

Pediatric/Parent

- • Treat the child with respect, give him or her the opportunity to talk about concerns, and answer questions honestly.
- • Listen to the child's expression of grief.
- • Consider giving the child a "memory bag" to have after experiencing a sudden death; contents include a teddy bear, a coloring book on working through grief for different ages, a journal for children to write in, and crayons.
- • Help parents recognize that the child does not have to be "fixed," instead he or she needs support going through an experience of grieving just as adults do.
- ▲ Refer grieving children and parents to a program to help facilitate grieving if desired, especially if the death was traumatic.

- Help the adolescent determine sources of support and how to use them effectively.
- ▲ Encourage parents to seek mental health services as needed, learn stress reduction, and take good care of their health.

Geriatric

- ▲ Monitor an older adult who has been treated for bereavement-related depression for relapse or recurrence.
- ▲ Use reminiscence therapy in conjunction with the expression of emotions. Refer to a reminiscence group if available.
- Provide support for the family when the loss is associated with dementia of the family member.

Multicultural

- Assess the influence of cultural beliefs, norms, and values on the client's grief and mourning practices.
- Empathy may be especially important in caring for women with pregnancy loss who live in patrilineal cultures in which producing children is a critical role for women.
- Validate the client's feelings regarding the loss.
- Teach clients to recognize grief responses.

Home Care

NOTE: **Grieving** may be encountered as the client comes to terms with his or her own loss or death, or as the family reacts to the client's death.

- The interventions previously described may be adapted for home care use.
- Actively listen as the client grieves for his or her own death or for real or perceived loss. Normalize the client's expressions of grief for himself or herself. Demonstrate a caring and hopeful approach.
- ▲ Refer the client to medical social services as necessary for losses not related to death.
- ▲ Refer the bereaved to hospice bereavement programs.
- ▲ Refer the bereaved spouse to an Internet self-help group if desired.
- Assess caregiver reaction to bereavement issues and caregiver burden. Suggest preventive intervention for potential bereavement maladjustment if indicated.

- • Modify expectations of the family's response according to the degree of anticipation of the loved one's death.
- ▲ After loss of a pregnancy, encourage the client and family to follow through on a counseling referral.

Complicated Grieving

NANDA Definition

A disorder that occurs after the death of a significant other in which the experience of distress accompanying bereavement fails to follow normative expectations and manifests in functional impairment.

Defining Characteristics

Decreased functioning in life roles; decreased sense of well-being; depression; experiencing somatic symptoms of the deceased; fatigue; grief avoidance; longing for the deceased; low levels of intimacy; persistent emotional distress; preoccupation with thoughts of the deceased; rumination; searching for the deceased; self-blame; separation distress; traumatic distress; verbalizes anxiety; verbalizes distressful feelings about the deceased; verbalizes feeling dazed; verbalizes feeling empty; verbalizes feeling in shock; verbalizes feeling stunned; verbalizes feelings of anger; verbalizes feelings of detachment from others; verbalizes feelings of disbelief; verbalizes feelings of mistrust; verbalizes lack of acceptance of the death; verbalizes persistent painful memories; verbalizes self-blame; yearning

Related Factors (r/t)

Death of a significant other; emotional instability; lack of social support; sudden death of a significant other

Client Outcomes

Client Will (Specify Time Frame):

- Express appropriate feelings of guilt, fear, anger, or sadness
- Identify somatic distress associated with grief (e.g., anxiety, changes in appetite, insomnia, nightmares, loss of libido, decreased energy, altered activity levels)
- Seek support in dealing with grief-associated issues
- Identify personal strengths and effective coping strategies

- Function at a normal developmental level and begin to successfully and increasingly perform activities of daily living

Nursing Interventions

- • Assess the client's state of grieving. Use a tool such as the Texas Revised Inventory of Grief (TRIG), Pathological Grief Items (PGI), Impact of Events Scale (IES), Hogan Grief Reaction Checklist (HGRC), Beck Depression Inventory (BDI-II), Hamilton Rating Scale for Depression or Social Adjustment Scale – Self Report (SAS-SR).
- ▲ Determine whether the client is experiencing depression, suicidal tendencies, or other emotional disorders. Refer the client for counseling or therapy as appropriate.
- • Identify problems of eating and sleeping; ensure that basic human needs are being met.
- • Develop a trusting relationship with the client by using presence and therapeutic communication techniques.
- • Educate the client and his or her support systems that grief resolution is not a sequential process and that the positive outcome of grief resolution is the integration of the deceased into the ongoing life of the griever.
- • Understand and support the client's expression of pain in his or her own way and in his or her own time. Encourage the client to create quiet and comfortable healing environments.
- ▲ Assess for spiritual distress; refer the client to an appropriate spiritual leader, if appropriate.
- • Focus on enhancing coping skills to alleviate life problems and distressing symptoms such as anxiety and depression.
- • Encourage the client to follow comforting grief rituals such as interacting with nature, lighting votive candles, saying a prayer, or whatever ritual brings spiritual comfort in dealing with the loss.
- ▲ Identify available community resources, including community and/or Web-based bereavement groups. Volunteers who provide bereavement support can also be effective.

Pediatric/Parent

- • If client is an adolescent exposed to a peer's suicide, watch for symptoms of traumatic grief as well as PTSD, which include numbness, preoccupation with the deceased, functional impairment, and poor adjustment to the loss.

- See the interventions in the care plan for **Grieving.**

Geriatric

▲ Use reminiscence therapy in conjunction with the expression of emotions. Refer to a reminiscence group if available.
- Identify previous losses and assess the client for depression.
- Monitor an older adult who has been treated for bereavement-related depression for relapse or recurrence.
- Evaluate the social support system of the elderly client. If the support system is minimal, help the client determine how to increase available support.

Multicultural

- See the interventions in the care plan for **Grieving**.
- Assess for the influence of cultural beliefs, norms, and values on the client's grief and mourning practices.
- Assess for the influence of cultural beliefs, norms, and values on the client's expressions of grief.
- Encourage discussion of the grief process.
- Identify whether the client had been notified of the health status of the deceased and was able to be present during illness and death.

Home Care

- See the interventions in the care plan for **Grieving.**

Risk for complicated Grieving

NANDA Definition

At risk for a disorder that occurs after the death of a significant other in which the experience of distress accompanying bereavement fails to follow normative expectations and manifests in functional impairment

Risk Factors

Death of a significant other; emotional instability; lack of social support

Client Outcomes

Client Will (Specify Time Frame):

- Express appropriate feelings of guilt, fear, anger, or sadness
- Identify somatic distress associated with grief (e.g., anxiety, changes in appetite, insomnia, nightmares, loss of libido, decreased energy, altered activity levels)
- Seek support in dealing with grief-associated issues
- Identify personal strengths and effective coping strategies
- Function at a normal developmental level and begin to successfully and increasingly perform activities of daily living

Nursing Interventions and Client Teaching

- Refer to care plan for **Complicated Grieving.**

Delayed Growth and development

NANDA Definition

Deviations from age-group norms

Defining Characteristics

Altered physical growth; decreased response time; delay in performing skills typical of age group; difficulty in performing skills typical of age group; inability to perform self-care activities appropriate for age; inability to perform self-control activities appropriate for age; flat affect; listlessness

Related Factors (r/t)

Effects of physical disability; environmental deficiencies; inadequate caretaking; inconsistent responsiveness; indifference; multiple caretakers; prescribed dependence; separation from significant others; stimulation deficiencies

Client Outcomes

Client/Parents/Primary Caregiver Will (Specify Time Frame):

- Describe realistic, age-appropriate patterns of growth and development

- Promote activities and interactions that support age-related developmental tasks
- Display consistent, sustained achievement of age-appropriate behaviors (social, interpersonal, and/or cognitive) and/or motor skills
- Achieve realistic developmental and/or growth milestones based on existing abilities, extent of disability, and functional age
- Exhibit limited temporary behavioral regression that reverses shortly after episode of illness or hospitalization
- Attain steady gains in growth patterns

G

Nursing Interventions

- • To determine risk for or actual deviations in normal development, consider the use of a screening tool.
- • Regularly compare height and weight measurements for the child or adolescent with established age-appropriate norms and previous measurements.
- ▲ Identify coexisting health or medical conditions that may be contributing to the alteration in growth and/or development, and refer the client to a specialist in the appropriate healthcare discipline for management.
- • Provide skin-to-skin contact for newborns and moms. Place the naked baby prone on the mother's bare chest at birth or soon afterwards (<24 hours).
- • Provide opportunities for mother-infant skin-to-skin contact (kangaroo care) for preterm infants.
- • Provide neonatal positioning procedures for preterm infants to prevent extremity malalignment, skull deformities, and gross motor delay.
- • Provide developmental care interventions to preterm infants.
- • Provide meaningful stimulation for hospitalized infants and children.
- • Provide support groups and education on human immunodeficiency virus (HIV) and caring for infants with this diagnosis.
- ▲ Engage the child in appropriate play activities. Refer the child to a play or recreational therapist (if available) for supplemental strategies.
- • Provide an environment that promotes additional sleep and rest opportunities.

Multicultural

- Assess the influence of cultural beliefs, norms, and values on the client's perceptions of child development.
- Assess and identify for possible environmental conditions, which may be a contributing factor to altered growth and development.
- Acknowledge racial and ethnic differences at the onset of care.
- Use a neutral, indirect style in addressing areas in which improvement is needed (such as a need for verbal stimulation) when working with Native American clients.
- Provide information on the effects of environmental risk exposure on growth and development.

Home Care

- The interventions previously described may be adapted for home care use.
- Assess whether exposure to community violence is contributing to developmental problems.
- ▲ Refer maternal drug users to home intervention programs.
- ▲ If possible, refer the family to a program of animal-assisted therapy.

Client/Family Teaching

- ▲ Encourage parents to take infants and children for routine health visits to the family physician or pediatrician.
- Provide parents and/or caregivers realistic expectations for attainment of growth and development milestones. Clarify expectations and correct misconceptions.
- Have parents and/or caregivers rehearse coping strategies for approaching developmental milestones and acknowledge positive actions and behaviors.
- Teach methods of providing meaningful stimulation for infants and children.
- Instruct the client regarding appropriate baby equipment.
- ▲ Elicit the involvement of parents and caregivers in social support groups and parenting classes.
- ▲ Furnish information about community resources.

Risk for disproportionate Growth

NANDA Definition

At risk for growth above the 97th percentile or below the third percentile for age, crossing two percentile channels

Risk Factors

G

Caregiver

Abuse; mental illness; mental retardation; or severe learning disability

Environmental

Deprivation; lead poisoning; natural disasters; poverty; teratogen; violence

Individual

Anorexia; caregiver maladaptive feeding behaviors; chronic illness; individual maladaptive feeding behaviors; infection; insatiable appetite; prematurity; malnutrition; substance abuse

Prenatal

Congenital/genetic disorders; maternal infection; maternal nutrition; multiple gestation; teratogen exposure; substance use/abuse

Client Outcomes

Client/Parents/Primary Caregiver Will (Specify Time Frame):

- State information related to possible teratogenic agents
- State information related to adequate nutrition
- Seek help from appropriate professionals for nutritional needs

Nursing Interventions

Preconception/Pregnancy

▲ Assess and limit exposure to all drugs (prescription, "recreational," and over the counter) and give the mother information on known teratogenic agents.

• All women of childbearing age who are capable of becoming pregnant should take 400 mcg of folic acid daily.

▲ Women with phenylketonuria should be referred to a nutritionist experienced in the dietary implications of phenylalanine restriction.

▲ Promote a team approach toward preconception and pregnancy glucose control for women with diabetes.

Infants/Children

- • Consider breast milk for extremely low birth weight infants in the neonatal intensive care unit.
- ▲ Provide tube feedings per physician's orders when appropriate for clients with neuromuscular impairment.
- ▲ Reduce the risk of TORCH infections (***t***oxoplasmosis, ***o***ther infections, ***r***ubella, ***c***ytomegalovirus infection, and ***h***erpes simplex) as follows:
  - ■ Varicella-zoster and rubella viruses: vaccinate nonimmune women before conception
  - ■ Cytomegalovirus: practice meticulous handwashing and secretion control and limit exposure to large numbers of infants and children
  - ■ *Toxoplasma gondii:* avoid exposure to cat litter and avoid work in the garden or areas where cat feces may be present; do not feed undercooked meats to cats
  - ■ Parvovirus: limit contact with persons with known fifth disease
  - ■ Herpes virus: practice meticulous handwashing and secretion control, especially in contact with young infants
- • Provide for adequate nutrition and nutritional monitoring in clients with developmental disorders.
- ▲ Adequate intake of vitamin D is set at 200 international units/day by the National Academy of Sciences. Because adequate sunlight exposure is difficult to determine, a supplement of 200 international units/day is recommended for the following groups to prevent rickets and vitamin D deficiency in healthy infants and children:
  - ■ All breastfed infants unless they are weaned to at least 500 mL/day of vitamin D–fortified formula or milk
  - ■ All non-breastfed infants who are ingesting less than 500 mL/day of vitamin D–fortified formula or milk
  - ■ Children and adolescents who do not receive regular sunlight exposure, do not ingest at least 500 mL/day of vitamin D–fortified milk, or do not take a daily multivitamin supplement containing at least 200 international units of vitamin D

- Provide adequate nutrition to clients with active intestinal inflammation.
- Provide for adequate nutrition for pediatric and adolescent clients on long-term oral glucocorticoid therapy (e.g., those treated for chronic severe asthma).
- Refer to the care plan for **Delayed Growth and development.**

Multicultural

- Assess the influence of cultural beliefs, norms, values, and expectations on parents' perceptions of normal growth and development.
- Assess for the influence of acculturation.
- Assess whether the parents are concerned about the amount of food eaten.
- Assess the influence of family support on patterns of nutritional intake.
- Negotiate with clients regarding which aspects of healthy nutrition can be modified while still honoring cultural beliefs.
- Encourage parental efforts at increasing physical activity and decreasing dietary fat for their children. Encourage limiting television viewing to <2 hours/day for children and discourage the consumption of sweetened soft drinks.

Home Care

- The interventions previously described may be adapted for home care use.

Client/Family Teaching

▲ Provide prenatal counseling for women with unintended pregnancies to evaluate if they have been exposed to teratogenic agents.
▲ Refer clients to a registered dietitian for nutritional counseling.
- Teach families the importance of taking measures to prevent lead poisoning.

Ineffective Health maintenance

NANDA Definition

Inability to identify, manage, and/or seek out help to maintain health

Defining Characteristics

Demonstrated lack of adaptive behaviors to environmental changes; demonstrated lack of knowledge regarding basic health practices; lack of expressed interest in improving health behaviors; history of lack of health seeking behavior; inability to take responsibility for meeting basic health practices; impairment of personal support systems

Related Factors (r/t)

Cognitive impairment; complicated grieving; deficient communication skills; diminished fine motor skills; diminished gross motor skills; inability to make appropriate judgments; ineffective family coping; ineffective individual coping; insufficient resources (e.g., equipment finances); lack of fine motor skills; lack of gross motor skills; perceptual impairment; spiritual distress; unachieved developmental tasks

Client Outcomes

Client Will (Specify Time Frame):

- Discuss fear of or blocks to implementing health regimen
- Follow mutually agreed on healthcare maintenance plan
- Meet goals for healthcare maintenance

Nursing Interventions

- • Assess the client's feelings, values, and reasons for not following the prescribed plan of care. See Related Factors.
- • Assess for family patterns, economic issues, and cultural patterns that influence compliance with a given medical regimen.
- • Help the client to choose a healthy lifestyle and to have appropriate diagnostic screening tests.
- • Assist the client in reducing stress.
- • Help the client determine how to manage complex medication schedules (e.g., HIV/AIDS regimens or polypharmacy).
- • Identify complementary healing modalities, such as herbal remedies, acupuncture, healing touch, yoga, or cultural shamans, that the client uses in addition to or instead of the prescribed allopathic regimen.
- ▲ Refer the client to appropriate services as needed.
- ▲ Refer the client to community agencies for appropriate follow-up care (e.g., day treatment or adult day health program).

- ▲ Identify support groups related to the disease process (e.g., Reach to Recovery for a woman who has had a mastectomy).
- ▲ Ensure that follow-up appointments are scheduled before the client is discharged; discuss a way to ensure that appointments are kept.

Geriatric

- ▲ Assess sensory deficits and psychomotor skills. Supply the appropriate assistive devices.
- • Recognize resistance to change in lifelong patterns of personal health care.
- • Discuss "symptoms of daily living" in addition to the major illness.
- • Discuss with the client and support person realistic goals for changes in health maintenance.
- • Educate the client about the symptoms of life-threatening illness, such as myocardial infarction (MI), and the need for timeliness in seeking care.
- • Consider the age of the client when suggesting screening for disease.

Multicultural

- • Assess influence of cultural beliefs, norms, and values on the client's ability to modify health behavior.
- • Assess the effect of fatalism on the client's ability to modify health behavior.
- • Assess access to health services.
- • Discuss with the client those aspects of health behavior and lifestyle that will remain unchanged by health status.

Home Care

- • The interventions described previously may be adapted for home care use.
- ▲ Include a health promotion focus for the client with disabilities, with the goals of reducing secondary conditions (e.g., obesity, hypertension, pressure sores), maintaining functional independence, providing opportunities for leisure and enjoyment, and enhancing overall quality of life.
- • Encourage a regular routine for health-related behaviors.
- • Provide sufficient outside supports (e.g., written notices, calen-

dars, planned ride shares) to assist with follow-through on the agreed-on actions.

- Assist client to develop confidence in ability to manage the health condition.
- Establish a written contract with the client to follow the agreed-upon healthcare regimen. Written agreements reinforce the verbal agreement and serve as a reference.
- Meet with the client following completion of the proposed actions to review the contract and determine the next course of action. Do this until the client is able to initiate and follow through independently.
- Using self-care management precepts, instruct the client about possible situations to which he or she may need to respond; include the use of role playing. Instruct in generating hypotheses from available evidence rather than solely from experience.

Client/Family Teaching

- Provide the family with website addresses where information can be obtained from the Internet. (Most libraries have Internet access with printing capabilities.)
- ▲ Develop collaborative multidisciplinary partnerships.
- Tailor both the information provided and the method of delivery of information to the specific client and/or family.
- Obtain or design educational material that is appropriate for the client; use pictures if possible.
- Teach the client about the symptoms associated with discontinuation of medications, such as a selective serotonin reuptake inhibitor (SSRI).
- Explain nonthreatening aspects before introducing more anxiety-producing information regarding possible side effects of the disease or medical regimen.
- Treat tobacco use as a chronic problem. Acknowledge the pleasure associated with smoking. Encourage the client to work towards a goal of permanent abstinence. Advise the client about possible relapse.

Health-seeking behaviors (specify)

NANDA Definition

Active seeking (by a person in stable health) of ways to alter personal health habits and/or the environment in order to move toward a higher level of health

Defining Characteristics

H

Demonstrated lack of knowledge about health promotion behaviors; expressed concern about current environmental conditions on health status; expressed desire for increased control of health practice; expressed desire to seek a higher level of wellness; observed unfamiliarity with wellness community resources; stated unfamiliarity with wellness community resources

Client Outcomes

Client Will (Specify Time Frame):

- Maintain ideal weight and be knowledgeable about nutritious diet
- Demonstrate ways to fit newly prescribed change in health habits into lifestyle
- List community resources available for assistance with achieving wellness
- List ways to include wellness behaviors in current lifestyle

Nursing Interventions

- Discuss the client's beliefs about health and his or her ability to maintain health.
- Identify barriers and benefits to being healthy.
- Identify environmental and social factors that the client perceives as health promoting.

Nutritional

- Assess the role that stress plays in overeating and weight cycling.
- Encourage use of the nutritional guidelines developed by the U.S. Department of Agriculture (USDA).
- Refer to care plan **Readiness for enhanced Nutrition** for additional interventions.

Exercise

- ▲ Advise the client to consult with a healthcare provider to determine the ability to tolerate a specific regimen.
- • Engage in regular physical activity and reduce sedentary activities to promote health, psychological well-being, and a healthy body weight.
  - ■ Engage in 30 or more minutes of moderate-intensity physical activity above usual activity level 4 or more days per week.
  - ■ Engagement in more vigorous physical activity or for longer periods generally provides greater health benefits.
  - ■ Engage in 60 minutes of moderate to vigorous activity on most days of the week to help manage body weight and prevent gradual, unhealthy body weight gain in adulthood.
  - ■ Engage in 60 to 90 minutes of daily moderate physical activity to sustain weight loss in adulthood.
  - ■ Engage in stretching exercises for flexibility, and resistance exercises or calisthenics for muscle strength and endurance.
- • Encourage appropriate exercise for individuals with chronic illnesses.
- • Set up a support and reward system.
- • Consider using music to help the client focus on the enjoyment of exercise.
- • Determine the exercises that the client prefers and encourage exercise at least three times per week (e.g., walking, jogging, aerobics, swimming, bicycling, yoga, tai chi).

Stress Management

- • Determine overall patterns of stress.
- • Determine the client's social support network.
- • Teach stress-relieving techniques (e.g., deep and slow breathing, progressive muscle relaxation, meditation, imagery, problem solving).
- • Implement nursing case management with chronic illness.

Smoking, Drinking, Self-Medication

- • Involve the client in mutual goal setting.
- • Refer a client who smokes to SmokEnders or a similar community-based program. Discuss ways in which the client can deal with a change in behavior.
- • Alcoholic beverages should be avoided by individuals engaging

in activities that require attention, skill, or coordination, such as driving or operating machinery.

- ▲ Refer a client who drinks alcohol excessively to Alcoholics Anonymous (AA). Identify a support person to help the client into the organization.
- ▲ Identify patterns of self medication with over-the-counter medications and herbal remedies, and excessive use of prescribed medications.
- • Refer to the care plans for **Dysfunctional Family processes: alcoholism, Ineffective Denial,** and **Defensive Coping.**

Health-Seeking Behaviors

- • Recognize and allow the client to discuss the choice of complementary therapies available, such as spiritual practice, relaxation, imagery, exercise, lifestyle, diet (e.g., macrobiotic, vegetarian), and nutritional supplementation.

Health Screening, Appropriate Health Care

- • Assess the frequency of illness-preventing practices, such as routine physical examinations, dental examinations, influenza immunization, breast self-examinations (BSEs), and mammograms, as recommended for women; testicular self-examinations (TSEs) and prostate examinations for men; and screening for familial diseases, such as glaucoma and elevated cholesterol level.
- • Tailor health-related messages to stress the benefits of adherence (gain framed) and the costs of nonadherence (loss framed).
- • Provide a phone call to remind the client of appointments.
- • Refer to the care plan for **Ineffective Health maintenance.**

Pediatric

- • Follow the recommended guidelines for childhood immunizations as laid out by the Centers for Disease Control and Prevention (CDC), available at http://www.cdc.gov/nip/recs/child-schedule.htm.

Geriatric

- • Assess the client's awareness of deficits that may result from normal aging (e.g., changes in sleep patterns or frequency of urination, loss of visual acuity in night driving, loss of hearing, changes in diet, changes in memory, loss of significant others).

- ▲ Find suitable housing that provides support, safety, protection, meals, and social events. Consider in-home care by adult children when possible.
- ▲ Give the client information about community resources for older adults (e.g., services providing transportation to appointments, Meals on Wheels, home visitation services, pets, American Association of Retired Persons [AARP], Elder Hostel, informational websites).
- ▲ Assess for signs of elder abuse and report as appropriate.
- ▲ Teach health-protecting behaviors to older adult clients: monitoring cholesterol intake, exercising, having the stool checked for occult blood, or undergoing a mammogram, Pap test, or prostate or skin evaluation.
- ▲ Consider the age of the client when suggesting screening for disease.
- • Teach the importance of exercise.
- ▲ Form collaborative, multidisciplinary partnerships with nurse-managed clinics for health promotion and chronic disease care management for community-residing older adults.

Multicultural

- • Assess for the influence of cultural beliefs, norms, and values on the client's beliefs about health behavior.
- • Negotiate with the client the aspects of health behavior that will require further modification.
- • Use a community focus intervention.

Home Care

NOTE: All the previously listed nursing interventions are applicable to the home care setting. For more information, see Home Care interventions in the care plan for **Ineffective Health maintenance.**

Client/Family Teaching

- • Discuss the role of environmental and social factors in supporting a healthy family life.
- • Use written, verbal, and video instruction to provide information about health-seeking opportunities and wellness, and provide the family with lists of addresses and where information can be found. Suggest use of the Internet. (Most libraries have Internet access with printing capabilities.)

▲ Teach the importance of receiving a flu vaccine. Offer vaccinations in convenient locations free of charge, and discuss perceived barriers with clients.
• Teach woman how to monitor ovarian health: monthly self-monitoring using a symptom checklist, including personal and family risks and early symptoms of gastrointestinal problems.

Impaired Home maintenance

NANDA Definition

Inability to independently maintain a safe and growth-promoting immediate environment

Defining Characteristics

Objective

Disorderly surroundings; inappropriate household temperature; insufficient clothes; insufficient linen; lack of clothes; lack of linen; lack of necessary equipment; offensive odors; overtaxed family members; presence of vermin; repeated unhygienic disorders; repeated unhygienic infections; unavailable cooking equipment; unclean surroundings

Subjective

Household members describe financial crises; household members describe outstanding debts; household members express difficulty in maintaining their home in a comfortable fashion; household members request assistance with home maintenance.

Related Factors (r/t)

Deficient knowledge; disease; inadequate support systems; injury; impaired functioning; insufficient family organization; insufficient family planning; insufficient finances; lack of role modeling; unfamiliarity with neighborhood resources

Client Outcomes

Client Will (Specify Time Frame):

• Wear clean clothing, eat nutritious meals, and have a sanitary and safe home

- Have the resources to cope physically and emotionally with the chronic illness process
- Use community resources to assist with treatment needs

Nursing Interventions

- • Assess the concerns of family members, especially the primary caregiver, about long-term home care.
- • Establish a plan of care with the client and family based on the client's needs and the caregiver's capabilities.
- • Set up a system of relief for the main caregiver in the home, and plan for sharing of household duties.
- • Consider the use of permethrin-impregnated mattress liners to control dust mites.
- ▲ Initiate referral to community agencies as needed, including housekeeping services, Meals on Wheels (MOW), wheelchair-compatible transportation services, and oxygen therapy services.
- ▲ Obtain adaptive equipment and telemedical equipment, as appropriate, to help family members continue to maintain the home environment.
- ▲ Ask the family to identify support people who can help with home maintenance.

Geriatric

- ▲ During the home visit, be alert for signs of elder abuse. Report any findings.
- ▲ Refer for telephone primary care management.
- ▲ Explore community resources to assist with home care (e.g., senior centers, Department of Aging, hospital case managers, the Internet, or church parish nurse).
- ▲ Provide assistive technology devices: barrier-free environment (home modification), daily living aids, mobility aids, seating and positioning devices, and sensory aids.
- • Encourage regular eye examinations.
- • The following interventions should be considered for clients with diminished or failing sight:
  - ■ **Reduce glare:** use nonglare light bulbs; remove wax from floors (to reduce glare); encourage the client to wear sunglasses; use sheer curtains or blinds.
  - ■ **Use proper lighting:** use night lights in the bedroom, bath-

room, and hallways; use dimmer switches and three-way bulbs to control light; put bright lights at the top and bottom of a staircase; use consistent lighting to minimize shadows.

- **Enhance color contrast:** use colored tape to define steps; paint walls and staircase to contrast with floor; put glow-in-the-dark tape on light switches and door knobs; use colored dishes.
- **Encourage the client to use low vision aids:** use magnifiers to improve near vision; hang magnifiers around the neck for convenience when sewing, doing crafts, or reading; request large-print medication labels, books, and phones; use handrails on stairs; keep flashlights in a convenient location.

• See the care plans for **Risk for Injury** and **Risk for Falls.**

Multicultural

• Acknowledge the stresses unique to racial/ethnic communities.

Home Care

• The previously mentioned interventions incorporate these resources.

▲ Refer clients with mental illness and medical conditions to in-home behavioral health case management.

▲ When the smart home becomes available, consider referral for use.

• See care plans **Contamination** and **Risk for Contamination.**

Client/Family Teaching

• Teach the caregiver the need to set aside some personal time every day to meet his or her own needs.

▲ Identify support groups within the community to assist families in the caregiver role.

▲ Provide counseling and support for caregivers of clients with Alzheimer's disease.

▲ Provide written instructions for medication management and side effects, written instructions for equipment brought to the home, and resource phone numbers for emergency needs.

▲ Promote food safety. Instruct client to avoid microbial food-borne illness by regularly washing hands, food contact surfaces, and fruits and vegetables. Meat and poultry should not be washed or rinsed. Separate raw, cooked, and ready-to-eat foods while shopping, preparing, or storing foods. Cook foods to a safe temperature to kill microorganisms. Chill (refrigerate) perishable food promptly and defrost foods properly. Avoid raw (unpasteurized) milk or any products made from unpasteurized milk, raw or partially cooked eggs, or foods containing raw eggs, raw or undercooked meat and poultry, unpasteurized juices, and raw sprouts.

▲ Teach clients to prevent exposure that could result in adverse health effects from disturbed mold. Avoid areas where mold contamination is obvious; use environmental controls; use personal protective equipment; and keep hands, skin, and clothing clean and free from mold-contaminated dust.

• See care plans **Risk for Infection, Contamination,** and **Risk for Contamination.**

H

Readiness for enhanced Hope

NANDA Definition

A pattern of expectations and desires that is sufficient for mobilizing energy on one's own behalf and can be strengthened

Defining Characteristics

Expresses desire to enhance: ability to set achievable goals; belief in possibilities; congruency of expectations with desires; hope; interconnectedness with others; problem solving to meet goals; sense of meaning to life; spirituality

Client Outcomes

Client Will (Specify Time Frame):

- Describe values, expectations, and meanings
- Set achievable goals that are consistent with values
- Design strategies to achieve goals
- Express belief in possibilities

Nursing Interventions

• Develop an open and caring relationship that enables the client to discuss hope.

- Screen the client for hope using a valid and reliable instrument as indicated.
- Focus on the positive aspects of hope, rather than the prevention of hopelessness.
- Provide emotional support.
- Promote the client's awareness of the existential meanings in life events.
- Help the person to identify his or her desires and expectations.
- Use a family-oriented approach when discussing hope.
- Review internal and external resources to enhance hope.
- Identify spiritual beliefs and practices.
- Assist the person to consider possible adaptations to changes.

Home Care

- Previously mentioned interventions may be adapted for home care use.

Client/Family Teaching

- Assess client and family hope before teaching.
- Incorporate client and family goal setting with teaching content.
- Provide information to the client and family regarding all aspects of the client's health condition.

Hopelessness

NANDA Definition

Subjective state in which an individual sees limited or no alternatives or personal choices available and is unable to mobilize energy on own behalf

Defining Characteristics

Closing eyes; decreased affect; decreased appetite; decreased response to stimuli; decreased verbalization; lack of initiative; lack of involvement in care; passivity; shrugging in response to speaker; sleep pattern disturbance; turning away from speaker; verbal cues (e.g., despondent content, "I can't," sighing)

Related Factors (r/t)

Abandonment; deteriorating physiological condition; lost belief in spiritual power; lost belief in transcendent values; long-term stress; prolonged activity restriction creating isolation

Client Outcomes

Client Will (Specify Time Frame):

- Verbalize feelings, participate in care
- Make positive statements (e.g., "I can" or "I will try")
- Set goals
- Make eye contact, focus on speaker
- Maintain appropriate appetite for age and physical health
- Sleep appropriate length of time for age and physical health
- Express concern for another
- Initiate activity

Nursing Interventions

▲ Monitor and document the potential for suicide. (Refer the client for appropriate treatment if a potential for suicide is identified.) Refer to the care plan **Risk for Suicide** for specific interventions.
- Be alert for symptoms of hopelessness in the general population.
- Assist in identifying sources of hope and hopelessness.
- Provide realistic feedback.
- Assess for pain and respond with appropriate measures for pain relief.
- Assist with problem solving and decision making.
- Determine appropriate approaches based on the underlying condition or situation that is contributing to feelings of hopelessness.
- Assist the client in looking at alternatives and setting goals that are important to him or her.
- In dealing with possible long-term deficits, work with the client to set small, attainable goals.
- Spend one-on-one time with the client. Use empathy; try to understand what the client is saying and communicate this understanding to the client and inspire hope.
- Encourage decision making in the daily schedule.
- Encourage expression of feelings and acknowledge acceptance of them.
- Give the client time to initiate interactions. After an appropri-

ate amount of time is allowed, approach the client in an accepting and nonjudgmental manner.
- • Encourage the client to participate in group activities.
- • Teach alternative coping strategies.
- • Review the client's strengths with the client.
- • Communicate clearly what the illness trajectory and/or course of treatment will involve.
- • Use humor as appropriate.
- • Involve family and significant others in the plan of care.
- • Encourage the family and significant others to express care, hope, and love for the client.
- ▲ Consider use of integrative therapies, such as omega-3 fatty acids, *Hypericum perforatum* (St. John's wort), *S*-adenosylmethionine, folate, 5-hydroxytryptophan, acupuncture, exercise, and light therapy.
- • Use touch to demonstrate caring, if culturally appropriate and with the client's permission, and encourage the family to do the same.
- • Facilitate access to resources to support a positive spirituality.
- • For additional interventions, see the care plans for **Readiness for enhanced Hope, Spiritual distress, Readiness for enhanced Spiritual well-being,** and **Disturbed Sleep pattern**.

Geriatric

- ▲ If depression is suspected, confer with the primary physician regarding referral for mental health services.
- • Take threats of self-harm or suicide seriously.
- • Identify significant losses that may be leading to feelings of hopelessness.
- • Discuss stages of emotional responses to multiple losses.
- • Use reminiscence and life-review therapies to identify past coping skills.
- • Express hope to the client and give positive feedback whenever appropriate.
- • Identify the client's past and current sources of spirituality. Help the client explore life and identify those experiences that are noteworthy. The client may want to read the Bible or other religious text or have it read to him or her.
- • Encourage visits from children.
- • Position the client by a window, take the client outside, or encourage such activities as gardening (if ability allows).

- Provide esthetic forms of expression, such as dance, music, literature, and pictures.

Multicultural

- Assess for the influence of cultural beliefs, norms, and values on the client's feelings of hopelessness.
- Assess the effect of fatalism on the client's expression of hopelessness.
- Assess for depression and refer to appropriate services.
- Encourage spirituality as a source of support for hopelessness.

Home Care

- Previously mentioned interventions may be adapted for home care use.
- ▲ Assess for isolation within the family unit. Encourage the client to participate in family activities. If the client cannot participate, encourage him or her to be in the same area and watch family activities. Refer for telephone support.
- Reminisce with the client about his or her life.
- Identify areas in which the client can have control. Allow the client to set achievable goals in these areas. Assist the client when necessary to negotiate desirable outcomes.
- Clearly explain potential benefits and risks of a proposed intervention.
- If illness precipitated the hopelessness, discuss knowledge of and previous experience with the disease. Help the client to identify past coping strengths.
- ▲ Provide plant or pet therapy if possible.

Client/Family Teaching

- Provide information regarding the client's condition, treatment plan, and progress.
- Provide positive reinforcement, praise, and acknowledgment of the challenges of caregiving to family members.
- Teach the use of stress-reduction techniques, relaxation, and imagery. Many cassette tapes and compact discs on relaxation and meditation are available. Assist the client and caregivers with relaxation based on their preference from the initial assessment.
- ▲ Refer the client to self-help groups, such as I Can Cope and Make Today Count.

▲ Refer the family to community support groups targeted to the specific needs of the family caregivers.

Hyperthermia

NANDA Definition

H

Body temperature elevated above normal range

Elevated body temperature can be either fever or hyperthermia. **Fever** is a regulated rise in the core body temperature or variation in the temperature set point. This elevation is in response to a chemical signal (endogenous pyrogen) released as part of an inflammatory response, with release of mediators such as interleukin-1B and interleukin-6. The immune system is enhanced by the fever, with lymphocyte proliferation and increased neutrophil activity. The client sleeps longer and deeper. The heart rate increases as well as the cardiac index. Also, the metabolic rate increases, and if the patient begins shivering, the rate may increase 200% or more.

Hyperthermia is an unregulated rise in body temperature, which is seen with heat illness, neurological disorders, or malignant hyperthermia, often with the temperature above 104° F (40° C). Hyperthermia is not adaptive and should be treated as a medical emergency.

Defining Characteristics

Flushed skin; increase in body temperature above normal range; tachycardia; tachypnea; warm to touch; seizures (convulsions)

Related Factors (r/t)

Anesthesia; decreased perspiration; dehydration; exposure to hot environment; inappropriate clothing; increased metabolic rate; illness; medications; trauma; vigorous activity

Client Outcomes

Client Will (Specify Time Frame):

- Maintain oral temperature within adaptive levels
- Remain free of complications of malignant hypertension (MH)
- Remain free of dehydration

Nursing Interventions

▲ Assess an afebrile hospitalized client's temperature per institutional policy, upon assessment of signs or symptoms of infection, if the client has chills, or at least once a day between 5 PM and 7 PM.

• Measure and record a febrile client's temperature using an oral or rectal thermometer at least every 4 to 6 hours or whenever a change in condition occurs (e.g., chills, change in mental status).

• Use the same site and method (device) for temperature measurement for a given client so that temperature trends are assessed accurately.

▲ Notify the physician of temperature according to institutional standards or written orders, or when temperature reaches 100.5° F (38° C) and above. Also notify the physician of the presence of a change in mental status.

▲ Work with the physician to help determine the cause of the temperature increase, which will often help direct appropriate treatment.

▲ Administer antipyretic medication per physician orders, when the cause of the temperature is not adaptive (neurological, heatstroke, or malignant hyperthermia), when infection-induced fever is greater than 39° C (102.2° F), and when the client cannot tolerate the increase in metabolic demand, such as when the client is the acutely ill or has cardiac or respiratory disease.

▲ Assess fluid loss and facilitate oral intake or administer intravenous fluids to replace fluids.

• When diaphoresis is present, assist the client with bathing and changing into dry clothing.

• Do not use external cooling measures, such as ice packs, tepid water baths, or removal of blankets and clothing for fever management; these measures cause shivering and are ineffective.

• Recognize that a hypothermia blanket is indicated for temperature reduction if the client's fever is above 104° F (40° C) and cannot be controlled with antipyretics, or if a high body temperature is related to a disorder of temperature regulation.

• When using a cooling blanket, choose a convective airflow system if possible, and set the temperature regulator to 1° to 2° F (0.6° to 1.1° C) below the client's current temperature.

• Use a nonsteroidal antipyretic (e.g., acetaminophen) as ordered instead of or in conjunction with a cooling blanket to improve fever reduction and decrease the duration of cooling blanket use.

▲ Recognize that shivering can be harmful and prevent shivering when possible. Wrap extremities in towels to decrease shivering before beginning use of the cooling blanket, or administer medications to prevent shivering as ordered.

Pediatric

- Assess risk factors of malignant hyperthermia, because this has an increased prevalence in the pediatric population.

▲ Administer dantrolene and oxygen as ordered.

- Avoid routine sponging—especially cold sponging—to reduce body temperature in children.

Geriatric

- Recognize that an increase in oral temperature of 1° F above their baseline temperature or above 99° F (37.2° C) should be considered a fever in older adults.
- Rectal temperature may be more accurate to diagnose fever in older clients. However, nursing judgment must be used to determine if rectal temperature measurement is acceptable to the client, especially a client with mental changes or dementia.
- Assess for other signs and symptoms of infection in addition to or in the absence of fever in older clients. Suspect infection when there has been a decline in function, including new or increased confusion, incontinence, falling, decreased mobility, or failure to cooperate.

▲ Help the client seek medical attention immediately if fever is present. To diagnose the fever source, assess for possible precipitating factors, including medication changes, environmental changes, and recent medical interventions or infectious exposures.

- In hot weather, encourage older adult clients to drink 8 glasses of fluid per day (within their cardiac and renal reserves) regardless of whether they are thirsty. Assess for the need for and presence of fans or air conditioning.
- In hot weather, monitor older adult clients for signs of heatstroke, which include body temperature of 100° to 102° F (37.8°-38.9° C), orthostatic blood pressure drop, weakness, restlessness, mental status changes, faintness, thirst, nausea, and

vomiting. If signs are present, move the client to a cool place, have the client lie down, give sips of water, check orthostatic blood pressure, spray with lukewarm water, cool with a fan, and seek medical assistance immediately.

Home Care

- • Some of the interventions described previously may be adapted for home care use.
- • Assess whether the client or family has a thermometer and knows how to use it.
- ▲ Teach the client and family to use ordered antipyretic medication safely.
- • Help the client and caregivers prevent and monitor for heatstroke/hyperthermia during times of high outdoor temperatures.
- • To prevent heat-related injury in athletes, laborers, and military personnel, instruct them to acclimate gradually to the higher temperatures, increase fluid intake, wear vapor-permeable clothing, and rest frequently.
- • If body temperature increases above the adaptive range, institute measures to decrease temperature (e.g., get the client out of the sun and into a cool place, remove excess clothing, have the client drink fluids, spray the client with lukewarm water, and fan with cool air).
- ▲ If the client is in hospice or is terminally ill, follow the client's wishes and the physician's orders in determining the management of fever.

Client/Family Teaching

- ▲ Teach that infection-induced fever generally enhances the immune system, so the client can participate in the decision of whether to treat the fever. If treatment is elected or appropriate for comfort, instruct in the use of antipyretics as ordered.
- • Teach the client that shivering with infection-induced fever has detrimental effects and that activities that can cause shivering (e.g., removing blankets, lowering the room temperature, taking tepid water baths, applying ice packs) should be avoided.
- • Instruct the client to increase fluids to prevent heat-induced hyperthermia and dehydration in the presence of fever.
- • Teach the client to stay in a cooler environment during periods of excessive outdoor heat or humidity. If the client does go out,

instruct him or her to avoid vigorous physical activity, wear lightweight, loose-fitting clothing, and wear a hat to minimize sun exposure.

Hypothermia

NANDA Definition

Body temperature below normal range

Defining Characteristics

Body temperature below normal range; cool skin; cyanotic nail beds; hypertension; pallor; piloerection; shivering; slow capillary refill; tachycardia

Related Factors (r/t)

Aging; consumption of alcohol; damage to hypothalamus; decreased ability to shiver; decreased metabolic rate; evaporation from skin in cool environment; exposure to cool environment; illness; inactivity; inadequate clothing; malnutrition; medications; trauma

Client Outcomes

Client Will (Specify Time Frame):

- Maintain body temperature within normal range
- Identify risk factors of hypothermia
- State measures to prevent hypothermia
- Identify symptoms of hypothermia and actions to take when hypothermia is present

Nursing Interventions

- • Remove the client from the cause of the hypothermic episode (e.g., cold environment, cold or wet clothing). Ensure that the client is in a warm environment.
- • Watch the client for signs of hypothermia: shivering, slurred speech, clumsy movements, fatigue, and confusion. As hypothermia progresses, the skin becomes pale, numb, and waxy. Muscles are tense, fatigue and weakness progress, and gradually there can be loss of consciousness with loss of a pulse and breathing.

- • Cover the client with warm blankets and apply a covering to the head and neck to conserve body heat.
- • Take the client's temperature at least hourly; if more than mild hypothermia is present (temperature lower than 95° F [35° C]), use a continuous temperature-monitoring device, preferably two of them, one in the rectum and the other in the esophagus.
- ▲ If the client is awake, measure the oral temperature, instead of the tympanic or axillary temperature. Use a pulmonary artery catheter temperature-measuring device if available; if not, consider using a bladder catheter that measures temperature. Monitor the client's vital signs every hour and as appropriate. Note changes associated with hypothermia, such as initially increased pulse rate, respiratory rate, and blood pressure with mild hypothermia, and then decreased pulse rate, respiratory rate, and blood pressure with moderate to severe hypothermia.
- ▲ Attach electrodes and a cardiac monitor. Watch for dysrhythmias.
- • Monitor for signs of coagulopathy (e.g., oozing of blood from open areas, intravascular catheter sites, or mucous membranes). Also note results of clotting studies as available.
- • For mild hypothermia (core temperature of 90°-95° F [32.2°-35° C]), rewarm client passively:
  - ■ Set room temperature to 70° to 75° F (21° to 24° C).
  - ■ Keep the client dry and remove damp or wet clothing.
  - ■ Layer clothing and blankets and cover the client's head; use insulated metallic blankets.
  - ■ Offer warm fluids, but no alcohol or caffeine.
- ▲ For moderate hypothermia (core temperature 82.4° to 90° F [28° to 32.2° C]) use active external rewarming methods. The rewarming rate should not exceed 1.8° F (1° C) per hour. Methods include the following:
  - ■ Forced-air warming blankets
  - ■ Carbon-fiber blanket
  - ■ Radiant heat lights
- ▲ For severe hypothermia (core temperature below 82.4° F [28° C]) use active core-rewarming techniques as ordered:
  - ■ Recognize that extracorporeal blood rewarming methods are most effective.
  - ■ Administer heated and humidified oxygen through the ventilator as ordered.

  - ■ Administer heated intravenous (IV) fluids at prescribed temperature.
  - ■ Perform peritoneal lavage and bladder irrigations as ordered.
- • Check blood pressure frequently when rewarming; watch for hypotension.
- ▲ Administer IV fluids, using a rapid infuser IV fluid warmer as ordered.
- • Determine the factors leading to the hypothermic episode; see Related Factors.
- ▲ Request a social service referral to help the client obtain the heat, shelter, and food needed to maintain body temperature.
- ▲ Encourage proper nutrition and hydration. Request a referral to a dietitian to identify appropriate dietary needs.

Pediatric

- • Recognize that pediatric clients have a decreased ability to adapt to temperature extremes. Take the following actions to maintain body temperature in the infant/child:
  - ■ Keep the head covered.
  - ■ Use blankets to keep the client warm.
  - ■ Keep the client covered during procedures, transport, and diagnostic testing.
  - ■ Keep the room temperature at 72° F (22.2° C).
- • For the preterm or low birth weight newborn, use specially designed bags, skin-to-skin care, and transwarmer mattresses to keep preterm infants warm.

Geriatric

- • Assess neurological signs frequently, watching for confusion and decreased level of consciousness.
- • Recognize that older adults can develop indoor hypothermia from air conditioning or ice baths.
- • Recognize that older adults often wear socks and sweaters to protect themselves from feeling cold, even in warmer weather.

Home Care

NOTE: Hypothermia is not a symptom that appears in the normal course of home care. When it occurs, it is a clinical emergency and the client/family should access emergency medical services immediately.

- • Some of the interventions described earlier may be adapted for home care use.
- • Before a medical crisis occurs, confirm that the client or family has a thermometer and can read it. Instruct as needed. Verify that the thermometer registers accurately.
- • Instruct the client or family to take the temperature when the client displays cyanosis, pallor, or shivering.
- ▲ Monitor temperature every hour, as noted previously. If the temperature of the client begins dropping below the normal range, apply layers of clothing or blankets, or adjust environmental heat to the comfort level. Do not overheat. Contact a physician.
- ▲ If temperature continues to drop, activate the emergency system and notify a physician.
- ▲ If the client is in hospice care or is terminally ill, follow advance directives, client wishes, and the physician's orders. Keep the client free of pain.

Client/Family Teaching

- • Teach the client and family signs of hypothermia and the method of taking the temperature (age-appropriate).
- • Teach the client methods to prevent hypothermia: wearing adequate clothing, including a hat and mittens; heating the environment to a minimum of 68° F (20° C); and ingesting adequate food and fluid.
- ▲ Teach the client and family about medications, such as sedatives, opioids, and anxiolytics, that predispose the client to hypothermia (as appropriate).

Disturbed personal Identity

NANDA Definition

Inability to distinguish between self and nonself

Client Outcomes

Client Will (Specify Time Frame):

- Show interest in surroundings
- Respond to stimuli with appropriate affect
- Perform self-care and self-control activities appropriate for age
- Acknowledge personal strengths
- Engage in interpersonal relationships
- Verbalize willingness to change lifestyle and use appropriate community resources

Nursing Interventions

- Assess carefully for a history of abuse.
- Assess for any history of seizure disorder; adhere to the diagnostic criteria for dissociative disorder in the Diagnostic and Statistical Manual of Mental Disorders, Fourth Edition (DSM-IV), and conduct a structured clinical interview.
- Avoid labeling the client with terms such as multiple personality disorder (MPD).
- Spend time communicating with the client.
- Provide time for one-on-one interactions to establish a therapeutic relationship.
- Work with the client on setting personal goals.
- Provide communication, clear rules and aims, and safety procedures.
- Work with the client to utilize their senses to deescalate problem behavior.
- Give the client permission to share his or her experiences.
- Use touch only after a thorough assessment and as appropriate.
- Encourage the client to verbalize feelings about self and body image. Have the client make a list of strengths.

▲ Support client's autonomy in a nurse-led shared care environment where the client is encouraged to participate in his or her care.

▲ Encourage participation in group therapy for building relationship skills and getting feedback from others with regard to behavior.

- Encourage the client to use a daily diary to set achievable and realistic goals and to monitor successes.

▲ Refer for rational emotive therapy to help dispel underlying irrational thinking.

Geriatric

- Address the client by his or her full name preceded by the proper title (i.e., Mr., Mrs., Ms., Miss); use a nickname or first name only if suggested by the client, and do not use terms of endearment (e.g., "honey").
- Practice reality orientation principles.
- Ask the client about important past experiences.

▲ If the client's symptoms are associated with a stroke, refer the client for longer rehabilitation that includes physical programs addressing psychological as well as neuromuscular issues.

Multicultural

- Assess for the influence of cultural beliefs, norms, and values on the family's perceptions of infant/child behavior.
- Use a neutral, indirect style when addressing areas in which improvement is needed, such as a need for verbal or oral stimulation, when working with Native-American clients.

Home Care

- The interventions described previously may be adapted for home care use.

Client/Family Teaching

- Teach stress reduction and relaxation techniques. These techniques can be used when the client becomes anxious about the loss of self.

▲ Refer to community resources or other self-help groups appropriate for the client's underlying problem (e.g., Adult Children of Alcoholics, parent effectiveness group).

▲ Refer to appropriate treatment as soon as signs of depression are noted.

Readiness for enhanced Immunization status

NANDA Definition

A pattern of conforming to local, national, and/or international standards of immunization to prevent infectious disease(s) that is sufficient to protect a person, family, or community and can be strengthened

Defining Characteristics

Expresses desire to enhance: behavior to prevent infectious disease; identification of possible problems associated with immunizations; identification of providers of immunizations; immunization status; knowledge of immunization standards; record-keeping of immunizations

Client Outcomes

Client/Caregiver Will (Specify Time Frame):

- Review appropriate recommended immunization schedule with provider
- Ask questions about the benefits and risks of immunizations
- Ask questions regarding the risk of choosing not to be immunized
- Accurately respond to provider's questions related to pertinent information regarding individual health status as it relates to contraindications for individual vaccines.
- Inform provider of the health status of close contacts and household members
- Evidence understanding of the risks and benefits of individual immunization decisions
- Evidence understanding of the benefits of community immunization
- Communicate decisions about immunization decision to provider in relation to personal preferences, values, and goals
- Communicate to provider ongoing personal record of immunization
- Evidence understanding of the client's responsibility to maintain an accurate record of immunization

Nursing Interventions

Psychosocial

- Assess barriers to immunization:
  - Anxiety related to injection/parenteral pharmacologic therapy
  - Anxiety related to immunization side effects
  - Knowledge of risk associated with disease
  - Cost of health care
- Assess client-provider relationship.
- Assess client/caregiver level of participation in decision making process.
- Assess sources of information client has previously turned to.
- Assist client/caregiver to find appropriate educational resources.
- Assess cultural or religious beliefs that may relate to either the decision making process or specific immunizations such as sexually transmitted disease.

Physiological

- Perform comprehensive interview to elicit information regarding the client's susceptibility to adverse reactions to specific vaccines according to the manufacturer guidelines.
- Identify clients for whom a specific vaccine is contraindicated.

▲ Report potential or actual adverse effects.

- Inform client/caregiver of the vaccine-specific risks to both women of childbearing age and the fetus.
- Discuss pregnancy planning with appropriate clients considering immunization.
- Identify high risk individuals for specific vaccine-preventable disease.
- Identify high risk groups for specific vaccine-preventable disease.
- Identify high risk populations for specific vaccine preventable disease.
- Assess client's recent travel history and future travel plans.
- Identify vulnerable populations and marginalized populations.
- Tailor educational programs specific to these marginalized and vulnerable populations.
- Adopt recommendations made by national and international professional groups advocating the use of Immunization Central Registries, Standing orders.

- Support access to health care that enables clients to access well preventive care on a walk-in basis during times that are consistent with client schedules.

Multicultural

- Assess cultural beliefs and practices that may have an impact on the educational and decision making process specific to immunization as well as vaccine-specific illness.
- Actively listen and be sensitive to how communication is shared culturally.
- Employ culturally sensitive educational strategies to maximize the individual, family, or community response.

Home Care

- Above interventions may be adapted for home care use.
- Develop clinical practice guidelines that include shared decision making.
- Implement home care strategies that will enhance decision making and ability to maintain current immunization status.
- Implement mechanisms to contact the client/caregiver at appropriate intervals with reminder literature or phone contact.

Client/Family Teaching

- Before teaching, evaluate the client preference for involvement with the decision making process.
- Use community-based and school-based interventions to teach school-age children and thereby provide vicarious education to the family.
- Develop curricula and media that enhance immunization education.
- Employ media and curricula in office waiting rooms.
- Develop and distribute client log books that provide record keeping and foster ownership of the responsibility of current immunization status.

Functional urinary Incontinence

NANDA Definition

Inability of usually continent person to reach toilet in time to avoid unintentional loss of urine. Impairment or loss of continence due to functional deficits, including altered mobility, dexterity, or cognition, or environmental barriers.

Defining Characteristics

Although functional limitations (impaired mobility, dexterity, and cognition) are risk factors for urinary incontinence (UI), the nature of their relationship is complex and only partly understood. For example, impaired cognition associated with Alzheimer's type dementia leads to detrusor overactivity. Whether or not detrusor overactivity leads to UI (either urge UI or UI without sensory awareness) depends on multiple factors, including mobility, the severity of cognitive impairment, among other factors. Thus, while functional impairment exacerbates the severity of urinary incontinence, the underlying factors that contribute to these functional limitations themselves also contribute to abnormal lower urinary tract function and impaired continence.

Related Factors (r/t)

Cognitive disorders (delirium, dementia, severe or profound retardation); neuromuscular limitations impairing mobility or dexterity; environmental barriers to toileting

Client Outcomes

Client Will (Specify Time Frame):

- Eliminate or reduce incontinent episodes
- Eliminate or overcome environmental barriers to toileting
- Use adaptive equipment to reduce or eliminate incontinence related to impaired mobility or dexterity
- Use portable urinary collection devices or urine containment devices when access to the toilet is not feasible

Nursing Interventions

▲ Perform a history taking and physical assessment focusing on bothersome lower urinary tract symptoms, cognitive status, functional status (particularly physical mobility and dexterity), frequency and severity of leakage episodes, and alleviating and aggravating factors.

▲ Consult with the client and family, the client's physician, and other healthcare professionals concerning treatment of incontinence in the elderly client undergoing detailed geriatric evaluation.

- Teach the client, the client's care providers, or the family to complete a voiding diary (bladder log) by recording voiding frequency, the frequency of urinary incontinent episodes, and their association with urgency (a sudden and strong desire to urinate that is difficult to defer) over a 3- to 7-day period. An electronic voiding diary may be kept whenever feasible. In addition to these parameters, the client may be asked to record voided volume and fluid intake.
- Assess the client for potentially reversible or modifiable causes of acute/transient urinary incontinence (e.g., urinary tract infection; atrophic urethritis; constipation or impaction; use of sedatives or narcotics, antidepressants or psychotropic medications interfering with efficient detrusor contractions, parasympatholytics, or alpha-adrenergic antagonists; polyuria caused by uncontrolled diabetes mellitus or insipidus).
- Assess the client in an acute care or rehabilitation facility for risk factors for functional incontinence.
- Assess the client for coexisting or premorbid urinary incontinence.
- Assess clients, regardless of frailty or age, residing in a long-term care facility for UI.
- Assess the home, acute care, or long-term care environment for accessibility to toileting facilities, paying particular attention to the following:
  - Distance of the toilet from the bed, chair, and living quarters
  - Characteristics of the bed, including presence of side rails and distance of the bed from the floor
  - Characteristics of the pathway to the toilet, including barriers such as stairs, loose rugs on the floor, and inadequate lighting
  - Characteristics of the bathroom, including patterns of use, lighting, height of the toilet from the floor, presence of handrails to assist transfers to the toilet, and breadth of the

door and its accessibility for a wheelchair, walker, or other assistive device

- • Assess the client for mobility, including the ability to rise from chair and bed, transfer to the toilet, and ambulate, and the need for physical assistive devices such as a cane, walker, or wheelchair.
- ▲ Assess the client for dexterity, including the ability to manipulate buttons, hooks, snaps, loop and pile closure, and zippers as needed to remove clothing. Consult a physical or occupational therapist to promote optimal toilet access as indicated.
- • Evaluate cognitive status with a Neecham Confusion Scale in cases of acute cognitive change or with a Folstein Mini-Mental State Examination or other tool as indicated.
- • Remove environmental barriers to toileting in the acute care, long-term care, or home setting. Assist the client in removing loose rugs from the floor and improving lighting in hallways and bathrooms.
- • Provide an appropriate, safe urinary receptacle such as a three-in-one commode, female or male hand-held urinal, no-spill urinal, or containment device when toileting access is limited by immobility or environmental barriers.
- ▲ Help the client with limited mobility to obtain evaluation by a physical therapist and to obtain assistive devices as indicated; assist the client in selecting shoes with a nonskid sole to maximize traction when arising from a chair and transferring to the toilet.
- • Assist the client in altering the wardrobe to maximize toileting access. Select loose-fitting clothing with stretch waistbands rather than buttoned or zippered waist; minimize buttons, snaps, and multilayered clothing; and substitute a loop and pile closure or other easily loosened systems for buttons, hooks, and zippers in existing clothing.
- • Begin a prompted voiding program or patterned urge response toileting program for the elderly client in the home or a long-term care facility who has functional incontinence and dementia:
  - ■ Determine the frequency of current urination using an alarm system or check-and-change device.
  - ■ Record urinary elimination and incontinent patterns in a bladder log to use as a baseline for assessment and evaluation of treatment efficacy.

I

- Begin a prompted toileting program based on the results of this program; toileting frequency may vary from every 1.5 to 2 hours to every 4 hours.
- Praise the client when toileting occurs with prompting.
- Refrain from any socialization when incontinent episodes occur; change the client and make her or him comfortable.

Geriatric

I

- Institute aggressive continence management programs for the cognitively intact, community-dwelling client in consultation with the client and family.
- Monitor the elderly client in a long-term care facility, acute care facility, or home for dehydration.

Home Care

- The interventions described previously may be adapted for home care use.
- Assess current strategies used to reduce urinary incontinence, including limitation of fluid intake, restriction of bladder irritants, prompted or scheduled toileting, and use of containment devices.
- Encourage a mind-set and program of self-care management.
- Implement a bladder-training program, including self-monitoring activities (e.g., reducing caffeine intake, adjusting amount and timing of fluid intake, decreasing long voiding intervals while awake, instituting dietary changes to promote bowel regularity); bladder training; and pelvic muscle exercise.
- For a memory-impaired elderly client, implement an individualized scheduled toileting program (on a schedule developed in consultation with the caregiver, approximately every 2 hours, with toileting reminders provided and existing patterns incorporated, such toileting before or after meals).
- Teach the family the general principles of bladder health, including avoidance of bladder irritants, adequate fluid intake, and a routine schedule of toileting. (Refer to the care plan for **Impaired Urinary elimination.**)
- Teach prompted voiding to the family and client for the client with mild to moderate dementia (refer to previous description).
- Inspect the perineal and perianal skin for evidence of incontinence-associated dermatitis, including inflammation, vesicles in

skin exposed to urinary leakage, and especially skin folds or denudation of the skin, particularly when incontinence is managed by absorptive pads or containment briefs.

- • Begin a preventive skin care regimen for all clients with urinary and/or fecal incontinence and treat clients with incontinence-associated dermatitis or related skin damage (Refer to the care plan for **Total Incontinence.**)
- • Advise the client about the advantages of using disposable or reusable insert pads, pad-pant systems, or replacement briefs specifically designed for urinary incontinence (or double urinary and fecal incontinence) as indicated.
- • Assist the family with arranging care in a way that allows the client to participate in family or favorite activities without embarrassment. Elicit discussion of the client's concerns about the social or emotional burden of incontinence.
- ▲ Refer to occupational therapy for help in obtaining assistive devices and adapting the home for optimal toilet accessibility.
- ▲ Consider the use of an indwelling catheter for continuous drainage in the client who is both homebound and bed bound and is receiving palliative or end-of-life care (requires a physician's order).
- ▲ When an indwelling urinary catheter is in place, follow prescribed maintenance protocols for managing the catheter, drainage bag, perineal skin, and urethral meatus. Teach infection control measures adapted to the home care setting.
- • Assist the client in adapting to the catheter. Encourage discussion of the client's response to the catheter.

Client/Family Teaching

- • Work with the client, family, and their extended support systems to assist with needed changes in the environment and wardrobe, and other alterations required to maximize toileting access.
- • Work with the client and family to establish a reasonable and manageable prompted voiding program using environmental and verbal cues to remind caregivers of voiding intervals, such as television programs, meals, and bedtime.
- • Teach the family to use an alarm system for toileting or to carry out a check-and-change program and to maintain an accurate log of voiding and incontinence episodes.

Overflow urinary Incontinence

NANDA Definition

Involuntary loss of urine associated with overdistention of the bladder

Defining Characteristics

Bladder distention; high post-void residual volume; nocturia; observed involuntary leakage of small volumes of urine; reports involuntary leakage of small volumes of urine

Related Factors (r/t)

Bladder outlet obstruction; detrusor external sphincter dyssynergia; detrusor hypocontractility; fecal impaction; severe pelvic prolapse; side effects of anticholinergic medications; side effects of calcium channel blockers; side effects of decongestant medications; urethral obstruction

Client Outcomes

Client Will (Specify Time Frame):

- Demonstrate consistent ability to urinate when desire to void is perceived or via timed schedule; measured urinary residual volume is <200-250 mL or 25% of total bladder capacity (voided volume plus urinary residual volume)
- Experience correction or relief from voiding and postvoid lower urinary tract symptoms (LUTS)
- Experience correction or alleviation of storage LUTS
- Be free of upper urinary tract distress (renal function remains sufficient; febrile urinary infections are absent)

Nursing Interventions

- Please refer to the care plan for **Urinary retention**

Reflex urinary Incontinence

NANDA Definition

Involuntary loss of urine at somewhat predictable intervals when a specific bladder volume is reached. Involuntary loss of urine caused by a defect in the spinal cord between the nerve roots at or below the first cervical segment and those above the second sacral segment. Urine elimination occurs at unpredictable intervals; micturition may be elicited by tactile stimuli, including stroking of inner thigh or perineum.

Defining Characteristics

Urinary incontinence caused by neurogenic detrusor overactivity; disruption of spinal pathways leads to absent or diminished awareness of the desire to void or the occurrence of an overactive detrusor contraction; incomplete bladder emptying caused by dyssynergia of striated sphincter mechanism, which produces functional outlet obstruction of bladder; reflex urinary incontinence may be associated with sweating and acute elevation in blood pressure and pulse rate in clients with spinal cord injury. Refer to the care plan for **Autonomic dysreflexia.**

Related Factors (r/t)

Paralyzing spinal disorder affecting spinal segments C1 to S2

Client Outcomes

Client Will (Specify Time Frame):

- Follow prescribed schedule for bladder evacuation
- Demonstrate successful use of triggering techniques to stimulate voiding
- Have intact perineal skin
- Remain clear of symptomatic urinary tract infection
- Demonstrate how to apply containment device or insert indwelling catheter or be able to provide caregiver with instructions for performing these procedures
- Demonstrate awareness of risk of autonomic dysreflexia, its prevention, and management

Nursing Interventions

- Assess the client's neurological status, including the type of neurological disorder, the functional level of neurological impairment, its completeness (effect on motor and sensory function), and the ability to perform bladder management tasks, including intermittent catheterization, application of a condom catheter, and so on.

- Knowledge of functional impairments related to a spinal cord injury, including upper extremity function, is essential because it determines the client's ability to manage the bladder by self-catheterization.
- Inspect the perineal and perigenital skin.
- Complete a bladder log to determine the pattern of urine elimination, incontinence episodes, and current bladder management program.
- ▲ Consult with the physician concerning current bladder function and the potential of the bladder to produce upper urinary tract distress (hydronephrosis, vesicoureteral reflux, febrile urinary tract infection, or compromised renal function).
- ▲ Determine a bladder management program in consultation with the client, family, and rehabilitation team.
- ▲ In consultation with the rehabilitation team, counsel the client and family concerning the merits and potential risks associated with each possible bladder management program, including spontaneous voiding, intermittent self-catheterization, reflex voiding with condom catheter containment, and indwelling catheterization.
- Teach the client with reflex incontinence to consume an adequate amount of fluids on a daily basis (approximately 30 mL/kg of body weight).
- Advise clients that while consumption of cranberry products or cranberry tablets is in no way harmful or contraindicated, it does not reduce the risk for urinary tract infection.
- ▲ Teach the client with reflex urinary incontinence that is managed by spontaneous voiding to self-administer an alpha-adrenergic blocking medication as directed and to recognize and manage potential side effects.
- ▲ Begin intermittent catheterization using a modified clean or sterile technique based on facility policies.
- ▲ Teach intermittent catheterization as the client approaches discharge as directed. Instruct the client and at least one family member, spouse, or partner in the performance of catheteriza-

tion using clean technique. Teach the client with quadriplegia how to instruct others to perform this procedure.

▲ Teach the client managed by intermittent catheterization to self-administer antispasmodic (parasympatholytic) medications as directed, and to recognize and manage potential side effects.

▲ Consult with the physician and occupational therapist concerning the use of a neuroprosthesis or other device designed to improve hand use for the quadriplegic client with partial hand function.

I

▲ For a male client with reflex incontinence who cannot manage the condition effectively with spontaneous voiding, does not choose to perform intermittent catheterization, or cannot perform catheterization, teach the client and his family to obtain, select, and apply a condom catheter with drainage bag. Assist them in choosing a product that adheres to the penile shaft without allowing seepage of urine onto surrounding skin or clothing, contains a material and adhesive that does not produce hypersensitivity reactions on the skin, and includes a leg bag that is easily concealed under the clothing and does not cause irritation to the skin of the thigh.

- Teach the client who uses a condom catheter to remove the condom device, inspect the skin, cleanse the penis thoroughly, and reapply a new catheter every day.
- Teach the client whose incontinence is managed by a condom catheter to routinely inspect the skin with each catheter change for evidence of lesions caused by pressure from the containment device or by exposure to urine.
- Teach the client managed by intermittent or indwelling catheter to recognize signs of significant urinary tract infection and to seek care promptly when these signs occur. The signs of significant infection are the following:
  - Discomfort over the bladder or during urination
  - Acute onset of urinary incontinence
  - Fever
  - Markedly increased spasticity of muscles below the level of the spinal lesion
  - Malaise, lethargy
  - Hematuria
  - Autonomic dysreflexia (hyperreflexia)

Geriatric

▲ If difficulties are encountered in client teaching, refer the elderly client to a nurse who specializes in care of the aging client with urinary incontinence.

Home Care

- The interventions described previously may be adapted for home care use. Teach the client what the complications of reflex incontinence are and when to report changes to a physician or primary nurse.

▲ If the client is taught intermittent self-catheterization, arrange for contingency care in the event that the client is unable to perform self-catheterization.

- Assess and instruct the client and family in care of the catheter and supplies in the home.
- Encourage a mind-set and program of self-care management.
- Assist the family with arranging care in a way that allows the client to participate in family or favorite activities without embarrassment. Elicit discussion of the client's concerns about the social or emotional burden of incontinence.

▲ If medications are ordered, instruct the family or caregivers and the client in medication administration, use, and side effects.

Client/Family Teaching

- Teach the client with a spinal injury the signs of autonomic dysreflexia, its relationship to bladder fullness, and management of the condition. Refer to the care plan for **Autonomic dysreflexia.**
- Teach the client and several significant others the techniques of intermittent catheterization, indwelling catheter care and removal, or condom catheter management as appropriate.
- Teach the client and family techniques to clean catheters used for intermittent catheterization, including washing with soap and water and allowing to air dry, and using microwave cleaning techniques.

Stress urinary Incontinence

NANDA Definition

State in which the individual experiences urine loss of less than 50 mL accompanied by increased intraabdominal pressure

NOTE: The value of less than 50 mL for the volume of urine loss may be exceeded by women and men with severe stress incontinence caused by incompetence of the urethral sphincter mechanism. This is sometimes classified as *total incontinence.* In this book, however, *total incontinence* will be used to refer exclusively to incontinence due to extra-urethral causes, and all forms of stress incontinence are reviewed under this diagnosis, regardless of severity.

Defining Characteristics

Observed urine loss with physical exertion (sign of stress incontinence); reported loss of urine associated with physical exertion or activity (symptom of stress incontinence); urine loss associated with increased abdominal pressure (urodynamic stress urinary incontinence)

Related Factors (r/t)

Urethral hypermobility/pelvic organ prolapse (genetic factors/familial predisposition, multiple vaginal deliveries, delivery of infant large for gestational age, forceps-assisted or breech delivery, obesity, changes in estrogen levels at climacteric, extensive abdominopelvic, or pelvic surgery); urethral sphincter mechanism incompetence (multiple urethral suspensions in women, radical prostatectomy in men, uncommon complication of transurethral prostatectomy or cryosurgery of prostate, spinal lesion affecting sacral segments 2 to 4 or cauda equina, pelvic fracture)

Client Outcomes

Client Will (Specify Time Frame):

- Report fewer stress incontinence episodes and/or a decrease in the severity of urine loss
- Experience reduction in grams of urine loss measured objectively by a pad test
- Experience reduction in frequency of urinary incontinence episodes as recorded on voiding diary (bladder log)

- Identify containment devices that assist in management of stress incontinence

Nursing Interventions

- Take a focused history addressing duration of urinary leakage and related lower urinary tract symptoms, including daytime voiding frequency, urgency, frequency of nocturia, frequency of urinary leakage, and factors provoking urine loss, focusing on the differential diagnosis of stress, urge or mixed stress and urge urinary symptoms. Consider using a symptom questionnaire that elicits relevant lower urinary tract symptoms and provides differentiation between stress and urge incontinence symptoms.
- ▲ Perform a focused physical assessment, including inspection of the perineal skin, vaginal examination to determine hypoestrogenic changes in the mucosa, pelvic examination to determine the presence of vaginal wall prolapse and uterine prolapse, and to reproduce the sign of stress urinary incontinence.
- Inspect the perineal and perianal skin for evidence of incontinence-associated dermatitis, including inflammation, vesicles in skin exposed to urinary leakage, and especially skin folds or denudation of the skin, particularly when incontinence is managed by absorptive pads or containment briefs.
- Attempt to reproduce the sign of stress urinary incontinence by asking the client to perform Valsalva maneuver or to cough while observing the urethral meatus for urine loss.
- ▲ Perform a focused pelvic examination, including visual inspection of the vaginal mucosa, observation of urethral hypermobility and related pelvic floor descent (prolapse), and digital assessment of pelvic floor muscle strength.
- Determine the client's current use of containment devices; evaluate the devices for their ability to adequately contain urine loss, protect clothing, and control odor. Assist the client in identifying containment devices specifically designed to contain urinary leakage.
- Teach the client to complete a voiding diary (bladder log) by recording voiding frequency, the frequency of urinary incontinent episodes, and their association with urgency (a sudden and strong desire to urinate that is difficult to defer) over a 3- to 7-day period. An electronic voiding diary may be kept whenever

feasible. In addition to these parameters, the client may be asked to record voided volume and fluid intake.

▲ With the client and in close consultation with the physician, review treatment options, including behavioral management; drug therapy; use of a pessary, vaginal device, or urethral insert; and surgery. Outline their potential benefits, efficacy, and side effects.

▲ Assess the client's pelvic muscle strength immediately prior to initiating a pelvic floor muscle rehabilitation using pressure manometry, a digital evaluation technique, or urine stop test.

- Begin a pelvic floor muscle rehabilitation program.
- Teach the client undergoing pelvic muscle rehabilitation to identify, contract, and relax the pelvic floor muscles without contracting distant muscle groups (e.g., abdominal muscles) using tactile, audible, or visual biofeedback techniques.
- Incorporate principles of exercise physiology into a pelvic muscle rehabilitation program using the following strategies:
  - Begin a graded exercise program, usually starting with 5 to 10 repetitions and advancing gradually to no more than 35 to 50 repetitions every day or every other day based on baseline and ongoing evaluation of maximal strength and endurance.
  - Continue exercise sessions over a period of 3 to 6 months.
  - Integrate muscle training into activities of daily living.
  - Assess progress every 2 weeks during the first month and every 4 to 6 weeks thereafter.
- Alternatively, female clients may be taught pelvic muscle rehabilitation using weighted vaginal cones.

▲ Begin transvaginal or transrectal electrical stimulation therapy in selected persons with stress incontinence in consultation with the client and physician.

- Teach the principles of bladder training to women with stress urinary incontinence:
  - Assist the client in completing a voiding diary over a period of a minimum of 3 days or up to 7 days.
  - Review the results with the client, determining typical voiding frequency and establishing goals for voiding frequency.
  - Using baseline voiding frequency, as determined by the diary, teach the client to urinate by the clock when awake, typically every 30 to 120 minutes.

- ■ Encourage adherence to the program with timing devices, as well as verbal encouragement and support, and address individual reasons for schedule interruption.
- ■ Gradually increase the time between urinations to the negotiated goal. Time intervals between voiding are typically increased in increments of 15 to 30 minutes for clients with a baseline frequency of less than every 60 minutes and increments of 25 to 30 minutes for clients with a baseline frequency of more than every 60 minutes.

I

▲ Teach the client to self-administer alpha-adrenergic agonist medications as ordered, imipramine, and topical estrogens as directed.

▲ Refer the female client with stress urinary incontinence and pelvic organ prolapse who wishes to employ a pessary, vaginal device, or urethral insert to manage stress incontinence to a nurse specialist or gynecologist with expertise in the placement and maintenance of these devices.

- Discuss potentially reversible or controllable risk factors with the client with stress incontinence and assist the client to formulate a strategy to alleviate or eliminate these conditions.

▲ Provide information about support resources such as the Simon Foundation for Continence or the National Foundation for Continence.

▲ Refer the client with persistent stress incontinence to a continence service, physician, or nurse who specializes in the management of this condition.

Geriatric

- Evaluate the elderly client's functional and cognitive status to determine the effect of functional limitations on the frequency and severity of urine loss and on plans for management.

Home Care

- The interventions described previously may be adapted for home care use.
- Elicit discussion of the client's concerns about the social or emotional burden of stress incontinence.
- Encourage a mind-set and program of self-care management.
- Implement a bladder-training program, including self-monitoring activities (reducing caffeine intake, adjusting amount and

timing of fluid intake, decreasing long voiding intervals while awake, making dietary changes to promote bowel regularity), bladder training, and pelvic muscle exercise.

- ▲ Consider the use of an indwelling catheter for continuous drainage in the client with severe stress urinary incontinence who is homebound, bed bound, and receiving palliative or end-of-life care (requires a physician's order).
- ▲ When an indwelling catheter is in place, follow the prescribed maintenance protocols for managing the catheter, drainage bag, and perineal skin and urethral meatus. Teach infection control measures adapted to the home care setting.
- • Assist the client in adapting to the catheter. Encourage discussion of the client's response to the catheter.
- • Begin a program of pelvic muscle rehabilitation in the homebound elderly client who is motivated to adhere to the program and has adequate cognitive function to understand and follow instructions.

Client/Family Teaching

- • Teach the client to perform pelvic muscle exercise using an audiotape or videotape if indicated.
- • Teach the client the importance of avoiding dehydration and instruct the client to consume fluid at the rate of 30 mL/kg of body weight daily (0.5 ounce/pound/day).
- • Teach the client the importance of avoiding constipation by a combination of adequate fluid intake, adequate intake of dietary fiber, and exercise.
- • Teach the client to apply and remove support devices such as a urethral insert.
- • Teach the client to select and apply urine containment devices.

Total urinary Incontinence

NANDA Definition

State in which the individual experiences continuous and unpredictable loss of urine

NOTE: In this book, the diagnosis **Total urinary Incontinence** will be used to refer to continuous urine loss due to an extraurethral cause, and the diagnosis **Stress urinary Incontinence** will be used to refer to leakage caused by urethral sphincter incompetence, regardless of severity.

Defining Characteristics

Continuous urine flow varying from dribbling incontinence superimposed on an otherwise identifiable pattern of voiding to severe urine loss without identifiable micturition episodes

Related Factors (r/t)

Ectopia (ectopic ureter opens into vaginal vault or cutaneously; bladder ectopia with exstrophy/epispadias complex); fistula (opening from bladder or urethra to vagina or skin that bypasses urethral sphincter mechanism, allowing continuous urine loss)

Client Outcomes

Client Will (Specify Time Frame):

- Experience urine loss that is adequately contained, with clothing remaining unsoiled and odor controlled
- Maintain intact perineal skin
- Maintain dignity, hide urine containment device in clothing, and minimize bulk and noise related to device

Nursing Interventions

- • Obtain a history of the duration and severity of urine loss, prior management, and aggravating or alleviating features.
- • Query the client about risk factors for a fistula.
- ▲ Perform a focused physical assessment, including inspection of the perineal skin, examination of the vaginal vault, reproduction of the sign of stress incontinence (refer to the care plan for **Stress urinary Incontinence**), and testing of bulbocavernosus reflex and perineal sensations.
- ▲ Consult a physician concerning the results of colposcopy, cystourethroscopy, intravenous urogram, cystogram, Pyridium pad test, methylene blue pad test, or pelvic examination.
- • Assist the client in selecting and applying a urine containment device. Review types of containment products with the client, including advantages and potential complications associated with each type of product.
- • Evaluate disposable versus reusable products for urine contain-

ment, considering the setting (home care versus acute care versus long-term care), preferences of the client and caregivers, and immediate versus long-term costs.

- Begin a structured skin care regimen that incorporates three essential steps: cleanse, moisturize, and protect. Select a cleanser with a pH range comparable to that of normal skin (usually labeled "pH balanced"), moisturize with an emollient to replace lipids removed with cleansing, and protect with a skin protectant containing a petrolatum, dimethicone, or zinc oxide base, or a no sting skin barrier. Skin that is exposed to urine and/or stool should be cleansed daily and following major incontinence episodes. Cleanse the skin gently with a soft cloth (either disposable or reusable). When feasible, select a product that combines two or all three of these processes into a single step. Ensure that products are available at the bedside when caring for a client with total incontinence in an inpatient facility.
- Apply a thin layer of ointment as a skin protectant when using absorbent incontinence products such as adult containment briefs.
- When cleansing a client with a moisture barrier containing zinc oxide, avoid vigorous scrubbing or use of a traditional washcloth to remove the paste. Instead, cleanse fecal materials away from the skin, leaving a clean layer of zinc oxide paste when cleansing after a single episode or gently removing the paste with mineral oil.

▲ Consult the physician or advanced practice nurse concerning use of a moisture barrier with active healing ingredients when incontinence-associated dermatitis exists. In addition, an antifungal powder may be applied underneath the ointment when perineal dermatitis is complicated by monilial infection. Teach the client to use the product sparingly when applying to affected areas.

▲ Consult the physician or advanced practice nurse concerning placement of an indwelling catheter when severe urine loss is complicated by urinary retention, when careful fluid monitoring or core body temperature monitoring is indicated in the critically ill client, or when urinary bypassing is required to promote healing of a stage III or IV pressure ulcer, or in the terminally ill client when use of absorbent products produces pain or distress.

▲ Refer the client with "intractable" or extraurethral incontinence to a continence service or specialist for further evaluation and management of urine loss.

Geriatric

- Provide privacy and support when changing incontinent devices in elderly clients.
- Avoid brisk scrubbing and use of a washcloth when cleansing the skin of an aging client.
- Employ meticulous infection control procedures when using an indwelling catheter.

Home Care

- The interventions described previously may be adapted for home care use.
- Encourage a mind-set and program of self-care management.
- Assist the family with arranging care in a way that allows the client to participate in family or favorite activities without embarrassment. Elicit discussion of the client's concerns about the social or emotional burden of incontinence.

▲ Consider the use of an indwelling catheter for continuous drainage in the client with severe urinary incontinence who is homebound, bed bound, and receiving palliative or end-of-life care (requires a physician's order).

▲ When an indwelling catheter is in place, follow the prescribed maintenance protocols for managing the catheter, drainage bag, and perineal skin and urethral meatus. Teach infection control measures adapted to the home care setting.

- Assist the client in adapting to the catheter. Encourage discussion of the client's response to the catheter.

Client/Family Teaching

- Teach the family to obtain, apply, and dispose of or clean and reuse urine containment devices.
- Teach the family a routine perineal skin care regimen, including daily or every other day hygiene and cleansing with containment product changes.
- Teach the client and family to recognize and manage perineal dermatitis, ammonia contact dermatitis, and monilial rash.
- Teach the client to maintain adequate fluid intake (30 mL/kg of body weight per day).
- Teach the client and family to recognize and manage urinary tract infection.

Urge urinary Incontinence

NANDA Definition

State in which the individual experiences involuntary passage of urine occurring with precipitous desire to urinate. *Urge incontinence* is defined within the context of overactive bladder syndrome. The overactive bladder is characterized by bothersome urgency (a sudden and strong desire to urinate that is not easily deferred). Overactive bladder is typically associated with frequent daytime voiding and nocturia, and approximately 37% will experience urge urinary incontinence.

Defining Characteristics

Diurnal urinary frequency (voiding more than once every 2 hours while awake); nocturia (awakening three or more times per night to urinate); voiding more than eight times within a 24-hour period as recorded on a voiding diary (bladder log); bothersome urgency (a sudden and strong desire to urinate that is not easily deferred); symptom of urge incontinence (urine loss associated with desire to urinate); enuresis (involuntary passage of urine while asleep)

Related Factors

Neurological disorders (brain disorders, including cerebrovascular accident, brain tumor, normal pressure hydrocephalus, traumatic brain injury); inflammation of bladder (calculi; tumor, including transitional cell carcinoma and carcinoma in situ; inflammatory lesions of the bladder; urinary tract infection); bladder outlet obstruction (see **Urinary retention**); stress urinary incontinence (mixed urinary incontinence; these conditions often coexist but relationship between them remains unclear); idiopathic causes (implicated factors include depression, sleep apnea/hypoxia)

Client Outcomes

Client Will (Specify Time Frame):

- Report relief from urge urinary incontinence or a decrease in the incidence or severity of incontinent episodes
- Identify containment devices that assist in the management of urge urinary incontinence

Nursing Interventions

- • Take a nursing history focusing on duration of urinary incontinence, diurnal frequency, nocturia, severity of symptoms, and alleviating and aggravating factors.
- ▲ In close consultation with a physician of advanced practice nurse, consider administering a symptom questionnaire that elicits relevant lower urinary tract symptoms and differentiates stress and urge incontinence symptoms.
- ▲ Perform a focused physical assessment, including inspection of the perineal skin, vaginal examination to determine hypoestrogenic changes in the mucosa, pelvic examination to determine the presence of vaginal wall prolapse and uterine prolapse, and to reproduce the sign of stress urinary incontinence.
- • Inspect the perineal and perianal skin for evidence of incontinence-associated dermatitis, including inflammation, vesicles in skin exposed to urinary leakage, and especially skin folds or denudation of the skin, particularly when incontinence is managed by absorptive pads or containment briefs.
- ▲ Perform a focused pelvic examination including visual inspection of the vaginal mucosa, observation of urethral hypermobility and related pelvic floor descent (prolapse), and digital assessment of pelvic floor muscle strength. Refer the woman with moderately severe to severe vaginal wall prolapse (descent to or beyond the introitus) to a female urologist or urogynecologist.
- ▲ Complete a urinalysis, examining for the presence of nitrites, leukocytes, glucose, or hemoglobin (red blood cells).
- • Teach the client to complete a voiding diary (bladder log) by recording voiding frequency, the frequency of urinary incontinent episodes and their association with urgency (a sudden and strong desire to urinate that is difficult o defer) over a 3- to 7-day period. An electronic voiding diary may be kept whenever feasible. In addition to these parameters, the client may be asked to record voided volume and fluid intake.
- ▲ Review all medications the client is receiving, paying particular attention to sedatives, opioid analgesics, diuretics, antidepressants, psychotropic drugs, and cholinergics. Consult the physician or nurse practitioner about altering or eliminating these medications if they are suspected of affecting incontinence.
- • Assess the client for urinary retention (see the care plan for **Urinary retention**).

- Assess the client for functional limitations (environmental barriers, limited mobility or dexterity, impaired cognitive function; refer to the care plan for **Functional urinary Incontinence**).

▲ Consult the physician concerning diabetic management and pharmacotherapy for urinary tract infection when indicated.

▲ Assess for signs and symptoms of atrophic vaginal changes in the perimenopausal or postmenopausal woman, including vaginal dryness, tenderness to touch, mucosal dryness, friability, and discomfort with gentle palpation. Specifically query the woman with atrophic vaginitis concerning associated lower urinary tract symptoms (usually voiding frequency, urgency, and dysuria). Refer the woman with atrophic vaginal changes and bothersome lower urinary tract symptoms to a gynecologist, urologist, or women's health nurse practitioner for further evaluation and management.

- Teach the principles of bladder training to women with urge urinary incontinence.
  - Assist the client in completing a voiding diary over a period of a minimum of 3 days or up to 7 days.
  - Review the results with the client, determining typical voiding frequency and establishing goals for voiding frequency.
  - Using baseline voiding frequency, as determined by the diary, teach the client to urinate by the clock when awake, typically every 30 to 120 minutes.
  - Encourage adherence to the program with timing devices and verbal encouragement and support, and address individual reasons for schedule interruption.
  - Gradually increase the time between urinations to the negotiated goal. Time intervals between voiding are typically increased in increments of 15 to 30 minutes for clients with a baseline frequency of less than every 60 minutes and increments of 25 to 30 minutes for clients with a baseline frequency of more than every 60 minutes.
- Review with the client the types of beverages consumed, focusing on the intake of caffeine, which is associated with a transient effect on lower urinary tract symptoms. Advise all clients to reduce or eliminate intake caffeinated beverages or over-the-counter medications of dietary aids containing caffeine.
- Review with the client the volume of fluids consumed and gradually adjust the fluid intake to meet the Adequate Intake rec-

ommendation of 3 L for the 19- to 30-year-old male and 2.2 L for the 19- to 30-year-old female.

- Instruct in techniques of urge suppression. Teach the client to identify, isolate, contract, and relax the pelvic floor muscles. When a strong or precipitous urge to urinate is perceived, teach the client to avoid running to the toilet. Instead, she or he should perform repeated, rapid pelvic muscle contractions until the urge is relieved. Relief is followed by micturition within 5 to 15 minutes, using non-hurried movements when locating a toilet and voiding.

- ▲ Begin transvaginal or transrectal electrical stimulation using a low-frequency current (5 to 20 Hz) in consultation with the physician.
- ▲ Teach the client to self-administer antimuscarinic (anticholinergic) drugs as directed. Teach dosage and administration of the medication and the importance of combining pharmacotherapy with scheduled voiding, adequate fluid intake, restriction of bladder irritants, and urge suppression techniques.
- ▲ Assist the client in selecting, obtaining, and applying a containment device for urine loss as indicated (refer to the care plan for **Total urinary Incontinence**).
- ▲ Provide the client with information about incontinence support groups such as the National Association for Continence and the Simon Foundation for Continence.

Geriatric

- Assess the functional and cognitive status of the elderly client with urge incontinence.
- Plan care in long-term or acute care facilities based on knowledge of the elderly client's established voiding patterns, paying particular attention to patterns of nocturia.
- ▲ Carefully monitor the elderly client for potential adverse effects of antispasmodic medications, including a severely dry mouth interfering with the use of dentures, eating, or speaking, or confusion, nightmares, constipation, mydriasis, or heat intolerance.

Home Care

- The interventions described previously may be adapted for home care use.
- Teach the importance of avoiding dehydration or excessive fluid

consumption and the paradoxical relationship between dehydration and symptoms of urgency.

- Teach the family and client to identify and correct environmental barriers to toileting within the home.
- Encourage a mind-set and program of self-care management.
- Implement a bladder-training program as appropriate, including self-monitoring activities (reducing caffeine intake, adjusting amount and timing of fluid intake, decreasing long voiding intervals while awake, making dietary changes to promote bowel regularity), bladder training, and pelvic muscle exercise.
- Help the client and family to identify and correct environmental barriers to toileting within the home.

I

Client/Family Teaching

- Teach the client and family to recognize foods and beverages that are likely to irritate the bladder.
- Teach the family and client to recognize and manage side effects of antispasmodic medications used to treat urge incontinence.
- Help the client and family to recognize and manage side effect of anticholinergic medications used to manage irritative lower urinary tract symptoms.

Risk for urge urinary Incontinence

NANDA Definition

At risk for involuntary loss of urine associated with a sudden, strong sensation or urinary urgency

Risk Factors

Overactive bladder dysfunction with associated detrusor overactivity; inflammation from urinary tract infection; inflammatory lesion; bladder or lower ureteral stone; bladder outlet obstruction; dietary risk factors; consumption of caffeine

Overactive bladder is a symptom syndrome characterized by bothersome urgency (a sudden and strong desire to urinate that is not easily deferred) typically associated with day and nighttime voiding frequency (more than eight urinations per day). Although urge urinary incontinence affects approximately 37% of patients with overactive bladder, 63% have an identifiable condition that is not adequately described by this diagnosis. It is hoped that **Risk for urge urinary Incontinence** will evolve in a manner that more clearly describes the underlying syndrome, overactive bladder.

Client Outcomes

Client Will (Specify Time Frame):

- Report relief from urge urinary incontinence or a decrease in the incidence or severity of incontinent episodes
- Identify containment devices that assist in the management of urge urinary incontinence

Nursing Interventions

- • Take a nursing history focusing on the following lower urinary tract symptoms: daytime voiding frequency, nocturia, presence of bothersome urgency (precipitous desire to urinate that interferes with activities of daily living [ADLs]), and presence of urine loss.
- ▲ In close consultation with a physician or advanced practice nurse, select and administer a validated questionnaire focusing on symptoms of overactive bladder.
- • Query the client about specific risk factors for urge urinary incontinence, such as childhood enuresis, depression, prostate enlargement with bladder outlet obstruction, and neurological disorders, including stroke or Parkinsonism.
- • Assess the client's functional status, focusing on mobility, dexterity, and cognitive status.
- ▲ Complete a urinalysis, focusing on the presence of nitrites, leukocytes, glucose, or hemoglobin (red blood cells).
- • Teach the client to complete a voiding diary (bladder log) by recording voiding frequency, the frequency of urgency episodes over a 3- to 7-day period. An electronic voiding diary may be kept whenever feasible. In addition to these parameters, the client may be asked to record voided volume and fluid intake.
- • Advise all clients to reduce or eliminate intake caffeinated beverages or over-the-counter medications of dietary aids containing caffeine.
- • Advise community-dwelling men that moderate consumption of beer may reduce the risk of developing overactive bladder dysfunction and the associated risk for urge urinary incontinence.

- • Advise community-dwelling women that intake of a balanced diet, and supplementation of vitamin D to ensure meeting daily recommended allowances may reduce the risk for of developing overactive bladder dysfunction and the associated risk for urge urinary incontinence.
- • Recognize that additional bladder irritants, including aspartame, carbonated drinks, decaffeinated coffee or tea, citrus juices, highly spiced foods, chocolates, and vinegar-containing foods, may be eliminated from the diet and added back singly to determine their impact on lower urinary tract symptoms and urgency.
- • Review with the client the volume of fluids consumed and gradually adjust the fluid intake to meet the adequate intake recommendation of 3 L for the 19- to 30-year-old male and 2.2 L for the 19- to 30-year-old female.
- ▲ Review all medications the client is receiving, paying particular attention to sedatives, opioid analgesics, diuretics, antidepressants, psychotropic drugs, and cholinergics. Consult the physician about altering or eliminating these medications if they are suspected of affecting incontinence.
- ▲ Consult the physician concerning diabetic management and pharmacotherapy for urinary tract infection when indicated.
- ▲ Assess for signs and symptoms of atrophic vaginal changes in the perimenopausal or postmenopausal woman, including vaginal dryness, tenderness to touch, dryness of mucosa on touch with friability, and discomfort with gentle palpation. Specifically query the client with atrophic vaginitis concerning storage lower urinary tract symptoms (voiding frequency, urgency, or dysuria). Refer the client with atrophic vaginal changes and bothersome lower urinary tract symptoms to a gynecologist, urologist, or women's health nurse practitioner for further evaluation and management.
- • Teach clients techniques of bladder training and pelvic muscle rehabilitation focusing on urge suppression.
- • Provide the client with information about incontinence support groups such as the National Association for Continence and the Simon Foundation for Continence.

Geriatric

- • Assess the functional and cognitive status of an elderly client with irritative lower urinary tract symptoms or urge incontinence.

▲ Advise a male client with bothersome lower urinary tract symptoms to see his physician or nurse practitioner, because these symptoms may be related to prostate enlargement.

▲ Carefully monitor the elderly client for potential adverse effects of anticholinergic medications, including severe dry mouth interfering with the use of dentures, eating, or speaking, or the occurrence of confusion, nightmares, constipation, mydriasis, or heat intolerance.

Home Care

- The interventions described previously may be adapted for home care use.
- Encourage a mind-set and program of self-care management.
- Implement a bladder-training program, including self-monitoring activities (reducing caffeine intake, adjusting amount and timing of fluid intake, decreasing long voiding intervals while awake, making dietary changes to promote bowel regularity), bladder training, and pelvic muscle exercise.
- Teach the client and family to recognize foods and beverages that are likely to irritate the bladder.
- Teach the importance of avoiding dehydration or excessive fluid consumption and the paradoxical relationship between dehydration and symptoms of urgency.
- Teach the family and client to recognize and manage side effects of anticholinergic medications used to treat irritative lower urinary tract symptoms.
- Teach the family and client to identify and correct environmental barriers to toileting within the home.
- Assist the family with arranging care in a way that allows the client to participate in family or favorite activities without embarrassment. Elicit discussion of the client's concerns about the social or emotional burden of incontinence.

Client/Family Teaching

- Teach the client and family to recognize foods and beverages that are likely to irritate the bladder.
- Teach the importance of avoiding dehydration or excessive fluid consumption and the paradoxical relationship between dehydration and symptoms of urgency.

Disorganized Infant behavior

NANDA Definition

Disintegrated physiological and neurobehavioral responses of infant to the environment

Defining Characteristics

Attention-Interaction System

Abnormal response to sensory stimuli (e.g., difficult to soothe, inability to sustain alert status)

Motor System

Altered primitive reflexes; changes to motor tone; finger splaying; fisting; hands to face; hyperextension of extremities; jittery; startles; tremors; twitches; uncoordinated movement

Physiological

Arrhythmias; bradycardia; desaturation; feeding intolerances; skin color changes; tachycardia; time-out signals (e.g., gaze, grasp, hiccough, cough, sneeze, sigh, slack jaw, open mouth, tongue thrust)

Regulatory Problems

Inability to inhibit startle; irritability

State-Organization System

Active-awake (fussy, worried gaze); diffuse sleep; irritable crying; state-oscillation; quiet-awake (staring, gaze aversion)

Related Factors (r/t)

Caregiver

Cue knowledge deficit; cue misreading; environmental stimulation contribution

Environmental

Lack of containment within environment; physical environment inappropriateness; sensory deprivation; sensory inappropriateness; sensory overstimulation

Individual

Gestational age; illness; immature neurological system; postconceptual age

Postnatal

Feeding intolerance; invasive procedures; malnutrition; motor problems; oral problems; pain; prematurity

Prenatal

Congenital disorders; genetic disorders; teratogenic exposure

Client Outcomes

Client Will (Specify Time Frame): Infant/Child

- Display physiologic/autonomic stability: cardiorespiratory, visceral, neurofunctional
- Display organized motor system
- Display signs of state organization: ability to maintain organized sleep and awake states
- Demonstrate progress toward effective self-regulation
- Display clear behavior cues that communicate approach/ engagement and stress/avoidance
- Demonstrate ability to engage in positive interactive experiences with parent(s)
- Demonstrate ability to process, organize, and respond to sensory information in an adaptive way

Parent/Significant Other

- Recognize infant/child behaviors as a unique way of communicating needs
- Recognize infant behaviors used to communicate stress/ avoidance and approach/engagement
- Recognize and support infant/child's coping behaviors used to self-regulate
- Read and respond to infant/child behavior cues in a way that facilitates autonomic/physiologic, motor, and state organization
- Recognize how the personal style of interactions can positively or negatively affect the infant/child's responses
- Recognize that following the infant's lead will help in fostering effective interactions

- Identify appropriate positioning and handling techniques that will enhance normal motor development and prevent positioning acquired abnormalities
- Promote infant/child's attention capabilities to orient to visual and auditory input
- Engage in pleasurable parent/infant/child interactions that encourage bonding and attachment
- Structure and modify the environment in response to infant/child's behavioral, personal, nurturing, medical, and sensory needs
- Identify available community resources that provide early intervention services, emotional support, community health nursing, and parenting classes

Nursing Interventions

- Identify infant/child's behavioral organization as unique way of communicating in five sub-systems of functioning (i.e., physiologic/autonomic, motor, state, self-regulatory, attention-interactional).
- Provide individualized developmental care for low-birth-weight, preterm infants that positively influences neurodevelopmental functioning and reduces the severity of medical illness.
- Identify appropriate positioning and handling techniques that enhance normal development and motor organization and prevent position-acquired abnormalities.
- Demonstrate ways to facilitate state organization and control.
- Support the infant's need for uninterrupted sleep periods. Cluster care whenever possible, allowing for longer periods of uninterrupted sleep.
- Structure and organize the environment.
- Identify and support the infant/child's use of self-regulatory/consoling behaviors needed for mastering the environment.
- Recognize behavior used to communicate stress/avoidance and approach/engagement.
- Correlate stress/disorganized behaviors to internal factors (e.g., pain, hunger, discomfort) and/or external factors (e.g., lights, noise, handling).
- Provide opportunities for physical closeness, loving touch, massage, cuddling, skin-to-skin (Kangaroo Care), and rocking.
- Provide opportunities for parent/caregiver to engage in positive parent-infant interactions.

- Encourage parents' competence by affirming their strengths and capabilities when caring for their infants.
- Identify and support infant/child's attention capabilities.
- Provide pleasurable experiences (i.e., visual, auditory, tactile, vestibular, proprioceptive) that enhance development of sensory pathways.

▲ Provide information or refer to community based follow-up programs for preterm/at-risk infants and their families.

Multicultural

- Assess for the influence of cultural beliefs, norms, and values on the family's perceptions of infant/child behavior.
- Use a neutral, indirect style when addressing areas where improvement is needed (such as a need for verbal or oral stimulation) when working with Native American clients. Use therapeutic communication techniques that emphasize acceptance, offer the self, validate the client's concerns, and convey respect when discussing the infant/child behavior.

Family Teaching

- Assist family's support systems in recognizing and responding to infant's unique behavioral cues.
- Demonstrate calming interventions to provide parents with tools for positive interactions with their infant/child.
- Nurture parents so that they in turn can nurture their infant/child.
- Establish a nurturing environment in which parents can interact with their infant/child.
- Have knowledge of community early intervention services and follow-up programs for preterm and at-risk infants and families.

Home Care

- Above interventions may be adapted for home care use.
- Educate families in preparing home environment.
- Prepare families for realistic challenges of caring for preterm and at-risk infants prior to discharge. Areas include corrected versus chronological age, feeding skills, poor endurance/easy fatiguability, shorter sleep-wake cycles, decreased alertness and increased fussiness, overstimulation, and so forth. Encourage families to teach friends/visitors to recognize and respond to infant's unique behavioral cues.

• Provide information about community resources, developmental follow-up services, and parent-to-parent support programs.

Risk for disorganized Infant behavior

NANDA Definition

Risk for alteration in integrating and modulation of the physiological and behavioral systems of functioning (i.e., autonomic, motor, state, organizational, self-regulatory, and attentional-interactional systems)

Risk Factors

Environmental overstimulation; invasive procedures; lack of containment within environment; motor problems; oral problems; pain; painful procedures; prematurity

Client Outcomes

Client Will (Specify Time Frame):
Infant/Child

- Display physiologic/autonomic stability: cardiorespiratory, visceral, neurofunctional
- Display organized motor system
- Display signs of state organization
- Demonstrate progress toward effective self-regulation: display range of effective self-regulatory behaviors
- Display clear behavior cues that communicate approach/ engagement and stress/avoidance
- Demonstrate ability to engage in positive interactive experiences with parent(s)
- Demonstrate ability to process, organize, and respond to sensory information in an adaptive way

Parent/Significant Other

- Recognize infant/child behaviors as a unique way of communicating needs
- Recognize infant behaviors used to communicate stress/ avoidance and approach/engagement
- Recognize and support infant/child's coping behaviors used to self-regulate

- Read and respond to infant/child behavior cues in a way that facilitates autonomic/physiologic, motor, and state organization
- Recognize how the personal style of interactions can positively or negatively affect the infant/child's responses
- Recognize that following the infant's lead will help in fostering effective interactions
- Identify appropriate positioning and handling techniques that will enhance normal motor development and prevent positioning acquired abnormalities
- Promote infant/child's attention capabilities to orient to visual and auditory input
- Engage in pleasurable parent/infant/child interactions that encourage bonding and attachment
- Structure and modify the environment in response to infant/child's behavioral, personal, nurturing, medical, and sensory needs
- Identify available community resources that provide early intervention services, emotional support, community health nursing, and parenting classes

Nursing Interventions

Refer to **Disorganized Infant behavior.**

Readiness for enhanced organized Infant behavior

NANDA Definition

A pattern of modulation of the physiological and behavioral systems of functioning (i.e., autonomic, motor, state-organizational, self-regulatory, and attentional-interactional systems) in an infant that is satisfactory but that can be improved

Defining Characteristics

Definite sleep-wake states; response to stimuli (e.g., visual, auditory); stable physiologic measures; use of some self-regulatory behaviors

Related Factors (r/t)

Pain, prematurity

Client Outcomes

Client Will (Specify Time Frame):
Infant/Child

- Display stable vital signs and skin color
- Display smooth, synchronous, and purposeful body movements
- Display range of clear sleep and awake states
- Display smooth transitions between sleep and wake states
- Demonstrate range of effective self-consoling behaviors
- Demonstrate smooth visceral/digestive functioning without feeding intolerances
- Ability to effectively attend and interact with the environment with minimal stress
- Enjoy engaging in reciprocal social play experiences
- Display pleasure with sensory-motor experiences
- Is not "over-" or "under reactive" to sensory-motor experiences (visual, auditory, tactile, movement, body awareness)
- Continue to demonstrate progressive growth and development

Parents/Significant Other

- Demonstrate ways to structure and modify the environment that enhances the infant/child's own adaptive capacity for achieving optimal physiologic and neurobehavioral functioning
- Identify their infant/child's behaviors that signal "stress/avoidance" or "approach"
- Demonstrate ways to facilitate motor organization and development by appropriate handling and positioning techniques
- Demonstrate care that is contingent with the state of the infant/child
- Demonstrate additional ways to facilitate state organization/development
- Support and expand infant's/child's self-regulatory skills
- Demonstrate ways to help infant/child achieve an attentive state that allows him/her to orient to visual and auditory sensory stimuli
- Support and expand infant/child's calm alert periods, the ideal state for learning and interacting
- Demonstrate ways to engage the infant/child in social interactions and allow the infant/child to lead the interaction
- Demonstrate contingent responses to the infant/child's approach/engagement and avoidance/disengagement cues

- Demonstrate ways to provide pleasurable and developmentally appropriate sensory-motor experiences (visual, auditory, tactile, movement, body awareness)

Nursing Interventions

Refer to care plans for **Disorganized Infant behavior** and **Risk for disorganized Infant behavior.**

NOTE: Interventions should be based on individual response of the infant/child to each intervention. Interventions appropriate for one infant/child may not be appropriate for another. In addition, a particular intervention that seems appropriate for one infant/child at a particular time may not be as effective with the same infant/child at another time. Carefully observe for the desired adaptive response or expected outcomes and continually reevaluate. Nursing care that is responsive and contingent with the state of the infant is ideal; however, if stressful events occur, provide appropriate interventions to minimize stress and facilitate self-regulation.

Ineffective Infant feeding pattern

NANDA Definition

Impaired ability of an infant to suck or coordinate the suck/swallow response resulting in inadequate oral nutrition for metabolic needs

Defining Characteristics

Inability to coordinate sucking, swallowing, and breathing; inability to initiate an effective suck; inability to sustain an effective suck

Related Factors (r/t)

Anatomic abnormality; neurological delay; neurological impairment; oral hypersensitivity; prematurity; prolonged NPO status

Client Outcomes

Infant Will (Specify Time Frame):

- Consume adequate calories that will result in appropriate weight gain and optimal growth and development
- Have opportunities for skin-to-skin (kangaroo care) experiences

- Have opportunities for "trophic" (i.e., small volume of breast-milk/formula) enteral feedings prior to full oral feedings
- Progress to stable, neurobehavioral organization (i.e., motor, state, self-regulation, attention-interaction)
- Demonstrate presence of mature oral reflexes that are necessary for safe feeding
- Progress to safe, self-regulated oral feedings
- Coordinate the suck-swallow-breathe sequence while nippling
- Display clear behavioral cues related to hunger and satiety
- Display approach/engagement cues, with minimal avoidance/disengagement cues
- Have opportunities to pace own feeding, taking breaks as needed
- Display evidence of being in the "quiet-alert" state while nippling
- Progress to and engage in mutually positive parent/caregiver-infant/child interactions during feedings

Parent/Family Will (Specify Time Frame):

- Recognize necessity of adequate calories for appropriate weight gain and optimal growth and development
- Learn to read and respond contingently to infant's behavioral cues (e.g., hunger, satiety, approach/engagement, stress/avoidance/disengagement)
- Learn strategies that promote organized infant behavior
- Learn appropriate positioning and handling techniques
- Learn effective ways to relieve stress behaviors during nippling
- Learn ways to help infant coordinate suck-swallow-breathe sequence (i.e., external pacing techniques)
- Engage in mutually positive interactions with infant during feeding
- Recognize ways to facilitate effective feedings: feed in quiet-alert state; keep length of feeding appropriate; burp; prepare/structure environment; recognize signs of sensory overload; encourage self-regulation; respect need for breaks and breathing pauses; avoid pulling and twisting nipple during pauses; allow infant to resume sucking when ready; provide oral support (cheek and/or jaw) as needed; use appropriate nipple hole size and flow rate

Nursing Interventions

- • Refer to care plans for **Disorganized Infant behavior** and **Risk for disorganized Infant behavior, Effective, Ineffective,** and **Interrupted Breastfeeding** and assess as needed.
- • Interventions follow a sequential pattern of implementation that can be adapted as appropriate.
- • Assess infant's functional oral reflexes (i.e., root, gag, suck, swallow, cough).
- • Assess infant's suck, swallow, and breathing coordination in a 1:1:1 ratio.
- • Assess infant's baseline cardiopulmonary parameters prior to, during, and 10 minutes after feeding.
- • Assess for attachment behaviors that can affect a feeding, negatively or positively.
- ▲ Provide developmentally supportive neonatal intensive care for preterm infants.
- • Provide opportunities for kangaroo (i.e., skin-to-skin) care.
- ▲ Before the infant is ready for oral feedings, implement gavage feedings (or other alternative) as ordered, using breast milk whenever possible.
- • Provide a naturalistic environment for tube feedings (naso-oro-gastric, gavage, or other) that approximates a pleasurable oral feeding experience: hold in semi-upright/flexed position; offer NNS; pace feedings; allow for semi-demand feedings contingent with infant cues; offer rest breaks; burp, as appropriate.
- • Provide 10 minutes of NNS prior to oral feeding.
- • Consider trophic (i.e., small volume) feedings for high-risk hospitalized infants if appropriate.
- • Structure the environment and modify sensory stimuli according to infant's physiologic and behavioral organization. Position preterm infant in semi-upright position, with head in neutral alignment, chin slightly tucked, back straight, shoulders/arms forward, hands in midline, hips flexed 90 degrees.
- • Feed infant in the quiet-alert state.
- • Determine the appropriate shape, size, and hole of nipple to provide flow rate for preterm infants that facilitates 1:1:1 ratio of suck-swallow-breathe sequence.
- • Implement external pacing for infants having difficulty coordinating breathing with sucking and swallowing.
- • Provide infants with jaw and/or cheek support, as needed.

I

- • Allow appropriate time for nipple feeding to ensure infant's safety.
- • Monitor length of feeding so that it does not exceed 30 minutes.
- • Encourage transitioning from scheduled to semi-demand feedings, contingent with infant behavior cues.
- • Progress to self-regulatory feedings based on the infant's hunger and satiety cues. Encourage the parents to engage other family members in the feeding process.
- ▲ Refer to a multidisciplinary team (e.g., neonatal/pediatric nutritionist, physical or occupational therapist, speech pathologist, lactation specialist, as needed.

I

Home Care

- • The above appropriate interventions may be adapted for home care use.
- ▲ Infants with risk factors and clinical indicators of feeding problems present prior to hospital discharge should be referred to appropriate community early-intervention service providers (e.g., community health nurses, Early-On, occupational therapy, speech pathologists, feeding specialists) to facilitate adequate weight gain for optimal growth and development.

Family Teaching

- • Provide anticipatory guidance for infant's expected feeding course.
- • Teach various effective feeding methods and strategies to parent(s).
- • Teach parents how to read, interpret, and respond contingently to infant cues.
- • Provide a family-focused caring environment that supports parents in their primary caregiving role.
- • Help parents identify support systems prior to hospital discharge.
- • Provide anticipatory guidance for the infant's discharge.

Risk for Infection

NANDA Definition

At increased risk for being invaded by pathogenic organisms

Risk Factors

Chronic disease; inadequate acquired immunity; inadequate primary defenses (broken skin, traumatized tissue, decrease in ciliary action, stasis of body fluids, change in pH secretions, altered peristalsis); inadequate secondary defenses (decreased hemoglobin, leucopenia, suppressed inflammatory response); increased environmental exposure to pathogens; immunosuppression; invasive procedures; insufficient knowledge to avoid exposure to pathogens; malnutrition; pharmaceutical agents (e.g., immunosuppressants); rupture of amniotic membranes; trauma; tissue destruction

Client Outcomes

Client Will (Specify Time Frame):

- Remain free from symptoms of infection
- State symptoms of infection of which to be aware
- Demonstrate appropriate care of infection-prone site
- Maintain white blood cell count and differential within normal limits
- Demonstrate appropriate hygienic measures such as hand washing, oral care, and perineal care

Nursing Interventions

▲ Consider targeted surveillance for methicillin-resistant Staphylococcus aureus (MRSA) (screen clients at risk for MRSA on admission).

▲ Observe and report signs of infection such as redness, warmth, discharge, and increased body temperature.

▲ Assess temperature of neutropenic clients; report a single temperature of greater than 38.05° C (100.5° F).

- Oral or tympanic thermometers may be used to assess temperature in adults and infants.
- The chemical (Tempa.DOT) thermometer may be used with intensive care unit (ICU) clients.

▲ Note and report laboratory values (e.g., white blood cell count and differential, serum protein, serum albumin, and cultures).
- Assess skin for color, moisture, texture, and turgor (elasticity). Keep accurate, ongoing documentation of changes.
- Carefully wash and pat dry skin, including skinfold areas. Use hydration and moisturization on all at-risk surfaces. Refer to care plan for **Risk for impaired Skin integrity.**
- Monitor weight loss, leaving 25% or more of food uneaten at most meals. Refer to care plan **Readiness for enhanced Nutrition** for additional interventions.
- Use strategies to prevent nosocomial pneumonia (NP): assess lung sounds, sputum; use sterile water rather than tap water for mouth care of immunosuppressed clients; provide a clean manual resuscitation bag for each client; use sterile technique when suctioning; suction secretions above tracheal tube before suctioning; drain accumulated condensation in ventilator tubing into a fluid trap or other collection device before repositioning the client; assess patency and placement of nasogastric tubes; elevate the client's head to 30 degrees or higher to prevent gastric reflux of organisms in the lung.
- Encourage fluid intake.
- Use appropriate "hand hygiene" (i.e., hand washing or use of alcohol-based hand rubs).
- When using an alcohol-based hand rub, apply product to palm of one hand and rub hands together, covering all surfaces of hands and fingers, until hands are dry. Note that the volume needed to reduce the number of bacteria on hands varies by product.
- Follow Standard Precautions and wear gloves during any contact with blood, mucous membranes, nonintact skin, or any body substance except sweat. Use goggles, powder-free gloves, and gowns when appropriate. Standard Precautions apply to all clients. You must assume all clients are carrying blood-borne pathogens. Standard Precautions exceed Universal Precautions.
- Follow Transmission-Based Precautions for airborne-, droplet-, and contact-transmitted microorganisms.
- Use alternatives to indwelling catheters whenever possible (external catheters, incontinence pads, bladder control techniques). Sterile technique must be used when inserting urinary catheters.
- If a urinary catheter is necessary, follow catheter management

practices: All indwelling catheters should be connected to a sterile closed drainage system (i.e., not broken), except for good clinical reasons. Cleanse the perineum and meatus twice daily using soap and water.

- Use evidence-based practices and education personal in care of peripheral catheters: use aseptic technique for insertion and care, label insertion sites and all tubing with date and time of insertion, inspect every 8 hours for signs of infection, record, and report.
- Use careful sterile technique wherever there is a loss of skin integrity.
- Use clean gloves for all high-risk hospitalized clients.
- Ensure the client's appropriate hygienic care with hand washing; bathing; and hair, nail, and perineal care performed by either the nurse or the client.

▲ Recommend responsible use of antibiotics; use antibiotics sparingly.

▲ Carefully screen and treat women with infertility who may have female genital tuberculosis.

Pediatric

NOTE: Many of the above interventions are appropriate for the pediatric client.

- Follow meticulous hand hygiene when working with premature infants.
- Cluster nursing procedures to decrease number of contacts with infants allowing time for appropriate hand hygiene.
- Avoid the prophylactic use of topical cream in premature infants.

Geriatric

- Suspect pneumonia when the client has symptoms of lethargy or confusion.
- Most clients develop NP by either aspirating contaminated substances or inhaling airborne particles. Refer to care plan for **Risk for Aspiration.**

▲ Carefully screen elderly women for salmonella with symptoms of urinary tract infections.

▲ Observe and report if the client has a low-grade temperature or new onset of confusion.

▲ Recommend that the geriatric client receive an annual influenza immunization and one-time pneumococcal vaccine.
• Recognize that chronically ill geriatric clients, particularly those with depression, have an increased susceptibility to infection; practice meticulous care of all invasive sites.
• Recognize that older adults are at risk for human immunodeficiency virus (HIV)/acquired immune deficiency syndrome (AIDS); institute Universal Precautions and appropriate instruction for all age groups.

Home Care

• Some of the above interventions may be adapted for home care use.
• Assess and treat wounds in the home.
• Review standards for surveillance of infections in home care.
• Maintain strong infection control policies.
▲ Monitor recurrent antibiotic use in infants. Instruct parents on appropriate indicators for medical visits and on the influence of breastfeeding and day care at home for avoiding increased need for antibiotics.
▲ Monitor for the occurrence of infectious exacerbation of chronic obstructive pulmonary disease (COPD); refer to physician for treatment.
▲ Refer for nutritional evaluation; implement dietary changes to support recovery and address antibiotic side effects.

Client/Family Teaching

• Teach the client risk factors contributing to surgical wound infection, smoking, and higher body mass index.
▲ Teach the client and family the symptoms of infection that should be promptly reported to a primary medical caregiver (e.g., redness, warmth, swelling, tenderness or pain, new onset of drainage or change in drainage from wound, increase in body temperature).
▲ Teach signs of HBV and AIDS symptoms: malaise, abdominal pain, vomiting or diarrhea, enlarged glands, rash; tuberculosis symptoms: cough, night sweats, dyspnea, changes in sputum, changes in breath sounds; insulin-dependent diabetes mellitus (IDDM) symptoms: sores or wounds that do not heal.
▲ Encourage high-risk persons, including healthcare workers, to have influenza vaccinations.

- Influenza: Teach frequent hand washing, limited contact with sick person, use of masks by caregiver and sick person, and keeping sick person in the "sick room."
- Assess whether the client and family know how to read a thermometer; provide instructions if necessary. Chemical dot thermometers are easy to use and decrease risk of infection. Clients need to know that the instructions should be followed carefully and that electronic thermometers may be the best choice for accuracy.

Risk for Injury

NANDA Definition

At risk of injury as a result of the interaction of environmental conditions interacting with the individual's adaptive and defensive resources

NOTE: This nursing diagnosis overlaps with other diagnoses such as **Risk for Falls, Risk for Trauma, Risk for Poisoning, Risk for Suffocation, Risk for Aspiration,** and if the client is at risk of bleeding, **Ineffective Protection.** Refer to care plans for these diagnoses if appropriate.

Risk Factors

External

Biological (e.g., immunization level of community, microorganism); chemical (e.g., poisons, pollutants, drugs, pharmaceutical agents, alcohol, nicotine, preservatives, cosmetics, dyes); human (e.g., nosocomial agents; staffing patterns; cognitive, affective, psychomotor factors); mode of transport; nutritional (e.g., vitamins, food types); physical (e.g., design, structure, and arrangement of community, building, and/or equipment)

Internal

Abnormal blood profile (leukocytosis/leukopenia, altered clotting factors, thrombocytopenia, sickle cell, thalassemia, decreased hemoglobin); biochemical dysfunction; developmental age (physiological, psychosocial); effector dysfunction; immune-autoimmune dysfunction; integrative dysfunction; malnutrition; physical (e.g., broken skin, altered mobility); psychological (affective orientation); sensory dysfunction; tissue hypoxia

Client Outcomes

Client Will (Specify Time Frame):

- Remain free of injuries
- Explain methods to prevent injury

Nursing Interventions

- Prevent iatrogenic harm to the hospitalized client by following the 2007 National Patient Safety goals:
  - ■ Accuracy of Patient Identification
    - ❏ Use at least two methods (e.g., client's name and medical record number or birth date) to identify the client before administering medications, blood products, treatments, or procedures.
    - ❏ Prior to beginning any invasive or surgical procedure, have a final verification to confirm the correct client, the correct procedure, and the correct site for the procedure using active communication techniques.
  - ■ Effectiveness of Communication among Care Staff
    - ❏ When taking verbal or telephone orders, the orders should be written down and then read back for verification to the individual giving the order.
    - ❏ Standardize use of abbreviations, acronyms, symbols, and dose designations that are used in the institution.
    - ❏ Make sure of timeliness of reporting and taking action of critical test results and values.
    - ❏ Utilize a standardized approach of "handing off" communications, including opportunities to ask and answer questions.
  - ■ Medication Safety
    - ❏ Standardize and limit the number of drug concentrations utilized by the institution (e.g., concentrations of medications such as morphine in patient controlled analgesia [PCA] pumps).
    - ❏ Label all medications and medication containers (e.g., syringes, medication cups, or other solutions on or off the surgical field).
    - ❏ Identify all of the client's current medications upon admission to a healthcare facility, and ensure that all healthcare staff have access to the information.
    - ❏ Reconcile all medication at discharge, and provide list to the client.

    - ❑ Improve the effectiveness of alarm systems in the clinical area.
  - ■ Reduce the risk of infections by following Centers for Disease Control (CDC) hand hygiene guidelines.
  - ■ Evaluate all clients for fall risk and take appropriate actions to prevent falls.
  - ■ Prevent pressure ulcer formation.
- • See care plan for **Risk for Falls.**
- ▲ Avoid use of restraints if at all possible. Restraint free is now the standard of care for hospitals and long-term care facilities. Obtain a physician's order if restraints are necessary.
- • In place of restraints, use the following:
  - ■ Well-staffed and educated nursing personnel with frequent client contact
  - ■ Continuity of care with familiar staff
  - ■ Nursing units designed to care for clients with cognitive or functional impairments
  - ■ Avoiding use of IVs or tubes that are susceptible to being removed
  - ■ Alarm systems with ankle, above the knee, or wrist sensors
  - ■ Bed or wheelchair alarms
  - ■ Increased observation of the client
  - ■ Providing exercise to diffuse and deflect client behavior
  - ■ Low or very low height beds
  - ■ Border-defining pillow/mattress to remind the client to stay in bed
- • For an agitated client, consider providing individualized music of the client's choice.
- • Review drug profile for potential side effects that may increase risk of injury.
- • Use one quarter– to one half–length side rails only, and maintain bed in a low position. Ensure that wheels are locked on bed and commode. Keep dim light in room at night.
- • If the client has a new onset of confusion (delirium), refer to the care plan for **Acute Confusion.** If the client has chronic confusion, see the care plan for **Chronic Confusion.**
- • Ask family to stay with the client to prevent the client from accidentally falling or pulling out tubes.
- • Remove all possible hazards in environment such as razors, medications, and matches.

- • Place an injury-prone client in a room that is near the nurses station.
- • Help clients sit in a stable chair with armrests. Avoid use of wheelchairs and geri-chairs except for transportation as needed.
- ▲ Refer to physical therapy for strengthening exercises and gait training to increase mobility.
- ▲ For the agitated psychotic client, use nonphysical forms of behavior management, such as verbal intervention or show of force. If medication is required, use oral medications if at all possible.

Pediatric

- • Teach parents the need for close supervision of all young children playing near water, including washing machines.
- • If child has epilepsy, recommend showers instead of tub baths, and no unsupervised swimming is ever allowed.
- • Assess the client's social economic status.
- • Never leave young children unsupervised around cooking areas.
- • Teach parents and children the need to maintain safety for the exercising child, including wearing helmets when biking and using breakaway bases for baseball.
- • Teach both parents and children the need for gun safety.

Geriatric

- • Encourage the client to wear glasses and hearing aids and to use walking aids when ambulating.
- • If the client experiences dizziness because of orthostatic hypotension when getting up, teach methods to decrease dizziness, such as rising slowly, remaining seated several minutes before standing, flexing feet upward several times while sitting, sitting down immediately if feeling dizzy, and trying to have someone present when standing.
- • Discourage driving at night.

Multicultural

- • Acknowledge racial/ethnic differences at the onset of care.
- • Assess for the influence of cultural beliefs, norms, and values on the client's perceptions of risk for injury.
- • Assess whether exposure to community violence is contributing to risk for injury.

- Use culturally relevant injury prevention programs whenever possible.
- Validate the client's feelings and concerns related to environmental risks.

Home Care/Client/Family Teaching

- For interventions and rationales see **Risk for Trauma.**

Risk for perioperative positioning Injury

NANDA Definition

At risk for inadvertent anatomical and physical changes as a result of posture or equipment used during an invasive/surgical procedure

Risk Factors

Disorientation; edema; emaciation; immobilization; muscle weakness; obesity; sensory/perceptual disturbances due to anesthesia

NOTE: The following systems are most frequently affected by surgical positioning: neurological, musculoskeletal, integumentary, respiratory, and cardiovascular. Risk factors contributing to the incidence of injury related to surgical positioning include, but are not limited to, the client's age; height; weight; nutritional status; skin condition; the presence of preexisting conditions such as diabetes, vascular, and/or respiratory disease; anemia; hypovolemia; immuno-compromise; impaired nerve function; physical mobility limitations such as arthritis, limited range of motion (ROM), presence of implants/prosthesis or malignancy; effects of anesthesia; staff's knowledge of the equipment; required position for the procedure; use of a heating blanket; extracorporeal circulation; and the duration of the procedure—3 hours or more. Studies have shown statistical significance between pressure ulcer development and length of surgical procedure. As a result of these factors, there is the potential for impaired tissue perfusion, impaired skin integrity, or neuromuscular or joint injury related to surgical positioning. The anesthetized client is at increased risk of injury due to positioning because anesthesia prevents the body's defense mechanism from warning the client of exaggerated stretching, twisting, or compression of his or her body.

Complications of Surgical Positioning

Complications of positioning include, but are not limited to, mechanical restriction of the rib cage, vasodilatation, hyper/hypotension, decreased cardiac output, inhibition of normal compensatory mechanisms, redistribution and congestion of the blood supply, and nerve and muscle trauma due to stretching and compression. Studies have shown that procedures lasting more than 2.5 to 3 hours significantly increase the risk for pressure ulcer formation. Studies have also shown that a normal capillary interface pressure of 32 mm Hg or less should be maintained due to higher pressures causing occlusion and subsequent restriction/blockage of blood flow and ultimately tissue breakdown/ischemia. Research has shown that pressure ulcers will develop in 8.5% of all surgical patients whose procedure lasted more than 3 hours.

Transient physiological reactions to surgical positioning include skin redness and/or bruising, lumbar backache, stiffness in the limbs and neck, numbness, and generalized muscle aches that usually resolve within 24 to 48 hours without treatment. Lumbar back pain, previously considered a transient physiological reaction to positioning, may be an indication of rhabdomyolysis.

More serious complications of surgical positioning include pressure ulcers, peripheral nerve injury, deep venous thrombosis, joint dislocation, compartment syndrome (impairment of microcirculation in soft tissue), rhabdomyolysis, and joint injury.

Client Outcomes

Client Will (Specify Time Frame):

- Demonstrate unchanged skin condition, with exception of the incision, between admission and discharge from the operating room
- Demonstrate redness of the skin for less than 30 minutes at points of pressure
- Be free of injury related to positioning during the surgical procedure, including intact skin and free from pain or numbness associated with surgical positioning
- Demonstrate unchanged or improved physical mobility from preoperative status
- Demonstrate unchanged or improved cardiovascular and respiratory status from preoperative status

- Demonstrate unchanged or improved peripheral sensory integrity from preoperative status
- Maintain sense of privacy and dignity

Nursing Interventions

General Interventions for Any Surgical Client

Prevention of Pressure Ulcers

I

- Identify clients at risk for pressure ulcer development so that cost-effective, evidence-based preventive measures can be instituted.
- Recognize that clients undergoing cardiac surgical procedures are at increased risk of developing a pressure ulcer, especially below the waist or in the occiput area. Use of pressure-reducing devices is necessary to prevent ulcer formation. Pad the operating room table well. Avoid use of gel overlays. Avoid using rolled towels and bolsters made using towels, sheets, and so on, as they tend to produce high and inconsistent pressures.
- Avoid covering positioning devices as the material used to cover the device reduces the effectiveness of the positioning device.
- Appropriate numbers of personnel should be present to assist in positioning the client.
- Monitor pressure being applied to the client intraoperatively by staff, equipment, and/or instruments. Pad all bony prominences. Reddened areas or areas injured by pressure should not be massaged.
- Keep linens on the OR table free of wrinkles. Lift rather than pull or slide the client when positioning. Recognize that the longer the surgery, the greater the chance of the client developing pressure ulcers.

Positioning the Perioperative Client

- Equipment should be checked to verify it is in good working order and it should be used according to manufacturer's instructions.
- Recognize that the nurse must demonstrate knowledge of not only the equipment, but also anatomy and the application of physiological principles in order to properly position the client.
- A preoperative assessment should be completed prior to the surgical procedure to "identify physical alterations that may require additional precautions for procedure-specific positioning."

- Lock the OR table, cart, or bed and stabilize the mattress before transfer/positioning of the client.
- Clients, especially those with limited range of motion/mobility, should be asked to position themselves under the nurse's guidance before induction of anesthesia so that he or she can verify that a position of comfort has been obtained.
- Ensure nerves are protected by positioning extremities carefully.
- Avoid hyperextension of joints.
- Movements during positioning should be slow and smooth.
- Reassess the client after positioning and periodically during the procedure for maintenance of proper alignment and skin integrity.
- Do not allow extremities to extend beyond/off the OR table.
- Monitor intraocular pressure when client is in prone position.
- Extended pressure on the scalp can cause localized alopecia in that area postoperatively.
- Avoid contact with metal when positioning the client.
- Position hips in proper alignment with knees flexed.
- Monitor vulnerable areas such as ulnar nerves, brachial plexus, occiput, and so on.
- To decrease the potential for a brachial plexus injury, position arms so that they don't extend beyond a 90-degree angle.
- When positioning arms at sides, place the arm on the sheet; pass the sheet over the top of the arm, and then have another person roll the client up so that the arm can be tucked under the client. Prevent pooling of preparative solutions, blood, irrigation, urine, and feces. Prior to initiating the skin prep, absorbent pads should be placed to collect any preoperative solutions that run off the area being prepped.
- Ensure that the airway and chest are free from obstruction, that is, arms not pressing on chest, gown not causing neck or chest constriction.
- Keep the client appropriately covered during the procedure. Reducing unnecessary exposure provides privacy and dignity for the client during positioning and also helps in the prevention of hypothermia.
- Implement measures to prevent inadvertent hypothermia.
- If the client is positioned in Trendelenburg/reverse Trendelenburg or with the head of the bed raised/lowered, every attempt should be made to lift the client for several seconds, prior to prepping and draping, to allow the skin to realign itself.

I

- Position the client's legs parallel and uncrossed.
- Maintain alignment of head with cervical, thoracic, and lumbar spine.
- Body supports and restraint straps (safety belt) should be loose and secured over waist or mid-thigh at least 2 inches above knees, avoiding bony prominences by placing a blanket between the strap and the client.
- Clients positioned in lithotomy should be kept in this position for as short a time as possible.
- Recognize that complete, concise, accurate documentation of client assessment and use of positioning devices is imperative.

For information on specific positioning—Supine, Prone, Lateral, Lithotomy, Trendelenburg, Reverse Trendelenburg—please refer to Phillips NF: *Berry & Kohn's Operating Room Technique*, ed 11, Philadelphia, 2007, Mosby.

Insomnia

NANDA Definition

A disruption in amount and quality of sleep that impairs functioning

Defining Characteristics

Observed changes in affect; observed lack of energy; increased work/school absenteeism; patient reports changes in mood; patient reports decreased health status; patient reports decreased quality of life; patient reports difficulty concentrating; patient reports difficulty falling asleep; patient reports difficulty staying asleep; patient reports dissatisfaction with sleep (current); patient reports increased accidents; patient reports lack of energy; patient reports nonrestorative sleep; patient reports sleep disturbances that produce next-day consequences; patient reports waking up too early

Related Factors (r/t)

Activity pattern (e.g., timing, amount); anxiety; depression; environmental factors (e.g., ambient noise, daylight/darkness exposure, ambient temperature/humidity, unfamiliar setting, fear, gender-related hormonal shifts, grief, inadequate sleep hygiene [current], intake of stimulants, intake of alcohol, impairment of normal sleep pattern (e.g., travel, shift work, parental responsibilities, interruptions for interventions); medications; physical discomfort (e.g., body temperature, pain, shortness of breath, cough, gastroesophageal reflux, nausea, incontinence/urgency); stress (e.g., ruminative presleep pattern)

Client Outcomes

Client Will (Specify Time Frame):

- Wake up less frequently during night
- Awaken refreshed and not be fatigued during day
- Fall asleep without difficulty
- Verbalize plan to implement sleep promoting routines

Nursing Interventions

- • Obtain a sleep history including bedtime routines, history of sleep problems, changes in sleep with present illness, and use of medications and stimulants.
- ▲ Assess level of pain and use available pharmacological and nonpharmacological approaches to pain management.
- • Provide pain relief shortly before bedtime and position the client comfortably for sleep.
- • Determine level of anxiety. If the client is anxious, use relaxation techniques. See Nursing Interventions for **Anxiety.**
- • Teach methods for calming the mind.
- ▲ Assess for signs of new onset of depression: depressed mood state, statements of hopelessness, poor appetite. Refer for counseling as appropriate.
- ▲ If the client is waking frequently during the night, consider the presence of sleep apnea problems and refer to a sleep clinic for evaluation.
- ▲ Monitor for presence of sleep disordered breathing as evidenced by loud snoring with periods of apnea, or other sleep disorders such as restless leg syndrome or periodic limb movement disorder. Refer to an accredited sleep disorder center.
- • Observe the client's medication, diet, and caffeine intake. Look for hidden sources of caffeine, such as over-the-counter medications.
- • Provide measures to take before bedtime to assist with sleep (e.g., quiet time to allow the mind to slow down, carbohydrates such as crackers).
- • Provide a back massage before bedtime.

- Provide pain relief shortly before bedtime and position the client comfortably for sleep.
- Keep environment quiet for sleeping (e.g., avoid use of intercoms, lower the volume on radio and television, keep beepers on nonaudio mode, anticipate alarms on intravenous [IV] pumps, talk quietly on unit).
- Use soothing sound generators with sounds of the ocean, rainfall, or waterfall to induce sleep, or use "white noise" such as a fan to block out other sounds. Also consider the use of earplugs.
- Encourage the client to use soothing music to facilitate sleep.
- For hospitalized stable clients, consider instituting the following sleep protocol to foster sleep:
  - Night shift: Give the client the opportunity for uninterrupted sleep from 1 AM–5 AM. Keep environmental noise to a minimum.
  - Evening shift: Limit napping between 4 PM and 9 PM. At 10 PM, lower intensity of room and unit lights, provide sleep medication according to individual assessment, and keep noise and conversation on the unit to a minimum.
  - Day shift: Encourage short naps before 11 AM. Enforce a physical activity regimen as appropriate. Schedule newly ordered medications to avoid waking the client between 1 AM and 5 AM.

Geriatric

- Determine if the client has new onset of a physiological problem that could result in insomnia, such as pain, cardiovascular disease, pulmonary disease, neurological problems such as dementia, or urinary problems.
- Assess urinary elimination patterns. Instruct the client to decrease fluid intake in the evening and take diuretics early in the morning unless contraindicated.
- Obtain a list of all medications including over-the-counter medications and alcohol intake.

▲ If the client is waking frequently during the night, consider the presence of sleep apnea problems and refer to a sleep clinic for evaluation.

▲ Evaluate the client for presence of depression or anxiety, which can result in insomnia. Refer for treatment as appropriate.

- Suggest light reading or TV viewing that does not excite as an evening activity.
- Recommend avoidance of hypnotics and alcohol to induce sleep.
- Reduce daytime napping in the late afternoon; limit naps to short intervals as early in the day as possible.
- Help the client recognize that changes in length of sleep occur with aging, as well as nature of sleep experience.

Home Care

- Previously discussed interventions may be adapted for home care use.
- Provide support to the family of the client with chronic sleep pattern disturbance.
- Instruct the client/family in expectations for normal sleep. Elicit expectations for sleep, previous sleep patterns; correct misconceptions that influence emotional responses to deviation from expectations.
- Assess the client for sleep apnea, particularly poststroke (e.g., interview partner regarding the client's sleep pattern and behaviors, have the client maintain sleep log).
- ▲ Assess the client for depression or other psychiatric disorder. Refer for mental health services as indicated.
- Have the client maintain a sleep diary, describing daily activity levels, use of stimulants, activities, or physical sensations around bedtime. Assess diary for potential areas of intervention.
- Assess environment for possible hazards to the client during periods of disturbance (e.g., appliances, stairs). Ensure that, if client awakens during the night, there will be sufficient light (consider a night light), with passageways clear of obstruction between bed and bathroom.
- Initiate nonpharmacological interventions for insomnia: control of environmental stimuli, sleep restriction, relaxation techniques, increasing sunlight exposure, acupuncture, cognitive and educational interventions to address dysfunctional attitudes about sleep.
- Use the scent of lavender. In the presence of a cognitive disorder, reassure family regarding sleep expectations for the client and address potential problems (e.g., enuresis will require frequent cleansing of client and changes of bed linens); procure-

ment of a hospital bed with side rails may be necessary to prevent falling out of bed.

▲ In the presence of a psychiatric disorder, refer for psychiatric home healthcare services for client reassurance and implementation of therapeutic regimen.

• Provide support to the family of the client with chronic sleep pattern disturbance.

Client/Family Teaching

I

• Encourage the client to avoid coffee and other caffeinated foods and liquids and also to avoid eating large high-protein or high-fat meals close to bedtime.
• Advise the client to avoid use of alcohol or hypnotics to induce sleep. Avoid alcohol ingestion 4 to 6 hours before bedtime.
• Ask the client to keep a sleep diary for several weeks.
• Teach somatic and cognitive relaxation techniques to induce the relaxation response and facilitate sleep.
• Teach the client need for increased exercise. Encourage to take a daily walk 5 to 6 hours before retiring.
• Encourage the client to develop a bedtime ritual that includes quiet activities such as reading, television, or crafts.
• Teach the following guidelines for good sleep hygiene to improve sleep habits:
  ■ Go to bed only when sleepy.
  ■ When awake in the middle of the night, go to another room, do quiet activities, and go back to bed only when sleepy.
  ■ Use the bed only for sleeping.
  ■ Avoid afternoon and evening naps.
  ■ Get out of bed at the same time every morning.
  ■ Recognize that not everyone needs 8 hours of sleep.
  ■ Move the alarm clock away from the bed so that it cannot be seen.
  ■ Do not associate lulls in performance with sleeplessness; sleeplessness should not be blamed for everything that goes wrong during the day.

Decreased Intracranial adaptive capacity

NANDA Definition

Intracranial fluid dynamic mechanisms that normally compensate for increases in intracranial volumes are compromised, resulting in repeated disproportionate increases in intracranial pressure (ICP) in response to a variety of noxious and non-noxious stimuli

Defining Characteristics

Baseline ICP greater than 10 mm Hg; disproportionate increases in ICP following a single environmental or nursing maneuver stimulus; elevated P2 component of ICP waveform; repeated increases in ICP of greater than 10 mm Hg for more than = minutes following any of a variety of external stimuli; volume-pressure response test variation (volume-pressure ratio of 2, pressure-volume index of less than 10); wide-amplitude ICP waveform.

Related Factors (r/t)

Brain injuries: decreased cerebral perfusion less than or equal to 50 to 60 mm Hg; sustained increase in ICP greater than 10 to 15 mm Hg; systemic hypotension with intracranial hypertension

Client Outcomes

Client Will (Specify Time Frame):

- Experience fewer than five episodes of disproportionate increases in intracranial pressure (DIICP) in 24 hours
- Have neurological status changes that are not triggered by episodes of DIICP
- Have cerebral perfusion pressure (CPP) remaining greater than 60 to 70 mm Hg in adults

Nursing Interventions

- To assess ICP and CPP effectively:
  - Maintain and display ICP and CPP continuously.
  - Maintain ICP <20 mm Hg and CPP >60 mm Hg.
  - Monitor neurological status frequently using the Glasgow Coma Scale (GCS), noting changes in eye opening, motor response to painful stimuli, and awareness of self, time, and place.

▲ To prevent harmful increases in ICP:
- Administer sedation per collaborative protocol.
- Administer pain medication per collaborative protocol.
- Maintain normothermia.
- Maintain optimal oxygenation and ventilation, applying positive end expiratory pressure (PEEP) as needed and avoiding hyperventilation.
- Limit endotracheal suction passes to two in order to limit ICP increases. Premedicate clients with adequate sedation, opiates, and/or neuromuscular blocking agents to prevent coughing and associated increases in ICP.
- Allow auditory stimuli (family voices and music).

• To prevent harmful decreases in CPP:
- Maintain euvolemia.
- Maintain head of bed flat or less than 30° in acute stroke clients.

• To treat sustained intracranial hypertension (ICP >20 mm Hg):
- Elevate head of bed at least 30° with head in midline position.
- Remove or loosen rigid cervical collars.

▲ Administer a bolus dose of mannitol and/or hypertonic saline per collaborative protocol.

▲ Drain CSF from an intraventricular catheter system per collaborative protocol.

▲ Administer barbiturates per collaborative protocol.

▲ Induce moderate hypothermia (32°-35° C) per collaborative protocol.

▲ To treat decreased CPP (sustained CPP <60 mm Hg):
- Administer norepinephrine to raise MAP per collaborative protocol.
- Administer hypertonic saline per collaborative protocol.

Deficient Knowledge (specify)

NANDA Definition

Absence or deficiency of cognitive information related to a specific topic

Defining Characteristics

Exaggerated behaviors; inaccurate follow through of instruction; inaccurate performance of test; inappropriate behaviors (e.g., hysterical, hostile, agitated, apathetic); verbalization of the problem

Related Factors (r/t)

Cognitive limitation; information misinterpretation; lack of exposure; lack of interest in learning; lack of recall; unfamiliarity with information resources

Client Outcomes

Client Will (Specify Time Frame):

- Explain disease state, recognize need for medications, and understand treatments
- Explain how to incorporate new health regimen into lifestyle
- State an ability to deal with health situation and remain in control of life
- Demonstrate how to perform health-related procedure(s) satisfactorily
- List resources that can be used for more information or support after discharge

Nursing Interventions

- Observe the client's ability and readiness to learn (e.g., mental acuity, ability to see or hear, no existing pain, emotional readiness, absence of language or cultural barriers) and previous knowledge.
- Assess personal context and meaning of illness (e.g., perceived change in lifestyle, financial concerns, cultural patterns, and lack of acceptance by peers or coworkers).
- Monitor the information needs of clients over time.
- Use approaches that support client priorities, preferences, and choice.
- Provide information to support self-efficacy, self-regulation, and self-management.
- Focus teaching on wellness versus "disease state."
- Consider the client's literacy skill when using written information. Tailor the delivery of instruction to the client's cognitive abilities.
- Provide visual aids to enhance learning.

- • Consider multifaceted methods of disbursing information.
- • Consider using phone calls to monitor and reinforce learning.
- ▲ Help the client identify community resources for continuing information and support.
- ▲ Consider using a group educational program.
- • Use computer- and web-based methods as appropriate.
- • Provide adequate time for mastery of content.
- • Evaluate learning outcomes.

Pediatric

- • Use family-centered approaches when teaching children and adolescents.
- • Use educational strategies that are interactive and engaging for younger children and toddlers.
- • Provide a developmentally appropriate environment when addressing the health education needs of adolescents.

Geriatric

- • Adapt the teaching process for the physical constraints of the aging process (e.g., speak clearly, use a variety of audio-visual-psychomotor methods, provide examples, and allow time for the client to repeat and review.
- • Ensure that the client uses necessary reading aids (e.g., eyeglasses, magnifying lenses, large-print text) or hearing aids.
- • Use printed material, videotapes, lists, diagrams, and Internet.
- • Repeat and reinforce information during several brief sessions.
- • Discuss healthy lifestyle changes that promote wellness for the older adult.
- • Offer opportunities for practice of psychomotor skills.
- • Deliver education within a social context and appropriate physical environment.
- • Consider health education programs using television and newspapers.
- • Consider using technology including interactive computer programs to disperse health education to older adults.

Multicultural

- • Acknowledge racial/ethnic differences at the onset of care.
- • Assess for the influence of cultural beliefs, norms, and values on the client's knowledge base.

- Provide written healthcare information to clients with limited English proficiency in their native language.
- Assess for cultural/ethnic self-care practices.
- Use teaching methods that are culturally sensitive and support client customs, values, and lifestyle.

Home Care

- All of the previously mentioned interventions are applicable to the home setting.
- Assess the client/family learning needs, information needs, and current level of knowledge.
- Monitor the appropriateness of using telehome health care as a teaching method for clients and family caregivers.
- Consider using an outreach home-based educational intervention.
- Encourage family and peer support.
- Assess for specific areas of learning that have the potential for strong emotional responses by the client or family/caregiver.

K

Readiness for enhanced Knowledge (specify)

NANDA Definition

The presence or acquisition of cognitive information related to a specific topic is sufficient for meeting health-related goals and can be strengthened

Defining Characteristics

Behaviors congruent with expressed knowledge; explains knowledge of the topic; expresses an interest in learning; describes previous experiences pertaining to the topic

Client Outcomes

Client Will (Specify Time Frame):

- Demonstrate knowledge of new information
- Meet personal health-related goals
- Explain how to incorporate new health regimen into lifestyle
- List sources to obtain information

Nursing Interventions

- ▲ Include clients as members of the healthcare team in mutual goal setting when providing education.
- • Use open-ended questions and encourage two-way communication.
- • Support client priorities, preferences, and choice.
- • Use strategies to promote client motivation and sustain learning.
- • Provide information to support self-efficacy, self-regulation, and self-management.
- • Seek teachable moments to encourage health promotion.
- • Consider the client's literacy skill when using written information.
- • Ensure that the client's literacy levels, including English as a second language, are considered when developing and selecting written health information for clients.
- • Use computer and web-based methods as appropriate.
- • Individualize health education interventions.
- • Assist clients to access the Internet, libraries, and schools to locate appropriate health resources and information.
- • Facilitate individualized proactive planning with clients before visits to their healthcare provider.
- • Provide appropriate healthcare information and screening for clients with physical disabilities.
- • Encourage group and peer support as appropriate to enhance learning.
- • Use a combination of teaching methods.
- • Reinforce learning through educational follow-up.
- • Refer to care plan for **Deficient Knowledge.**

Pediatric

- • Consider the delivery of alternative settings for teaching parents of children with chronic conditions.
- • Use educational strategies that are interactive and engaging for younger children and toddlers.
- • Provide a developmentally appropriate environment when addressing the health education needs of adolescents.
- • Refer to **Deficient Knowledge** care plan.

Geriatric and Multicultural

- • Refer to **Deficient Knowledge** care plan.

Home Care

- Consider high-tech options for delivery of home-based instruction.

Sedentary Lifestyle

NANDA Definition

Reports a habit of life that is characterized by a low physical activity level

Defining Characteristics

Chooses a daily routine lacking physical exercise; demonstrates physical deconditioning; verbalizes preference for activities low in physical activity

L

Related Factors

Deficient knowledge of health benefits of physical exercise; lack of training for accomplishment of physical exercise; lack of resources (time, money, companionship, facilities); lack of motivation; lack of interest

Client Outcomes

Client Will (Specify Time Frame):

- Increase physical activity to minimum of 10,000 steps per day
- Meet mutually defined goals of increased exercise
- Verbalize feeling of increased strength and ability to move

Nursing Interventions

- Observe the client for cause of sedentary lifestyle. Determine whether cause is physical or psychological. See care plan for **Ineffective Coping** or **Hopelessness.**
- ▲ Assess for reasons why the client would be unable to participate in an exercise program; refer for evaluation by a primary care practitioner as needed.
- Use the Outcome Expectation for Exercise Scale to determine client's self-efficacy expectations and outcomes expectations toward exercise.
- Recommend the client enter an exercise program with a friend.

- Recommend the client begin a walking program using the following criteria:
  - Purchase a pedometer
  - Determine common times when walking can be incorporated into usual lifestyle
  - Set goal of walking 10,000 steps per day, which equals = 4 miles per day
  - If, after coming home from work, does not have required number of steps, go for a walk until reach designated goal of 10,000 steps per day

Pediatric

- Encourage child to increase the amount of walking done per day; if child is willing, ask him or her to wear a pedometer to measure number of steps.
- Encourage the adolescent to increase exercise to help feel better.

Geriatric

- Assess ability to move using the Get Up and Go test. Ask the client to rise from a sitting position, walk 10 feet, turn, and return to the chair to sit.
- Recommend the client begin a regular exercise program, even if generally active.

▲ Refer the client to physical therapy for resistance exercise training as able including abdominal crunch, leg press, leg extension, leg curl, calf press, and more.

- Use the WALC Intervention (**W**alk; **A**ddress pain, fear, fatigue during exercise; **L**earn about exercise; **C**ue by self-modeling) to improve exercise adherence in the older adult.
- Recommend the client begin a Tai Chi practice.
- If client is frail, ensure good nutrition, appropriate medications, attention to vision and hearing deficits, and increase social support along with exercise.
- If client is scheduled for an elective surgery that will result in admission into the intensive care unit (ICU) and immobility, or recovery from a knee replacement, initiate a prehabilitation program that includes a warm-up, aerobic strength, flexibility, and functional task work.

▲ Evaluate the client for signs of depression (flat affect, insomnia, anorexia, frequent somatic complaints) or cognitive impairment (use Mini-Mental State Exam [MMSE]). Refer for treatment or counseling as needed.

Home Care

- • Above interventions may be adapted for home care use.
- ▲ Assess home environment for factors that create barriers to mobility. Refer to occupational therapy services if needed to assist the client in restructuring home and daily living patterns.

Client/Family Teaching

- • Work with the client using the Transtheoretical Model of behavior change and determine if the client is in the precontemplation, contemplation, preparation, action, or maintenance state of behavior change about exercise. Provide appropriate strategies to support change to exercising based on determined state of change.
- • Develop a series of contracts with mutually agreed on goals of increased activity. Include measurable landmarks of progress, consequences for meeting or not meeting goals, and evaluation dates. Sign the contracts with the client.

Risk for impaired Liver function

NANDA Definition

At risk for liver dysfunction

Risk Factors

Hepatotoxic medications (e.g., acetaminophen, statins); HIV co-infection; substance abuse (e.g., alcohol, cocaine); viral infection (e.g., hepatitis A, B, C, D, E, Epstein-Barr); chronic biliary obstruction and infection; right heart failure; acute fatty liver of pregnancy; Reye's syndrome, nutritional deficiencies

Client Outcomes

Client Will (Specify Time Frame):

- State the upper limit of the amount of acetaminophen can safely take per day

- Have normal liver enzymes, serum and urinary bilirubin levels, white blood cell count (WBC), red blood cell count (RBC)
- Be free of jaundice, pruritus, bruising, petechiae, gastrointestinal bleeding, hemorrhage
- Have coagulation studies within normal limits
- Report abdominal girth of normal dimensions
- Be oriented to time, place, and person
- Be able to eat frequent small meals per day without nausea and/or vomiting
- State rationale for seeking medical attention for gallbladder/biliary disease
- If alcohol abuse is factor, state relationship between abuse and worsening gastrointestinal and liver disease
- Be free of cardiovascular and/or renal compromise: fluid retention, peripheral edema, ascites, decreased urinary output, changes in serum blood urea nitrogen (BUN) and creatinine levels
- Be free of abdominal tenderness/pain and have normal colored stool

Nursing Interventions

- Watch for signs of liver dysfunction including: jaundice of the eyes or skin, pruritus, gastrointestinal bleeding, coagulopathy, infections, increasing abdominal girth, fluid overload, shortness of breath, and mental status changes, changes in the color of the stool, changes in urinary function concurrent with increased serum and urinary bilirubin levels.
- Evaluate liver function tests.
- Evaluate coagulation studies such as international normalized ratio (INR), prothrombin time (PT), and partial thromboplastin time (PTT), especially with concurrent bleeding of mouth/gums.
- Monitor for signs and symptoms of electrolyte and acid-base imbalances, especially hyperkalemia, hypoglycemia, and metabolic acidosis.
- Instruct client about possibility of a liver biopsy if he or she has other symptoms of possible liver problems, such as abnormal liver function tests, bleeding, jaundice, and nutritional deficits.

▲ Determine the total amount of acetaminophen the client is taking per day and administer medications for an overdose as ordered. The amount of acetaminophen ingested should not exceed 4 g per day as a limit.

- • Evaluate the serum acetaminophen-protein adducts in the client with possible liver failure from excessive intake of acetaminophen.
- ▲ If the client is an alcoholic, refer to a cessation program. See care plan for **Ineffective Denial** and **Dysfunctional Family processes: alcoholism.**
- • Recognize that severe malnutrition may result in acute liver failure, which is reversible with improved nutrition.
- • Encourage vaccinations for hepatitis A and B for all ages.
- • Measure abdominal girth if individual presents with abdominal distention and pain.
- • Assess for tenderness and/or pain level in the right upper quadrant.
- • Recognize that new onset of symptoms of liver dysfunction such as jaundice, fatigue, and nausea may be caused by infection with hepatitis C.
- • Provide frequent smaller meals for easier digestion. Provide diet with optimal carbohydrates, proteins, and fats.
- • Observe for signs and symptoms of mental status changes such as confusion from encephalopathy. Assess ammonia level if mental changes occur.

Pediatric

- • Encourage vaccinations for hepatitis A and B for all ages.
- • Recognize that children can develop fatty liver disease, which can result in liver failure. Most children are asymptomatic, but others complain of malaise, fatigue, or vague recurrent abdominal pain.

Geriatric

- • The interventions above are appropriate for the elderly.

Home Care

- • Encourage rest, optimal nutrition (high carbohydrates, low protein, essential vitamins and minerals) during initial inflammatory processes of the liver.
- • Watch for liver dysfunction in the client receiving long-term parenteral nutrition.

Client/Family Teaching

- Teach the client and family to examine all medications the client is taking, looking for acetaminophen as an ingredient, and reinforce the 4 GM upper limit of intake of acetaminophen to protect liver function.
- For the caregiver and client with hepatitis A, B, and C, teach the need for careful handwashing, use of gloves, and other precautions to prevent spread of any of these diseases.
- Teach avoidance of high-risk behaviors that cause hepatitis and ways to avoid those behaviors.
- Educate clients and their caregivers about treatment options and interventions for hepatitis.
- Teach client and family to report signs and symptoms that may indicate further complications including increased abdominal girth, bleeding, bruising, petechiae, jaundice, pruritus, confusion, rapid weight gain, or weight loss (fluid overload versus anorexia and nausea/vomiting), shortness of breath.

Risk for Loneliness

NANDA Definition

At risk for experiencing discomfort associated with a desire or need for more contact with others

Risk Factors

Affectional deprivation; cathectic deprivation; physical isolation; social isolation

Client Outcomes

Client Will (Specify Time Frame):

- Maintain one or more meaningful relationships (growth enhancing versus codependent or abusive in nature)—relationships allowing self-disclosure—and demonstrate a balance between emotional dependence and independence
- Participate in ongoing positive and relevant social activities and interactions that are personally meaningful
- Demonstrate positive use of time alone when socialization is not possible

Nursing Interventions

- Assess the client's perception of loneliness. (Is the person alone by choice, or do others impose the aloneness?) Refer to care plan for **Social isolation.**
- Assess the client's ability and/or inability to meet physical, psychosocial, spiritual, and financial needs and how unmet needs further challenge the ability to be socially integrated. NOTE: See care plan for **Disturbed Body image** if loneliness is associated with impaired skin integument.

▲ Assess the bereaved client who is alone for suicide and make appropriate referrals. Refer to care plan **Risk for Suicide.**

▲ Assess the client who is alone for substance abuse and make appropriate referrals.

- Evaluate the client's desire for social interaction in relation to actual social interaction.
- Use active listening skills. Establish therapeutic relationship and spend time with the client.

▲ Assist the client with identifying loneliness as a feeling and the causes related to loneliness; make appropriate referrals.

- Explore ways to increase the client's support system and participation in groups and organizations.
- Encourage the client to be involved in meaningful social relationships and support personal attributes.
- Encourage the client to develop closeness in at least one relationship.

Adolescents

- Assess the client's social support system.
- Evaluate the family stability of younger and middle adolescent clients and advocate and encourage healthy, growth-producing relationships with family and support systems.
- Evaluate peer relationships.
- Encourage social support for clients with visual impairments.
- For older adolescents, encourage close relationships with peers and involvement with groups and organizations.
- Consider use of pets to cope with loneliness.

Geriatric

- Refer to care plan **Social isolation** for additional interventions.
- Assess the client's adaptive sensory functions or any other

health deviations that may limit or decrease his or her ability to interact with others.

- • Assess caregivers for Alzheimer's disease clients for depression related to loneliness.
- ▲ Identify community support systems specific to elderly populations.
- • To keep older people independent, interventions to prevent loneliness should be explored. Consider using art as an intervention.
- • Consider a retirement village.
- • Encourage support by friends and family when the decision to stop driving must be made.
- • Provide opportunities for indoor gardening.
- • Provide reading materials for clients who are able to read.

Multicultural and Home Care

- • Refer to care plan **Social isolation**.

Home Care

- • Refer to care plan **Social isolation** for additional interventions.
- ▲ Above interventions may be adapted for home care use. Assess for depression with lonely elderly client and make appropriate referrals.
- ▲ If the client is experiencing somatic complaints, evaluate client complaints to ensure physical needs are being met, and then identify relationship between somatic complaints and loneliness.
- • Identify alternatives to being alone (e.g., telephone contact).
- • Consider using computers and the Internet to alleviate or reduce loneliness and social isolation.

Client/Family Teaching

- • Refer to care plan **Social isolation** for additional interventions.
- • Encourage positive use of solitude to prevent loneliness (e.g., reading, listening to music, enjoying nature and art).
- • Include the family in all client-teaching activities, and give them accurate information regarding the illness severity.
- • Give family members something to do such as holding a hand, applying lotion, or assisting with feeding.
- • Encourage family members to express caring by telling the client where they will be and sending messages when they cannot be present.

▲ Provide appropriate education for clients and their support persons about hepatitis C: transmission and treatment.

Impaired Memory

NANDA Definition

Inability to remember or recall bits of information or behavioral skills; impaired memory may be attributed to pathophysiological or situational causes that are either temporary or permanent

Defining Characteristics

Experience of forgetting; forgets to perform a behavior at a scheduled time; inability to determine if a behavior was performed; inability to learn new information; inability to learn new skills; inability to perform a previously learned skill; inability to recall events; inability to recall factual information; inability to retain new information; inability to retain new skills

Related Factors (r/t)

Anemia; decreased cardiac output; excessive environmental disturbances; fluid and electrolyte imbalance; hypoxia; neurological disturbances

Client Outcomes

Client Will (Specify Time Frame):

- Demonstrate use of techniques to help with memory loss
- State has improved memory for everyday concerns

Nursing Interventions

- Assess overall cognitive function and memory. The emphasis of the assessment is everyday memory, the day-to-day operations of memory in real-world ordinary situations. Use an assessment tool such as the Mini-Mental State Examination (MMSE) and/or the Metamemory in Adulthood (MIA) questionnaire.
- Assess for memory complaints since memory loss may be the earliest manifestation of mild cognitive impairment (MCI).

▲ Determine whether onset of memory loss is gradual or sudden.

If memory loss is sudden, refer the client to a physician or neuropsychologist for evaluation.

- • Determine amount and pattern of alcohol intake.
- • Note the client's current medications and intake of any mind-altering substances such as benzodiazepines, ecstasy, marijuana, cocaine, or glucocorticoids.
- • Note the client's current level of stress. Ask if there has been a recent traumatic event.
- ▲ If stress is associated with memory loss, refer to a stress reduction clinic. If not available, suggest that the client meditate, receive massages, and participate in moderate physical activity, all of which may promote stress reduction and reduce anxiety and depression. Encourage the client to develop an aerobic exercise program.
- • Determine the client's sleep patterns. If insufficient, refer to care plan for **Insomnia.**
- ▲ Determine the client's blood sugar levels. If they are elevated, refer to physician for treatment and encourage healthy diet and exercise to improve memory.
- ▲ If signs of depression such as weight loss, insomnia, or sad affect are evident, refer the client for psychotherapy.
- ▲ Perform a nutritional assessment. If nutritional status is marginal, confer with a dietitian and primary care practitioner to evaluate whether the client needs supplementation with foods or vitamins. Teach the client the need to eat a healthy diet with adequate intake of whole grains, fruits, and vegetables to decrease cerebrovascular infarcts.
- ▲ Question the client about cholesterol level. If it is high, refer to physician or dietitian for help in lowering. Encourage the client to eat a healthy diet, avoiding saturated fats and *trans*-fatty acids.
- • Suggest clients use cues, including alarm watches, electronic organizers, calendars, lists, or pocket computers, to trigger certain actions at designated times.
- • Encourage the client to use external memory devices, such as a calendar for appointments, keep reminder lists, place a string around finger or rubber band around wrist as reminders, or enlist someone else to remind him or her of important events.
- • Help the client set up a medication box that reminds the client to take medication at needed times; assist the client with refilling the box at intervals if necessary.

- If safety is an issue with certain activities (e.g., the client forgets to turn off stove after use or forgets emergency telephone numbers), suggest alternatives such as using a microwave or whistling teakettle for heating water and programming emergency numbers in telephone so that they are readily available.
- ▲ Refer the client to a memory clinic (if available), a neuropsychologist, or an occupational therapist. Memory clinics can help the client learn ways to improve memory.
- For clients with memory impairments associated with dementia, see care plan for **Chronic Confusion.**

Geriatric

- Assess for signs of depression.
- Evaluate all medications that the client is taking to determine whether they are causing the memory loss.
- Evaluate all herbal and/or nutraceutical products that the individual might be using to improve their memory function.
- Recommend that elderly clients maintain a positive attitude and active involvement with the world around them and that they maintain good nutrition.
- Encourage the elderly to believe in themselves and to work to improve their memory.
- ▲ Refer the client to a memory class that focuses on helping older adults learn memory strategies.
- Help family develop a memory aid booklet or wallet that contains pictures and labels from the client's life, or develop a video movie that includes familiar pictures with narration.
- Help family label items such as the bathroom or sock drawer to increase recall.

Multicultural

- Assess for the influence of cultural beliefs, norms, and values on the family or caregiver's understanding of impaired memory.
- Use bias-free instruments when assessing memory in the culturally diverse client.
- Inform the client's family or caregiver of meaning of and reasons for common behavior observed in the client with impaired memory.
- Validate family members' feelings regarding the impact of the client's behavior on family lifestyle.

Home Care

- Above interventions may be adapted for home care use.
- Arrange cues for medication taking that are focused around daily events (e.g., meals and bedtimes).
- Assess the client's need for outside assistance with recall of treatment, medications, and willingness/ability of family to provide needed support. Identify a checking-in support system (e.g., Lifeline or significant others).
- Keep furniture placement and household patterns consistent.
- ▲ In the presence of a medical disorder, institute case management of frail elderly to support continued independent living.

Client/Family Teaching

- When teaching the client, determine what the client knows about memory techniques and then build on that knowledge.
- When teaching a skill to the client, set up a series of practice attempts. Begin with simple tasks so that the client can be positively reinforced and progress to more difficult concepts.
- Teach clients to use memory techniques such as repeating information they want to remember, making mental associations to remember information, and placing items in strategic places so that they will not be forgotten.

M

Impaired bed Mobility

NANDA Definition

Limitation of independent movement from one bed position to another

Defining Characteristics

Impaired ability to: move from supine to sitting; to move from sitting to supine; to move from supine to prone; to move from prone to supine; to move from supine to long sitting; to move from long sitting to supine; to "scoot" or reposition self in bed; to turn from side to side

Related Factors (r/t)

Cognitive impairment; deconditioning; deficient knowledge; environmental constraints (i.e., bed size, bed type, treatment equipment, restraints); insufficient muscle strength; musculoskeletal impairment; neuromuscular impairment; obesity; pain; sedating medications. NOTE: specify level of independence using a standardized functional scale

Client Outcomes

Client Will (Specify Time Frame):

- Demonstrate optimal independence in positioning, exercising, and performing functional activities in bed
- Demonstrate ability to direct others on how to do bed positioning, exercising, and functional activities

Nursing Interventions

- Assess/determine client's risk for intracranial pressure (ICP)/aspiration/pressure ulcer/pain and for respiratory/cardiovascular/muscle tone abnormalities.
- Critically think/set priorities to use most therapeutic bed positions/frequency of turns based on client's history, risk profile, preventative needs; realize positioning for one condition may negatively affect another.
- Raise HOB 30° for clients with acute increased ICP and 0° to 15° for those with acute cerebral ischemia. Refer to care plan for **Decreased Intracranial adaptive capacity.**
- Turn clients at high risk for pressure/shear/friction frequently.
- Tilt clients 30° or less while lying on side.
- Assist client to sit as upright as possible during meals/ingestion of pills if dysphagic. Refer to care plan for **Impaired Swallowing.**
- Periodically sit client as upright as tolerated in bed, if vital signs/oxygen saturation levels remain stable. Dangle client's legs at the bedside if possible.
- Maintain HOB at lowest elevation that is medically possible to prevent pressure ulcers; check sacrum often.
- Position bed flat at intervals unless medically contraindicated.
- Place pillows under legs of immobile supine-lying clients unless contraindicated, for example, after total knee replacement.
- Therapeutically (re)position joints/limbs in neutral alignment; safely pad pressure points/body parts needing support preoperatively/intraoperatively.
- Use static/dynamic bed surfaces and assess for "bottoming out"

M

under susceptible bony areas (body sinks onto mattress, thus the recommended 1 inch between mattress/bones is absent). Refer to care plan for **Risk for impaired Skin integrity.**

- Place clients with stage III or IV pressure ulcers on low-air-loss surface or air-fluidized bed or consult enterostomal therapy nurse to determine appropriate surfaces.
- Recognize and actively prevent complications associated with immobility.
- Use a formalized screening tool to identify persons at high risk for deep vein thrombosis (DVT).
- Assess clients for venous thromboembolism and implement prophylaxis as ordered, for example, anticoagulants, antiembolic stockings, elastic wraps, sequential compression devices, feet/ankle exercises, and hydration. Refer to care plan for **Ineffective Tissue perfusion.**
- Start oxygen/manage airway/follow protocols for clients with unexplained acute cardiopulmonary problems.
- Implement the following interventions during bed mobility activities:
  - Place positioning devices such as pillows/foam wedges between bony prominences (knees, etc.).
  - Use transferring devices such as trapeze, draw sheet, mechanical lateral transfer aid, ceiling-mounted lifts to move (rather than drag) dependent/obese persons.
- Use special beds/equipment to move bariatric (very obese) clients, such as mattress overlay, sliding/roller board, trapeze, stirrup, and pulley attached to overhead traction system (holds one leg up during pericare).
- Place bariatric beds along a corner wall.
- Logroll and tilt dependent bariatric clients (avoid full side-lying position) until familiar with his or her ability to help turn in bed.
- Apply elbow pads to comatose/restrained clients and to those who use elbows to prop/scoot up in bed; apply nocturnal elbow splint if ulnar nerve palsy exists or if painful elbow with paresthesia in ulnar side of fourth/fifth fingers develops.
- Range/exercise joints and apply padded foot splints/boots on a rotating schedule.
- Explain importance of exhaling (versus holding one's breath/straining) during bed activities.

M

- • If bed movement intensifies pain, administer analgesics and accept clients' rating of pain.
- • Assess for effects of antispasmodic medications.
- ▲ Assess for increased joint resistance, spasms, and related pain/sensations.
- ▲ Recognize benefits of continuous intrathecal baclofen infusion (CITB) via an implanted pump in the spinal canal as ordered.
- • Assist clients to splint incisions/wounds/painful abdominal areas with a pillow as they change positions, cough, or perform functional activities in bed.
- ▲ Refer clients to dietitian or provide dietary information to promote normal weight.
- • Identify/modify hospital beds with large gaps within the side rail/mattress system that potentially create an entrapment hazard. Act to ensure mattresses fit the bed, and instill gap fillers, rail inserts/pads/covers, and bumper wedges; monitor their effectiveness.

Exercising

- • Perform passive range of motion (ROM) at least twice a day to immobile joints; support limb above/below joint being ranged.
- • Perform ROM slowly/rhythmically. Do not range beyond point of pain. Range only to point of resistance in those with loss of sensation/mentation.
- • Range a hemiplegic arm with the shoulder slightly externally rotated.
- ▲ Reinforce self-initiated practice of exercises taught by therapists (muscle setting, strengthening, and contraction against resistance, and weight lifting).
- • Intervene for misalignment, flaccidity, spasticity, reduced sensation, and excessive effort while moving.
- • Allow clients to do as many bed activities as they can; help with light manual guidance and verbal cues if needed.

Bed Positioning

- • Incorporate the following measures to promote normal tone and prevent complications.
  - ■ Position head and neck in midline.
  - ■ Use a flat head pillow when clients are supine if their neck tends to flex forward; use a small pillow behind

the head and/or between shoulder blades if extension occurs.

- Lay a sandbag under the pillow along one or both sides of the head when clients with lateral neck rotation are supine, and one thick/two thin pillows under the head, when they are side-lying.
- Change the position of clients' shoulders/arms frequently. Abduct the shoulders of persons with high paraplegia or quadriplegia horizontally to 90° briefly twice a day.
- Position a hemiplegic shoulder fairly close to the client's body.
- Apply resting forearm, wrist, and hand splints. Strictly adhere to on/off orders. Routinely check underlying skin for signs of pressure/poor circulation.
- Use hard hand cone or splint as ordered.
- Periodically elevate paralyzed arms on pillows and apply isotoner gloves.
- Place a thin pillow under the weak pelvis/hip/upper thigh of persons with hemiplegia and a trochanter roll along the outside of a hemiplegic leg or paralyzed legs.
- Strictly maintain leg abduction in persons with a surgical hip pinning or replacement by placing an abductor splint/pillow between legs.
- Apply foot splints, boots, or high-top tennis shoes as recommended by the physical therapist; routinely assess underlying skin for signs of pressure.
- Assist clients to lie prone/semiprone periodically unless contraindicated (cardiopulmonary disturbances or increased intracranial pressure).
- Tilt hemiplegics onto both unaffected/affected sides with the affected shoulder slightly forward (move/lift the affected shoulder, <u>not</u> the forearm/hand).

• Components of normal bed mobility include rolling, bridging, scooting, long sitting, and sitting upright. Most movements start with the client supine, flat in bed. Normal movements are bilateral, segmental, well-timed, and effortless. They involve set positions, weight bearing and shifting, trunk centering, and stabilization against gravity.

Geriatric

• Discriminately raise bed side rails; instead try body pillows, low beds, bed alarms, and antislip floor mats next to beds.

- Assess caregivers' strength, health history, and cognitive status to predict ability/risk for assisting bed-bound clients at home. Explore alternatives if risk is too high.
- Assess the client's stamina and energy level during bed mobility/activities; if limited, spread out activities and allow rest breaks.

Home Care

▲ Utilize nurse case managers, care coordinators, or social workers to assess support systems and identify need for durable medical equipment, assistive technology, and home health services.
- Encourage use of the client's bed unless contraindicated. Raise HOB with commercial blocks or grooved-out pieces of wood under legs; set bed against walls in a corner.
- Suggest rearranging furniture for accessibility and to meet sleeping/toileting/living needs on one level.
- Stress psychological/physical benefits of clients being as self-sufficient as possible with bed mobility/cares even though it may be time-consuming.
- Prepare family for potential regression in clients' self-care during the transition from hospital to home.
- Offer emotional support and suggest community support systems to help with adjustment and coping issues.
- Discuss support systems available for caregivers to help them cope.

▲ In the presence of medical disorders, institute case management for the frail elderly to support continued independent living.
- Refer to the Home Care interventions of the care plan for **Impaired physical Mobility.**

Client/Family Teaching

- Use various sensory modalities to teach client/caregivers correct techniques for ROM, exercises, repositioning, self-care activities, and using devices.
  - ■ Provide visual information such as demonstrations, sketches, instructional videos, written directions, stickems, or other notes.
  - ■ Encourage/offer auditory information such as verbal instructions/cueing, audio recorded tapes, timers, audiovisual tapes, reading aloud written directions, and self-talk during activities.

M

- ■ Use tactile stimulation such as motor task practice/repetition, return demonstrations, note taking, manual guidance, or hand-on-hand technique as needed.
- • Schedule time with family/caregivers for education and practice. Suggest they come prepared with questions and wear comfortable, safe clothing/shoes.
- • Implement ergonomic approaches and reinforce sound body mechanics during bed mobility/exercises/hygiene.
- • Use memory aids/strategies such as written schedules, directions, sketches, and timers for bed mobility and exercises with clients with cognitive decline.

Impaired physical Mobility

NANDA Definition

A limitation in independent, purposeful physical movement of the body or of one or more extremities

Defining Characteristics

Decreased reaction time; difficulty turning; engages in substitutions for movement (e.g., increased attention to other's activity, controlling behavior, focus on pre-illness disability/activity); exertional dyspnea; gait changes; jerky movements; limited ability to perform gross motor skills; limited ability to perform fine motor skills; limited range of motion; movement-induced tremor; postural instability; slowed movement; uncoordinated movements

Related Factors

Activity intolerance; altered cellular metabolism; anxiety; body mass index above 75th age-appropriate percentile; cognitive impairment; contractures; cultural beliefs regarding age-appropriate activity; deconditioning; decreased endurance; depressive mood state; decreased muscle control; decreased muscle mass; decreased muscle strength; deficient knowledge regarding value of physical activity; developmental delay; discomfort; disuse; joint stiffness; lack of environmental supports (e.g., physical or social); limited cardiovascular endurance; loss of integrity of bone structures; malnutrition; medications;

musculoskeletal impairment; neuromuscular impairment; pain; prescribed movement restrictions; reluctance to initiate movement; sedentary lifestyle; sensoriperceptual impairments

Suggested functional level classifications include the following:

0—Completely independent
1—Requires use of equipment or device
2—Requires help from another person for assistance, supervision, or teaching
3—Requires help from another person and equipment device
4—Dependent (does not participate in activity)

Client Outcomes

Client Will (Specify Time Frame):

- Increase physical activity
- Meet mutually defined goals of ambulation
- Verbalize feeling of increased strength and ability to move
- Demonstrate use of adaptive equipment (e.g., wheelchairs, walkers) to increase mobility

M

Nursing Interventions

- • Screen for mobility skills in the following order: (1) bed mobility; (2) supported and unsupported sitting; (3) transition movements such as sit to stand, sitting down, and transfers; and (4) standing and walking activities. Use a tool such as the Assessment Tool for Safe Patient Handling and Movement. Additional measures of physical function include: unassisted leg stand, use of a balance platform, elbow flexion and knee extension strength, grip strength, timed chair stands, and the 6-minute walk.
- • Observe the client for cause of impaired mobility. Determine whether cause is physical or psychological. Refer to care plan for **Ineffective Coping** or **Hopelessness.**
- • Monitor and record the client's ability to tolerate activity and use all four extremities; note pulse rate, blood pressure, dyspnea, and skin color before and after activity. Refer to the care plan for **Activity intolerance.**
- ▲ Before activity, observe for and, if possible, treat pain. Ensure that the client is not oversedated.
- ▲ Consult with physical therapist for further evaluation, strength training, gait training, and development of a mobility plan.

- ▲ Obtain any assistive devices needed for activity, such as gait belt, walker, cane, crutches, or wheelchair, before the activity begins.
- • If the client is immobile, perform passive range of motion (ROM) exercises at least twice a day unless contraindicated; repeat each maneuver three times.
- ▲ If the client is immobile, consult with physician for a safety evaluation before beginning an exercise program; if program is approved, begin with the following exercises:
  - ■ Active ROM exercises using both upper and lower extremities (e.g., flexing and extending at ankles, knees, hips)
  - ■ Chin-ups and pull-ups using a trapeze in bed (may be contraindicated in clients with cardiac conditions)
  - ■ Strengthening exercises such as gluteal or quadriceps sitting exercises
- • If client is immobile, consider use of a transfer chair, a chair that becomes a stretcher.
- • Help the client achieve mobility and start walking as soon as possible if not contraindicated.
- • Use a gait-walking belt when ambulating the client.
- • Apply any ordered brace before mobilizing the client.
- • Initiate a "No Lift" policy where appropriate assistive devices are utilized for manual lifting.
- • Increase independence in activities of daily living (ADLs), encouraging self-efficacy and discouraging helplessness as the client gets stronger.
- ▲ If the client has osteoarthritis or rheumatoid arthritis, ask for a referral to a physical therapist to begin an exercise program that includes aerobic exercise, resistance exercise, and gentle stretching.
- • If client has had a cerebrovascular accident (CVA) with hemiparesis, consider use of constraint-induced movement therapy (CIMT), where the functional extremity is purposely constrained and the client is forced to use the involved extremity.
- • If the client has had a CVA, recognize that balance is likely impaired and protect from falling.
- • If the client does not feed or groom self, sit side-by-side with the client, put your hand over the client's hand, support the client's elbow with your other hand, and help the client feed self; use the same technique to help the client comb hair.

M

Geriatric

- Assess ability to move using the "Get Up and Go" test. Ask the client to rise from a sitting position, walk 10 feet, turn, and return to the chair to sit.
- Help the mostly immobile client achieve mobility as soon as possible, depending on physical condition.
- If client is frail, ensure good nutrition, appropriate medications, attention to vision and hearing deficits, and increase social support along with exercise.
- Use the Outcome Expectation for Exercise Scale to determine client's self-efficacy expectations and outcomes expectations toward exercise.
- For a client who is mostly immobile, minimize cardiovascular deconditioning by positioning the client in the upright position several times daily.

▲ Refer the client to physical therapy for resistance exercise training as able, including abdominal crunch, leg press, leg extension, leg curl, calf press, and more.

- Use the WALC Intervention (**W**alk; **A**ddress pain, fear, fatigue during exercise; **L**earn about exercise; **C**ue by self-modeling) to improve exercise adherence in the older adult.

▲ If client is scheduled for an elective surgery that will result in admission into an intensive care unit (ICU) and immobility, or recovery from a knee replacement, initiate a prehabilitation program that includes a warm-up, aerobic strength, flexibility, and functional task work.

▲ Evaluate the client for signs of depression (flat affect, insomnia, anorexia, frequent somatic complaints) or cognitive impairment (use Mini-Mental State Exam [MMSE]). Refer for treatment or counseling as needed.

- Watch for orthostatic hypotension when mobilizing elderly clients. Have the client dangle legs at the side of the bed with legs hanging over the edge of the bed, flex and extend feet several times after sitting up, then stand up slowly with someone holding the client. If client becomes light-headed or dizzy, return them to bed immediately.
- Be very careful when getting a mostly immobile client up. Be sure to lock the bed and wheelchair and have sufficient personnel to protect the client from falls.

M

- Do not routinely assist with transfers or bathing activities unless necessary.
- Use gestures and nonverbal cues when helping clients move if they are anxious or have difficulty understanding and following verbal instructions.
- Recognize that wheelchairs are not a good mobility device and often serve as a mobility restraint.
- Ensure that chairs fit clients. Chair seat should be 3 inches above the height of the knee. Provide a raised toilet seat if needed.
- If the client is mainly immobile, provide opportunities for socialization and sensory stimulation (e.g., television and visits). Refer to the care plan for **Deficient Diversional activity.**
- Recognize that immobility and a lack of social support and sensory input may result in confusion or depression in the elderly. Refer to nursing interventions for **Acute Confusion** or **Hopelessness** as appropriate.

Home Care

- • Above interventions may be adapted for home care use.
- ▲ Begin discharge planning as soon as possible with case manager or social worker to assess need for home support systems, assistive devices, and community or home health services.
- ▲ Assess home environment for factors that create barriers to physical mobility. Refer to occupational therapy services if needed to assist the client in restructuring home and daily living patterns.
- ▲ Refer to home health aide services to support the client and family through changing levels of mobility. Reinforce need to promote independence in mobility as tolerated.
- ▲ Refer to physical therapy for gait training, strengthening, and balance training.
- • Discuss with client and caregiver the possibility of a service dog to support the more immobile client.
- • Assess skin condition at every visit. Establish a skin care program that enhances circulation and maximizes position changes.
- • Once the client is able to walk independently, suggest the client enter an exercise program, or walk with a friend.
- • Provide support to the client and family/caregivers during long-

term impaired mobility. Refer to the care plan for **Caregiver role strain.**

▲ Institute case management of frail elderly to support continued independent living.

Client/Family Teaching

- Teach the client to get out of bed slowly when transferring from the bed to the chair.
- Teach the client relaxation techniques to use during activity.
- Teach the client to use assistive devices such as a cane, a walker, or crutches to increase mobility.
- Teach family members and caregivers to work with clients during self-care activities such as eating, bathing, grooming, dressing, and transferring rather than having the client be a passive recipient of care.
- Work with the client using self-efficacy interventions using single or multiple methods.
- Work with the client using the Transtheoretical Model of behavior change and determine if the client is in the precontemplation, contemplation, preparation, action, or maintenance state of behavior change about exercise. Provide appropriate strategies to support change to exercising based on determined state of change.

Impaired wheelchair Mobility

NANDA Definition

Limitation of independent operation of wheelchair within environment

Defining Characteristics

Impaired ability to operate: manual or power wheelchair on curbs; manual or power wheelchair on even surface; manual or power wheelchair on an uneven surface; manual or powered wheelchair on an incline; manual or powered wheelchair on a decline

Related Factors (r/t)

Intolerance to activity; decreased strength and endurance; pain or discomfort; perceptual or cognitive impairment; neuromuscular im-

pairment; musculoskeletal impairment; depression; severe anxiety. Suggested functional level classifications include the following:
0—Completely independent
1—Requires use of equipment or device
2—Requires help from another person for assistance, supervision, or teaching
3—Requires help from another person and equipment or device
4—Dependent—does not participate in activity

Client Outcomes

Client Will (Specify Time Frame):

- Demonstrate independence in operating and moving a wheelchair or other device with wheels
- Demonstrate the ability to direct others in operating and moving a wheelchair or other device
- Demonstrate therapeutic positioning, pressure relief, and safety principles while operating and moving wheelchair or other device equipped with wheels

Nursing Interventions

- • Assist client to put on and take off equipment (e.g., braces, orthoses, abdominal binders) in bed.
- • Inspect skin where orthoses, braces, and so on rested, once they are removed.
- ▲ Obtain referrals for physical and occupational therapy, or wheelchair seating clinic.
- • Keep the right cushion and wheelchair with the right client.
- • Use of properly contoured surfaces/cushions/supports, and continence management, nutrition, hydration, and repositioning help prevent sitting-acquired pressure ulcers.
- ▲ Obtain physical therapist (PT), occupational therapist (OT), or wheelchair clinic referral for cushion reevaluation if signs of pressure exist.
- • Emphasize importance of weight shifts every 15 minutes with safety belts in place (leaning and pushups).
- • Activate passive standing position of wheelchair (if available) or, if applicable, stand client briefly.
- • Place both feet on floor when clients are passively sitting in a wheelchair.

- Routinely assess client's sitting posture and frequently reposition him/her into sound alignment as needed.
- Place client's feet securely on foot rests and fasten seat belts across the top of the thighs before propelling the wheelchair.
- Implement use of friction-coated projection hand rims and leather gloves as clients propel manual wheelchairs.
- Manually guide or explain to push forward on both wheel rims to move ahead, push the right rim to turn left and vice versa, and pull backward on both wheel rims to back up.
- Recommend that clients back wheelchairs into an elevator. If entering face first, instruct them to turn chair around to face the elevator doors.
- Reinforce principle of descending a curb backward ("popping a wheelie") if balance, trunk control, strength, and timing are adequate.
- Ascend curbs in a forward position by popping a wheelie or having aid tilt chair back, place front wheels over curb, and roll chair up. If surface is muddy or sandy, ascend backwards.
- During assisted wheelies, helper must hold wheelchair until all four wheels are back on the ground and client has control of wheelchair.
- Reinforce compensatory strategies for unilateral neglect and agnosia (visual scanning, self-talk, self-questioning as to what could be wrong) as clients propel wheelchair through doorways and around obstacles.
- Sit dysphagic clients as upright as possible in individualized wheelchair versus geri-chair when eating.

▲ Follow therapist recommendations as to how clients should propel manual wheelchairs to prevent upper extremity pain and joint degeneration.
  - Stress that clients maintain normal versus extra body weight.
  - Reinforce use of long/smooth strokes to limit high force on the pushrim, and let the hand "naturally drift down" when letting go of the pushrim.
  - Remind clients to press with length of arm (not elbows) during repositioning and weight shifts. Nocturnal splints, elbow pads, and use of ultra lightweight, pushrim-activated, power-assisted, or electric wheelchair may relieve tendonitis.

- Recognize value systems of clients/nurses regarding use of a wheelchair may differ and create tension.

M

- ▲ Offer support/referrals to help clients cope with issues related to physical disability and loss.
- • Suggest and help clients transition from a manual to a powered wheelchair or device if progressive physical disability occurs.
- ▲ Reduce floor clutter and establish safety rules for drivers of power mobility devices; make referrals to PT or OT for driver reevaluations if accidents occur or client's health deteriorates.
- • Request and receive clients' permission before moving unoccupied wheelchair in room or out to hallway.

Geriatric

- • Alternate wheelchair mobility with rest periods.
- • Avoid using restraints on fidgeting clients who slide down in a wheelchair; rather, assess for deformities, spinal curvatures, abnormal tone, discomfort, and limited joint range.
- • Ensure proper seat depth leg positioning when elders are sitting up and use custom foot rests (not elevated leg rests) to prevent sliding down in wheelchairs.
- ▲ Assess for side effects of medications and potential need for dosage readjustments to increase wheelchair tolerance.
- • Allow client to propel wheelchair independently at his or her own speed.

Home Care

- • Assess home environment for barriers and for a support system for emergency and contingency care (e.g., Lifeline).
- • Arrange traffic patterns so they are wide enough to maneuver a wheelchair.
- • Explain a 5-foot turning space is necessary to maneuver wheelchairs, doorways need to be 32 to 36 inches wide, and entrance ramps/paths should slope 1 inch per foot.
- • Suggest simple changes such as replacing door hardware with fold-back hinges, removing doorway encasements (if too narrow), and removing or replacing thresholds (if too high).
- • Suggest rearranging room functions, furniture, and storage so that toileting, sleeping, bathing, and preparing and eating meals can safely take place on one level of the home.
- ▲ Request PT/OT referrals to evaluate wheelchair skills and safety, to suggest home modifications and ways to propel

wheelchairs on irregular surfaces and get back into a chair after a fall.

- ▲ Provide support to clients and teach about pertinent local support groups and internet resources.
- ▲ Provide client with information about advocacy, resources, accessibility, assistive technology, potential funding, and issues under the Americans with Disabilities Act.
- ▲ Suggest community resources for servicing and tuning up wheelchairs and/or locating parts so clients can service their own chairs, since an annual tune-up is recommended.

Client/Family Teaching

- • Suggest that the client test-drive wheelchairs and try out cushions and postural supports before purchasing them.
- • Assess pain levels of long-term wheelchair users and make referrals to therapists or wheelchair clinics for modifications.
- • Instruct and have client return demonstrate re-inflation of pneumatic tires; encourage client to monitor tire pressure every 2 to 3 weeks.
- • Instruct clients to remove large wheelchair parts when lifting wheelchair into car for transport; when reassembling it, check that all parts are fastened securely and temperature is tepid.
- ▲ Make social service referral to educate clients on financial coverage/regulations of third-party payors and Health Care Financing Association for equipment.
- • Teach the importance of using seatbelts or chair tie-downs when riding in motor vehicles; if unavailable, clients in wheelchairs should be transported in large heavy vehicles only.
- • For further information, refer care plans for **Impaired Transfer ability** and **Impaired bed Mobility.**

Nausea

NANDA Definition

A subjective, unpleasant, wavelike sensation in the back of the throat, epigastrium, or the abdomen that may lead to the urge or need to vomit

Defining Characteristics

Aversion to food; gagging sensation; increased salivation; increased swallowing; report of nausea; sour taste in mouth

Related Factors (r/t)

Biophysical

Biochemical disorders (e.g., uremia, diabetic ketoacidosis, pregnancy); esophageal disease; gastric distention; gastric irritation; increased intracranial pressure; intraabdominal tumors; labyrinthitis; liver capsule stretch; localized tumors (e.g., acoustic neuroma, primary or secondary brain tumors, bone metastases at base of skull); meningitis; Meniere's disease; motion sickness; pain; pancreatic disease; splenetic capsule stretch; toxins (e.g., tumor-produced peptides, abnormal metabolites due to cancer)

Situational

Anxiety; fear; noxious odors; noxious taste; pain; psychological factors; unpleasant visual stimulation

Treatment Related

Gastric distention; gastric irritation: pharmaceuticals

Client Outcomes

Client Will (Specify Time Frame):

- State relief of nausea
- Explain methods they can use to decrease nausea and vomiting (N&V)

Nursing Interventions

- Determine cause of N&V (e.g., medication effects, viral illness, food poisoning, extreme anxiety, anesthetic agents, pregnancy).
- Provide distraction from the sensation of nausea, using soft music, television, and videos per the client preference.
- Apply a cold washcloth to the forehead of a nauseated client.
- Maintain a quiet, well-ventilated environment free of strong odors from food, perfume or cleaning solutions.
- Avoid sudden movement of the client; allow the client to lie still.
- If nausea is associated with frequent vomiting, assess client for fluid and electrolyte imbalances.
- Keep a clean emesis basin and tissues within the client's reach.

- Provide oral care after the client vomits.
- Stay with the client to give support, place hand on shoulder, and hold the emesis basin.
- After vomiting is controlled and nausea abates, begin offering the client small amounts of clear fluids, such as water, clear soda, or preferably ginger ale, and then bland foods, such as crackers or dry toast; progress to a soft diet.
- Remove cover of food tray before bringing it into the client's room.
- ▲ Refer clients with HIV for management of antiretroviral-related nausea.

Nausea in Pregnancy

- Recommend that the woman eat dry crackers or dry toast in bed before arising and then get up slowly. Also advise to chew gum or suck hard candies, eat small frequent meals, avoid foods with offensive odors, and avoid preparing food or shopping when nauseated.
- ▲ Discuss with the primary care practitioner the possibility of using transcutaneous electrical stimulation in the form of Relief Band Device to help relieve nausea.
- ▲ Consider the use of continuous acupressure applied by Sea-Bands with acupressure buttons or by hand to P6 on both wrists.
- ▲ Refer client for acupuncture.

Nausea Following Surgery

- ▲ Medicate the client for nausea as ordered.
- ▲ Alleviate postoperative pain using ordered analgesic agents (refer to care plan for **Acute Pain**).
- Ensure that the nauseated client is not hypotensive. Check blood pressure and note signs of postural hypotension.
- Consider use of a recliner chair postoperatively for clients who have had laparoscopy if not contraindicated.
- Recommend that the client sit down when experiencing nausea.
- ▲ Consider use of isopropyl alcohol (IPA) inhalation for treatment of PONV for clients who have general anesthesia for a surgical procedure.
- ▲ Consult with primary care practitioner for use of nonpharmacological techniques, such as acupuncture, electroacupuncture, or transcutaneous electrical nerve stimulation as an adjunct for controlling PONV.

N

• Teach the use of acupressure on two points on the wrist, or use of bands providing pressure to prevent or relieve nausea in some kinds of surgery.
• Use relaxation, imagery, and distraction techniques for nausea; encourage the client to take slow, deep breaths.

Nausea Following Chemotherapy

▲ Consult with physician regarding need for antiemetic medications, either prophylactic or when N&V occurs.
▲ Use antiemetics and a nursing intervention program of increased access to support and increased information.
▲ If nausea is associated with the use of opioids, consult with the primary care practitioner for possible use of alternative pain medication.
• Help the client learn how to use acupressure for nausea, applying pressure bilaterally at P6 points using fingers or bands to decrease the amount and severity of nausea.
▲ For clients who continue to experience nausea after antiemetic drugs or other treatments, consult with the primary care practitioner regarding the possibility of using acupuncture to help control nausea. Such devices as the Relief Band are not effective.
• Recognize that the use of ginger root may relieve nausea.
• Work with the client, using guided imagery and progressive muscle relaxation to reduce nausea.
• Offer the nauseated client a 10-minute foot massage.
• If client has anticipatory nausea, use such interventions as education, relaxation therapy, and imagery to help client decrease nausea associated with the event.

Geriatrics

▲ Administer antiemetic drugs carefully; watch for side effects.
▲ Evaluate nonsteroidal antiinflammatory drugs (NSAIDs) as a possible cause of nausea.

Home Care

• Previously mentioned interventions may be adapted for home care use.
▲ In hospice care clients, assess for causes of nausea, such as con-

stipation, bowel obstruction, adverse effects of medications, and onset of increased intracranial pressure. Refer the client to a primary care practitioner if needed.
- Assist the client and family with identifying and avoiding irritants in the home that exacerbate nausea (e.g., strong odors from food, plants, perfume, and room deodorizers).

Client/Family Teaching

- Teach the client techniques to use when uncomfortable, including relaxation techniques, guided imagery, hypnosis, and music therapy.

Unilateral Neglect

NANDA Definition

Impairment in sensory and motor response, mental representation, and spatial attention of the body and the corresponding environment characterized by inattention to one side and overattention to the opposite side. Left side neglect is more severe and persistent than right side neglect.

Defining Characteristics

Appears unaware of positioning of neglected limb; difficulty remembering details of internally represented familiar scenes that are on the neglected side; displacement of sounds to the nonneglected side; distortion of drawing on the half of the page on the neglected side; failure to cancel lines on the half of the page on the neglected side; failure to eat food from portion of the plate on the neglected side; failure to dress neglected side; failure to groom neglected side; failure to move eyes, head, limbs, trunk in the neglected hemispace, despite being aware of a stimulus in that space; failure to notice people approaching from the neglected side; lack of safety precautions with regard to the neglected side; marked deviation of the eyes to the nonneglected side to stimuli and activities on that side; marked deviation of the head to the nonneglected side to stimuli and activities on that side; marked deviation of the trunk to the nonneglected side to stimuli and activities on that side; omission of drawing on the half of the page on the neglected side; perseveration of visual motor tasks on nonneglected side; substitution of letters to form alternative words that are similar to the original in length when reading; transfer of pain sensation to the nonneglected side; use of only vertical half of page when writing

Related Factors (r/t)

Brain injury from cerebrovascular problems; brain injury from neurological illness; brain injury from trauma; brain injury from tumor; left hemiplegia from CVA of the right hemisphere; hemianopsia
NOTE: Because the right hemisphere is dominant in directing attention, unilateral neglect is more common if neurological pathology occurs in the right hemisphere of the brain, which results in left-sided neglect. Also, unilateral neglect often occurs with damage to the right parietal lobe, the right frontal lobe, the thalamus, and basal ganglia.

Client Outcomes

N

Client Will (Specify Time Frame):

- Use techniques that can be used to minimize unilateral neglect
- Care for both sides of the body appropriately and keep affected side free from harm
- Return to the highest functioning level possible based on personal goals and abilities
- Remain free from injury

Nursing Interventions

- Assess the client for signs of unilateral neglect (e.g., not washing, shaving, or dressing one side of the body; sitting or lying inappropriately on affected arm or leg; failing to respond to environmental stimuli contralateral to the side of lesion; eating food on only one side of plate; or failing to look to one side of the body).
- It is strongly recommended that stroke recovery is assessed using the National Institutes of Health Stroke Scale (NIHSS) at the time of admission or within the first 24 hours.
- It is practical to postpone evaluation for unilateral neglect until a couple of weeks after a stroke.
- Provide a safe, well-lighted, and clutter-free environment. Place call light and other personal items (such as a urinal) on the unaffected side. Cue the client to environmental hazards when mobile.

▲ Refer to a rehabilitation team (including, but not limited to, rehabilitation clinical nurse specialist, physical medicine and rehabilitation physician, neuropsychologist, occupational therapist, physical therapist, and speech and language pathologist) for continued help in dealing with unilateral neglect.

• Use the principles of rehabilitation to progressively increase the client's ability to compensate for unilateral neglect by using assistive devices, feedback, and support, depending on phase of recovery:
  - **Stage I** (Stabilization) Focus attention mainly on non-neglected side.
    - ❑ Set up environment so that most activity is on unaffected side.
    - ❑ Place the client's personal items within view and on unaffected side.
    - ❑ Position the bed so that client is approached from the unaffected side.
    - ❑ Monitor and assist the client to achieve adequate food and fluid intake.
  - **Stage II** (Early recovery): Help the client develop an awareness of neglected side.
    - ❑ Gradually focus the client's attention on affected side.
    - ❑ Gradually move personal items and activity to affected side.
    - ❑ Stand on the client's affected side when assisting with ambulation or ADLs.
  - **Stage III** (Rehabilitation): Help the client compensate for neglect.
    - ❑ Use cues and anchors to promote attention to the neglected side and help the client develop compensatory mechanisms to deal with the neglect syndrome (Kalbach, 1991). Use reminders to keep the client scanning the entire environment.
    - ❑ Use bright yellow or red stickers on outer margins in reading or writing exercises. Have the client look for the sticker while reading or writing. Similar markers can be applied to a meal tray or plate to encourage scanning of the entire meal.
    - ❑ Encourage the client to bathe and groom the affected side first.

- ❑ Focus touch and talking on affected side; use a positive approach (e.g., "Mary, turn your head to the left and you'll see your daughter").
- Recognize that unilateral neglect can improve following a stroke.

Home Care

- Many of the previously listed interventions may be adapted for use in the home care setting.
- Position bed at home so that client gets out of bed on unaffected side.

Client/Family Teaching

- Explain pathology and symptoms of unilateral neglect to both the client and family.
- Teach the client how to scan regularly to check the position of body parts and to regularly turn head from side to side for safety when ambulating, using a wheelchair, or doing self-care tasks. Recommend the client think of self like a horizon-illuminating lighthouse.
- Teach caregivers to cue the client to the environment.

Noncompliance

NANDA Definition

Behavior of person and/or caregiver that fails to coincide with a health-promoting or therapeutic plan agreed on by the person (and/or family and/or community) and healthcare professional; in the presence of an agreed-on, health-promoting, or therapeutic plan, person's or caregiver's behavior is fully or partially nonadherent and may lead to clinically ineffective or partially ineffective outcomes

Defining Characteristics

Behavior indicative of failure to adhere (directly observed or verbalized by patient or significant others) (critical); objective tests (e.g., physiological measures, detection of physiological markers); evidence of development of complications; evidence of exacerbation of symptoms; failure to keep appointments; failure to progress

Related Factors (r/t)

Healthcare plan

Duration; significant others; cost; intensity; complexity; financial flexibility of plan

Individual Factors

Cultural influences; developmental abilities; health beliefs; individual's value system; knowledge relevant to the regimen behavior; motivational forces; personal abilities; significant others; skill relevant to the regimen behavior; spiritual values

Health System

Access to care; client/provider relationships; communication skills of the provider; convenience of care; credibility of provider; individual health coverage; provider continuity; provider regular follow-up; provider reimbursement; satisfaction with care; teaching skills of the provider

Network

Involvement of members in health plan; social value regarding plan; perceived beliefs of significant others

NOTE: The nursing diagnosis **Noncompliance** is judgmental and places blame on the client. The authors recommend use of the diagnosis **Ineffective Therapeutic regimen management** in place of the diagnosis **Noncompliance.** The diagnosis **Ineffective Therapeutic regimen management** has interventions that are developed by both the healthcare providers and the client. It is a more respectful and efficacious nursing diagnosis than **Noncompliance.**

Client Outcomes

Client Will (Specify Time Frame):

- Describe consequence of continued noncompliance with treatment regimen
- State goals for health and the means by which to obtain them
- Communicate an understanding of disease and treatment
- List treatment regimens and expectations and agree to follow through
- List alternative ways to meet goals
- Describe the importance of family participation to help achieve goals

Nursing Interventions

- Ask the client why he or she has not complied with the prescribed treatment. Have the client "tell his or her story." Listen nonjudgmentally.
- Make the client an active partner in his or her own healthcare management. Recognize that the client has absolute control over whether he or she follows the healthcare regimen. Always treat the client with respect, and develop mutual outcomes for treatment.
- Instruct the client about the purpose, action, side effects, and administration of medications.
- Assess the likelihood of medication-related problems and noncompliance with medication regimen.
- Determine the client's ability to obtain required medications.
- Instruct the client on self-monitoring and self-regulation of medications as appropriate.
- Provide structured education tailored to the individual.
- Provide written educational materials at an appropriate reading level.
- Work with the client to determine how he or she will handle the illness and need for medications or prescribed care.
- Arrange for follow-up via telephone.
- If the client is in denial, provide information, communicate unconditional positive regard, avoid distancing yourself, and look for opportunities for authentic contact with your client, being present psychologically and physically. See care plan for **Ineffective Denial.**
- Observe for cause of noncompliance (see Related Factors). Recognize that noncompliance is very common.
- Recognize that behavioral change comes slowly and often in stages:
  - Precontemplation: change is not contemplated; unaware of problem or risk
  - Contemplation: aware that problem exists; no specific plans or commitment to change
  - Preparation: plan to take action within the next 30 days
  - Action: now taking action to improve health; often behavior not consistently carried out
  - Maintenance: consistently engages in healthful behavior for more than 6 months

N

- • Determine the client's and family's knowledge of illness and treatment. Teach them about the illness and purpose of the treatment regimen if necessary.
- ▲ Monitor the client for signs of depression that may cause noncompliance. Refer for treatment if appropriate.
- • Monitor the client's ability to follow directions, solve problems, concentrate, and read.
- • Avoid using threats, pressure, and inappropriate fear arousal to increase compliance.
- • Determine whether the client's support system helps or hinders therapy. Bring family members and significant others into the educational process as desired by the client.
- • Listen to the client's descriptions of abilities; encourage the client to use these abilities in self-care. When dealing with complex healthcare regimens, start the client with small behavioral changes (e.g., have a client receiving chemotherapy rinse mouth with a saliva substitute twice daily). When one step has been accomplished, add another step.
- • Work with the client to develop cues that trigger needed healthcare behaviors (e.g., checking blood sugar level before putting on makeup each morning), including weekends, holidays, and vacations.
- • Work with the client to develop an instruction and reminder sheet that fits medications and treatments into the client's lifestyle.
- • Observe the noncompliant client for possibility of secondary gain, such as increased attention, if the client continues to be ill and noncompliant.
- ▲ Consult with the primary care practitioner about simplifying the healthcare regimen so that it more easily fits into the client's lifestyle (e.g., taking medications once daily versus four times daily).
- ▲ Refer the client for compliance therapy (motivational interviewing and cognitive behavioral therapy) for medication management for clients with schizophrenia.

Geriatric

- • Make the client an explicit medication instruction using bulleted lists and simple icons.
- ▲ If the client has sensory and coordination deficits, use a medica-

tion organizer and have the home health nurse or family place the client's medications in daily compartments.

- • Assess for cognitive ability to understand medication use.
- ▲ Ask clients if they can afford medications. Refer clients for financial help from social worker or case manager if needed.
- ▲ Monitor the client for signs of depression associated with noncompliance (e.g., refusing to eat or take medications). Refer the client for treatment of depression as needed.
- • Use repetition, verbal cues, and memory aids, such as pictures, schedules, or reminder sheets, when teaching the healthcare regimen. Use events, such as meals, bedtime, and so on, as reminders when to take medications.
- • Consider assistive medication technology, such as talking reminders and pill dispensers.

Multicultural

- • Assess for the influence of cultural beliefs, norms, and values on the client's ability to modify health behavior.
- • Discuss with the client those aspects of their health behavior/lifestyle that will remain unchanged by their health status.
- • Negotiate with the client regarding the aspects of health behavior that will need to be modified.
- • Assess the role of fatalism on the client's ability to modify health behavior.
- • Validate the client's feelings regarding the impact of health status on current lifestyle.
- • Use mechanical reminders to cue clients and improve adherence.

Home Care

NOTE: Because the home care nurse enters the client's home as a guest, the ability of the nurse to establish a supportive, therapeutic relationship is especially important. A paradigm shift in nurses' view of noncompliance has been proposed, to include the recognition of clients as experts on their own lives, and the assessment of client social context to determine possible rationales for not following professional advice.

- • Previously mentioned interventions may be adapted for home care use.
- • Before providing any care, review the Home Health Care Bill of Rights with the client, including the right to refuse treatment.

- • If included in agency policies and procedures, also review client responsibilities with the client, which is often part of a printed Bill of Rights.
- • When the client is noncompliant, redefine personal and health priorities (contract for services) with the client to determine alternative motivational strategies or health actions to meet health goals.
- ▲ Institute self-care management to maximize client responsibility for own care. Refer to the care plan for **Powerlessness.**
- • Elicit and answer questions respectfully regarding illness and treatment, correcting any misconceptions and highlighting the importance of assisting the client to incorporate treatment plan into daily lifestyle. Do not use medical jargon in explanations.
- • Explore barriers to medical regimen adherence. Review medications and treatment regularly for needed modifications. Take complaints of side effects seriously and serve as the client advocate to address changes as indicated.
- ▲ If noncompliance compromises the client's health status, refer for psychiatric home healthcare services to assess the client's motivation and implement therapeutic regimen.
- ▲ If noncompliant behavior continues and the client chooses not to cooperate with medical regimen, the home healthcare agency cannot continue to provide services.
- • If care is to be terminated, identify all possible alternatives for the client, and assist with making an informed choice about future health actions.
- • Respect the wishes of terminally ill clients to refuse selected aspects of medical regimen. With terminally ill clients, do not terminate care. Provide those aspects of care that the client and family or caregivers will accept.

Client/Family Teaching

- ▲ Teach clients about medication side effects (e.g., mental changes, sexual dysfunction) so that they understand them and feel comfortable discussing them.
- • Teach clients to control their "self-talk" by giving themselves positive messages to promote desired behaviors, such as taking medications and controlling food intake.

N

Imbalanced Nutrition: less than body requirements

NANDA Definition

Intake of nutrients insufficient to meet metabolic needs

Defining Characteristics

Abdominal cramping; abdominal pain; aversion to eating; body weight 20% or more under ideal; capillary fragility; diarrhea; excessive loss of hair; hyperactive bowel sounds; lack of food; lack of information; lack of interest in food; loss of weight with adequate food intake; misconceptions; misinformation; pale mucous membranes; perceived inability to ingest food; poor muscle tone; reported altered taste sensation; reported food intake less than RDA (recommended daily allowance); satiety immediately after ingesting food; sore buccal cavity; steatorrhea; weakness of muscles required for swallowing or mastication

Related Factors (r/t)

Biological factors; economic factors; inability to absorb nutrients; inability to digest food; inability to ingest food; psychological factors

Client Outcomes

Client Will (Specify Time Frame):

- Progressively gain weight toward desired goal
- Weigh within normal range for height and age
- Recognize factors contributing to underweight
- Identify nutritional requirements
- Consume adequate nourishment
- Be free of signs of malnutrition

Nursing Interventions

▲ Utilize a nutritional screening tool to determine possibility of malnutrition on admission into any healthcare facility. Watch for recent weight loss of over 10 pounds; 10% under healthy weight; not eating for more than three days; half of normal eating for more than five days; Body Mass Index (BMI) of less than 20; presence of large wound or surgical area; multiple trauma; or other reasons why the client may be malnourished, and refer client to a dietitian for a complete nutritional assessment.

- • Monitor for signs of malnutrition, including brittle hair that is easily plucked, bruises, dry skin, pale skin and conjunctiva, muscle wasting, smooth red tongue, cheilosis, "flaky paint" rash over lower extremities, and disorientation.
- • Recognize that severe protein calorie malnutrition can result in septicemia from impairment of the immune system, organ failure including heart failure, liver failure, respiratory dysfunction, especially in the critically ill client.
- ▲ Note laboratory test results as available: serum albumin, prealbumin, serum total protein, serum ferritin, transferrin, hemoglobin, hematocrit, and electrolytes.
- • Weigh the client daily in acute care, weekly in extended care, at the same time of day (usually before breakfast) and with same amount of clothing.
- ▲ Monitor food intake; record percentages of served food that is eaten (25%, 50%); consult with dietitian for actual calorie count if needed.
- • Observe the client's relationship to food. Attempt to separate physical from psychological causes for eating difficulty.
- • Compare usual food intake with the Food Guide Pyramid, noting slighted or omitted food groups.
- • If the client is a vegetarian, evaluate vitamin B_{12} and iron intake. Strict vegetarians may be at particular risk for vitamin B_{12} and iron deficiencies.
- • Observe the client's ability to eat (time involved, motor skills, visual acuity, and ability to swallow various textures). If the client needs to be fed, allocate *at least 35 minutes* to feeding.

NOTE: If the client is unable to feed self, refer to Nursing Interventions for **Feeding Self-care deficit.** If the client has difficulty swallowing, refer to Nursing Interventions for **Impaired Swallowing.** If the client is receiving tube feedings, refer to the Nursing Interventions for **Risk for Aspiration.**

- ▲ If the client has a minimally functioning gastrointestinal tract and is on a diet of clear fluids, consult with a dietitian regarding use of a clear liquid product that contains increased amounts of protein and calories, such as Citrotein, Boost Breeze, or Resource Fruit Beverage.

N

- For the client with anorexia who will not eat foods, consider offering 30 mL of a nutritional supplement in a medication cup every hour.
- For the client who is malnourished and can eat, offer small quantities of energy-dense and protein-enriched food, served in an appetizing fashion, at frequent intervals.
- If the client lacks endurance, schedule rest periods before meals, open packages, and cut up food for the client.
- When the client is malnourished, watch carefully for signs of infection and maintain every action possible to protect the client from infection.
- If the client is pregnant, ensure that she is receiving adequate folic acid by eating a balanced diet and taking prenatal vitamins as ordered.
- Provide companionship at mealtime to encourage nutritional intake.
- Monitor state of oral cavity (gums, tongue, mucosa, teeth). Provide good oral hygiene before and after meals.
- If a client has anorexia and dry mouth from medication side effects, offer sips of fluids throughout the day, along with sugarless hard candy and chewing gum to stimulate saliva formation.
- Determine relationship of eating and other events to onset of nausea, vomiting, diarrhea, or abdominal pain.
- Determine time of day when the client's appetite is the greatest. Offer highest calorie meal at that time.

▲ Administer antiemetics and pain medications as ordered and needed before meals.

- Prepare the client for meals. Clear unsightly supplies and excretions. Avoid invasive procedures before meals.
- If client is nauseated, remove cover of food tray before bringing it into the client's room.
- Work with the client to develop a plan for increased activity.
- If the client is anemic, offer foods rich in iron and vitamins B_{12}, C, and folic acid.
- For the agitated pacing client, offer finger foods (sandwiches, fresh fruit) and fluids.

▲ If a client has been malnourished for a significant length of time, consult with a dietitian and refeed carefully after correcting electrolyte balance. Watch for heart and respiratory failure.

N

Pediatric

- Watch for symptoms of malnutrition, including short stature, thin arms and legs, poor condition of skin and hair, visible vertebrae and rib cage, wasted buttocks, wasted facial appearance, lethargy, and in extreme cases, edema.
- Weigh and measure the length (height) of the child and use a growth chart to help determine growth pattern, which reflects nutrition.
- Determine the child's BMI after the age of 3 years.

▲ Refer to a physician and a dietician a child who is underweight for any reason.

▲ Work with parents of the underweight child to improve the child's nutritional status as needed by:
  - Referring to a breast feeding specialist if needed
  - Teaching how to select, prepare, and handle appropriate food for the age of the child
  - Teaching when to introduce solid foods and progress weaning
  - Advising on the appropriate range of food and portion sizes for children
  - Advising the parent to accept the child's natural size and shape, because the child needs the parents' unconditional love
  - Make family meals a priority
  - Involving the child in menu planning, cooking, and preparing food, as appropriate for the child's age
  - Encouraging children to love their bodies

- Work with the child and parent to develop an appropriate weight gain plan.
- Recognize that a large percentage of girls and teenagers are dieting, which can result in nutritional problems.

Geriatric

- Assess for protein-energy malnutrition in older adult clients regardless of setting. Use a screening tool, such as the Nutritional Risk Screening (NRS) if in acute care, or the Mini Nutritional Assessment (MNA) if in long term care or living in the community.
- Assess for factors contributing to a current acute illness, such as dehydration and the presence of diarrhea.

N

- ▲ Interpret laboratory findings cautiously.
- • Offer high-protein supplements based on individual needs and capabilities.
- • Recognize that constipation is a common problem with older clients, therefore they avoid many types of food for fear of problems with their bowel regimen.
- • Give the client a choice of supplements, including a taste test, to increase personal control. If the client is unwilling to drink a glass of liquid supplement, offer 30 mL/hr in a medication cup.
- • Offer liquid energy supplements.
- • Unless medically contraindicated, permit self-selected seasonings and foods.
- • Serve food in a restaurant style manner if possible.
- • Encourage physical activity and toileting assistance before meals.
- • Assess components of bone health: older adults need 1200 mg calcium daily and adequate vitamin D.
- • Recognize that older women may continue their younger preoccupation with weight and recurrent dieting, despite being at normal weight.
- • Assess for psychological and mental factors that impact nutrition. Watch for signs of depression.
- • Provide soothing music during meals.
- ▲ Provide appropriate diet for ability to chew food. Insert dentures (if needed) before meals. Assess the fit of dentures. Refer the client for dental consultation if needed.

NOTE: If the client is unable to feed self, refer to Nursing Interventions for **Feeding Self-care deficit.** If the client has impaired physical function, malnutrition, depression and cognitive impairment, please refer to care plan on **Adult Failure to thrive.**

Multicultural

- • Assess for dietary intake of essential nutrients.
- • Assess for the influence of cultural beliefs, norms, and values on the client's nutritional knowledge.
- • Discuss with the client those aspects of their diet that will remain unchanged. Negotiate with the client regarding the aspects of his or her diet that will need to be modified.
- • Encourage family meals.

Home Care

- • Previously mentioned interventions may be adapted for home care use.
- • Monitor food intake. Instruct the client in intake of small frequent meals of foods with increased calories and protein.
- • Assess a client's willingness to eat; fashion interventions accordingly.
- ▲ Assess the client for depression. Refer for mental health services as indicated.
- • Consider social factors that may interfere with nutrition (e.g., lack of transportation, inadequate income, lack of social support).
- ▲ Monitor the effect of total parenteral nutrition (TPN) as ordered by physician, and use appropriate interventions including weight, blood glucose levels, electrolytes, symptoms of fluid overload or deficit, and symptoms of infection at entry site of catheter.
- ▲ In the presence of a diagnosis of depression, refer the client for psychiatric home healthcare services for client reassurance and implementation of therapeutic regimen.

Client/Family Teaching

- • Help the client/family identify the area to change that will make the greatest contribution to improved nutrition.
- • Build on the strengths in the client's/family's food habits. Adapt changes to their current practices.
- • Select appropriate teaching aids for the client's/family's background.
- • Implement instructional follow-up to answer the client's/family's questions.
- • Suggest community resources as suitable (food sources, counseling, Meals on Wheels, senior centers).
- • Teach the client and family how to manage tube feedings or parenteral therapy at home.

N

Imbalanced Nutrition: more than body requirements

NANDA Definition

Intake of nutrients that exceeds metabolic needs

Defining Characteristics

Concentrating food intake at the end of the day; dysfunctional eating pattern (e.g., pairing food with other activities); eating in response to external cues (e.g., time of day, social situation); eating in response to internal cues other than hunger (e.g., anxiety); sedentary activity level; triceps skin fold >25 mm in women, >15 mm in men; weight 20% over ideal for height and frame

Related Factors (r/t)

N

Excessive intake in relation to metabolic need

Client Outcomes

Client Will (Specify Time Frame):

- State pertinent factors contributing to weight gain
- Identify behaviors that remain under client's control
- Design dietary modifications to meet individual long-term goal of weight control
- Lose weight in a reasonable period (1 to 2 lb per week)
- Incorporate appropriate activities requiring energy expenditure into daily life

Nursing Interventions

- Ask the client to keep a food diary for 1-3 days, where everything ingested (food and drink) is recorded.
- Advise the client to measure food periodically. Help the client learn usual portion sizes.
- Help the client determine their body mass index (BMI).
- Recommend the client follow the U.S. Dietary Guidelines, which can be found at www.healthierus.gov/dietaryguidelines.
- Recommend the client use the interactive Food Guide Pyramid site at www.MyPyramid.gov to determine the number of calories to eat, and gain more information on how to eat in a healthy fashion. Recommend that the client lose

weight slowly, no more than 1-2 pounds per week, based on a healthy eating pattern and increased exercise. The number of calories consumed should be at least 1600 for men, and 1300 for women.

- Demonstrate the use of food labels to make healthful choices. Alert the client/family to focus on serving size, total fat, and simple carbohydrates.
- Weigh the client twice a week under the same conditions.
- Watch the client for signs of depression, such as flat affect, poor sleeping habits, or lack of interest in life.

Pattern of Dietary Intake

- Recommend the client eat a healthy breakfast every morning.
- Recommend the client avoid eating in fast food restaurants.
- ▲ Obtain a thorough history. Refer to a dietitian if the client has a medical condition.

Recommended Foods/Fluids

- Encourage the client to increase intake of vegetables and fruits to at least five servings per day, preferably 9 servings per day.
- Encourage the client to eat at least 3 servings of whole grains per day, preferably more.
- Evaluate the client's usual intake of fiber.
- Discuss the possibility of using a primarily plant-based or vegetarian diet to lose weight.
- Encourage the client to decrease intake of sugars, including soft drinks, desserts, and candy.
- Recommend client increases intake of water to at least 2000 mL, or 2 quarts per day. A guideline is 1-1.5 mL of fluid per each calorie needed, so an average intake would be between 2000 and 3000 mL/day, or at least 8 cups of fluid.
- For more information on healthy eating, refer to nursing interventions for **Readiness for enhanced Nutrition.**

Behavioral Methods for Weight Loss

- Familiarize the client with the following behavior modification techniques:
  - ■ Self-monitoring of food intake, including keeping a food and exercise diary

- Graphing weight weekly
- Controlling stimuli that causes overeating, such as watching television with frequent food-related commercials
- Limiting food intake to one site in the home
- Sitting down at the table to eat
- Planning food intake for each day
- Rearranging the schedule to avoid inappropriate eating
- Avoiding boredom that results in eating; keeping a list of activities on the refrigerator
- For a party, eating before arriving, sitting away from the snack foods, and substituting lower-calorie beverages for alcoholic ones
- Deciding beforehand what to order in a restaurant
- Bringing only healthy foods into the house to decrease temptation
- Slowing mealtime by swallowing food before putting more food on the utensil, pausing for a minute during the meal and attempting to increase the number of pauses, and trying to be the last one to finish eating
- Drinking a glass of water before each meal; taking sips of water between bites of food
- Charting one's progress
- Making an agreement with oneself or a significant other for a meaningful reward and not rewarding oneself with food
- Changing one's mindset, as in control of eating behavior
- Viewing exercise as a means of controlling hunger
- Practicing relaxation techniques
- Visualizing oneself enjoying a fresh apple in preference to apple pie

Physical Activity

▲ Assess for reasons why the client would be unable to participate in an exercise program; refer the client for evaluation by a primary care practitioner as needed.

• Use the Outcome Expectation for Exercise Scale to determine the client's self-efficacy expectations and outcomes expectations toward exercise.

• Recommend the client enter an exercise program with a friend.

• Recommend the client begin a walking program using the following guidelines:

- Buy a pedometer
- Determine times when walking can be incorporated into usual lifestyle
- Set a goal of walking 10,000 steps per day, or 5 miles per day.
- If the client does not have required number of steps when he or she comes home from work, go for another walk until the designated goal of 10,000 steps per day is reached.

Pediatric

- Work with parents of the overweight child by encouraging the following behaviors:
  - Emphasize providing good food, not depriving children of food.
  - Accept the child's natural size and shape, because the child needs the parents' unconditional love
  - Make family meals a priority
  - Involve the child in planning menus, cooking, and preparing foods as appropriate for the child's age
  - Educate parents to participate in activities with children
  - Encourage children to love their bodies
- Determine the child's BMI after the child is 3 years old.
- Work with the child and parent to develop an appropriate weight maintenance plan, including behavioral methods of weight loss as well as increased activity.
- Encourage children to increase the amount of walking done per day, if they are willing, and ask them to wear a pedometer to measure number of steps.
- Do not use food as a reward for good behavior, especially foods that are concentrated sources of sugar or fat.
- Recommend the child decrease television viewing, watching movies, and playing video games. Ask parents to limit television to 1 to 2 hours per day maximum.

Geriatric

- Assess changes in lifestyle and eating patterns.
- Assess fluid intake. Recommend routine drinks of water regardless of thirst.
- Observe for socioeconomic factors that influence food choices (e.g., inadequate funds or cooking facilities).
- Suggest a variety of seasonings.

Multicultural

- Assess for the influence of cultural beliefs, norms, acculturation, and values on the client's nutritional knowledge and practices.
- Encourage parental efforts at increasing physical activity and decreasing dietary fat for their children.
- Assess for the influence of cultural beliefs, norms, and values on the client's idea of acceptable body weight and body size.
- Discuss with the client those aspects of his or her diet that will remain unchanged, and work with the client to adapt cultural core foods.
- Negotiate with the client regarding the aspects of his or her diet that will need to be modified.
- Validate the client's feelings regarding the impact of current lifestyle, finances, and transportation on the ability to obtain and prepare nutritious food.
- Limit television viewing and consumption of soft drinks. Encourage family meals.

Client/Family Teaching

- Provide the client and family with information regarding the treatment plan options.
- Inform the client about the health risks associated with obesity, which include cancer, diabetes, heart disease, strokes, hypertension, gastroesophageal reflux, gallstones, osteoarthritis, and venous thrombosis.
- Inform the client and family of the disadvantages of trying to lose weight by dieting alone.
- Teach the importance of exercise in a weight control program.
- Recommend the client receive adequate amounts of sleep.
- Teach stress reduction techniques as alternatives to eating.

Readiness for enhanced Nutrition

NANDA Definition

A pattern of nutrient intake that is sufficient for meeting metabolic needs and can be strengthened

Defining Characteristics

Attitude toward drinking is congruent with health goals; attitude toward eating is congruent with health goals; consumes adequate fluid; consumes adequate food; eats regularly; expresses knowledge of health fluid choices; expresses knowledge of health food choices; expresses willingness to enhance nutrition; follows an appropriate standard for intake (e.g., the food pyramid or American Diabetic Association guidelines); safe preparation for fluids; safe preparation for food; safe storage for food and fluids

Client Outcomes

Client Will (Specify Time Frame):

- Explain how to eat according to the *Dietary Guidelines for Americans 2005*
- Design dietary modifications to meet individual long-term goal of health, using principles of variety, balance, and moderation
- Weigh within normal range for height and age

Nursing Interventions

- See the Nursing Interventions for **Imbalanced Nutrition: more than body requirements.**
- Ask the client to keep a food diary for 1-3 days, where everything consumed (food or drink) is recorded. Analyze the quality, quantity, and pattern of food intake.
- Advise the client to measure food periodically. Help the client learn usual portion sizes.
- Help the client determine their body mass index (BMI). Use a chart or a website such as: *http://www.bcm.edu/cnrc/caloriesneed.htm*
- Recommend the client use the interactive Food Pyramid site at www.MyPyramid.gov to determine the number of calories to eat and gain more information on how to eat in a healthy fashion.
- Recommend the client follow the Dietary Guidelines for Americans which can be found at www.healthierus.gov/dietaryguidelines. Use the Food Guide Pyramid to analyze the quality of the diet.
- Recommend the client eat a healthy breakfast every morning.
- Recommend the client avoid eating in fast food restaurants.

▲ Review the client's current exercise level. With the client and primary healthcare provider, design a long-term exercise program. Encourage the client to adopt an exercise program that involves walking 3-5 hours per week at an average pace.

- Demonstrate the use of food labels to make healthful choices. Alert the client/family to focus on serving size, total fat, and simple carbohydrate.
- Determine the client's knowledge of the need for supplements. Discourage the client from taking excessive amounts of vitamins unless prescribed by a physician.

Carbohydrates

- Encourage the client to decrease intake of sugars, including soft drinks, desserts, and candy. Limit sugar intake to 12 teaspoons of added sugar daily.
- Recommend the client eat whole grains whenever possible, and explain how to find whole grains using the food label.
- Evaluate the client's usual intake of fiber. Recommended intake is 25 grams per day.
- Recommend the client eat five to nine fruits and vegetables per day, with a minimum of two servings of fruit and three servings of vegetables. Encourage client to eat a rainbow of fruits and vegetables, because bright colors are associated with increased nutrients.

Fats

- Recommend the client limit intake of saturated fats and *trans*-fatty acids; instead increase intake of vegetable oils, such as canola oil and olive oil. Limit fat intake to around 30% of total calories per day.
- Recommend client use low-fat choices when selecting and cooking meat, and also when selecting dairy products.
- Recommend that the client eat cold-water fish, such as salmon, tuna, or mackerel, at least two times per week to ensure adequate intake of omega-3 fatty acids. If the client is unwilling to eat fish, suggest other sources, such as flaxseed, soy, or walnuts. NOTE: Fish oil capsules should be taken cautiously; some brands can be contaminated with mercury or pesticides.

Protein

- Recommend the client decrease intake of red meat and processed meats, instead eat more poultry, fish, and dairy sources of protein.

- Recommend the client eat meatless meals at intervals and try alternative sources of protein, including nuts, especially almonds (one handful), and nut butters.
- Recommend the client eat beans and especially soybeans as an alternative to animal proteins at intervals. Introduce the client to soy products, such as flavored soy milk.

Fluid and Electrolytes

- Recommend the client choose and prepare foods with less salt, aiming for a maximum of 2300 mg per day, which is approximately 1 teaspoon.
- If the client drinks alcohol, encourage him or her to drink in moderation—no more than one drink per day for women and two drinks per day for men.
- Recommend that the client increase intake of water to at least 2000 mL or 2 quarts per day. A guideline is 1 to 1.5 mL of fluid per each calorie needed, so an average intake would be between 2000 and 3000 mL/day, or at least 8 cups of fluid.

Pediatric

- Provide appropriate nutrition for children.

Geriatric

- Use a nutritional screening tool designed for older adults, such as the Mini Nutrition Assessment (MNA), the Malnutrition Universal Screening Tool (MUST), or the Nutrition Risk Screening (NRS). Assess changes in lifestyle and eating patterns.
- ▲ Recommend the client discuss the need for a low-dose balanced multiple vitamin and mineral supplement with physician.
- Assess fluid intake. Recommend routine drinks of water regardless of thirst.
- Observe for socioeconomic factors that influence food choices (e.g., finances, cooking facilities).
- Suggest a variety of seasonings.

Multicultural

- Assess for dietary intake of essential nutrients.
- Assess for the influence of cultural beliefs, norms, and values on the client's nutritional knowledge.

- Discuss with the client those aspects of their diet that will remain unchanged.
- Determine the motivational factors operating within the client at the present time.
- Negotiate with the client regarding the aspects of his or her diet that will need to be modified.
- Validate the client's feelings regarding the impact of current lifestyle, finances, and transportation on ability to obtain nutritious food.
- Encourage family meals.

Client/Family Teaching

- The majority of interventions previously described involve teaching.
- Work with the family members regarding information on how to improve nutritional status.
- Teach the importance of exercise in a weight control program.

Risk for imbalanced Nutrition: more than body requirements

NANDA Definition

At risk for intake of nutrients that exceeds metabolic needs

Risk Factors

Concentrating food at the end of day; dysfunctional eating patterns; eating in response to external cues (e.g., time of day, social situation); eating in response to internal cues other than hunger (e.g., anxiety); higher baseline weight at beginning of each pregnancy; observed use of food as comfort measure; observed use of food as reward; pairing food with other activities; parental obesity; rapid transition across growth percentiles in children; reported use of solid food as major food source before 5 months of age

Client Outcomes

Client Will (Specify Time Frame):

- Explain concept of a balanced diet
- Compare current eating pattern with recommended healthy one

- Design dietary modifications to meet individual long-term goal of weight control, using principles of variety, balance, and moderation
- Identify role of exercise in weight control

Nursing Interventions

- Refer to care plan for **Imbalanced Nutrition: more than body requirements.**

Impaired Oral mucous membrane

NANDA Definition

Disruptions of lips and soft tissues of oral cavity

Defining Characteristics

Bleeding; cheilitis; coated tongue; desquamation; difficult speech; difficulty eating; difficulty swallowing; diminished taste; edema; enlarged tonsils; fissures; geographic tongue; gingival hyperplasia; gingival pallor; gingival recession; halitosis; hyperemia; macroplasia; mucosal denudation; mucosal pallor; nodules; oral discomfort; oral lesions; oral pain; oral ulcers; papules; pocketing deeper than 4 mm; presence of pathogens; purulent drainage; purulent exudates; red or bluish masses (e.g., hemangiomas); reports bad taste in mouth; smooth atrophic tongue; spongy patches; stomatitis; vesicles; white curdlike exudates; white patches/plaques; xerostomia

Related Factors (r/t)

Barriers to oral self-care; barriers to professional care; chemotherapy; chemical irritants (e.g., alcohol, tobacco, acidic foods, drugs, regular use of inhalers or other noxious agents); cleft lip; cleft palate; decreased platelets; decreased salivation; deficient knowledge of appropriate oral hygiene; dehydration; depression; diminished hormone levels (women); ineffective oral hygiene; infection; immunocompromised; immunosuppression; loss of supportive structures; malnutrition; mechanical factors (e.g., ill-fitting dentures); braces; tubes (endotracheal/nasogastric); surgery in oral cavity; medication side effects; mouth breathing; NPO for more than 24 hours; radiation therapy; stress; trauma

Client Outcomes

Client Will (Specify Time Frame):

- Maintain intact, moist oral mucous membranes that are free of ulceration and debris
- Demonstrate measures to regain or maintain intact oral mucous membranes

Nursing Interventions

▲ Inspect the oral cavity at least once daily and note any discoloration, lesions, edema, bleeding, exudate, or dryness. Refer to a physician or dental specialist as appropriate.

- Assess for mechanical agents such as ill-fitting dentures and chemical agents such as frequent exposure to tobacco that could cause or increase trauma to oral mucous membranes.
- Monitor the client's nutritional and fluid status to determine if it is adequate. Refer to the care plan for **Deficient Fluid volume** or **Imbalanced Nutrition: less than body requirements** if applicable.
- Encourage fluid intake of up to 3000 mL/day if not contraindicated by the client's medical condition.
- Determine the client's mental status. If the client is unable to care for himself or herself, oral hygiene must be provided by nursing personnel. The nursing diagnosis **Bathing/hygiene Self-care deficit** is then applicable.
- Determine the client's usual method of oral care and address any concerns regarding oral hygiene.
- If the client does not have a bleeding disorder and is able to swallow, encourage the client to brush the teeth with a soft toothbrush using fluoride-containing toothpaste at least twice per day.
- Encourage the client to brush the tongue with the toothbrush or use a tongue scraper twice a day.
- If the client does not have a bleeding disorder, encourage the client to floss once per day or use an interdental cleaner.

Client Receiving Chemotherapy/Radiation

- Ensure that the client receives a comprehensive oral examination before initiation of chemotherapy or radiation, with aggressive preventative dental care given as needed.
- Provide instructions about the need for and method of providing frequent oral care to the client 1 week before radiation therapy.

- For measurement of presence or severity of mucositis, use the Oral Mucositis Assessment Scale (OMAS).
- Use cryotherapy with ice chips dissolved in the client's mouth before, during, and after bolus administration of fluorouracil to reduce the severity of mucositis. Also use cryotherapy for clients receiving bolus edatrexate and melphalan.
- Give the client frequent sips of water, and ask client to rinse the mouth with water regularly.
- If client has a dry mouth (xerostomia):
  - ■ Provide saliva substitutes as ordered.
  - ■ Suggest the client chew sugarless gum or sugarless sour candy to promote salivary flow.
  - ■ Provide ice chips frequently to keep the mouth moist.
- Help client use a mouth rinse of salt and soda every 1 to 2 hours for prevention and treatment of stomatitis.

▲ If the mouth is severely inflamed and it is painful to swallow, contact the physician for a topical anesthetic or analgesic order. Modification of oral intake (e.g., soft or liquid diet) may also be necessary to prevent friction trauma. The nursing diagnosis **Imbalanced Nutrition: less than body requirements** may apply.

- If the client's platelet count is lower than 50,000/mm^3 or the client has a bleeding disorder, use a specially made toothbrush designed for sensitive or diseased tissue, or a toothette that is not soaked in glycerin or flavorings; if the client cannot tolerate a toothbrush or a toothette, a piece of gauze wrapped around a finger can be used to remove plaque and debris.
- Use tap water or normal saline to provide oral care; do not use commercial mouthwashes containing alcohol or hydrogen peroxide. Also do not use lemon-glycerin swabs.
- Use foam sticks to moisten the oral mucous membranes, clean out debris, and swab out the mouth of the edentulous client. Do not use foam sticks to clean the teeth unless the platelet count is very low and the client is prone to bleeding gums.
- Keep the lips well lubricated by using a lip balm that is water or aloe based.

Client on a Ventilator

- Use a child-sized toothbrush to brush teeth; use suction to remove secretions.
- Use water as a rinsing agent and mouthwash.

▲ Apply chlorhexidine gluconate in the oral cavity by swab or spray early after intubation and at intervals if ordered.
• Refer to the care plan for **Impaired Dentition** if the client has problems with the teeth.

Geriatric

• Determine the functional ability of the client to provide his or her own oral care. Refer to **Bathing/hygiene Self-care deficit.**
• Provide appropriate oral care to the elderly with a self-care deficit by brushing the teeth after every meal.
• Carefully observe the oral cavity and lips for abnormal lesions such as white or red patches, masses, ulcerations with an indurated margin, or a raised granular lesion.
• Ensure that dentures are removed and scrubbed at least once daily, removed and rinsed thoroughly after every meal, and removed and kept in an appropriate solution at night.
• If the client has xerostomia, evaluate medications to see if they could be the cause, provide synthetic saliva products to moisten the oral cavity as ordered, and offer frequent sips of water and sugarless gum or candy to provide lubrication.

O

Home Care

• The interventions previously described may be adapted for home care use.
▲ If dryness is a side effect of the client's medication(s), instruct the client in the use of artificial saliva.
• Instruct the client to avoid alcohol-based or hydrogen peroxide–based commercial products for mouth care and to avoid other irritants to the oral cavity (e.g., tobacco, spicy foods).
• Instruct the client in ways to soothe the oral cavity (e.g., cool beverages, ice pops, viscous lidocaine).
• If the client often breathes by mouth, add humidity to the room unless contraindicated.
▲ If necessary, refer for home health aide services to support the family in oral care and observation of the oral cavity.

Client/Family Teaching

• Teach the client how to inspect the oral cavity and monitor for signs and symptoms of infection or complications as well as when to call the healthcare practitioner.

- Teach the client and family how to perform appropriate mouth care if necessary.
- Recommend the client use a powered toothbrush for removal of dental plaque and prevention of gingivitis.

Acute Pain

NANDA Definition

Pain is whatever the experiencing person says it is, existing whenever the person says it does. Unpleasant sensory and emotional experience arising from actual or potential tissue damage or described in terms of such damage; sudden or slow onset of pain of any intensity from mild to severe with anticipated or predictable end and a duration of less than 6 months.

Defining Characteristics

Subjective

Pain is always subjective and cannot be proved or disproved. A client's report of pain is the most reliable indicator of pain. A client with cognitive ability who can speak or point should use a pain rating scale (e.g., 0 to 10) to identify the current level of pain intensity (self-report) and determine a comfort-function goal. Establishment of a comfort-function goal involves helping the client to select a pain rating level that will allow the client to easily perform identified functional goals (e.g., a pain rating of 3 on a scale of 0 to 10 to cough, deep breathe, and ambulate).

Objective

Expressions of pain are extremely variable and cannot be used in lieu of self-report. Neither behavior nor vital signs can substitute for the client's self-report. However, observable responses to pain may be helpful in assessing clients who cannot or will not use a self-report pain rating scale. Observable responses may be loss of appetite and inability to deep breathe, ambulate, sleep, or perform ADLs. Clients may show guarding, self-protective behavior, self-focusing or narrowed focus, distraction behavior ranging from crying to laughing, and muscle tension or rigidity. In sudden and severe pain, autonomic responses such as diaphoresis, blood pressure and pulse changes, pupillary dilation, or increases or decreases in respiratory rate and depth may be present, but physiologic indicators are considered the least sensitive for pain as they may be a sign of other pathology, such as hypovolemia and anxiety. Physiological indicators may be used to confirm other findings; however, the absence of any physiological or behavioral indicator does not mean the absence of pain. A hierarchy of pain measures is recommended for the assessment of pain in patients who cannot report pain: (1) attempt to obtain self-report; (2) consider the presence of underlying painful pathology or condition and assume pain is present if appropriate; (3) observe behaviors that may indicate the presence of pain in patients who cannot report pain; (4) obtain a proxy (parent, caregiver, or significant other who knows patient very well) report of behaviors that might indicate pain; (5) attempt an analgesic trial whereby a dose of analgesia is administered and any reduction in pain behaviors is noted. From this analgesic trial a pain treatment plan can be developed.

Related Factors (r/t)

Injury agents (biological, chemical, physical, psychological)

Client Outcomes

Client Will (Specify Time Frame):

- Use pain rating scale to identify current pain intensity and determine comfort/function goal (if client has cognitive abilities)
- Describe how unrelieved pain will be managed
- Report that pain management regimen relieves pain to satisfactory level with acceptable and manageable side effects
- Perform activities of recovery with reported acceptable level of pain (if pain is above comfort-function goal, take action that decreases pain or notify a member of the health care team)
- If cognitively impaired, demonstrate a reduction in pain behaviors, have manageable and tolerable side effects, and perform recovery activities satisfactorily
- State ability to obtain sufficient amounts of rest and sleep
- Describe nonpharmacological method that can be used to help control pain

Nursing Interventions

▲ Determine whether the client is experiencing pain at the time of the initial interview. If so, intervene at that time to provide pain relief. Assess and document the intensity, character, onset, duration, and aggravating and relieving factors of pain during the initial evaluation of the client.

- Assess pain in a client by using a self-report such as the 0 to 10 numerical pain rating scale, Wong-Baker FACES Scale, or the Faces Pain Scale.
- Question the client regarding pain at frequent intervals, often at the same time as taking vital signs.
- Ask the client to describe past experiences with pain and the effectiveness of methods used to manage pain, including experiences with side effects, typical coping responses, and the way the client expresses pain.
- Establish a comfort-function goal with the client. Question the client regarding the level of pain that he or she believes is appropriate to achieve a state of comfort and appropriate function. Attempt to keep pain at a level that will allow the client to achieve functional and quality-of-life goals with relative ease.
- Describe the adverse effects of unrelieved pain.
- Assess and document the intensity of the pain and discomfort after any known pain-producing procedure, with each new report of pain, and at regular intervals.
- If the client is cognitively impaired and unable to report pain or use a pain rating scale, assess and document behaviors that may indicate pain (e.g., change in activity, loss of appetite, guarding, grimacing, moaning). A hierarchy of pain assessment is recommended in these clients: (1) attempt to obtain self-report because it is the single most reliable indicator of pain; (2) consider the presence of underlying painful pathology or condition and assume pain is present; (3) observe behaviors that may indicate the presence of pain; (4) obtain a proxy (parent, caregiver, or significant other who knows client very well) report of behaviors that might indicate pain; (5) attempt an analgesic trial in which a dose of analgesia is administered and any reduction in pain behaviors is noted.
- Assume that pain is present and treat accordingly in a client who has a pathological condition or who is undergoing a procedure thought to be painful.
- Attempt an analgesic trial in clients who are unable to report pain but have an underlying pathology or condition that is thought to be painful or have behaviors that may indicate the

presence of pain. Administer a nonopioid if pain is thought to be mild and an opioid if pain is thought to be moderate to severe. Observe for any change in behavior. Prevent pain when possible during procedures such as venipuncture, nasogastric tube insertion, and male Foley catheter insertion. Use a topical local anesthetic such as EMLA cream.

- • Determine the client's current medication use.
- ▲ Explore the need for both opioid (narcotic) and nonopioid analgesics.
- • Use a multimodal analgesic approach.
- ▲ Obtain a prescription to administer an opioid analgesic if indicated, especially for severe pain.
- ▲ Administer opioids orally or IV. Provide client-controlled analgesia (PCA), perineural infusions, and intraspinal analgesia as ordered and when appropriate and available.
- • Avoid giving pain medication intramuscularly (IM).
- • Explain to the client the pain management approach that has been ordered, including therapies, medication administration, side effects, and complications.
- • Plan nursing care when the client is comfortable based on the reality that oral opioid medications begin to work in approximately 1 hour and IV medications work in 5 to 30 minutes depending on the medication. Most transdermal medications become effective in 12 to 16 hours, with steady blood levels within 48 hours.
- • Discuss the client's fears of undertreated pain, overdose, and addiction.
- ▲ When opioids are administered, assess pain intensity, sedation, and respiratory status at regular intervals. Assess sedation and respiratory status at least every 2 hours for the first 24 hours of opioid therapy in opioid-naive clients (those who have not been taking regular daily doses of opioids). Awaken sleeping clients for further assessment if they have an inadequate respiratory rate; shallow, irregular, or noisy (snoring) respirations; or apneic episodes. Decrease the opioid dose immediately if the client is excessively sedated.
- • Review the client's flow sheet and medication records to determine overall degree of pain relief, side effects, and analgesic requirements during the previous 24 hours.
- ▲ Administer supplemental opioid doses as ordered to keep pain ratings at or below the comfort-function goal.

P

▲ Obtain prescriptions to increase or decrease opioid doses as needed; base prescriptions on the client's report of pain severity and response to the previous dose in terms of relief, side effects, and ability to perform the activities of recovery.

▲ When the client is able to tolerate oral analgesics, obtain a prescription to change to the oral route; use an equianalgesic chart to determine initial dose.

• In addition to administering analgesics, support the client's use of nonpharmacological methods to help control pain, such as distraction, imagery, relaxation, and application of heat and cold.

• Teach and implement nonpharmacological interventions when pain is relatively well controlled with pharmacological interventions.

▲ Ask the client to describe appetite, bowel elimination, and ability to rest and sleep. Administer medications and treatments to improve these functions. Obtain a prescription for a stool softener plus a peristaltic stimulant to prevent opioid-induced constipation if needed.

Pediatric

• As with adults, use complementary therapies to supplement, not replace, pharmacological interventions. For the neonate, use oral sucrose for pain of short duration such as heel stick or venipuncture.

• Recognize that breastfeeding has been shown to reduce behavioral indicators of pain. Use a topical local anesthetic such as EMLA cream or LMX-4 before performing venipuncture in an infant or child.

• For the neonate experiencing moderate to severe pain, use opioid analgesics and anesthetics in appropriate dosages.

• For the young child (age 4 years and older), use the Wong-Baker FACES Scale or the Faces Pain Scale to determine the level of pain present.

Geriatric

▲ Always take the older client's reports of pain seriously and ensure that the pain is relieved.

• When assessing pain, speak clearly, slowly, and loudly enough for the client to hear, and if the client uses a hearing aid, be sure it is in place; repeat information as needed. Be sure the client can see well enough to read the pain scale (use an enlarged scale) and written materials.

- • Handle the client's body gently. Allow the client to move at his or her own speed.
- ▲ Use acetaminophen and nonsteroidal antiinflammatory drugs (NSAIDs) with low gastrointestinal side effect profiles, such as the selective COX-2 selective NSAID celecoxib or the nonselective NSAID naproxen may be the safest, in clients with cardiovascular risk. Watch for side effects such as gastrointestinal and cardiovascular disturbances and renal dysfunction.
- ▲ Avoid or use with caution drugs with a long half-life, such as the NSAID piroxicam (Feldene) and the opioids methadone (Dolophine) and levorphanol (LevoDromoran).
- ▲ Use opioids with caution in the older client.
- ▲ Avoid the use of opioids with toxic metabolites, such as meperidine (Demerol) and propoxyphene (Darvon, Darvocet), in older clients.

Multicultural

- • Assess for the influence of cultural beliefs, norms, and values on the client's perception and experience of pain.
- • Assess for the effect of fatalism on the client's beliefs regarding the current state of comfort.
- • Assess for pain disparities among racial and ethnic minorities.
- • Incorporate safe and effective folk healthcare practices and beliefs into care whenever possible.
- • Use a family-centered approach to care.
- • Teach information about pain medications and their side effects and how to work with healthcare providers to manage pain, and encourage clients to use religious faith to cope with pain.
- • Use culturally relevant pain scales to assess pain in the client.
- • Ensure that directions for medication use are available in the client's language of choice and are understood by the client and caregiver.

Home Care

- • Develop the treatment plan with the client and caregivers.
- ▲ Develop a full medication profile, including medications prescribed by all physicians and all over-the-counter medications.

Assess for drug interactions. Instruct the client to refrain from mixing medications without physician approval.

- Assess the client's and family's knowledge of side effects and safety precautions associated with pain medications (e.g., use caution in operating machinery when opioids are first taken or dosage has been significantly increased).
- If medication is administered by using highly technological methods, assess the home for the necessary resources (e.g., electricity) and ensure that responsible caregivers will be available to assist the client with administration.

▲ Assess the knowledge base of the client and family with regard to highly technological medication administration. Teach as necessary. Be sure the client knows when, how, and whom to contact if analgesia is unsatisfactory.

Client/Family Teaching

NOTE: To avoid the negative connotations associated with the words *drugs* and *narcotics,* use the term *pain medicine* when teaching clients.

- Provide written materials on pain control.
- Discuss the various discomforts encompassed by the word *pain* and ask the client to give examples of previously experienced pain. Explain the pain assessment process and the purpose of the pain rating scale.

▲ Teach the client to use the pain rating scale to rate the intensity of past or current pain. Ask the client to set a comfort-function goal by selecting a pain level on the rating scale that makes it easy to perform recovery activities (e.g., turn, cough, deep breathe). If pain is above this level, the client should take action that decreases pain or notify a member of the healthcare team. (See information on teaching clients to use the pain rating scale.)

▲ Demonstrate medication administration and the use of supplies and equipment. If PCA is ordered, determine the client's ability to press the appropriate button. Remind the client and staff that the PCA button is for client use only.

- Reinforce the importance of taking pain medications to keep pain under control.
- Reinforce that taking opioids for pain relief is not addiction and that addiction is not likely to occur.

P

- Demonstrate the use of appropriate nonpharmacological approaches in addition to pharmacological approaches for helping control pain, such as application of heat and/or cold, distraction techniques, relaxation breathing, visualization, rocking, stroking, music listening, and television watching.

Chronic Pain

NANDA Definition

Pain is whatever the experiencing person says it is, existing whenever the person says it does.

Pain is an unpleasant sensory and emotional experience arising from actual or potential tissue damage or described in terms of such damage; sudden or slow onset of pain of any intensity from mild to severe, constant or recurring, without anticipated or predictable end and a duration of greater than six months; state in which the individual experiences pain that persists for a period beyond the usual course of acute illness or a reasonable duration for the injury to heal, is associated with a chronic pathological process, or recurs at intervals for months or years.

Defining Characteristics

Subjective

Pain is always subjective and cannot be proved or disproved. The client's report of pain is the most reliable indicator of pain. Clients with cognitive abilities who can speak or point should use a pain rating scale (e.g., 0 to 10) to identify their current level of pain intensity (self-report) and determine a comfort-function goal. Establishment of a comfort-function goal involves assisting clients in selecting a pain rating that will allow them to easily perform identified functional goals (e.g., a pain rating of 3 on a scale of 0 to 10 to work or walk the dog).

Objective

Expressions of pain are extremely variable and cannot be used in lieu of self-report. Neither behavior nor vital signs can substitute for the client's self-report. However, observable responses to pain may be helpful in pain assessment, especially in clients who cannot or will not use a self-report pain rating scale. Observable responses may be loss of appetite or the inability to ambulate, perform ADLs, work, or sleep. Clients may show guarding, self-protective behavior, self-focusing or narrowed focus, distraction behavior ranging from crying to laughing, and muscle tension or rigidity. In sudden severe pain, autonomic responses such as diaphoresis, blood pressure and pulse changes, pupillary dilation, and increase or decrease in respiratory rate and depth may be present but are usually not seen with chronic pain that is relatively stable. A hierarchy of pain measures is recommended for the assessment of pain in clients who cannot report pain: (1) attempt to obtain self report, (2) consider the presence of underlying painful pathology or condition and assume pain is present if appropriate, (3) observe behaviors that may indicate the presence of pain, (4) obtain a proxy (parent, caregiver, or significant other who knows patient very well) report of behaviors that might indicate pain, (5) attempt an analgesic trial whereby a dose of analgesia is administered and any reduction in pain behaviors is noted. From this analgesic trial a pain treatment plan can be developed. Clients with chronic or persistent cancer or nonmalignant pain may experience threats to self-image; a perceived lack of options for coping; and worsening helplessness, anxiety, and depression. Chronic pain may affect almost every aspect of the client's daily life, including concentration, work, and relationships.

Related Factors (r/t)

Actual or potential tissue damage; tumor progression and related pathology; diagnostic and therapeutic procedures; central or peripheral nerve injury (neuropathic pain). NOTE: The cause of chronic nonmalignant pain may not be known because pain study is a new science and an area encompassing diverse types of problems.

Client Outcomes

Client Will (Specify Time Frame):

- Use pain rating scale to identify current level of pain intensity, determine comfort/function goal, and maintain a pain diary (if client has cognitive abilities)
- Describe total plan for pharmacological and nonpharmacological pain relief, including how to safely and effectively take medicines and integrate nondrug therapies
- Demonstrate ability to pace self, taking rest breaks before they are needed

- Function on acceptable ability level with minimal interference from pain and medication side effects (if pain is above comfort-function goal, take action that decreases pain or notify a member of healthcare team)
- If cognitively impaired, demonstrate a reduction in pain behaviors, have manageable and tolerable side effects, and perform ADLs satisfactorily

Nursing Interventions

▲ Determine whether the client is experiencing pain at the time of the initial interview. If so, intervene at that time to provide pain relief. Assess and document the intensity, character, onset, duration, and aggravating and relieving factors of pain during the initial evaluation of the client.

- Assess pain in a client by using a self-report 0 to 10 numerical pain rating scale, Wong-Baker FACES scale, or Faces Pain Scale.
- Question the client regarding pain at frequent intervals, such as while taking vital signs.
- Tell the client to report pain location, intensity, and quality when experiencing pain. Assess and document the intensity of pain and discomfort after any known pain-producing procedure, with each new report of pain, and at regular intervals.
- Question the client regarding the level of pain that he or she believes is appropriate to achieve a state of comfort and appropriate function. Attempt to keep pain level no higher than that level, preferably much lower.
- Ask the client to describe past and current experiences with pain and the effectiveness of the methods used to manage the pain, including experiences with side effects, typical coping responses, and the way the client expresses pain.
- Describe the adverse effects of unrelieved pain.
- Ask the client to maintain a diary (if able) of pain ratings, timing, precipitating events, medications, treatments, and steps that work best to relieve pain.
- If the client is cognitively impaired and unable to report pain or use a pain rating scale, assess and document behaviors that might be indicative of pain (e.g., change in activity, loss of appetite, guarding, grimacing, moaning). Use a hierarchy of pain measures to assess pain in clients who cannot report pain: (1) attempt to obtain a self-report, (2) consider the presence of

underlying painful pathology or condition and assume pain is present if appropriate, (3) observe behaviors that may indicate the presence of pain, (4) obtain a proxy (parent, caregiver, or significant other who knows client very well) report of behaviors that might indicate pain, (5) attempt an analgesic trial in which a dose of analgesia is administered and any reduction in pain behaviors is noted. Develop a treatment plan based on the analgesic trial.

▲ Assume that pain is present and treat accordingly in clients who have a pathological condition or are undergoing a procedure thought to be painful.

• Obtain a complete history of medications the client is taking, including over-the-counter medications, or has taken to prevent drug-drug interactions and toxicity problems that can occur when incompatible drugs are combined or when allergies are present.

▲ Explore the need for medications from the three classes of analgesic: opioids (narcotics), nonopioids (acetaminophen, nonsteroidal antiinflammatory drugs), and adjuvant medications. For chronic neuropathic pain, consider adjuvant medications that are analgesic, such as anticonvulsants and antidepressants.

▲ For persistent mild cancer pain, obtain a prescription to administer nonopioid analgesics.

▲ For persistent chronic nonmalignant pain, discuss the use of opioid analgesics with the healthcare team and obtain a prescription to administer if appropriate.

▲ The oral route for pain medication administration is preferred. If the client is receiving parenteral analgesia, use an equianalgesic chart to convert to a controlled release, long-acting oral medication as soon as possible.

▲ Avoid the IM route for administration of pain medication.

▲ Establish around-the-clock dosing and administer supplemental opioid doses for breakthrough pain as needed to keep pain ratings at or below the comfort-function goal.

▲ Ask the client to describe appetite and bowel elimination. Always obtain a prescription for a stool softener and a peristaltic stimulant daily to prevent opioid-induced constipation in clients taking regular daily doses of opioids.

• Question the client about any disruption in sleep.

• Watch for signs of depression in clients with chronic pain, in-

P

cluding sleeplessness, not eating, flat affect, statements of depression, or suicidal ideation.

- • Explain to the client the pain management approach that has been ordered, including therapies, medication administration, side effects, and complications. Discuss the client's fears of undertreated pain, addiction, and overdose.
- • Review the client's pain diary, flow sheet, and medication records to determine the overall degree of pain relief, side effects, and analgesic requirements for an appropriate period (e.g., 1 week).
- ▲ Obtain prescriptions to increase or decrease analgesic doses when indicated. Base prescriptions on the client's report of pain severity and the comfort-function goal and response to previous dose in terms of relief, side effects, and ability to perform ADLs and comply with the prescribed therapeutic regimen.
- ▲ If opioid dose is increased, monitor sedation and respiratory status for a brief time.
- ▲ In addition to the use of analgesics, support the client's use of nonpharmacological methods to help control pain, such as physical therapy, group therapy, distraction, imagery, relaxation, massage, and application of heat and cold.
- • Teach and implement nonpharmacological interventions when pain is relatively well controlled with pharmacological means.
- • Encourage the client to plan activities around periods of greatest comfort whenever possible.
- • Explore appropriate resources for management of pain on a long-term basis (e.g., hospice, pain care center).
- • If the client has progressive cancer pain, assist the client and family with handling issues related to death and dying.
- • Assist the client and family in minimizing the effects of pain on interpersonal relationships and daily activities such as work and recreation.

P

Pediatric

- • For the young child (4 years of age and older) use the Wong-Baker FACES Scale or the Faces Pain Scale to determine the level of pain present.
- • Help children and adolescents learn and use techniques such as relaxation and cognitive-behavioral techniques to handle pain.

Geriatric

- ▲ Always take an older client's reports of pain seriously and ensure that the pain is relieved.
- • When assessing pain, speak clearly, slowly, and loudly enough for the client to hear. If the client uses a hearing aid, be sure it is in place; repeat information as needed. Be sure the client can see well enough to read the pain scale (use an enlarged scale) and written materials.
- • In the absence of the client's report of pain in situations where pain is expected (e.g., anesthetized, critically ill, or cognitively impaired client), the clinician should assume pain is present and treat accordingly.
- • Handle the client's body gently. Allow the client to move at his or her own speed.
- ▲ Use acetaminophen and NSAIDs with low gastrointestinal side effect profiles, such as celecoxib (Celebrex), choline magnesium trisalicylate (Trilisate), and diflunisal (Dolobid). Naproxen may be the best choice for long term treatment. Watch closely for side effects, such as cardiovascular and gastrointestinal disturbances and bleeding and renal problems.
- ▲ Avoid or use with caution drugs with a long half-life, such as the NSAID piroxicam (Feldene) and the opioids methadone (Dolophine) and levorphanol (LevoDromoran).
- ▲ Use opioids cautiously in the older client with moderate to severe pain unrelieved by NSAIDs. Reduce initial doses by 25% to 50%. After titrating to comfort with a short-acting opioid, switch to an extended-release opioid for persistent pain treatment.
- ▲ Avoid the use of opioids with toxic metabolites, such as meperidine (Demerol) and propoxyphene (Darvon, Darvocet), in older clients.
- ▲ Monitor for signs of depression in elders and refer for treatment if needed.

Multicultural

- • Assess for the influence of cultural beliefs, norms, and values on the client's perception and experience of pain.
- • A representational approach offers a flexible framework for nurses to get cancer clients to delve deeply into their own belief

systems about health, disease, and pain and to add sound concepts that work for their pain management. The program is called Representational Intervention to Decrease Cancer Pain (RIDcancerPain) and has the following 6 steps:

1. Representational assessment: the client describes beliefs about cancer pain along five dimensions (identity, cause, timeline, consequences, and cure/control)
2. Exploring misconceptions, with emphasis on their origins
3. Creating conditions for conceptual change by discussing the limitations of holding beliefs that are misconceptions (i.e., what one loses by maintaining those beliefs)
4. Introducing replacement information
5. Summarizing and discussing benefits of adopting beliefs that are credible replacements
6. Developing a plan and strategies

- • Assess for the effect of fatalism on the client's beliefs regarding the current state of comfort.
- • Assess for pain disparities among racial and ethnic minorities.
- • Incorporate safe and effective folk healthcare practices and beliefs into care whenever possible.
- • Use a family-centered approach to care.
- • Teach information about pain medications and their side effects and how to work with health care providers to manage pain, and encourage the use of religious faith to cope with pain.
- • Use culturally relevant pain scales to assess pain in the client.
- • Ensure that directions for medication use are available in the client's language of choice and are understood by the client and caregiver.

P

Home Care

- • Develop the treatment plan with the client and caregivers.
- ▲ Develop a full medication profile, including medications prescribed by all physicians and all over-the-counter medications. Assess for drug interactions. Instruct the client to refrain from mixing medications without physician approval.
- • Assess the client's and family's knowledge of side effects and safety precautions associated with pain medications (e.g., use caution if operating machinery when opioids are first taken or dosage has been significantly increased).
- ▲ Collaborate with the healthcare team (including the client and

family) on an ongoing basis to determine an optimal pain control profile. Identify the most effective interventions and the medication administration routes most acceptable to the client and family.

- If medication is administered by highly technological methods, assess the home for necessary resources (e.g., electricity) and ensure that responsible caregivers will be available to help the client with administration.
- ▲ Assess the knowledge base of the client and family for highly technological medication administration. Teach as necessary. Be sure the client knows when, how, and whom to contact if analgesia is unsatisfactory.
- Support the client and family in the use of opioid analgesics.

Client/Family Teaching

NOTE: To avoid the negative connotations associated with the words *drugs* and *narcotics,* use the term *pain medicine* when teaching clients.

- Provide written materials on pain control.
- Discuss the various discomforts encompassed by the word pain and ask the client to give examples of previously experienced pain. Explain the pain assessment process and the purpose of the pain rating scale.
- ▲ Ask the client to set a comfort-function goal by selecting a pain level on the rating scale that makes it easy to perform recovery activities (e.g., turn, cough, deep breathe). If pain is above this level, the client should take action that decreases pain or notify a member of the healthcare team. (See information on teaching clients to use the pain rating scale.)
- Discuss the total plan for pharmacological and nonpharmacological treatment, including the medication plan for around-the-clock administration and supplemental doses, the maintenance of a pain diary, and the use of supplies and equipment.
- Reinforce the importance of taking pain medications to keep pain under control.
- Reinforce that taking opioids for pain relief is not addiction and that addiction is highly unlikely.
- Explain to a client with chronic neuropathic pain the process of taking adjuvant analgesics (e.g., tricyclic antidepressants).
- Suggest the client with cancer try having a massage, with aromatherapy if desired.

P

- • Emphasize to the client the importance of pacing himself or herself and taking rest breaks before they are needed.
- ▲ Demonstrate the use of appropriate nonpharmacological approaches in addition to pharmacological approaches for helping to control pain (e.g., physical therapy, group therapy, distraction, imagery, and application of heat and cold).
- • Teach and implement nonpharmacological interventions when pain is relatively well controlled with pharmacological means.

Readiness for enhanced Parenting

NANDA Definition

A pattern of providing an environment for children or other dependent person(s) that is sufficient to nurture growth and development and can be strengthened.

Defining Characteristics

Children or other dependent person(s) express(es) satisfaction with home environment, emotional support of children; evidence of attachment; exhibits realistic expectations of children; expresses willingness to enhance parenting; needs of children are met (e.g., physical and emotional)

Client Outcomes

Client/Family Will (Specify Time Frame):

- Affirm desire to improve parenting skills to further support growth and development of children
- Demonstrate loving relationship with children
- Provide a safe, nurturing environment
- Assess risks in home/environment and takes steps to prevent possibility of harm to children
- Meet physical, psychosocial, and spiritual needs or seek appropriate assistance

Nursing Interventions

- • Use family-centered care and role modeling for holistic care of families.

- • Assess parents' feelings when dealing with a child who has a chronic illness.
- • Encourage positive parenting: respect for children, understanding of normal development, and use of creative and loving approaches to meet parenting challenges.
- • Promote low-technology interventions, such as massage and multisensory interventions (maternal voice, eye-to-eye contact, and rocking) to reduce maternal and infant stress and improve mother-infant relationship.
- • Provide opportunities for mother-infant skin-to-skin contact (kangaroo care) for preterm infants.
- • Provide the parent with the opportunity to assist in the newborn's first bath, allowing a flexible bath time.
- • When the person who is ill is the parent, use family-centered assessment skills to determine the impact of an adult's illness on the child and then guide the parent through those topics that are most likely to be of concern.
- ▲ Have family members participate in client conferences that involve all members of the healthcare team.
- ▲ Help parents develop realistic expectations of their child's development.
- • Provide practical and psychological assistance for parents of clients with psychiatric diagnoses, such as schizophrenia.

Multicultural

- • Assess the influence of cultural beliefs, norms, and values on the client's perception of parenting.
- • Acknowledge racial and ethnic differences at the onset of care.
- • Clarify parents' feelings, expectations, perceptions, and availability regarding participation in the care of their sick child. Acknowledge that value conflicts from acculturation stresses may contribute to increased anxiety and significant conflict with children.
- • Acknowledge and praise parenting strengths noted.

Home Care

- • The nursing interventions previously described should be used in the home environment with adaptations as necessary.
- ▲ Refer to a parenting program to facilitate learning of parenting skills.

P

Client/Family Teaching

- Refer to Client/Family Teaching for **Impaired Parenting** and **Risk for impaired Parenting** for suggestions that may be used with minor adaptations.
- Teach parents home safety: reduction of hot water temperature, proper poison storage, use of smoke alarms, and installation of safety gates for stairs.
- Teach parents and young teens conflict resolution by using a hypothetical conflict solution with and without a structured conflict resolution guide.
- ▲ Refer mothers of children with type 1 diabetes for community support in babysitting, child care, or respite.
- Support empowerment of parents of children with asthma and other chronic diseases.
- Parent training is one of the most effective interventions for behavior problems in young children. Teach families the importance of monitoring television viewing and limiting exposure to violence.
- Consider individual- and/or group-based parenting programs for teenage mothers.
- Consider group-based parenting programs for parents of children younger than 3 years with emotional and behavioral problems.
- Consider group-based parenting programs for parents with anxiety, depression, and/or low self-esteem.
- ▲ Refer adolescent parents for comprehensive psychoeducational parenting classes.
- Promotion of better-quality relationships between parents and children is an effective strategy that can lead to enhanced learning. Good-quality parenting leads to improved cognitive and social skills for the children.

P

Impaired Parenting

NANDA Definition

Inability of the primary caretaker to create, maintain, or regain an environment that promotes the optimum growth and development of the child.

Defining Characteristics

Infant or Child

Behavioral disorders; failure to thrive; frequent accidents; frequent illness; incidence of abuse; incidence of trauma (e.g., physical and psychological); lack of attachment; lack of separation anxiety; poor academic performance; poor cognitive development; poor social competence; runaway

Parental

Abandonment; child abuse; child neglect; frequently punitive; hostility to child; inadequate attachment; inadequate child health maintenance; inappropriate caretaking skills; inappropriate stimulation (e.g., visual, tactile, auditory); inappropriate child care arrangements; inconsistent behavior management; inconsistent care; inflexibility in meeting needs of child; little cuddling; maternal-child interaction deficit; negative statements about child; poor parent-child interaction; rejection of child; statements of inability to meet child's needs; unsafe home environment; verbalization of inability to control child; verbalization of frustration; verbalization of role inadequacy

Related Factors (r/t)

Infant/Child

Altered perceptual abilities; attention deficit–hyperactivity disorder; developmental delay; difficult temperament; handicapping condition; illness; multiple births; not desired gender; premature birth; separation from parent; temperamental conflicts with parental expectations

Knowledge

Deficient knowledge about child development; deficient knowledge about child health maintenance; deficient knowledge about parenting skills; inability to respond to infant cues; lack of cognitive readiness for parenthood; lack of education; limited cognitive functioning; poor communication skills; preference for physical punishment; unrealistic expectations

Physiological

Physical illness

Psychological

Closely spaced pregnancies; depression; difficult birthing process; disability; high number of pregnancies; history of mental illness; history of substance abuse; lack of prenatal care; sleep deprivation; sleep disruption; young parental age

Social

Change in family unit; chronic low self-esteem; father of child not involved; financial difficulties; history of being abused; history of being abusive; inability to put child's needs before own; job problems; lack of family cohesiveness; lack of parental role model; lack of resources; lack of social support networks; lack of transportation; lack of valuing of parenthood; legal difficulties; low socioeconomic status; maladaptive coping strategies; marital conflict; mother of child not involved; single parent; social isolation; poor home environment; poor parental role model; poor problem-solving skills; poverty; presence of stress (e.g., financial, legal, recent crisis, cultural move); relocations; role strain; situational low self-esteem; unemployment; unplanned pregnancy; unwanted pregnancy

Client Outcomes

Client Will (Specify Time Frame):

- Initiate appropriate measures to develop a safe, nurturing environment
- Acquire and display attentive, supportive parenting behaviors and child supervision
- Identify appropriate strategies to manage a child's inappropriate behaviors
- Identify strategies to protect child from harm and/or neglect and initiate action when indicated

Nursing Interventions

- Refer to **Readiness for enhanced Parenting** for additional interventions.
- Use the Parenting Risk Scale to assess parenting.
- Examine the characteristics of parenting style and behaviors, including the following: emotional climate at home, attribution of negative traits to the child, failure to support the child's increases in autonomy, type of interaction with the infant or child, competition with the child for attention of spouse/significant

other, lack of knowledge or concern about health maintenance or behavioral problems, other behaviors or concerns.

▲ Institute abuse/neglect protection measures if evidence exists of an inability to cope with family stressors or crisis, signs of parental substance abuse are observed, or a significant level of social isolation is apparent.

▲ For a mother with a toddler, assess maternal depression, perceptions of difficult temperament in the toddler, and low maternal self-efficacy. Make appropriate referral.

- Appraise the parent's resources and the availability of social support systems. Determine the single mother's particular sources of support, especially the availability of her own mother and partner. Encourage the use of healthy, strong support systems.
- Provide education to at-risk parents on behavioral management techniques such as looking ahead, giving good instructions, providing positive reinforcement, redirecting, planned ignoring, and instituting time-outs.
- Promotion of better-quality relationships between parents and children is an effective strategy that can lead to enhanced learning. Good-quality parenting leads to improved cognitive and social skills for the children. Support parents' competence in appraising their infant's behavior and responses.
- Aim supportive interventions at minimizing parents' experience of strain.
- Encourage kangaroo care by parents of preterm infants.
- Model age-appropriate and cognitively appropriate caregiver skills by doing the following: communicating with the child at an appropriate cognitive level of development, giving the child tasks and responsibilities appropriate to age or functional age/level, instituting safety considerations such as the use of assistive equipment, and encouraging the child to perform activities of daily living as appropriate.
- Encourage mothers to understand and capitalize on their infants' capacity to interact, particularly in the early months of life.

▲ Provide programs for homeless mothers with severe mental illness who have lost physical custody of their children.

▲ Provide a recovery program that includes instruction in parenting skills and child development for mothers who are addicted to cocaine.

P

Multicultural

- Acknowledge racial and ethnic differences at the onset of care.
- Approach individuals of color with respect, warmth, and professional courtesy.
- Clarify parents' feelings, expectations, perceptions, and availability regarding participation in the care of their sick child. Use a neutral, indirect style when addressing areas in which improvement is needed, such as a need for verbal stimulation when working with Native-American clients.
- Provide support for Chinese families caring for children with disabilities.
- Validate the client's feelings regarding parenting.
- Facilitate modeling and role playing to help the family improve parenting skills.

Home Care

- The interventions previously described may be adapted for home care use.
- Assess parenting stress at each home visit to provide appropriate support and anticipatory guidance to families of children with a chronic disease.

▲ Assess the single mother's history regarding childhood and partner abuse and current status regarding depressive symptoms, abusive parenting attitudes (lack of empathy, favorable opinion of corporal punishment, parent-child role-reversal, inappropriate expectations). Refer for mental health services as indicated.

▲ Implement behavioral parent training, including enhancement of skills in child-directed play, effective use of commands, use of discipline measures such as imposing time-outs and providing immediate and natural consequences, problem solving, and communication strategies.

Client/Family Teaching

- Consider individual and/or group-based parenting programs for teenage mothers.
- Consider group-based parenting programs for parents of children younger than 3 years with emotional and behavioral problems.

▲ Refer adolescent parents for comprehensive psychoeducational parenting classes.

- Explain individual differences in children's temperaments and compare them with the parents' expectations. Help parents determine and understand the implications of their child's temperament.

- Support empowerment of parents of children with asthma and other chronic diseases.
- Parent training is one of the most effective interventions for behavior problems in young children. Discuss sound disciplinary techniques, which include catching children being good, listening actively, conveying positive regard, ignoring minor transgressions, giving good directions, using praise, and imposing time-outs.
- Encourage positive parenting: respect for children, understanding of normal development, and creative and loving approaches to meet parenting challenges.
- Plan parental education directed toward the following age-related parental concerns. Birth to 2 years: transition, sleep, aggression; 3 to 5 years: transition, parent-child relationship, sleep; 6 to 10 years: school, parent-child relationship, divorce; 11 to 18 years: parent-child relationship, divorce, school.

▲ Initiate referrals to community agencies, parent education programs, stress management training, and social support groups.

▲ Provide information regarding available telephone counseling services.

- Refer to the care plan for **Delayed Growth and development** and **Risk for impaired parent/child Attachment** for additional teaching interventions.

Risk for impaired Parenting

NANDA Definition

Risk for inability of the primary caretaker to create, maintain, or regain an environment that promotes the optimum growth and development of the child.

Risk Factors

Infant/Child

Altered perceptual abilities; attention deficit–hyperactivity disorder; developmental delay; difficult temperament; handicapping condition; illness; multiple births; not gender desired; premature birth;

prolonged separation from parent; temperamental conflicts with parental expectation

Knowledge

Deficient knowledge about child development; deficient knowledge about child health maintenance; deficient knowledge about parenting skills; inability to respond to infant cues; lack of cognitive readiness for parenthood; low cognitive functioning; low educational level or attainment; poor communication skills; preference for physical punishment; unrealistic expectations of child

Physiological

Physical illness

Psychological

Closely spaced pregnancies; depression; difficult birthing process; disability; high number of pregnancies; history of mental illness; history of substance abuse; sleep deprivation; sleep disruption; young parental age

Social

Change in family unit; chronic low self-esteem; father of child not involved; financial difficulties; history of being abused; history of being abusive; inadequate child care arrangements; job problems; lack of access to resources; lack of family cohesiveness; lack of parental role model; lack of prenatal care; lack of resources; lack of social support network; lack of transportation; lack of valuing of parenthood; late prenatal care; legal difficulties; low socioeconomic class; maladaptive coping strategies; marital conflict; mother of child not involved; parent-child separation; poor home environment; poor parental role model; poor problem-solving skills; poverty; role strain; single parent; situational low self esteem; social isolation; stress; relocation; unemployment; unplanned pregnancy; unwanted pregnancy

Client Outcomes

Client Will (Specify Time Frame):

- Successfully establish a nurturing parenting role
- Affirm desire to acquire and maintain constructive parenting skills to support infant/child growth and development

- Maintain appropriate measures to develop a safe, nurturing environment
- Display attentive, supportive parenting behaviors
- Have knowledge of strategies to protect child from harm and/or neglect

Nursing Interventions

Refer to care plans **Readiness for enhanced Parenting** and **Impaired Parenting.**

Risk for Peripheral neurovascular dysfunction

NANDA Definition

At risk for disruption in circulation, sensation, or motion of an extremity

Risk Factors

Burns; fractures; immobilization; mechanical compression (e.g., tourniquet, cane, cast, brace, dressing, restraint); orthopedic surgery; trauma; vascular obstruction

Client Outcomes

Client Will (Specify Time Frame):

- Maintain circulation, sensation, and movement of an extremity within client's own normal limits
- Explain signs of neurovascular compromise and ways to prevent venous stasis

Nursing Interventions

- Perform neurovascular assessment every 1 to 4 hours or every 15 minutes as ordered.
- Use the six Ps of assessment:
  - **Pain:** Assess severity (on a scale of 1 to 10), quality, radiation, and relief by medications.
  - **Pulses:** Check the pulses distal to the injury.
  - **Pallor/Poikilothermia:** Check color and temperature changes below the injury site. Check capillary refill.

- **Paresthesia** (change in sensation): Check by lightly touching the skin proximal and distal to the injury. Ask if the client has any unusual sensations such as hypersensitivity, tingling, prickling, decreased feeling, or numbness.
- **Paralysis:** Ask the client to perform appropriate range-of-motion exercises in the unaffected and then the affected extremity.
- **Pressure:** Check by feeling the extremity; note new onset of firmness of the extremity.

• Monitor the client for symptoms of compartment syndrome evidenced by pain greater than expected, pain with passive movement, decreased sensation, weakness, loss of movement, absence of pulse, and tension in the skin that surrounds the muscle compartment.

• Monitor appropriate application and function of corrective device (e.g., cast, splint, traction) every 1 to 4 hours as needed.

• Position the extremity in correct alignment with each position change; check every hour to ensure appropriate alignment.

P

▲ Get the client out of bed and mobilize the client as soon as possible after consultation with the physician.

▲ Monitor for signs of DVT, especially in high-risk populations, including persons older than 40 years; persons with immobility or obesity; persons taking estrogen or oral contraceptives; persons with a history of trauma, surgery, or previous DVT; and persons with a cerebrovascular accident, varicose veins, malignancy, or cardiovascular disease.

▲ Apply graduated compression stockings if ordered; measure carefully to ensure proper fit, removing at least daily to assess circulation and skin condition.

• Watch for and report signs of DVT as evidenced by pain, deep tenderness, swelling in the calf and thigh, and redness in the involved extremity. Take serial leg measurements of the thigh and leg circumferences. In some clients, a tender venous cord can be felt in the popliteal fossa. Do not rely on Homans' sign.

▲ Help the client perform prescribed exercises every 4 hours as ordered.

• Provide a nutritious diet and adequate fluid replacement.

Geriatric

• Use heat and cold therapies cautiously.

Home Care

- • Assess the knowledge base of the client and family after any institutional care.
- • Teach about the disease process and care as necessary.
- • If risk is related to fractures and cast care, teach the family to complete a neurovascular assessment; it may be performed as often as every 4 hours but is more commonly done two to three times per day.
- • If the fracture is peripheral, position the limb for comfort and change position frequently, avoiding dependent positions for extended periods.
- ▲ Refer to physical therapy services as necessary to establish an exercise program and safety in transfers or mobility within limitations of physical status.
- • Establish an emergency plan.

Client/Family Teaching

- • Teach the client and family to recognize signs of neurovascular dysfunction and report signs immediately to the appropriate person.
- • Emphasize proper nutrition to promote healing.
- ▲ If necessary, refer the client to a rehabilitation facility for instruction in proper use of assistive devices and measures to improve mobility without compromising neurovascular function.

P

Risk for Poisoning

NANDA Definition

Accentuated risk of accidental exposure to, or ingestion of, drugs or dangerous products in doses sufficient to cause poisoning

Risk Factors

External

Availability of illicit drugs potentially contaminated by poisonous additives; dangerous products placed within reach of children; dangerous products placed within reach of confused individuals; large supplies of drugs in house; medicines stored in unlocked cabinets; medicines stored in unlocked cabinets accessible to confused individuals

Internal

Cognitive difficulties; emotional difficulties; lack of drug education; lack of proper precaution; lack of safety education; reduced vision; verbalization that occupational setting is without adequate safeguards

Client Outcomes

Client Will (Specify Time Frame):

- Prevent inadvertent ingestion of or exposure to toxins or poisonous substances
- Explain and undertake appropriate safety measures to prevent ingestion of or exposure to toxins or poisonous substances

Nursing Interventions

- When a client comes to the hospital with possible poisoning, begin care following the ABCs and administer oxygen if needed.
- Obtain a thorough history of what was ingested, how much, and when, and ask to look at the container. Note the client's age, weight, medications, and any medical conditions.
- Carefully inspect for signs of ingestion of poisons, including an odor on the breath, a trace of the substance on the clothing, burns or redness around the mouth and lips, as well as signs of confusion, vomiting, or dyspnea.
- Note results of toxicology screens, arterial blood gasses, blood glucose levels, and any other ordered laboratory tests.

▲ Initiate any ordered treatment for poisoning quickly.

- Prevent iatrogenic harm to the hospitalized client by following these guidelines for administering medications:
  - Use at least two methods to identify the client before administering medications or blood products, such as the client's name and medical record number or birth date.
  - When taking verbal or telephone orders, the orders should be written down and then read back for verification to the individual giving the order.
  - Standardize use of abbreviations and eliminate those that are prone to cause errors.
  - Take high-alert medications off the nursing unit, such as potassium chloride. Standardize concentrations of medications such as morphine in PCA pumps.

- Use only IV pumps that prevent free flow of IV solution when the tubing is taken out of the pump.
- Identify all the client's current medications on admission to a healthcare facility and ensure that all healthcare staff have access to the information.

• Detect possible interactions and cumulative or other adverse effects among prescribed medications, self-administered over-the-counter products, culturally based home treatments, herbal remedies, and foods.

Pediatric

▲ Evaluate lead exposure risk and consult the healthcare provider regarding lead screening measures as indicated (public/ambulatory health).

• Supply "Mr.Yuk" labels for families with children.

• Provide guidance for parents and caregivers regarding age-related safety measures, including the following:
  - Store potentially harmful substances in the original containers with safety closures intact.
  - Recognize that no container is completely childproof.
  - Do not store medications or toxic substances in food containers.
  - Remove poisonous houseplants from the home. Teach children not to put leaves or berries in their mouths.
  - Keep cleaning agents, disinfectants, and other hazardous materials out of sight and out of children's reach; keep them locked up.
  - Do not take medications in front of children; children mimic parents' behaviors.
  - Do not suggest that medications such as aspirin and children's vitamins are candy.
  - If interrupted when using a harmful product, take it with you; children can get into it within seconds.
  - Use extreme caution with pesticides and gardening materials close to children's play areas.
  - Keep perfume and makeup out of reach of children.

• Teach the family to keep the home safe for children by keeping harmful cleaning products and all liquids containing hydrocarbons away from children and using child-resistant packaging as available.

- Advise families that syrup of ipecac is no longer recommended to be kept and used in the home.

Geriatric

- Caution the client and family to avoid storing medications with similar appearances close to one another (e.g., nitroglycerin ointment near toothpaste or denture creams).
- Place medications in a medication box that indicates when they are to be taken.
- Remind the older client to store medications out of reach when young children come to visit.
- Perform medication reconciliation on all elderly clients entering the healthcare system as well as on discharge.

Home Care

- The interventions previously described may be adapted for home care use.
- Provide the client and/or family with a poison control poster to be kept on the refrigerator or a bulletin board. Ensure that the telephone number for local poison control information is readily available.
- Prepour medications for a client who is at risk of ingesting too much of a given medication because of mistakes in preparation. Delegate this task to the family or caregivers if possible.
- Identify poisonous substances in the immediate surroundings of the home, such as a garage or barn, including paints and thinners, fertilizers, rodent and bug control substances, animal medications, gasoline, and oil. Label with the name, a poison warning sign, and a poison control center number. Lock out of the reach of children.
- Identify the risk of toxicity from environmental activities such as spraying trees or roadside shrubs. Contact local departments of agriculture or transportation to obtain material substance data sheets or to prevent the activity in desired areas.
- Avoid carbon monoxide poisoning. Instruct the client and family in the importance of using a carbon monoxide detector in the home, having the chimney professionally cleaned each year, having the furnace professionally inspected each year, ensuring that all combustion equipment is properly vented, and

installing a chimney screen and cap to prevent small animals from moving into the chimney.

Multicultural

- Assess housing for pathways of lead poisoning.
- Prompt caregivers to take action to prevent lead poisoning.
- Inform minority parents of children who present for treatment of a poisoning episode of poisoning prevention education as part of the medical encounter.
- Poison control centers should offer information in bilingual and bicultural manner.

Client/Family Teaching

- Counsel the client and family members regarding the following points of medication safety:
  - Avoid sharing prescriptions.
  - Always use good light when preparing medication.
  - Read the label before you open the bottle, after you remove a dose, and again before you give it.
  - Always use child-resistant caps and lock all medications away from your child or confused elder.
  - Give the correct dose. NEVER guess.
  - Do not increase or decrease the dose without calling the physician.
  - Always follow the weight and age recommendations on the label.
  - Avoid making conversions. If the label calls for 2 tsp and you have a dosing cup labeled only with ounces, do not use it.
  - Be sure the physician knows if you are taking more than one medication at a time.
  - Never let young children take medication by themselves.
  - Read and follow labeling instructions on all products; adjust dosage for age.
  - Avoid excessive amounts and/or frequency of doses. ("If a little does some good, a lot should do more.")
- Advise the family to post first-aid charts and poison control center instructions in an accessible location. Poison control center telephone numbers should be posted close to each telephone and the number programmed into cell phones.

P

- Advise family when calling the poison control center to do the following:
  - Give as much information as possible, including your name, location, and telephone number, so that the poison control operator can call back in case you are disconnected or to summon help if needed.
  - Give the name of the potential poison ingested and, if possible, the amount and time of ingestion. If the bottle or package is available, give the trade name and ingredients if they are listed.
  - Be prepared to tell the person the child's height, weight, and age.
  - Describe the state of the poisoning victim. Is the victim conscious? Does he or she have any symptoms? What is the person's general appearance, skin color, respiration, breathing difficulties, mental status (alert, sleepy, unusual behavior)? Is the person vomiting? Having convulsions?
- Encourage the client and family to take first-aid and other types of safety-related programs.

▲ Initiate referrals to peer group interventions, peer counseling, and other types of substance abuse prevention/rehabilitation programs when substance abuse is identified as a risk factor.

Post-trauma syndrome

NANDA Definition

Sustained maladaptive response to a traumatic, overwhelming event

Defining Characteristics

Aggression; alienation; altered mood state; anger and/or rage; anxiety; avoidance; compulsive behavior; denial; depression; detachment; difficulty in concentrating; enuresis (in children); exaggerated startle response; fear; flashbacks; gastric irritability; grieving; guilt; headaches; hopelessness; horror; hypervigilance; intrusive dreams; intrusive thoughts; irritability; neurosensory irritability; nightmares; palpitations; panic attack; psychogenic amnesia; rape; reports feeling numb; repression; shame; substance abuse

Related Factors (r/t)

Abuse (physical and psychosocial); being held prisoner of war; criminal victimization; disasters; epidemics; events outside range of usual human experience; serious accidents (e.g., industrial, motor vehicle); serious injury/threat to self or loved ones; sudden destruction of one's home or community; torture; tragic occurrence involving multiple deaths; wars; witnessing of mutilation/violent death

Client Outcomes

Client Will (Specify Time Frame):

- Return to pretrauma level of functioning as quickly as possible
- Acknowledge traumatic event and begin to work with the trauma by talking about the experience and expressing feelings of fear, anger, anxiety, guilt, and helplessness
- Identify support systems and available resources and be able to connect with them
- Return to and strengthen coping mechanisms used in previous traumatic event
- Acknowledge event and perceive it without distortions
- Assimilate event and move forward to set and pursue life goals

Nursing Interventions

- Observe for a reaction to a traumatic event in all clients regardless of age or sex.
- Provide a safe and therapeutic environment.
- Remain with the client and provide support during periods of overwhelming emotions.
- Help the individual try to comprehend the trauma if possible.
- Use touch with the client's permission (e.g., a hand on the shoulder, holding a hand).
- Explore and enhance available support systems.
- Help the client regain previous sleeping and eating habits.

▲ Provide the client pain medication if he or she has physical pain.

▲ Assess the need for pharmacotherapy.

- Help the client use positive cognitive restructuring to reestablish feelings of self-worth.
- Provide the means for the client to express feelings through therapeutic drawing.

- Encourage the client to return to the normal routine as quickly as possible.
- Talk to and assess the client's social support after a traumatic event.

Pediatric

Refer to nursing care plan **Risk for Post-trauma syndrome.**

Geriatric

- Carefully screen elderly for signs of PTSD, especially after a disaster. Consider using the Horwitz Impact of Event Scale, which is an appropriate instrument to measure the subjective response to stress in the senior population. Allow the client more time to establish trust and express anger, guilt, and shame about the trauma. Review past coping skills and give the client positive reinforcement for successfully dealing with other life crises.
- ▲ Monitor the client for clinical signs of depression and anxiety; refer to a physician for medication if appropriate.
- Instill hope.

Multicultural

- Assess the influence of cultural beliefs, norms, and values on the client's ability to cope with a traumatic experience.
- Acknowledge racial and ethnic differences at the onset of care.
- Use a family-centered approach when working with Latino, Asian, African-American, and Native-American clients.
- When working with Asian-American clients, provide opportunities by which the family can save face.
- Validate the client's feelings regarding the trauma.
- Incorporate cultural traditions as appropriate.

Home Care

- ▲ Assess family support and the response to the client's coping mechanisms. Refer the family for medical social services or other counseling as necessary.
- Provide a stable routine of day-to-day activities consistent with pretrauma experience. Do not force a new routine on the client.
- ▲ Assess the impact of the trauma on significant others (e.g., a father may have to take over his partner's parenting responsibility after she has been raped and injured). Provide empathy and caring to significant others. Refer for additional services as necessary.

Client/Family Teaching

• Explain to the client and family what to expect the first few days after the traumatic event and in the future.
• Teach positive coping skills and avoidance of negative coping skills.
• Teach stress reduction methods such as deep breathing, visualization, meditation, and physical exercise. Encourage their use especially when intrusive thoughts or flashbacks occur.
• Encourage other healthy living habits of proper diet, adequate sleep, regular exercise, family activities, and spiritual pursuits.
▲ Refer the client to peer support groups.
• Instruct the family in ways to be helpful to and supportive of the traumatized person. Emphasize the importance of listening and being there. Also emphasize that no magic phrases are capable of easing the person's emotional suffering.
▲ Consider the use of complementary and alternative therapies.

P

Risk for Post-trauma syndrome

NANDA Definition

At risk for sustained maladaptive response to a traumatic, overwhelming event

Risk Factors

Diminished ego strength; displacement from home; duration of event; exaggerated sense of responsibility; inadequate social support; nonsupportive environment; occupation (e.g., police, fire, rescue, corrections, emergency department, mental health worker); perception of event; survivor's role in the event

Client Outcomes

Client Will (Specify Time Frame):

• Identify symptoms associated with PTSD and seek help
• Identify the event in realistic, cognitive terms
• State that he or she is not to blame for the event

Nursing Interventions

- • Assess for PTSD in a client who has chronic illness, anxiety, or personality disorder; was a witness to serious injury or death; or experienced sexual molestation.
- • Consider the use of a self-reported screening questionnaire.
- • Assess for ongoing symptoms of dissociation, avoidant behavior, hypervigilance, and reexperiencing.
- • Assess for past experiences with traumatic events.
- • Consider screening for PTSD in a client who is a high user of medical care.
- ▲ Provide peer support to contact co-workers experiencing trauma to remind them that others in the organization are concerned about their welfare.
- • Provide posttrauma debriefings. Effective posttrauma coping skills are taught, and each participant creates a plan for his or her recovery. During the debriefing, the facilitators assess participants to determine their needs for further services in the form of posttrauma counseling. For maximal effectiveness, the debriefing should occur within 2 to 5 days of the incident.
- • Provide posttrauma counseling. Counseling sessions are extensions of debriefings and include continued discussion of the traumatic event and posttrauma consequences and the further development of coping skills.
- • Instruct the client to use the following critical incident stress management techniques:

P

Things to Try: Critical Incident Stress Debriefing

- ■ Within the first 24 to 48 hours, engaging in periods of appropriate physical exercise alternated with relaxation to alleviate some of the physical reactions.
- ■ Structure your time; keep busy.
- ■ You are normal and are having normal reactions; do not label yourself as "crazy."
- ■ Talk to people; talk is the most healing medicine.
- ■ Be aware of numbing the pain with overuse of drugs or alcohol; you do not need to complicate the stress with a substance abuse problem.
- ■ Reach out; people do care
- ■ Maintain as normal a schedule as possible.
- ■ Spend time with others.

- Help your co-workers as much as possible by sharing feelings and checking out how they are doing.
- Give yourself permission to feel rotten and share your feelings with others.
- Keep a journal; write your way through those sleepless hours.
- Do things that feel good to you.
- Realize that those around you are under stress.
- Do not make any big life changes.
- Do make as many daily decisions as possible to give you a feeling of control over your life (e.g., if someone asks you what you want to eat, answer the person even if you are not sure).
- Get plenty of rest.
- Reoccurring thoughts, dreams, or flashbacks are normal; do not try to fight them because they will decrease over time and become less painful.
- Eat well-balanced and regular meals (even if you do not feel like it).

• Assess for a history of life-threatening illness such as cancer and provide appropriate counseling.

Pediatric

• Children with cancer should continue to be assessed for PTSD into adulthood.

• Provide protection for a child who has witnessed violence or who has had traumatic injuries. Help the child acknowledge the event and express grief over the event. The children in Iraq are particularly vulnerable.

• Assess for a medical history of anxiety disorders.

• Consider implementation of a school-based program for children to decrease PTSD after catastrophic events.

Geriatric/Multicultural

• Refer to the care plan for **Post-trauma syndrome.**

Home Care

▲ Assess the client's ability to meet primary needs of shelter, nourishment, and safety. Refer to medical social services, state departments of human services, or other organizations as appropriate.

- Identify other losses or stressors that may affect coping ability (e.g., role or relationship changes, deaths).
- ▲ Assess the family's response to the client's risk. Refer the family to medical social services, mental health services, or support groups as necessary. Provide nursing support.
- ▲ If the client is on medication, assess its effectiveness and the client's compliance with the regimen. Identify who administers the medication.
- Help the client in the home identify and establish daily patterns that have meaning for the client.
- For a client who is displaced from the home, identify internal values that can be maintained while the client is displaced, such as respite, contact with specific persons, and honesty.
- ▲ Encourage the client to verbalize feelings of risk and trauma to therapeutic staff or other supportive persons. Refer to medical social services or mental health/support group services as appropriate.
- ▲ Evaluate the client's response to a traumatic or critical event. If screening warrants, refer to a therapist for counseling/treatment.
- Refer to the care plan for **Post-trauma syndrome.**

Client/Family Teaching

- Instruct family and friends to use the following critical incident stress management techniques:
  - Listen carefully.
  - Spend time with the traumatized person.
  - Offer your assistance and a listening ear, even if the person has not asked for help.
  - Help the person with everyday tasks such as cleaning, cooking, caring for the family, and minding children.
  - Give the person some private time.
  - Do not take the individual's anger or other feelings personally, and do not tell the person that he or she is "lucky it wasn't worse"; such statements do not console traumatized people. Instead, tell the person that you are sorry such an event has occurred and you want to understand and assist him or her.
- Teach the client and family to recognize symptoms of PTSD and seek treatment when the client does the following:
  - Relives the traumatic event by thinking or dreaming about it often.

- Is unsettled or distressed in other areas of his or her life such as in school, at work, or in personal relationships.
- Avoids any situation that might cause him or her to relive the trauma.
- Demonstrates a certain amount of generalized emotional numbness.
- Shows a heightened sense of being on guard.

• Provide education to explain that acute stress disorder symptoms are normal reactions that are likely to resolve. Instruct to seek help if the symptoms persist.

Readiness for enhanced Power

NANDA Definition

A pattern of participating knowingly in change that is sufficient for well-being and can be strengthened

Defining Characteristics

Expresses readiness to enhance awareness of possible changes to be made; freedom to perform actions for change; identification of choices that can be made for change; involvement in creating change; knowledge for participation in change; participation in choices for daily living and health; power

Client Outcomes

Client Will (Specify Time Frame):

- Evaluate power resources
- Identify perceptions of control
- Select options to support health
- Seek assistance as needed
- Participate with health providers in relation to health issues and concerns

Nursing Interventions

• Support and enhance the client's inherent power.
• Focus on the positive aspects of power rather than the prevention of powerlessness.
• Follow the client's agenda.

- Develop partnerships with clients for shared power.
- Listen with intent.
- Affirm emotions.
- Help the client create images that support and sustain self-care, such as identification of people or events that provided encouragement and meaning.
- Collaborate with the person to identify resources to put a plan into action.
- Assess the meaning of health-related issues to the person.
- Facilitate the person's trust in self and others.
- Help the client mobilize social supports.
- Identify and support beliefs of power and perceptions of behavioral control.
- Promote optimal level of functioning.
- Change organizational and management patterns to support clients' power.

Home Care

P

- Above interventions may be adapted for home care use.
- Work with families to support the power of individual family members.

Client/Family Teaching

- When conducting any client or family teaching, support the client's power by working in partnership to identify learning needs, learning styles, health literacy, and desired objectives and content.

Powerlessness

NANDA Definition

Perception that one's own actions will not significantly affect an outcome; perceived lack of control over current situation or immediate happening

Defining Characteristics

Low

Expressions of uncertainty about fluctuating energy levels; passivity

Moderate

Anger; dependence on others that may result in irritability; does not defend self-care practices when challenged; does not monitor progress; expressions of dissatisfaction over inability to perform previous tasks/activities; expressions of doubt regarding role performance; expressions of frustration over inability to perform previous tasks/activities; fear of alienation from caregivers; guilt; inability to seek information regarding care; nonparticipation in care when opportunities are provided; nonparticipation in decision making when opportunities are provided; passivity; reluctance to express true feelings; resentment

Severe

Apathy; depression over physical deterioration; verbal expressions of having no control (e.g., over self-care, situation, outcome)

Related Factors (r/t)

Healthcare environment; illness-related regimen; interpersonal interactions; lifestyle of helplessness

Client Outcomes

Client Will (Specify Time Frame):

- State feelings of powerlessness and other feelings related to powerlessness (e.g., anger, sadness, hopelessness)
- Identify factors that are uncontrollable
- Participate in planning and implementing care; make decisions regarding care and treatment when possible
- Ask questions about care and treatment
- Verbalize hope for the future and sense of participation in planning and implementing care

Nursing Interventions

NOTE: Before implementation of interventions in the face of client powerlessness, nurses should examine their own philosophies of care to ensure that control issues or lack of faith in client capabilities will not bias the ability to intervene sincerely and effectively.

- • Observe for factors contributing to powerlessness (e.g., immobility, hospitalization, unfavorable prognosis, lack of support system, misinformation about situation, inflexible routine, chronic illness).

- Assess for **ineffective Therapeutic regimen management** or **Noncompliance.** Be alert to client behaviors that attempt to assert power, even if they seem confrontational. Help clients channel their behaviors in an effective manner.
- Assess the client's locus of control related to his or her health.
- Establish a therapeutic relationship with the client by spending one-on-one time with him or her, assigning the same caregiver, keeping commitments (e.g., saying, "I will be back to answer your questions in the next hour"), providing encouragement and support, and being empathetic.
- Encourage the client to share his or her beliefs, thoughts, and expectations about his or her illness.
- Have the client assist in planning care whenever possible (e.g., determining what time to bathe, taking pain medication before uncomfortable procedures, expressing food and fluid preferences). Document specifics in the care plan.
- Help the client specify the health goals he or she would like to achieve, prioritizing those goals with regard to immediate concerns and identifying actions that will achieve the goals. Goals may need to be small to be attainable (e.g., dangle legs at bedside for 2 days, then sit in chair 10 minutes for 2 days, then walk to window).
- Support clients' efforts to regain control of their lives by learning everything they can about their illnesses and treatment regimen.
- Encourage the client in goal-directed activities that promote a sense of accomplishment, especially regular exercise.
- Recognize the client's need to experience a sense of reciprocity in dealing with others. Negotiate actions that the client can contribute to the caregiving partnership with both family and nurse (e.g., have the client prepare a cup of tea for the nurse during visits if the client is able).
- Allow time for questions (15 to 20 minutes each shift). Have the client write down questions, and encourage the client to record a summary of answers received if desired or practicable or provide written material that reinforces answers.
- Encourage the client to take control of as many ADLs as possible; keep the client informed of all care that will be given. Keep items the client uses and needs, such as a urinal, tissues, telephone, and television controls, within reach.

- Give realistic and sincere praise for accomplishments.
- While the client's perspective is paramount, family members' powerlessness in assisting with client care must also be addressed to enhance family support.
- In evaluating outcomes implemented to address powerlessness, look to changes in the client, changes in relationships with others, and changes in behavior. Refer to the care plans for **Hopelessness** and **Spiritual distress.**

Pediatric

Two key issues that lead to powerlessness for children and their families are hospitalization and peer victimization or bullying.

- Encourage emotional expression through processes that are appropriate to the child's level of development.
- Recognize that a sense of powerlessness can prevent children and adolescents from reporting peer victimization. Be supportive, encourage disclosure without pressure, and help the child or adolescent problem solve options to deal with their stressors.
- Provide instruction and visual aids to family members so they may better understand a child's illness and how the family members can help.

Geriatric

In addition to the above interventions as appropriate:

- Initiate focused assessment questioning and education regarding syndromes common in the elderly.
- Assess for the presence of elder abuse. Initiate referral to Adult Protective Services and help client regain a sense of safety and control.
- Explore feelings of powerlessness—the feeling that the client's behavior will not affect outcomes.
- Explore personality resources and inner strengths that the client has used in the past. Incorporate these into the treatment plan.
- Establish therapeutic relationships by listening; participate with the client in generating choices and incorporate his or her statement of limitations.

▲ Monitor the use of alternative therapies but do not intervene unless the therapy interacts negatively with the existing therapeutic regimen. Ensure that all healthcare providers involved with the client are aware of the alternative therapies being used.

- Instruct caregivers in effective means of managing the behavior of clients with dementia.

Multicultural

- Assess the influence of cultural beliefs, norms, and values on the client's feelings of powerlessness.
- Assess the effect of fatalism on the client's expression of powerlessness.
- Encourage spirituality as a source of support to decrease powerlessness.
- Validate the client's feelings regarding the impact of health status on current lifestyle.
- For inner-city clients, help the client redefine behaviors as ways of coping with a hostile environment and reconnecting with community supports.
- Use an empowerment approach when working with African-American women.

Home Care

- Include an initial and ongoing assessment and evaluation of potential abuse and neglect. Photograph evidence of abuse or neglect when possible.
- ▲ If neglect or abuse is suspected, identify an emergency plan that addresses the problem immediately, ensures client safety, and includes a report to the appropriate authorities.
- Develop a therapeutic relationship in the home setting that respects the client's domain.
- Develop a written contract with the client that designates what care will be given and who has responsibility for care elements. Focus should be on care that is controlled by the client. Enable the client to develop his or her own resources actively.
- Empower the client by encouraging the client to guide specifics of care such as wound care procedures and dressing and grooming details. Confirm the client's knowledge and document in the chart that the client is able to guide procedures. Document in the home and in the chart the preferred approach to procedures. Orient the family and caregivers to the client's role.
- Identify the client's concerns and implement interventions to address the consequences of disability in clients with medical illness.

- Enhance self-efficacy by creating an environment that supports physical activities; provide support in the form of encouragement, anticipatory guidance, sharing of how others perform, and realistic assessment of the client's abilities.
- Respect the client's choices regarding desired assistance. Identify knowledge deficits and provide education to ensure that the client's choice is accurately informed.
- Assess the affective climate within the family and family support system, including other caregivers. Instruct the family in appropriate expectations of the client and in the specifics of the client's illness. Encourage the family and client in efforts toward educating friends and co-workers regarding appropriate expectations for the client.
- Evaluate the powerlessness of caregivers to ensure they continue their ability to care for the client. Provide assistance using interventions from this care plan.
- Be aware of and assist clients with potential needs for help in negotiating the healthcare system.
- ▲ Refer for homemaker or psychiatric home healthcare services for respite, client reassurance, and implementation of a therapeutic regimen.
- Explain all relevant symptoms, procedures, treatments, and expected outcomes.
- Provide written instructions for treatments and procedures for which the client will be responsible.
- Continually assess the client for signs of inappropriate exercise of self-care. Confront such applications of self-care; instruct the client in the dangers that inappropriate care may present and in alternatives for care that would be more effective.
- Teach stress reduction, relaxation, and imagery. Many audio recordings are available on relaxation and meditation. Assist the client with relaxation based on the client's preference indicated in the initial assessment.
- Teach cognitive-behavioral activities, such as active problem solving, reframing (reappraising the situation from a different perspective), or thought stopping (in response to a negative thought, such as picturing a large stop sign and replacing the image with a prearranged positive alternative). Teach the client to confront his or her own negative thought patterns (cognitive distortions).

P

- • Help the client practice assertive communication techniques.
- • Role play (e.g., say, "Tell me what you are going to ask your doctor").
- • Identify the strengths of the caregiver and efforts to gain control of unpredictable situations. Help the caregiver stay connected with a client who may be behaving differently than usual to make life as routine as possible, help the client set goals and sustain hope, and allow the client space to experience progress.
- ▲ Refer the client to support groups, pastoral care, or social services.

Risk for Powerlessness

NANDA Definition

At risk for perceived lack of control over a situation and/or one's ability to significantly affect an outcome

Risk Factors (r/t)

Physiological

Acute injury; aging; dying; illness; progressive debilitating disease process (e.g., spinal cord injury, multiple sclerosis)

Psychosocial

Absence of integrality (e.g., essence of power); chronic low self-esteem; deficient knowledge (e.g., of illness or healthcare system); disturbed body image; inadequate coping patterns; lifestyle of dependency; situational low self-esteem

Client Outcomes

Client Will (Specify Time Frame):

- State feelings of powerlessness and other feelings related to powerlessness (e.g., anger, sadness, hopelessness)
- Identify factors that are uncontrollable
- Participate in planning and implementing care; make decisions regarding care and treatment when possible
- Ask questions about care and treatment
- Verbalize hope for the future and sense of participation in planning and implementing care

Nursing Interventions

See the care plan for **Powerlessness.**

Ineffective Protection

NANDA Definition

Decrease in ability to guard self from internal or external threats such as illness or injury

Defining Characteristics

Altered clotting; anorexia; chilling; cough; deficient immunity; disorientation; dyspnea; fatigue; immobility; impaired healing; insomnia; itching; maladaptive stress response; neurosensory alteration; perspiring; pressure ulcers; restlessness; weakness

Related Factors (r/t)

Abnormal blood profiles (e.g., leukopenia, thrombocytopenia, anemia, coagulation); alcohol abuse; cancer; drug therapies (e.g., antineoplastic, corticosteroid, immune, anticoagulant, thrombolytic); extremes of age; immune disorders; inadequate nutrition; treatments (e.g., surgery, radiation)

Client Outcomes

Client Will (Specify Time Frame):

- Remain free of infection
- Remain free of any evidence of new bleeding
- Explain precautions to take to prevent infection
- Explain precautions to take to prevent bleeding

Nursing Interventions

- • Take temperature, pulse, and blood pressure (e.g., every 1 to 4 hours).
- ▲ Observe nutritional status (e.g., weight, serum protein and albumin levels, muscle mass, usual food intake). Work with the dietitian to improve nutritional status if needed. All clients diagnosed with HIV should have a dietary consult.
- • Observe the client's sleep pattern; if altered, see Nursing Interventions for **Insomnia.**

- • Determine the amount of stress in the client's life. If stress is uncontrollable, see Nursing Interventions for **Ineffective Coping.**

Prevention of Infection

- • Refer to care plan **Risk for Infection.**
- ▲ Monitor for and report any signs of infection (e.g., fever, chills, flushed skin, drainage, edema, redness, abnormal laboratory values, and pain) and notify the physician promptly.
- ▲ If the client's immune system is depressed, notify the physician of elevated temperature, even in the absence of other symptoms of infection.
- • If white blood cell count is severely decreased (i.e., absolute neutrophil count of <1000/mm^3), initiate the following precautions:
    - ■ Take vital signs every 4 hours.
    - ■ Complete a head-to-toe assessment twice daily, including inspection of oral mucosa, invasive sites, wounds, urine, and stool; monitor for onset of new reports of pain.
    - ■ Avoid any invasive procedures, including catheterization, injections, or rectal or vaginal procedures.
- • Consider warming the client before elective surgery.
- ▲ Administer granulocyte growth factor therapy as ordered.
- • Take meticulous care of all invasive sites; use chlorhexidine gluconate for cleansing.
- • Provide frequent oral care.
- ▲ Refer for prophylactic medication to prevent oral candidiasis.
- ▲ Refer for appropriate prophylactic antifungal treatment and avoid pathogen exposure (through air filtration, regular hand hygiene, avoidance of plants and flowers).
- • Have the client wear a mask when leaving the room.
- • Limit and screen visitors to minimize exposure to contagion.
- • Help the client bathe daily.
- • Practice food safety; a neutropenic diet may not be necessary (www.foodsafety.gov).
- ▲ Ensure that the client is well nourished. Provide food with protein and consider vitamin supplements. If appetite is suppressed, institute a dietary referral. Keep track of serum albumin levels as well as transferrin and prealbumin levels.
- • Refer to care plan **Readiness for enhanced Nutrition** for additional interventions.

- • Help the client to cough and practice deep breathing regularly. Maintain an appropriate activity level.
- • Obtain a private room for the client. Use high-energy particulate air filters if available and appropriate. Protective isolation is not recommended. Recognize that cotton cover gowns may not be effective in decreasing infection.
- ▲ Watch for signs of sepsis, including change in mental status, fever, shaking, chills, and hypotension. If present, notify the physician promptly.

Pediatric

- • Suggest kangaroo care, frequent and exclusive or nearly exclusive breastfeeding, and early discharge from hospital for low birth weight infants.
- • Treat postoperative fever in pediatric oncology clients promptly.
- • For hand hygiene with low birth weight infants, use alcohol hand rub and gloves.

Geriatric

- • If not contraindicated, promote exercise to strengthen the immune system in the elderly.
- • Give elderly clients with imbalanced nutrition a nutritional supplement to enhance immune function.
- • Refer to the care plan for **Risk for Infection** for more interventions related to the prevention of infection.

Prevention of Bleeding

- • Monitor the client's risk for bleeding; evaluate results of clotting studies and platelet counts.
- • Watch for hematuria, melena, hematemesis, hemoptysis, epistaxis, bleeding from mucosa, petechiae, and ecchymoses.
- ▲ Give medications orally or IV only; avoid giving them IM, subcutaneously, or rectally. Apply pressure for a longer time than usual to invasive sites such as venipuncture or injection sites.
- • Take vital signs often; watch for changes associated with fluid volume loss.
- • Monitor menstrual flow if relevant; have the client use pads instead of tampons.
- • Have the client use a moistened toothette or a very soft child's

toothbrush instead of an adult toothbrush. Have the client use alcohol-free dental products and avoid flossing.
- Ask the client either not to shave or to use an electric razor only.
- To decrease risk of bleeding, avoid administering salicylates or nonsteroidal antiinflammatory drugs (NSAIDs) if possible.

Home Care

- Some of the interventions previously described may be adapted for home care use.

▲ Consider institution of a nurse-administered mobile care unit for monitoring anticoagulant therapy.

▲ For terminally ill clients, teach and institute all of the aforementioned noninvasive precautions that maintain quality of life. Discuss with the client, family, and physician the consequences of contracting infection. Determine which precautions do not maintain quality of life and should not be used (e.g., physical assessment twice daily, multiple vital sign assessments).

Client/Family Teaching

Depressed Immune Function

- Teach precautions to take to decrease the chance of infection (e.g., avoiding uncooked fruits and vegetables, using appropriate self-care, ensuring a safe environment).
- Teach the client and family how to take a temperature. Encourage the family to take the client's temperature between 3 PM and 7 PM at least once daily.
- Teach the client to avoid crowds and contact with persons who have infections. Teach the need for good nutrition, avoidance of stress, and adequate rest to maintain immune system function.

Bleeding Disorder

▲ Teach the client to wear a medical alert bracelet and notify all healthcare personnel of the bleeding disorder.

▲ Teach the client and family the signs of bleeding, precautions to take to prevent bleeding, and action to take if bleeding begins. Caution the client to avoid taking over-the-counter medications without the permission of the physician. Medications containing salicylates can increase bleeding.

- Teach the client to wear loose-fitting clothes and avoid physical activity that might cause trauma.

Pruritus

Definition (NOTE: This is not a NANDA-I Diagnosis)

State in which an individual experiences an uncomfortable itching sensation in response to a noxious stimulus

Defining Characteristics

Verbalization of itching sensation; observed behaviors of itching; irritated skin from scratching

Related Factors (r/t)

Reaction to irritants, including allergies, dry skin, chronic illness, stress; medication side effect

Client Outcomes

Client Will (Specify Time Frame):

- State he or she is comfortable
- State that his or her itching is relieved to an acceptable level
- Explain methods to decrease itching
- Have intact skin

Nursing Interventions

- • Perform a complete assessment to determine the cause of pruritus (e.g., dry skin, contact with irritating substance, medication side effect, insect bite, infection, healing burns, underlying systemic disease). Implement soaks with cool or cold washcloths or offer cool baths if appropriate.
- ▲ Apply topical agents as ordered to decrease itching. Include cooling agents, topical anesthetics, topical antihistamines, capsaicin, and topical corticosteroids.
- • Recognize that a common cause of itching is dry skin (xerosis), especially in the elderly, during winter months, and in people who take frequent baths or showers with hot water. Apply creams or ointments to keep the skin well hydrated immediately after bathing. At times it may be necessary to use both a heavy ointment followed by an oil to adequately moisturize the skin.
- • Keep the client's fingernails short; have the client wear mitts if necessary. Leave pruritic area open to the air if possible.

P

- • Cleanse the body using nonallergenic, low-pH cleansing agents on the perineum and axilla; avoid use of regular soap.
- • Use behavior modification to help reduce self-injury caused by scratching and improve quality of life.
- ▲ Advocate altering or substituting medications if pruritus is potentially a side effect of the current medication regimen.
- • Assess for sleep disturbances.
- ▲ Consult the physician for appropriate medications to relieve itching. Be aware of current research regarding medications best suited to relieving the pruritus associated with different causes.

Multicultural

- • Assess black skin for ashy appearance for signs of dry skin.
- • Encourage the use of lanolin-based lotions for African-American clients with dry skin.
- • Offer hair oil and lanolin-based lotion for dry scalp and skin.
- • Use soap sparingly if the skin is dry.

P

Client/Family Teaching

- • Teach techniques to alleviate dry skin:
  - ■ Decrease time in the shower or bath.
  - ■ Add oil to the bathwater.
  - ■ Use lukewarm water only.
  - ■ Apply emollients immediately after bathing to slightly damp skin to "seal in" the moisture.
  - ■ Use low-pH cleansers; wash in essential areas only.
  - ■ Use a humidifier to put more moisture in the air in winter.
- • Teach techniques to deal with itching sensation:
  - ■ Keep skin well hydrated with emollients and good fluid intake.
  - ■ Use rubbing, massage, pressure, or vibration for scratching when itching is severe and irrepressible.
  - ■ Wear cool clothing and keep the ambient temperature cooler.
  - ■ Avoid hot or spicy foods, hot liquids, and alcohol, which can stimulate the histamine response resulting in itching.
  - ■ Keep fingernails short.
- • Teach techniques to use when the client is uncomfortable, including relaxation techniques, guided imagery, hypnosis, and music therapy.

- • Teach the client and the family correct application or administration of prescribed medications or therapies.
- ▲ Instruct the client to see the primary care practitioner if itching persists and no cause is found.

Rape-trauma syndrome

NANDA Definition

Sustained maladaptive response to forced, violent sexual penetration against the victim's will and consent

Defining Characteristics

Aggression; agitation; anger; anxiety; change in relationships; confusion; denial; dependence; depression; disorganization; dissociative disorders; embarrassment; fear; guilt; helplessness; humiliation; hyperalertness; impaired decision making; loss of self-esteem; mood swings; muscle spasms; muscle tension; nightmares; paranoia; phobias; physical trauma; powerlessness; revenge; self-blame; sexual dysfunction; shame; shock; sleep disturbances; substance abuse; suicide attempts; vulnerability

R

Related Factor (r/t)

Rape

Client Outcomes

Client Will (Specify Time Frame):

- Share feelings, concerns, and fears
- Recognize that the rape or attempt was not client's own fault
- State that, no matter what the situation, no one has the right to assault another
- Describe medical/legal treatment procedures and reasons for treatment
- Report absence of physical complications or pain
- Identify support people and be able to ask them for help in dealing with this trauma
- Function at same level as before crisis, including sexual functioning
- Recognize that it is normal for full recovery to take a minimum of 1 year

Nursing Interventions

- • Observe the client's responses, including anger, fear, self-blame, sleep pattern disturbances, and phobias.
- • Monitor the client's verbal and nonverbal psychological state (e.g., crying, hand wringing, avoidance of interactions or eye contact with staff, silence, and denial).
- ▲ Stay with (or have a trusted person stay with) the client initially. If a law enforcement interview is permitted, provide support by staying with the client, but only at the client's request.
- • Explain the entire medical/legal examination to the client before beginning any procedures.
- • Do not wait for the client to ask questions; explain everything you are doing, clarify why it must be done, and describe when and where you will touch.
- ▲ Observe for signs of physical injury as you are asking the client to undress and collecting the client's clothing for evidence. Ask the client where it hurts without asking leading questions. Do not ask specific questions but allow the client to give you a history of the sexual assault in the client's own words. If the examiner needs further clarification, ask the client to point to areas that were injured or touched. Inform the client that photographs of any injuries are necessary for forensic evidence. Obtain specific written permission for photographs to be taken and released to law enforcement personnel.
- • Documentation of a sexual assault examination is critical to evidentiary reports. It is important to document the client's exact description of the assault and then to collect evidence and photographs that validate the history the client reports.
- • It is also very important for the examiner not to offer any opinions in the documentation about whether or not the assault occurred according to the physical findings.
- ▲ Document a one- or two-sentence summary of what happened. The chief complaint of the client reporting sexual assault should always be listed as "reported sexual assault"; obtaining the details of the sequence of events is the police officer's job.
- • Encourage the client to verbalize feelings.
- • Escort the client to the treatment room immediately to remove the client from the general population; do not question the client in the triage area. Close curtains and door, and avoid

R

other interruptions during contact with the client (e.g., telephone calls, absence from the room, outside stimuli such as radios).

- ▲ Provide a sexual assault response team (SART) that includes a SANE, rape counseling advocate, and representative of law enforcement.
- ▲ The rape crisis center advocate should be part of the SART and respond when the SANE responds.
- • Provide items for self-care after examination (e.g., for cleansing the vaginal and rectal area).
- ▲ Most states provide sexual assault evidence collection kits that have been reviewed by the SART members to provide adequate evidence for analysis by the forensic laboratory. Explain to the client that all or some of the client's clothing may be kept for evidential purposes.
- ▲ Discuss the possibility of pregnancy and sexually transmitted diseases (STDs) and the treatments available.
- ▲ Encourage the client to report the rape to a law enforcement agency.
- • Discuss the client's support system. Involve the support system if appropriate and if the client grants permission.
- ▲ Obtaining blood alcohol levels or levels of any drug should be discussed thoroughly with the medical director of your facility and the SART members.

Geriatric

- • Build a trusting relationship with the client.
- ▲ Explain reporting and encourage the client to report.
- • Observe for psychosocial distress (e.g., memory impairment, sleep disturbances, regression, changes in bodily functions).
- ▲ All examinations should be done on the elderly as they would be done on any adult client after sexual assault. Evidence should be collected, and consent for collection, photography, and law enforcement contact should be obtained as in all cases. Special attention should be given to the explanation of the genital examination, especially as it relates to the use of a speculum.
- • Modify the rape protocol to promote comfort for the geriatric client. Consider positioning female clients with pillows rather than stirrups and consider using a smaller speculum.

R

- Assess for mobility limitations and cognitive impairment.
- Respect the client's need for privacy.

▲ Consider arrangements for temporary housing.

Male Rape

- Reactions to male rape are often either disbelief or an assumption that the man who was raped is gay.

Multicultural

- Assess for the influence of cultural beliefs, norms, and values on the client's ability to cope with the trauma of the rape experience.
- Assess to determine if physically abused women are also victims of sexual assault.
- Provide opportunities by which the family and individual can save face when working with Asian-American clients.
- Assure the client of confidentiality.
- Validate the client's feelings regarding the rape and allow the client to tell his or her rape story.
- A culturally sensitive approach should be part of the training of all SARTs and members of SARTs.

Home Care

- Some of the interventions described previously may be adapted for home care use.
- Interact with the client supportively and nonjudgmentally; this supports the client's self-worth.
- Assist the client with realistically assessing the home setting for safety and/or selecting a safe environment in which to live.

▲ Ensure that the client has a support system in place for long-term support. Instruct the family that recovery may take a long time. Refer for medical social work services to assist in setting up a support system if necessary. Refer for counseling if necessary.

▲ Make sure that physical symptoms from the rape or other physical conditions are followed up. Follow-up should include a visit to the primary care physician or the local health department in 3 to 4 weeks for repeat pregnancy testing and STD testing. Explain to the client that additional medication may be necessary for the treatment of STDs or pregnancy.

▲ If the client is homebound, refer for psychiatric home healthcare services for client reassurance and implementation of a therapeutic regimen.

Client/Family Teaching

- ▲ Provide information on prophylactic antibiotic therapy, hepatitis B vaccination, and tetanus prophylaxis for nonimmunized clients with trauma.
- • Discharge instructions should be written out for the client.
- • Give instructions to significant others.
- • Explain the purpose of the "morning-after pill."
- ▲ Explain the potential for common side effects related to treatment with norgestrel, such as breast swelling or nausea and vomiting. (Call the emergency department if the client vomits within 1 hour of taking the pill because the pill may need to be taken again.) (Discuss any issues about prophylactic medications at the follow-up visit in 3 to 4 weeks.) It may take 3 to 30 days for the menstrual period to start; if menstruation has not begun in 30 days, contact a physician.
- ▲ Explain the potential for severe side effects related to treatment with norgestrel, such as severe leg or chest pain, trouble breathing, coughing up of blood, severe headache or dizziness, and trouble seeing or talking.
- • Advise the client to call or return if new problems develop.
- • Discuss practical lifestyle changes within the client's control to reduce the risk of future attacks.
- ▲ Teach the client to use self-defense techniques to surprise an attacker and create an opportunity to run for help. Refer the client to a self-defense school.
- • Teach the client appropriate outlets for anger.
- • Emphasize the vulnerability of the client and ensure that reactions are appropriate for the victim of sexual assault.

Rape-trauma syndrome: compound reaction

NANDA Definition

Forced violent sexual penetration against the victim's will and consent. The trauma syndrome that develops from this attack or attempted attack includes an acute phase of disorganization of victim's lifestyle and a long-term process of reorganization of lifestyle.

Defining Characteristics

Change in lifestyle (e.g., changes in residence, dealing with repetitive nightmares and phobias, seeking family support, seeking social network support in long-term phase); emotional reaction (e.g., anger, embarrassment, fear of physical violence and death, humiliation, revenge, self-blame in acute phase); multiple physical symptoms (e.g., gastrointestinal irritability, genitourinary discomfort, muscle tension, sleep pattern disturbance in acute phase); reactivated symptoms of previous conditions (e.g., physical illness, psychiatric illness in acute phase); substance abuse (acute phase)

Client Outcomes

Client Will (Specify Time Frame):

- Share feelings, concerns, and fears
- Recognize that the rape or attempt was not client's own fault
- State that, no matter what the situation, no one has the right to assault another
- Describe medical/legal treatment procedures and reasons for treatment
- Report absence of physical complications or pain
- Identify support people and be able to ask them for help in dealing with this trauma
- Function at same level as before crisis, including sexual functioning
- Recognize that it is normal for full recovery to take a minimum of 1 year

Nursing Interventions

- Refer to the care plans for **Rape-trauma syndrome, Powerlessness, Ineffective Coping, Dysfunctional Grieving, Anxiety, Fear, Risk for self-directed Violence,** and **Sexual dysfunction.**

Geriatric

- A new subgroup of rape victims resides in nursing homes. Treatment is necessary.

Risk for Compound Reaction

- See the care plan for **Rape-trauma syndrome.**

Home Care

▲ If the client has pursued psychiatric counseling, monitor and encourage attendance.

▲ If the client is receiving medication, assess the client's knowledge of its purpose, side effects, and interactions with medications for other diagnoses. Monitor for effectiveness, side effects, and interactions.

▲ Establish an emergency plan including use of hotlines. Contract with the client to use the emergency plan. Roleplay using the hotlines.

- For other home care and hospice considerations, refer to the care plan for **Rape-trauma syndrome.**

Client/Family Teaching

- Teach the client what reactions to expect during the acute and long-term phases: acute phase-anger, fear, self-blame, embarrassment, vengeful feelings, physical symptoms, muscle tension, sleeplessness, stomach upset, genitourinary discomfort; long-term phase-changes in lifestyle or residence, nightmares, phobias, seeking of family and social network support.

▲ Encourage psychiatric consultation if the client is suicidal, violent, or unable to continue activities of daily living (ADLs).

▲ Discuss any of the client's current stress-relieving medications that may result in substance abuse.

R

Rape-trauma syndrome: silent reaction

NANDA Definition

Forced violent sexual penetration against the victim's will and consent. The trauma syndrome that develops from this attack or attempted attack includes an acute phase of disorganization of the victim's lifestyle and a long-term process of reorganization of lifestyle.

Defining Characteristics

Abrupt changes in relationships with men; increase in nightmares; increased anxiety during interview (e.g., blocking of associations, long periods of silence, minor stuttering, physical distress); no verbalization of the occurrence of rape; pronounced changes in sexual behavior; sudden onset of phobic reactions

Related Factors (r/t)

To be developed

Client Outcomes

Client Will (Specify Time Frame):

- Resume previous level of relationships with significant others
- State improvement in sleep and fewer nightmares
- Express feelings about and discuss the rape
- Return to usual pattern of sexual behavior
- Remain free of phobic reactions

Refer to the care plan for **Rape-trauma syndrome.**

Nursing Interventions

R

- Refer to the care plans for **Rape-trauma syndrome, Powerlessness, Ineffective Coping, Dysfunctional Grieving, Anxiety, Fear, Risk for self-directed Violence, Sexual dysfunction,** and **Impaired verbal Communication.**
- Observe for disruptions in relationships with significant others.
- Monitor for signs of increased anxiety (e.g., silence, stuttering, physical distress, irritability, unexplained crying spells).
- Focus on the client's coping strengths.
- Observe for changes in sexual behavior.
- Identify phobic reactions to persons or objects in the environment (e.g., strangers, doorbells, groups of people, knives).
- Provide support by listening when the client is ready to talk.
- Remain with an anxious client even if the client is silent. Use gentle speech and actions; move slowly.
- Evaluate somatic complaints.

Geriatric

- A new subgroup of rape victims resides in nursing homes. Treatment is necessary.
- Refer to the care plan for **Rape-trauma syndrome.**

Multicultural

- Allow the client to tell his or her rape story without probing.

Home Care

Refer to the care plan for **Rape-trauma syndrome.**

Client/Family Teaching

- ▲ Refer the client to a sexual assault counselor. Long-term counseling may be necessary.
- • Refer to the care plan for **Rape-trauma syndrome.**

Impaired Religiosity

NANDA Definition

Impaired ability to exercise reliance on beliefs and/or participate in rituals of a particular faith tradition

Defining Characteristics

Difficulty adhering to prescribed religious beliefs and rituals (e.g., religious ceremonies, dietary regulations, clothing, prayer, worship/religious services, private religious behaviors/reading religious material/media, holiday observances, meetings with religious leaders); expresses emotional distress because of separation from faith community; expresses a need to reconnect with previous belief patterns; expresses a need to reconnect with previous customs; questions religious belief patterns; questions religious customs

Related Factors (r/t)

Developmental and Situational: Aging; end-stage life crises; life transitions

Physical: Illness; pain

Psychological: Anxiety; fear of death; ineffective coping; ineffective support; lack of security; personal crisis; use of religion to manipulate

Sociocultural: Cultural barriers to practicing religion; environmental barriers to practicing religion; lack of social integration; lack of sociocultural interaction

Spiritual: Spiritual crises; suffering

NOTE: The DDC recognizes that the term *religiosity* may be culture specific; however, the term is useful in the U.S. and is well-supported in the U.S. literature.

Client Outcomes

Client Will (Specify Time Frame):

- Express satisfaction with the ability to express religious practices
- Express satisfaction with access to religious materials and rituals
- Demonstrate balance between religious practices and healthy lifestyles
- Avoid high-risk, controlling religious relationships that inflict physical, sexual, or emotional harm and/or exploitation

Nursing Interventions

- • Identify client's concerns regarding religious expression.
- • Encourage and/or coordinate the use of and participation in usual religious rituals or practices that are not detrimental to health.
- • Encourage the use of prayer or meditation as appropriate.
- • Determine family's religious practices and encourage use of religious practices (if used) to help cope with loss.
- • Coordinate or provide transportation to worship site, particularly for the elderly and in meeting the needs of the disabled or ill.
- ▲ Identify individuals at risk for an excessive dependence upon religion, religious leaders, or religious practices.
- ▲ Refer to religious leader, professional counseling, or support group as needed.

Geriatric

- • Promote established religious practices in the elderly.

Multicultural

- • Promote religious practices that are culturally appropriate.

R

Readiness for enhanced Religiosity

NANDA Definition

Ability to exercise reliance on beliefs and/or participate in rituals of a particular faith tradition

Defining Characteristics

Expresses desire to strengthen religious belief patterns that had provided comfort in the past; expresses desire to strengthen religious belief patterns that had provided religion in the past; expresses desire to strengthen religious customs that had provided comfort in the past; expresses desire to strengthen religious customs that had provided religion in the past; questions belief patterns that are harmful; questions customs that are harmful; rejects belief patterns that are harmful; rejects customs that are harmful; requests assistance expanding religious options; request for assistance to increase participation in prescribed religious beliefs (e.g., religious ceremonies, dietary regulations/rituals, clothing prayer, worship/religious services, private religious behaviors, reading religious materials/media, holiday observances); requests forgiveness; requests meeting with religious leaders/facilitators; requests reconciliation; requests religious experiences; requests religious materials

NOTE: The DDC recognizes that the term "*religiosity*" may be culture specific; however, the term is useful in the U.S. and is well-supported in the U.S. literature.

Client Outcomes

R

Client Will (Specify Time Frame):

- Express satisfaction with an enhanced ability to express religious practices
- Express satisfaction with access to religious materials and rituals
- Demonstrate balance between religious practices and healthy lifestyles
- Avoid high-risk, controlling religious relationships that inflict physical, sexual, or emotional harm and/or exploitation

Nursing Interventions

See care plan for **Impaired Religiosity.**

Pediatric

- Provide spiritual care for children based on developmental level.
  - **Infants:** Have the same nurse care for the child on a daily basis. Encourage holding, cuddling, rocking, playing with, and singing to the infant.

- **Toddlers:** Provide consistency in care and familiar toys, music, stories, clothing blankets, pillows, and any other individual object of contentment. Schedule home religious routines into the plan of care and support home routines regarding good and bad behavior.
- **School-age children and adolescents:** Encourage both groups to express their feelings regarding spirituality. Ask them, "Do you wish to pray and what do you want to pray about?" Offer age-appropriate complimentary therapies such as music, art, videos, and connectedness with peers through cards, letters, and visits.

Risk for impaired Religiosity

NANDA Definition

At risk for an impaired ability to exercise reliance on religious beliefs and/or participate in rituals of a particular faith tradition

Related Factors (r/t)

R

Developmental: Life transitions

Environmental: Barriers to practicing religion; lack of transportation

Physical: Hospitalization; illness; pain

Psychological: Depression; ineffective caregiving; ineffective coping; ineffective support; lack of security

Sociocultural: Cultural barrier to practicing religion; lack of social interaction; social isolation

Spiritual: Suffering

NOTE: The DDC recognizes that the term "religiosity" may be culture specific; however, the term is useful in the U.S. and is well-supported in the U.S. literature.

Client Outcomes

Client Will (Specify Time Frame):

- Express satisfaction with the ability to express religious practices
- Express satisfaction with access to religious materials and rituals
- Demonstrate balance between religious practices and healthy lifestyles

- Avoid high-risk, controlling religious relationships that inflict physical, sexual, or emotional harm and/or exploitation

Nursing Interventions

See care plan for **Impaired Religiosity.**

Relocation stress syndrome

NANDA Definition

Physiological and/or psychosocial disturbances that result from transfer from one environment to another

Defining Characteristics

Temporary and/or permanent move; voluntary and/or involuntary move; aloneness, alienation, or loneliness; depression; anxiety (e.g., separation); sleep disturbance; withdrawal; anger; loss of identity, self-worth, or self-esteem; increased verbalization of needs, unwillingness to move or concern over relocation; increased physical symptoms/illness (e.g., gastrointestinal disturbance, weight change); dependency; insecurity; pessimism; frustration; worry; fear

R

Related Factors (r/t)

Unpredictability of experience/isolation from family/friends; passive coping; language barrier; decreased health status; impaired psychosocial health; past, concurrent, and recent losses; feeling of powerlessness; lack of adequate support system/group; lack of predeparture counseling

Client Outcomes

Client Will (Specify Time Frame):

- Recognize and know the name of at least one staff member
- Express concern about move when encouraged to do so during individual contacts
- Carry out activities of daily living (ADLs) in usual manner
- Maintain previous mental and physical health status (e.g., nutrition, elimination, sleep, social interaction)

Nursing Interventions

- Begin relocation planning as early in the decision process as possible.
- Obtain a history, including the reason for the move, the client's usual coping mechanisms, history of losses, and family support for the client.
- Identify to what extent the client can participate in the relocation decisions and advocate for this participation.
- Assess family members' perceptions of clients' ability to participate in relocation decisions.
- Consider the clients' and families' cultural and ethnic values as much as possible when choosing roommates, foods, and other aspects of care.
- Promote clear communication between all participants in the relocation process.
- Observe the following procedures if the client is being transferred to an extended care facility or assisted living facility:
  - Facilitate the client's participation in decisions and choice of placement and arrange a preadmission visit if possible.
  - If the client cannot visit the new facility, arrange for a visit or telephone call by a member of the staff to welcome the client and show a videotape or at least provide pictures of the new care facility.
  - Have a familiar person accompany the client to the new facility.
  - Recommend that the caregiver write a journal of thoughts and feelings regarding the relocation of their loved one.
- Validate the caregiver's feelings of difficulty with deciding to relocate a loved one to a different environment.
- Identify previous routines for ADLs. Try to maintain as much continuity with the previous schedule as possible.
- Bring in familiar items from home (e.g., pictures, clocks, afghans).
- Establish the way the client would like to be addressed (Mr., Mrs., Miss, first name, nickname).
- Thoroughly orient the client and the family to the new environment and routines; repeat directions as needed.
- Spend one-to-one time with the client. Allow the client to express feelings and convey acceptance of them; emphasize that

the client's feelings are real and individual and that it is acceptable to be sad or angry about moving.

- Assign the same staff members to the client if compatible with client; maintain consistency in the personnel the client interacts with.
- Ask the client to state one positive aspect of the new living situation each day.
- Monitor the client's health status and provide appropriate interventions for problems with social interaction, nutrition, sleep, new onset of infection, or elimination problems.
- If the client is being transferred within a facility, have staff members from the new unit visit the client before transfer.
- Work with the caregivers & family members helping them deal with stages of "making the best of it," "making the move," and "making it better."
- If a client is being transferred from the intensive care unit (ICU), have previous staff make occasional visits until the client is comfortable in the new surroundings. Ensure that the family is told relevant information.
- Watch for coping problems (e.g., withdrawal, regression, angry behavior, impaired sleeping, refusal to eat, flat affect) and intervene immediately.
- Encourage the client to express grief for the loss of the old situation; explain that it is normal to feel sadness over change and loss.
- Encourage the client to participate in care as much as possible and make own decisions when possible (e.g., placement of the bed, choice of roommate, bathing routines).
- Make an effort to accommodate the client.

R

Pediatric

- Provide support for a child and family who must relocate to be near a transplant center.
- Encourage child to verbalize concerns in divorce situations when they and/or a parent relocate. If the client is an adolescent, try to avoid a move in the middle of the school year, find a newcomers' club for the adolescent to join, and refer for counseling if needed.
- Assess adolescents' perceptions of their acceptance by peers.

Geriatric

- Monitor the need for transfer and transfer only when necessary.
- Implement discharge planning early so that it is not rushed.
- Protect the client from injuries such as falls.
- After the transfer, determine the client's mental status.

▲ Facilitate visits from companion animals.

▲ Encourage reminiscence of happy times. Refer for music therapy. Monitor neuroleptic prescriptions.

Client/Family Teaching

- Teach family members and remind direct care staff about relocation stress syndrome. Encourage them to monitor for signs of the syndrome.
- Help significant others learn how to support the client in the move by setting up a schedule of visits, arranging for holidays, bringing familiar items from home, and establishing a system for contact when the client needs support.

Risk for Relocation stress syndrome

NANDA Definition

At risk for physiological and/or psychosocial disturbances that result from transfer from one environment to another

Risk Factors

Decreased health status; feelings of powerlessness; lack of adequate support system; lack of predeparture counseling; losses; moderate to high degree of environmental change; moderate mental competence; move from one environment to another; passive coping; unpredictability of experiences

Client Outcomes, Nursing Interventions and Client/Family Teaching

Refer to the care plan for **Relocation stress syndrome.**

Ineffective Role performance

NANDA Definition

Patterns of behavior and self-expression that do not match the environmental context, norms, and expectations

Defining Characteristics

Altered role perceptions; anxiety; change in capacity to resume role; change in other's perception of role; change in self-perception of role; change in usual patterns of responsibility; deficient knowledge; depression; discrimination; domestic violence; harassment; inadequate adaptation to change; inadequate confidence; inadequate coping; inadequate external support for role enactment; inadequate motivation; inadequate opportunities for role enactment; inadequate role competency; inadequate self-management; inadequate skills; inappropriate developmental expectations; pessimism; powerlessness; role ambivalence; role conflict; role confusion; role denial; role dissatisfaction; role overload; role strain; system conflict; uncertainty

Related Factors (r/t)

Knowledge

Inadequate role model; inadequate role preparation (e.g., role transition, skill rehearsal, validation); lack of education; lack of role model; unrealistic role expectations

Physiological

Body image alteration; cognitive deficits; depression; fatigue; low self-esteem; mental illness; neurological defects; pain; physical illness; substance abuse

Social

Conflict; developmental level; domestic violence; inadequate role socialization; inadequate support system; inappropriate linkage with the healthcare system; job schedule demands; lack of resources; lack of rewards; low socioeconomic status; stress; young age

Client Outcomes

Client Will (Specify Time Frame):

- Identify realistic perception of role
- State personal strengths
- Acknowledge problems contributing to inability to carry out usual role
- Accept physical limitations regarding role responsibility and consider ways to change lifestyle to accomplish goals associated with role performance
- Demonstrate knowledge of appropriate behaviors associated with new or changed role
- State knowledge of change in responsibility and new behaviors associated with new responsibility
- Verbalize acceptance of new responsibility

Nursing Interventions

Social

- • Ask the client direct questions regarding new roles and how the health care system can help him or her continue in roles.
- • Allow the client to express feelings regarding the role change.
- • Reinforce the client's strengths and internalized values.
- • Have the client make a list of strengths that are needed for the new role. Acknowledge which strengths the client has and which strengths need to be developed. Work with the client to set goals for desired role.
- • Support the client's religious practices.

Physiological

- ▲ Identify ways to compensate for physical disabilities (e.g., have a ramp built to provide access to house, put household objects within the client's reach from wheelchair) and provide technological assistance when available.
- • Refer to the care plans for **Readiness for enhanced family Coping, Readiness for enhanced Decision making, Impaired Home maintenance, Impaired Parenting, Risk for Loneliness, Readiness for enhanced community Coping, Readiness for enhanced Self-care,** and **Ineffective Sexuality patterns.**

Pediatric

- • Assist new parents to adjust to changes in workload associated with childbirth.
- • Assist parents in coping with infants with colic, a condition common in infants.
- ▲ Refer to home health agency for home visits when there is an infant who has excessive crying.
- • Provide parents with coping skills when the role change is associated with a critically ill child.
- ▲ Assist families how to manage day-to day needs of a child with cerebral palsy (CP). Teach family members to value the small things children do, connect with other families, locate community resources, and understand the short- and long-term needs of the child.
- ▲ Consider the use of media-based behavioral treatments for children with behavioral disorders.

Geriatric

- ▲ Provide support for grandparents raising grandchildren.
- • Provide support for spouses and families of clients with strokes.
- ▲ Support the client's religious beliefs and activities and provide appropriate spiritual support persons.
- • Encourage the use of humor by family caregivers to describe their role reversal.
- • Explore community needs after assessing the client's strengths. Encourage elders to participate in volunteer programs.
- ▲ Refer to appropriate support groups for adjustment to role changes.
- ▲ Refer to therapy to improve memory for clients with Alzheimer's disease.

Multicultural

- • Assess for the influence of cultural beliefs, norms, values, and expectations on the individual's role.
- • Assess for conflicts between the caregiver's cultural role obligations and competing factors like employment or school.
- • Negotiate with the client regarding the aspects of their role that can be modified and still honor cultural beliefs.

• Encourage family to use support groups or other service programs to assist with role changes.

Home Care

• Above interventions may be adapted for home care use.
▲ Offer a referral to medical social services to assist with assessing the short- and long-term impacts of role change.

Client/Family Teaching

• Provide educational materials to family members on client behavior management plus caregiver stress-coping management.
• Help the client identify resources for assistance in caring for a disabled or aging parent (e.g., adult day care).
▲ Refer to appropriate community agencies to learn skills for functioning in the new or changed role (e.g., vocational rehabilitation, parenting classes, hospice, respite care).

Readiness for enhanced Self-care

NANDA Definition

S

A pattern of performing activities for oneself that helps to meet health-related goals and can be strengthened

Defining Characteristics

Expresses desire to enhance independence in monitoring life; expresses desire to enhance independence in maintaining health; expresses desire to enhance independence in maintaining personal development; expresses desire to enhance independence in maintaining well-being; expresses desire to enhance knowledge of strategies for self-care; expresses desire to enhance responsibility for self-care; expresses desire to enhance self-care

Client Outcomes

Client Will (Specify Time Frame):

- Assess current level of self-care activities as acceptable
- Express the need or desire to enhance level of self-care
- Seek out health-related information as needed
- Identify strategies to enhance self-care

- Perform appropriate interventions as needed
- Monitor level of self-care
- Evaluate effectiveness of self-care interventions at regular intervals

Nursing Interventions

- • Assess client's current level of self-care.
- • Educate clients that enhanced self-care is an achievable, desirable, and positive life goal.
- • Promote trust and enhanced communication between clients and their healthcare provider.
- • Promote opportunities for spiritual care and growth.
- • Increase social support and family involvement.
- • Identify what information clients will need to enhance self-care activities and provide educational opportunities as needed.
- • As needed, promote a wide range of intervention strategies to enhance self-care, such as client empowerment, early intervention, and hope instillment.
- • Evaluate the effectiveness of all self-care activities, and intervene or adjust as needed.

Pediatrics

- • Assess and evaluate a child's level of self-care and adjust strategies as needed.
- ▲ Assist families to engage in and maintain social support networks.
- • Encourage activities that support or enhance spiritual care.

Multicultural

- • Identify cultural beliefs, values, lifestyle practices, and problem-solving strategies when assessing clients' level of self-care.
- • Enhance cultural knowledge by seeking out information regarding different cultural or ethnic groups.
- • Recognize the impact of culture on self-care behaviors.
- • Provide culturally competent care.

Home Care

- • The nursing interventions described previously can be used in the home care setting with adaptation as needed.
- • Identify discharge planning needs.

- ▲ Make appropriate referrals as needed to enhance self-care activities.
- • Assess the need for financial assistance.
- ▲ Provide an interdisciplinary approach to health care.
- • Evaluate regularly if enhanced self-care is attainable in the home setting.

Client/Family Teaching

- Teach clients how to regularly assess their level of self-care.
- Instruct clients that a variety of interventions may be needed to enhance self-care.
- Help clients to understand that enhanced self-care is an achievable goal.
- Empower clients.
- Teach clients about the decision-making process and self-care activities needed to manage their illness state and promote well being.
- Continuously stress that all self-care activities must be regularly evaluated to ensure that enhanced levels of self-care can be maintained.

Bathing/hygiene Self-care deficit

NANDA Definition

Impaired ability to perform or complete bathing/hygiene activities for oneself

Defining Characteristics

Inability to access bathroom; inability to dry body; inability to get bath supplies; inability to obtain water source; inability to regulate bath water; inability to wash body

Related Factors (r/t)

Cognitive impairment; decreased motivation; environmental barriers; inability to perceive body part; inability to perceive spatial relationship; musculoskeletal impairment; neuromuscular impairment; pain; perceptual impairment; severe anxiety; weakness

NOTE: Specify level of independence using a standardized functional scale.

Client Outcomes

Client Will (Specify Time Frame):

- Remain free of body odor and maintain intact skin
- State satisfaction with ability to use adaptive devices to bathe
- Use methods to bathe safely with minimal difficulty
- Bathe with assistance of caregiver as needed and report sense of dignity is maintained
- Bathe with assistance of caregiver as needed without exhibiting defensive (aggressive) behaviors

Nursing Interventions

- Establish the goal of client's bathing as being a pleasant experience, especially for cognitively impaired clients, without the symptoms of unmet needs—hitting, biting, kicking, screaming, resisting—and plan for client preferences in timing, type and length of bathing, water temperature, and with silence or music.
- Use and teach client-centered bathing: foster development of an understanding relationship with client, plan for client's comfort and preferences, personalize care, show respect in communications, critically think to solve issues that arise, and use a gentle approach.
- Ask the client for input on bathing habits and cultural bathing preferences.
- Develop a bathing care plan based on the client's own history of bathing practices that addresses skin needs, self-care needs, client response to bathing, and equipment needs.
- Individualize bathing by identifying the function of bathing (e.g., odor, urine removal), frequency required to achieve function, and best bathing form (e.g., towel bathing, tub, shower) to meet client preferences, preserve client dignity, make bathing a soothing experience, and reduce client aggression.
- Bathe cognitively impaired or older adult clients before bedtime.
- Provide pain relief measures, such as ice packs, heat, and analgesics for sore joints 45 minutes before bathing; move extremities slowly and carefully; and inform the client before movements associated with pain. These movements include walking; transferring to a new location; moving joints; and washing genitals, face, and between toes and under arms. Have the client wash painful areas, recognize indicators of pain, and apologize for any pain caused.

S

- Consider environmental and human factors that may limit bathing ability, such as bending to get into the tub, reaching for bathing items, grasping faucets, and lifting oneself. Adapt environment by placing items within easy reach, lowering faucets, and using a hand held shower.
- Use a comfortable padded shower chair with foot support, (or adapt a chair: pad it with towels/washcloths, cover the cold back with dry towels, and cover the arms with foam pipe insulation).
- Provide privacy. Have only one trusted, consistent caregiver assist with bathing, encourage a traffic-free bathing area, and post privacy signs.
- Ensure bathing assistance preserves client dignity through conveyance of honor and recognition of the deservedness of respect and esteem of all persons, regardless of their dependency and infirmity.
- If the client is bathing alone, place the assistance call light within reach.
- Keep the client warmly covered.
- For cognitively impaired clients, avoid upsetting factors associated with bathing: instead of using the terms *bath, shower,* or *wash,* use comforting words, such as *warm, relaxing,* or *massage.* Start at the client's feet and bathe upward; bathe the face last after washing hands and using a clean cloth. Use a beautician/barber or wash hair at another time to avoid water dripping in the face.
- Use towel bathing especially when other forms of bathing are distressing to client. Bathe client in bed using no-rinse soap, a bath blanket, and warm towels to keep the client covered the entire time. Warm and moisten towels/washcloths with no rinse soap and place in plastic bags to keep them warm. Use warm, moist towels to massage large areas (front, back) and one washcloth for facial areas and another one for genital areas. No rinsing or drying is needed.
- For shower bathing, use client-centered techniques: allow client to have choices, keep client covered with towels and cleanse under the towels, use no-rinse products, use favorite bathing items, and use a hand-held shower with adjustable spray.
- Allow the client to participate as able in bathing. Smile and provide praise for accomplishments in a relaxed manner.
- Inspect skin condition during bathing.

S

Geriatric

- Assess for grieving resulting from loss of function.
- Develop the client's muscle strength building plan through exercising and walking to build the client's physiological capacity and prevent decline in ADLs.
- Emphasize how the client experiences the bathing setting with a secondary focus on ways the environment can support the caregiver.
- ▲ Design the bathing environment for comfort: *Visual.* Reduce clutter and use partitions to hide equipment storage. Laminate and put artwork or decorative objects in bather's view, or place cue cards to bathing process (wall, ceiling, shower). Stand or sit in bather's position to experience what he/she sees. Decrease glare from tiles, white walls, and artificial lights. Use contrasting colors and soft but adequate lighting on a dimming switch for adjustment.
- Arrange the bathing environment to promote sensory comfort: *Auditory.* Reduce noise of voices and water. Do not allow traffic into bathing room. Add fabric to absorb sound (three to four times the width of the opening for sound absorbing folds). Play soft music.
- Design the bathing environment for comfort: *Tactile.* Use heat lamps or radiant heat panels to keep the room warm. Use powder-coated grab bars in decorative colors with nonslip grip. Provide a soft rug to stand on. Ensure that flooring is not slippery (a high coefficient of friction, ideally above 80, is desired and obtained through flooring coatings).
- When bathing a cognitively impaired client, have all bathing items ready for the client's needs before bathing begins.
- Teach caregivers to use behaviors that validate the client's feelings, reassure the client, and segment tasks. Teach them to explain the care process while bathing clients with Alzheimer's disease.
- Train caregivers bathing clients with dementia to avoid behaviors that can trigger assault: confrontational communication, invalidation of the resident's feelings, failure to prepare a resident for a task, initiating shower spray or touch during bathing without verbal prompts beforehand, washing the hair/face, speaking disrespectfully to the client, and hurrying the pace of the bath.

S

- Limit total body bathing using tepid water to once a week; provide a towel bath at other times.
- Test water temperature before use with a thermometer.
- Use a gentle touch when bathing a client; avoid vigorous scrubbing motions.
- Teach caregiver to use gentle massage for frail older adult clients during bathing.
- Add hydrating bath oils to tub bath water 15 minutes after the client immerses in water.
- Allow the client or caregiver adequate time to complete the bathing activity.

Home Care

- If in a typical bathing setting for the client, assess the client's ability to bathe self via direct observation using physical performance tests for ADLs.
- ▲ Request referrals for occupational and physical therapy if client has difficulty showering or getting into a tub.
- ▲ Based on functional assessment and rehabilitation capacity, refer for home health aide services to assist with bathing and hygiene.
- Recommend use of a water temperature–sensing shower valve to prevent scalding.
- Turn down temperature of hot water heater.
- Show caregiver a videotape of caregiver self-care activities (organizing the day, talking when frustrated, taking time for self, and talking to a nonjudgmental person) followed by a discussion.
- Cue cognitively impaired clients in the steps of hygiene.
- Respect the preference of terminally ill clients to refuse or limit hygiene care.
- If a terminally ill client requests hygiene care, make an extra effort to meet the request and provide care when the client and family will most benefit (e.g., before visitors arrive, at bedtime, in the early morning).

Client/Family Teaching

- Teach the client and family how to use adaptive devices for bathing (e.g., long-handled brushes, soap-on-a-rope, washcloth mitt, wall bars, tub bench, padded shower chair, commode chair without pan), and teach bathing techniques that promote safety and prevent burns (e.g., getting into tub before filling it with

S

water if a temperature sensor valve is used; testing water with a thermometer; emptying water before getting out; using an anti-slip mat, wall-grab bars, and tub bench).

- Teach the client and family an individualized bathing routine that includes a frequency schedule, privacy, skin inspection, no-rinse products, skin lubricants, chill prevention, and bathing options, such as sponge or towel.

Dressing/grooming Self-care deficit

NANDA Definition

Impaired ability to perform or complete dressing and grooming activities for self

Defining Characteristics

Inability to choose clothing; inability to put clothing on lower body; inability to maintain appearance at a satisfactory level; inability to pick up clothing; inability to put clothing on upper body; inability to put on shoes; inability to put on socks; inability to remove clothes; inability to use assistive devices; inability to use zippers; impaired ability to fasten clothing; impaired ability to obtain clothing; impaired ability to put on necessary items of clothing; impaired ability to take off necessary items of clothing

S

Related Factors (r/t)

Cognitive impairment; decreased motivation; discomfort; environmental barriers; fatigue; musculoskeletal impairment; neuromuscular impairment; pain perceptual impairment; severe anxiety; weakness

NOTE: Specify level of independence using a standardized functional scale.

Client Outcomes

Client Will (Specify Time Frame):

- Dress and groom self to optimal potential
- Use adaptive devices to dress and groom
- Explain and use methods to enhance strengths during dressing and grooming
- Dress and groom with assistance of caregiver as needed

Nursing Interventions

- Observe the client's ability to dress and groom self through direct observation and from the client/caregiver report, noting specific deficits and their causes.
- Assess client for symptoms of general weakness, arm paralysis, and fatigue for planning methods to promote self-care in dressing.
- Determine the client's personal preferences for dressing and grooming to maintain autonomy, personal routine, and quality of life of older client by using the Self-maintenance Habits and Preferences in Elderly (SHAPE) questionnaire and focus on items most preferred by the client.
- Encourage older clients to dress and groom rather than completing the tasks for them.
- Consider and remove environmental barriers and human factors that may limit dressing/grooming ability, such as having to reach for clothes or grooming aids in closets or drawers. Help the client arrange clothing and grooming devices within easy reach. Installing turntables, closet rods, or drawers between eye and hip level is helpful.
- Ask the client for input on clothing choices and how to increase the ease of dressing.

▲ Request referrals for occupational and physical therapy.

▲ Provide medication for pain 45 minutes before dressing and grooming as needed.

- Provide privacy and limit the number of people/caregivers in the room.
- Select clothing in larger sizes; clothing with elastic waistbands, wide sleeves, and pant legs; dresses that open down the back (for wheelchair-bound women), and clothing with Velcro fasteners or larger buttons.
- Use adaptive dressing and grooming equipment as needed (e.g., long-handled brushes, grasping devices, Velcro closures, zipper pulls, button hooks, elastic shoelaces, large buttons, soap-on-a-rope, suction holders).
- Lay clothing out in the order that it will be put on by the client. Dress bottom half, then top half of body.
- Encourage the client to dress appropriately for time of day. Perform dressing and grooming activities in a consistent sequence each day.

- Teach caregivers to see dressing as an opportunity to promote independence for clients who are able and as a time to increase social talk for others.
- Teach Certified Nursing Assistants to use graduated verbal prompting for clients with dementia to complete dressing task and provide positive reinforcement immediately for accomplished steps of task.
- For clients with dementia, maintain a specific routine for dressing to prevent increase in dressing time required.
- Encourage participation; guide the client's hand through task if necessary.
- If the client does not groom self, sit side by side with the client, put your hand over the client's hand, support the client's elbow with your other hand, and help the client comb his or her hair.
- Nurture personal attributes, such as humor, positive attitude, faith, and hope, and control of stress for clients with multiple sclerosis.
- Allow clients with a spinal cord injury to maximize control over activities and teach them how to direct their caregivers.
- If the client has had a cerebrovascular accident (CVA) with hemiparesis, consider use of constraint-induced movement therapy (CIMT), where the functional extremity is purposely constrained and the client is forced to use the involved extremity.

S

Geriatric

- Assess for grieving resulting from loss of function.
- ▲ Provide medication for pain if needed, and plan activities to prevent fatigue before dressing/grooming.
- Assess tasks the client can complete, noting areas of independence and difficulty to make adaptations.
- Allow the client or caregiver adequate time to complete dressing (e.g., do not insist that the client is dressed at an early hour).
- ▲ Request referral for older women with cardiac disease to rehabilitation programs for strength training.

Home Care

- Involve the client in planning of informal care and provide access to health professionals and financial support for the care.

- ▲ Based on functional assessment and rehabilitation capacity, refer for home health services for rehabilitation and to assist with dressing and grooming.
- • Have caregivers view a videotape showing caregiver self-care activities (organizing the day, talking when frustrated, taking time for self, and talking to a nonjudgmental person) followed by a discussion.
- • Cue cognitively impaired clients in steps of dressing and grooming.
- • Respect the preference of the terminally ill client to refuse dressing and limit grooming.
- • If terminally ill clients request dressing and grooming, make an extra effort to meet the request and provide care when the client and family will most benefit (e.g., before visitors, in early morning).
- • Maintain the temperature of the home at a comfortable level when dressing a terminally ill client.

Client/Family Teaching

- • Teach the client to dress the affected side first, then the unaffected side.
- • Teach the simplest step in a task until mastered, and then proceed to more complicated steps. Give praise.
- • Teach the client how to use adaptive devices for dressing and grooming.

S

Feeding Self-care deficit

NANDA Definition

Impaired ability to perform or complete feeding activities

Defining Characteristics

Inability to bring food from a receptacle to the mouth; inability to chew food; inability to complete a meal; inability to get food onto utensil; inability to handle utensils; inability to ingest food in a socially acceptable manner; inability to ingest food safely; inability to ingest sufficient food; inability to manipulate food in mouth; inability to open containers; inability to pick up cup or glass; inability to prepare food for ingestion; inability to swallow food; inability to use assistive device

Related Factors (r/t)

Cognitive impairment; decreased motivation; discomfort; environmental barriers; fatigue; musculoskeletal impairment; neuromuscular impairment; pain; perceptual impairment; severe anxiety; weakness

NOTE: Specify level of independence using a standardized functional scale.

Client Outcomes

Client Will (Specify Time Frame):

- Feed self safely
- State satisfaction with ability to use adaptive devices for feeding
- Use assistance with feeding when necessary (caregiver)

Nursing Interventions

- • Assess the client's ability to feed self and note specific deficits.
- • Ask the client for input on methods to facilitate eating and feeding (e.g., cultural foods, other food and fluid preferences developed during a lifetime), and provide four entrée choices, including ethnic choice.
- ▲ Consult speech-language pathologist for individualized feeding care plans.
- ▲ Request referral for occupational and physical therapy; request a dietician.
- • Use any necessary adaptive feeding equipment (e.g., rocker knives, plate guards, suction mats, built-up handles on utensils, scoop dishes, large-handled cups).
- • Before feeding the client with brain trauma or dementia, provide oral hygiene: for dry mouth, give tart or sour foods/fluids before meals; give proteolytic enzymes before meals if thick oral secretions are a problem.
- • Position the client with brain trauma or dementia for feeding: help the client sit upright with hips and knees flexed, feet supported, trunk and head in midline position, and head slightly flexed with chin down; for an immobilized client in bed, use high Fowler's position and support the head and neck with

S

neck slightly flexed; for a client with unilateral paralysis, tilt the head slightly to unaffected side and rotate the head toward the affected side.

- Provide small portions of favorite foods, one entrée at a time, at proper serving temperature, with unnecessary items and utensils removed.
- To increase oral intake, use a feeding assistance intervention protocol: individual assistance, proper positioning, dining location preferences, and meal tray substitutions; use graduated prompting to enhance self-feeding ability as needed: (1) social stimulation and encouragement, (2) nonverbal cueing, (3) verbal cueing, (4) physical guidance, and (5) full physical assistance.
- To increase oral intake, include between-meal snacks three times a day alone or if intake is not increased 15% with the feeding assistance intervention protocol (discussed previously) delivered to the client on a movable cart with a variety of food/fluid choices.
- The caregiver should sit beside the client (on the client's unaffected side) at eye level.
- Presentation of feeding: provide ½-1 teaspoon of solid food or 10-15 mL of liquid at a time; wait until client has swallowed prior food/liquid.
- Provide the client with a pleasant, quiet meal environment with no distractions.
- Keep the environment free of toileting devices and odors, avoid painful procedures before meals, remove lids from tray, and provide clean utensils for separate courses.
- Do not mix different foods together when assisting the client with eating.
- Encourage the client to keep food on the unaffected side of mouth with a rocking motion to deposit the food, if applicable.
- Be prepared to intervene if choking occurs; have suction equipment readily available and know the Heimlich maneuver.
- For clients with conditions such as Parkinson's disease or myasthenia gravis, ensure that their medications are given so that peak drug action occurs during meal times.
- ▲ Clients who have had a stroke should continue rehabilitation efforts long-term to achieve optimal functioning.
- If client has had a cerebrovascular accident (CVA) with hemiparesis, consider use of constraint-induced movement therapy

(CIMT), where the functional extremity is purposely constrained and the client is forced to use the involved extremity.

- If the client does not feed self, sit side by side with the client, put your hand over the client's hand, support the client's elbow with your other hand, and help the client feed self.
- Provide oral hygiene after every meal and check for pocketing of food.

Geriatric

- Provide nutrition care that honors the individual client and enhances rather than detracts from each client's quality of life.
- Use aromatherapy to increase appetite and pleasure in eating.
- ▲ Implement Hospital Elder Life Program, a model of care to prevent functional and cognitive decline of older persons during hospitalization.
- ▲ Implement the Wellspring model, which advocates education and empowerment of CNAs to solve problems without direct administrative oversight.
- ▲ Ensure CNAs know the signs/symptoms of dysphagia, such as choking, coughing, oral/chewing problems, throat clearing, wet voice, gurgling voice, or pneumonia; if any of these are exhibited during feeding, report them promptly.
- ▲ Seek CNA input on feeding concerns during discussion of possible actions and share techniques that are beneficial to specific clients.
- ▲ Ensure CNA feeding training includes the need to decrease command statements to clients being fed and instead offer encouraging statements.
- ▲ Suggest that CNAs learn 3-5 personal details about their client during the feeding.
- ▲ Provide medication for pain before meals if needed, and plan activities to prevent fatigue before meals.
- Upon admission to long-term care, assess and maintain documentation about eating and nutrition (include weight) for clients who have had a stroke.
- Serve meals family style, with food in serving bowls and an empty plate to be filled by the client.
- Obtain and incorporate the client's view of the agency's food selection and presentation into agency food service.
- ▲ Ensure adequate staffing at meal times.

- Choose soft foods rather than liquids, or use dietary thickeners.
- Assess for intolerance to food texture and, if found, reverse food texture pattern as tolerated, progressing finally to the texture stage of thick liquids.
- Provide finger foods for clients with Alzheimer's disease and place the food in their hands as needed to cue.
- Provide a dignified assisted dining experience: create a home-like dining room; provide leisurely pace, which allows the client with dentures adequate time to chew; and support choices and independence.
- Provide emotionally neutral, nonverbal cues to improve table-sitting behavior if the client rises from table early; for example, place a firm hand on the dominant shoulder, indicating that the client should sit.

Home Care

▲ Based on functional assessment and rehabilitation capacity, refer for home health aide services to assist with feeding.
- Cue cognitively impaired clients when feeding them.
- Respect the preference of terminally ill clients to refuse nutrition or assistance with eating. Refer to the care plans for **Imbalanced Nutrition: less than body requirements** and **Impaired Swallowing.**
- If a terminally ill client requests nutrition, take special care to provide foods and assistive devices that protect the client from aspiration, minimize energy requirements, and meet the client's taste preferences.

Client/Family Teaching

- Teach the client how to use adaptive devices.
- Teach the client with hemianopsia to turn the head so that the plate is in the line of vision.
- Teach visually impaired clients to locate foods according to numbers on a clock.
- Teach the caregiver feeding techniques that prevent choking (e.g., sitting beside the client on the unaffected side, feeding the client slowly, checking food temperature, providing fluid between bites, establishing a method to communicate readiness for next bite, limiting conversation while chewing).

Toileting Self-care deficit

NANDA Definition

Impaired ability to perform or complete own toileting activities

Defining Characteristics

Inability to carry out proper toilet hygiene; inability to flush toilet or commode; inability to get to toilet or commode; inability to manipulate clothing for toileting; inability to rise from toilet or commode; inability to sit on toilet or commode

Related Factors (r/t)

Cognitive impairment; decreased motivation; environmental barriers; fatigue; impaired mobility status; impaired transfer ability; musculoskeletal impairment; neuromuscular impairment; pain; perceptual impairment; severe anxiety; weakness

Client Outcomes

Client Will (Specify Time Frame):

- Remain free of incontinence and impaction with no urine or stool on skin
- State satisfaction with ability to use adaptive devices for toileting
- Explain and use methods to be safe and independent in toileting

Nursing Interventions

- • Provide privacy.
- • Assess ability to toilet; note specific deficits.
- • Assess the client's usual bowel and bladder toileting patterns and the terminology used for toileting.
- • Observe cause of inability to toilet independently (see Related Factors).
- • Ask the client for input on toileting methods and timing and how to better provide toileting activity assistance.
- • Assess barriers to implementation of a toileting program.
- • Make assistance call button readily available to the client and answer call light promptly.
- • Use any necessary assistive toileting equipment (e.g., raised

S

toilet seat, bedside commode, suction mats, spill-proof urinals, support rails next to toilet, toilet safety frames, Sanifems [allows a woman to void standing], fracture bedpans, long-handled toilet paper holders).

- If a client's voiding patterns are consistent, place them on an individualized toileting schedule that is documented and allows the client to use the toilet/commode.
- Develop toileting schedule using clocks, written schedules, or verbal prompting as cues for the client, and provide assistance at scheduled times.
- Schedule toileting to occur when the defecation urge is strongest or voiding is likely (e.g., in the morning, every 2 hours, after meals, at bedtime). Assist the client until self-care ability increases.
- Keep toilet paper and hand-washing items within easy reach of the client. Provide prompt skin care and linen changes after incontinence episodes.

Geriatric

- Assess the client's functional ability to manipulate clothing for toileting, and if necessary modify clothing with Velcro fasteners and elastic waists.
- Monitor clients with dementia for behavioral toileting cues (e.g., pacing, restlessness, fidgeting) and assist with prompt toileting, or use an individualized scheduled toileting for memory-impaired older adults.
- ▲ Remove barriers to toileting, support client's cultural beliefs, and preserve dignity.
- ▲ Include regular exercise and a walking program in plan of care.
- ▲ Assist client (especially frail older clients) to exercise (walk 2 minutes, push wheelchair, sit-stand repetitions) for several minutes every time he or she gets up to toilet.
- ▲ Implement Hospital Elder Life Program, a model of care to prevent functional and cognitive decline of older persons during hospitalization.
- After hip fracture, focus on hospital-based multidisciplinary interventions and discharge planning.
- Provide a small footstool in front of the toilet or commode.
- Avoid the use of indwelling catheters if possible, and use condom catheters in men without dementia.

Home Care

- ▲ Request referral for occupational and physical therapy to identify barriers and suggest strategies for safe toileting.
- ▲ Based on functional assessment and rehabilitation capacity, refer for home health aide services to assist with toileting.
- ▲ Avoid the use of medications that place undue toileting stress on the client who is terminally ill.
- ▲ Provide pain medication for terminally ill clients 20-45 minutes before toileting in anticipation of possible pain (e.g., in coordination with a bowel stimulation program). See the care plan for **Constipation.**
- ▲ Consider use of an indwelling catheter for terminally ill clients in too much pain to move when hygiene and skin integrity are difficult to maintain.

Client/Family Teaching

- • Teach the client and family about bladder control and how to toilet the client with adaptive and safety devices.
- • Have the family install a toilet seat of a contrasting color.
- • Prepare the client for toileting needs by teaching the action of medications, such as diuretics.
- • Help the visually impaired client to develop a plan for locating bathrooms in new environments.

S

Readiness for enhanced Self-concept

NANDA Definition

A pattern of perceptions or ideas about the self that is sufficient for well-being and can be strengthened

Defining Characteristics

Accepts limitations; accepts strengths; actions are congruent with verbal expression; expresses confidence in abilities; expresses satisfaction with body image; expresses satisfaction with personal identity; expresses satisfaction with role performance; expresses satisfaction with sense of worthiness; expresses satisfaction with thoughts about self; expresses willingness to enhance self-concept

Client Outcomes

Client Will (Specify Time Frame):

- State willingness to enhance self-concept
- State satisfaction with thoughts about self, sense of worthiness, role performance, body image, and personal identity
- Demonstrate actions that are congruent with expressed feelings and thoughts
- State confidence in abilities
- Accept strengths and limitations

Nursing Interventions

- • Assess and support activities that promote self-concept developmentally.
- ▲ Refer to nutritional and exercise programs to support weight loss
- ▲ Clients with cancer often use massage therapy as an adjunct treatment.
- ▲ Support establishing a church-based community health promotion programs (CBHPPs) with the following key elements: partnerships, positive health values, availability of services, access to church facilities, community-focused interventions, health behavior change, and supportive social relationships.
- ▲ For clients who have had breast surgery and need a prosthesis, provide the appropriate prosthesis before the client leaves the health care facility.

Pediatric

- ▲ Consider the development of a Healthy Kids mentoring program that has four components: (1) relationship building, (2) self-esteem enhancement, (3) goal setting, and (4) academic assistance (tutoring).
- ▲ Assess and provide referrals to mental health professionals for clients with unresolved worries associated with terrorism.
- ▲ Provide an alternative school-based program for pregnant and parenting teenagers.

Geriatric

- ▲ Encourage clients to consider a Web-based support program when they are in a caregiving situation.

▲ Consider a strength, mobility, balance, and endurance training program.

Multicultural

- Carefully assess each client and allow families to participate in providing care that is acceptable based on the client's cultural beliefs.
- Provide support for health-promoting behaviors and self-concept for clients from diverse cultures.
- Refer to the care plans **Disturbed Body image**, **Readiness for enhanced Coping**, **Chronic low Self-esteem**, and **Readiness for enhanced Spiritual well-being.**

Home Care

- Previously discussed interventions may be used in the home care setting.

Chronic low Self-esteem

S

NANDA Definition

Long-standing negative self-evaluation/feelings about self or self-capabilities

Defining Characteristics

Dependent on others' opinions; evaluates self as unable to deal with events; exaggerates negative feedback about self; excessively seeks reassurance; expressions of guilt; expressions of shame; frequent lack of success in life events; hesitant to try new things/situations; indecisive; lack of eye contact; nonassertive; overly conforming; passive; rejects positive feedback about self; self-negating verbalization

Client Outcomes

Client Will (Specify Time Frame):

- Demonstrate improved ability to interact with others (e.g., maintains eye contact, engages in conversation, expresses thoughts/feelings)

- Verbalize increased self-acceptance through positive self-statements about self
- Identify personal strengths, accomplishments, and values
- Identify and work on small, achievable goals
- Improve independent decision-making and problem-solving skills

Nursing Interventions

- Actively listen to and respect the client.
- Assess the client's environmental and everyday stressors, including physical health concerns and the potential of abusive relationships.
- Assess existing strengths and coping abilities, and provide opportunities for their expression and recognition.
- Reinforce the personal strengths and positive self-perceptions that a client identifies.
- Identify client's negative self-assessments.
- Encourage realistic and achievable goal setting and resources and identify impediments to achievement.
- Demonstrate and promote effective communication techniques; spend time with the client.
- Encourage independent decision making by reviewing options and their possible consequences with client.
- Assist client to challenge negative perceptions of self and performance.
- Use failure as an opportunity to provide valuable feedback.
- Promote maintaining a level of functioning in the community.
- Assist client with evaluating the effect of family and peer group on feelings of self-worth.
- Support socialization and communication skills.
- Encourage journal/diary writing as a safe way of expressing emotions.

S

Geriatric

- Support client in identifying and adapting to functional changes.
- Use reminiscence therapy to identify patterns of strength and accomplishment.

- Encourage participation in peer group activities.
- Encourage activities in which a client can support/help others.

Multicultural

- Assess for the influence of cultural beliefs, norms, and values on the client's sense of self-esteem.
- Assess for evidence of client financial strain.
- Assess for drug and alcohol use in individuals with low self-esteem.
- Validate the client's feelings regarding ethnic or racial identity.

Home Care

- Assess a client's immediate support system/family for relationship patterns and content of communication.
- Encourage the client's family to provide support and feedback regarding client value or worth.

▲ Refer to medical social services to assist the family in pattern changes that could benefit the client.

▲ If a client is involved in counseling or self-help groups, monitor and encourage attendance. Help the client identify the value of group participation after each group encounter.

▲ If a client is taking prescribed psychotropic medications, assess for knowledge of medication side effects and reasons for taking medication. Teach as necessary.

▲ Assess medications for effectiveness and side effects and monitor client for compliance.

Client/Family Teaching

▲ Refer to community agencies for psychotherapeutic counseling.

▲ Refer to psychoeducational groups on stress reduction and coping skills.

▲ Refer to self-help support groups specific to needs.

S

Situational low Self-esteem

NANDA Definition

Development of a negative perception of self-worth in response to a current situation (specify)

Defining Characteristics

Evaluation of self as unable to deal with situations or events; expressions of helplessness; expressions of uselessness; indecisive behavior; nonassertive behavior; self-negating verbalizations; verbally reports current situational challenge to self-worth

Related Factors (r/t)

Behavior inconsistent with values; developmental changes; disturbed body image; failures; functional impairment; lack of recognition; loss; rejections; social role changes

Client Outcomes

Client Will (Specify Time Frame):

- State effect of life events on feelings about self
- State personal strengths
- Acknowledge presence of guilt and not blame self if an action was related to another person's appraisal
- Seek help when necessary
- Demonstrate self-perceptions are accurate given physical capabilities
- Demonstrate separation of self-perceptions from societal stigmas

Nursing Interventions

▲ Assess the client for signs and symptoms of depression and potential for suicide and/or violence. If present, immediately notify the appropriate personnel of symptoms. See care plans for **Risk for other-directed Violence** and **Risk for Suicide.**

- Actively listen to, demonstrate respect for, and accept client.
- Assist in the identification of problems and situational factors that contribute to problems, offering options for resolution.
- Mutually identify strengths, resources, and previously effective coping strategies.

- Have client list strengths.
- Accept client's own pace in working through grief or crisis situations.
- Accept the client's own defenses in dealing with the crisis.
- Assess for unhealthy coping mechanisms, such as substance abuse.
- Provide information about support groups of people who have common experiences or interests.
- Teach the client mindfulness techniques to cope more effectively with strong emotional responses.
- Support problem-solving strategies but discourage decision making when in crisis.
- Assess the client's environmental and everyday stressors, including evidence of abusive relationships.
- Encourage objective appraisal of self and life events and challenge negative or perfectionist expectations of self.
- Provide psychoeducation to client and family.
- Validate confusion when feeling ill but looking well.
- Acknowledge the presence of societal stigma. Teach management tools.
- Validate the effect of negative past experiences on self-esteem and work on corrective measures.
- See care plan for **Chronic low Self-esteem.**

S

Geriatric and Multicultural

- See care plan for **Chronic low Self-esteem.**

Home Care

- Establish an emergency plan and contract with the client for its use.
- Access supplies that support a client's success at independent living.
- See care plan for **Chronic low Self-esteem**.

Client/Family Teaching

- Assess the person's support system (family, friends, and community) and involve them if desired.
- Educate client and family regarding the grief process.
- Teach client and family that the crisis is temporary.
- ▲ Refer to appropriate community resources or crisis intervention centers.

▲ Refer to resources for handicap and/or disability services.
▲ Refer to illness-specific consumer support groups.
▲ Refer to self-help support groups specific to needs.

Risk for situational low Self-esteem

NANDA Definition

At risk for developing negative perception of self-worth in response to a current situation (specify)

Risk Factors

Behavior inconsistent with values; decreased control over environment; developmental changes; disturbed body image; failures; functional impairment; history of abandonment; history of abuse; history of learned helplessness; history of neglect; lack of recognition; loss; physical illness; rejections; social role changes; unrealistic self-expectations

Client Outcomes

S

Client Will (Specify Time Frame):

- State accurate self-appraisal
- Demonstrate the ability to self-validate
- Demonstrate the ability to make decisions independent of primary peer group
- Express effects of media on self-appraisal
- Express influence of substances on self-esteem
- Identify strengths and healthy coping skills
- State life events and change as influencing self-esteem

Nursing Interventions

- Identify environmental and/or developmental factors that increase risk for low self-esteem, especially in children/adolescents, to make needed referrals.
- Assess the client's previous experiences with health care and coping with illness to determine the level of education and support needed.
- Assess for low and negative affect (expression of feelings).

- • Encourage client to maintain highest level of community functioning.
- • Treat the client with respect and as an equal to maintain positive self-esteem.
- • Help the client to identify the resources and social support network available at this time.
- • Assess for unhealthy coping mechanisms, such as substance abuse.
- • Encourage the client to find a self-help or therapy group that focuses on self-esteem enhancement.
- • Teach the client mindfulness techniques to cope with strong emotional responses and to prevent decreases in self-esteem.
- • Encourage the client to create a sense of competence through short-term goal setting and goal achievement.
- ▲ Assess the client for symptoms of depression and anxiety. Refer to specialist as needed.
- • Teach client a systematic problem-solving process.
- • See care plans for **Disturbed personal Identity** and **Situational low Self-esteem.**

Geriatric

- • Help the client to identify age-related and/or developmental factors that may be affecting self-esteem.
- • Assist the client in life review and identifying positive accomplishments.
- • Help client to establish a peer group and structured daily activities.

Home Care

- • Assess current environmental stresses and identify community resources.
- • Encourage family members to acknowledge and validate the client's strengths.
- • Assess the need for establishing an emergency plan.
- • See care plans for **Situational low Self-esteem** and **Chronic low Self-esteem.**

Client/Family Teaching

- ▲ Refer the client/family to community-based self-help and support groups.

S

▲ Refer the client to educational classes on stress management, relaxation training, and so on.
▲ Refer the client to community agencies that offer support and environmental resources.

Self-mutilation

NANDA Definition

Deliberate self-injurious behavior causing tissue damage with the intent of causing nonfatal injury to attain relief of tension

Defining Characteristics

Abrading; biting; constricting a body part; cuts on body; hitting; ingestion of harmful substances; inhalation of harmful substances; insertion of object into body orifice; picking at wounds; scratches on body; self-inflicted burns; severing

Related Factors (r/t)

Adolescence; autistic individual; battered child; borderline personality disorder; character disorder; childhood illness; childhood sexual abuse; childhood surgery; depersonalization; developmentally delayed individual; dissociation; disturbed body image; disturbed interpersonal relationships; eating disorders; emotionally disturbed; family alcoholism; family divorce; family history of self-destructive behaviors; feels threatened with loss of significant relationship; history of inability to plan solutions; history of inability to see long-term consequences; history of self-injurious behavior; impulsivity; inability to express tension verbally; incarceration; ineffective coping; irresistible urge to cut/damage self; isolation from peers; labile behavior; lack of family confidant; living in nontraditional setting (e.g., foster, group institutional care); low self-esteem; mounting tension that is intolerable; needs quick reduction of stress; negative feelings (e.g., depression, rejection, self-hatred, separation anxiety, guilt, depersonalization); peers who self-mutilate; perfectionism; poor communication between parent and adolescent; psychotic state (e.g., command hallucinations); sexual identity crisis; substance abuse; unstable body image; unstable self-esteem; use of manipulation to obtain nurturing relationship with others; violence between parental figures

Client Outcomes

Client Will (Specify Time Frame):

- Have injuries treated
- Refrain from further self-injury
- State appropriate ways to cope with increased psychological or physiological tension
- Express feelings
- Seek help when having urges to self-mutilate
- Maintain self-control without supervision
- Use appropriate community agencies when caregivers are unable to attend to emotional needs

Nursing Interventions

NOTE: Before implementation of interventions in the face of self-mutilation, nurses should examine their own emotional responses to incidents of self-harm to ensure that interventions will not be based on countertransference reactions.

▲ Provide medical treatment for injuries. Use careful aseptic technique when caring for wounds. Care for the wounds in a matter-of-fact manner.

• Assess for risk of suicide or other self-damaging behaviors. Refer to the care plan for **Risk for Suicide.**

• Assess for signs of depression, anxiety, and impulsivity.

• Assess for presence of hallucinations. Ask specific questions such as, "Do you hear voices that other people do not hear? Are they telling you to hurt yourself?"

▲ Assure the client that he or she will not be alone and will be safe during hallucinations. Provide referrals for medication.

▲ Assess for the presence of medical disorders, mental retardation, medication effects, or psychiatric disorders that may include self-mutilation. Initiate referral for evaluation and treatment as appropriate.

▲ Case finding and referral by school nurses for psychological or psychiatric treatment is critical. Monitor the client's behavior, using 15-minute checks at irregular times so that the client does not notice a pattern.

• Establish trust.

• Recognize that self-mutilation may serve a variety of functions for the person. Be extremely cautious about touching the client when he or she is experiencing an abreaction (reenactment of

S

precipitating trauma). Sometimes physically holding a client is necessary to prevent self-injury.

- • Assess the client's ability to enter into a no-suicide contract. Secure a written or verbal contract from the client to notify staff when experiencing the desire to self-mutilate.
- ▲ Use a collaborative approach for care.
- ▲ Refer for medication, such as clozapine.
- ▲ Consider partial hospitalization with individual and group therapy.
- • Refer to the care plan for **Risk for Self-mutilation** for additional information.

Home Care and Client/Family Teaching

See the care plan for **Risk for Self-mutilation.**

Risk for Self-mutilation

NANDA Definition

At risk for deliberate self-injurious behavior causing tissue damage with the intent of causing nonfatal injury to attain relief of tension

S

Risk Factors

Adolescence; autistic individuals; battered child; borderline personality disorders; character disorders; childhood illness; childhood sexual abuse; childhood surgery; depersonalization; developmentally delayed individuals; dissociation; disturbed body image; disturbed interpersonal relationships; eating disorders; emotionally disturbed child; family alcoholism; family divorce; family history of self-destructive behaviors; feels threatened with loss of significant relationship; history of inability to plan solutions; history of inability to see long-term consequences; history of self-injurious behavior; impulsivity; inability to express tension verbally; inadequate coping; incarceration; irresistible urge to damage self; isolation from peers; living in nontraditional setting (e.g., foster group, or institutional care); loss of control over problem-solving situations; low self-esteem; loss of significant relationship(s); mounting tension that is intolerable; needs quick reduction of stress; negative feelings (e.g., depression, rejection, self-hatred, separation anxiety, guilt); peers who self-mutilate; perfectionism; psychotic state (e.g., command hallucinations); sexual identity crisis; substance abuse; unstable self-esteem; use of manipulation to obtain nurturing relationship with others; violence between parental figures

Client Outcomes

Client Will (Specify Time Frame):

- Refrain from self-injury
- Identify triggers to self-mutilation
- State appropriate ways to cope with increased psychological or physiological tension
- Express feelings
- Seek help when having urges to self-mutilate
- Maintain self-control without supervision
- Use appropriate community agencies when caregivers are unable to attend to emotional needs

Nursing Interventions

- Refer to the care plan for **Self-mutilation**
- Assessment data from the client and family members may have to be gathered at different times; allowing a family member or trusted friend with whom the client is comfortable to be present during the assessment may be helpful.
- Assess for risk factors of self-mutilation, including categories of psychiatric disorders (particularly borderline personality disorder, psychosis, eating disorders, autism); psychological precursors (e.g., low tolerance for stress, impulsivity, perfectionism); psychosocial dysfunction (e.g., presence of sexual abuse, divorce or alcoholism in the family, manipulative behavior to gain nurturing, chaotic interpersonal relationships); coping difficulties (e.g., inability to plan solutions or see long-term consequences of behavior); personal history (e.g., childhood illness or surgery, past self-injurious behavior); and peer influences (e.g., friends who mutilate, isolation from peers).
- Assess for co-occurring disorders that require response, specifically childhood abuse, substance abuse, and suicide attempts. Assess family dynamics and the need for family therapy and community supports.
- Assess for a possible genetic disorder that results in severe and involuntary self-mutilation.

S

- Be alert to other risk factors of self-mutilation in clients with psychosis, including acute intoxication, dramatic changes in body appearance, preoccupation with religion and sexuality, and anticipated or perceived object loss.
- Monitor clients with obsessive-compulsive disorder for possible self-mutilation.
- Assess clients who have issues with gender identity or men who were molested as children for possible self-mutilation.
- Maintain ongoing surveillance of the client and environment. Monitor the client's behavior, using 15-minute checks at irregular times so that the client does not notice a pattern.
- When the client is experiencing extreme anxiety, use one-to-one staffing. Offer activities that will serve as a distraction.
- Implement active listening and early intervention.

▲ Refer to mental health counseling. Multiple therapeutic modalities are available for treatment.

- When working with self-mutilative clients who have borderline personality disorder, develop an effective therapeutic relationship by avoiding labeling, seeking to understand the meaning of the self-mutilation, and advocating for adequate opportunities for care.
- When working with self-mutilative clients with a diagnosis of a Cluster B Personality Disorder (borderline, antisocial, narcissistic, or histrionic), carefully assess suicidal ideation.
- Maintain a consistent relational distance from the client with borderline personality disorder who self-mutilates: neither too close nor too distant, neither rewarding unacceptable behavior nor trying to control or avoid the client.
- Inform the client of expectations for appropriate behavior and consequences within the unit. Emphasize that the client must comply with the rules. Contract with the client for no self-harm. Give positive reinforcement for compliance and minimize attention paid to disruptive behavior while setting limits.
- Clients need to learn to recognize distress as it occurs and express it verbally rather than as a physical action against the self.
- Assist the client to identify the motives/reasons for self-mutilation that have been perceived as positive.
- Help the client identify cues that precede impulsive behavior.
- Give praise when the client identifies urges and delays self-destructive behavior.

- Assist clients to identify ways to sooth themselves and generate hopefulness when faced with painful emotions.
- Reinforce alternative ways of dealing with depression and anxiety, such as exercise, engaging in unit activities, or talking about feelings.
- Keep the environment safe; remove all harmful objects from the area. Use of unbreakable glass is recommended for the client at risk for self-injury.
- Encourage the client to seek out care providers to talk with as the urge to harm oneself occurs. Develop a positive therapeutic relationship.
- Anticipate trigger situations and intervene to assist the client in applying alternatives to self-mutilation.
- Reduce or eliminate use of caffeine, alcohol, and street drugs.
- If self-mutilation does occur, use a calm, nonpunitive approach. Whenever possible, assist the client to assume responsibility for consequences (e.g., dress self-inflicted wound). Refer to the care plan for **Self-mutilation.**
- If the client is unable to control self-mutilation behavior, provide interactive supervision, not isolation.

▲ Refer for medication, such as clozapine.

- Involve the client in planning their care and problem solving, and emphasize that the client makes choices.

▲ Involve the client in group therapy.

▲ Use group therapy to exchange information about methods of coping with loneliness, self-destructive impulses, and interpersonal relationships as well as housing, employment, and health-care system issues directly and noninterpretively.

▲ Refer to protective services if evidence of abuse exists.

▲ Discharge planning: provide follow-up to ensure clients attend mental health appointments.

- Monitor the client for self-harm impulses that may progress to suicidal ideation.

Pediatrics

- Be aware of increasing incidence of self-mutilation, especially among teens and young adults.
- Conduct a thorough physical examination, being alert for superficial scars that may be patterned, although in most cases scabbing or infection is not evident.

- Maintaining a therapeutic relationship with teens requires explicit assurances of confidentiality, consistency of clinical routines, and a nonjudgmental communication style.
- Attend to behavioral clues of self-mutilation; a brief self-report assessment can be useful.
- Assess for the presence of an eating disorder or substance abuse. Attend to the themes that preoccupy teens with eating disorders who self-mutilate.
- Evaluate for suicidal ideation/suicide risk. Refer to the care plan for **Risk for Suicide** for additional information.
- Be aware that there is not complete overlap between self-mutilation and suicidal behavior. The motivation may be different (coping with difficult feelings rather than ending life), and the method is usually different.
- Use treatment approaches detailed previously, with modifications as appropriate for this age group.

Geriatric

- Provide hand or back rubs and calming music when elderly clients experience anxiety.
- Provide soft objects for elderly clients to hold and manipulate when self-mutilation occurs as a function of delirium or dementia. Apply mitts, splints, helmets, or restraints as appropriate.
- Older adults who show self-destructive behaviors should be evaluated for dementia.

Home Care

- Communicate degree of risk to family/caregivers; assess the family and caregiving situation for ability to protect the client and to understand the client's self-mutilative behavior. Provide family and caregivers with guidelines on how to manage self-harm behaviors in the home environment.
- Establish an emergency plan, including when to use hotlines and 911. Develop a contract with the client and family for use of the emergency plan. Role play access to the emergency resources with the client and caregivers.
- Assess the home environment for harmful objects. Have family remove or lock objects as able.

▲ If client behaviors intensify, institute an emergency plan for mental health intervention.

▲ Refer for homemaker or psychiatric home healthcare services for respite, client reassurance, and implementation of therapeutic regimen.
▲ If the client is on psychotropic medications, assess client and family knowledge of medication administration and side effects. Teach as necessary.
▲ Evaluate the effectiveness and side effects of medications.

Client/Family Teaching

- Explain all relevant symptoms, procedures, treatments, and expected outcomes for self-mutilation that is illness based (e.g., borderline personality disorder, autism).
- Assist family members to understand the complex issues of self-mutilation. Provide instruction on relevant developmental issues and on actions parents can take to avoid media that glorify self-harm behaviors.
- Provide written instructions for treatments and procedures for which the client will be responsible.
- Instruct the client in coping strategies (assertiveness training, impulse control training, deep breathing, progressive muscle relaxation).
- Role play (e.g., say, "Tell me how you will respond if someone ignores you").
- Teach cognitive-behavioral activities, such as active problem solving, reframing (reappraising the situation from a different perspective), or thought-stopping (in response to a negative thought, picture a large stop sign and replace the image with a prearranged positive alternative). Teach the client to confront his or her own negative thought patterns (or cognitive distortions), such as catastrophizing (expecting the very worst), dichotomous thinking (perceiving events in only one of two opposite categories), or magnification (placing distorted emphasis on a single event).

▲ Provide the client and family with phone numbers of appropriate community agencies for therapy and counseling.
▲ Give the client positive things on which to focus by referring to appropriate agencies for job-training skills or education.

Disturbed Sensory perception (specify: visual, auditory, kinesthetic, gustatory, tactile, olfactory)

NANDA Definition

Change in the amount or patterning of incoming stimuli accompanied by a diminished, exaggerated, distorted, or impaired response to such stimuli

Defining Characteristics

Change in behavior pattern; change in problem-solving abilities; change in sensory acuity; change in usual response to stimuli; disorientation; hallucinations; impaired communication; irritability; poor concentration; restlessness; sensory distortions

Related Factors (r/t)

Altered sensory integration; altered sensory reception; altered sensory transmission; biochemical imbalance; electrolyte imbalance; excessive environmental stimuli; insufficient environmental stimuli; psychological stress

Client Outcomes

Client Will (Specify Time Frame):

- Demonstrate understanding by a verbal, written, or signed response
- Demonstrate relaxed body movements and facial expressions
- Explain plan to modify lifestyle to accommodate visual or hearing impairment
- Remain free of physical harm resulting from decreased balance or a loss of vision, hearing, or tactile sensation
- Maintain contact with appropriate community resources

Nursing Interventions

Visual—Loss of Vision

- • Identify name and purpose when entering the client's room.
- • Orient to time, place, person, and surroundings. Provide a radio or talking books.
- • Keep doors completely open or closed. Keep furniture out of path to bathroom and do not rearrange furniture.

- • Feed the client at mealtimes if blindness is temporary.
- • Keep side rails up using half rails, maintain bed in a low position, keep call light readily available, and designate client a Fall Risk.
- • Converse with and touch the client frequently during care if frequent touch is within the client's cultural norm.
- • Walk the client by having the client grasp the nurse's elbow and walk partly behind the nurse.
- • Walk a frightened or confused client by having the client put both hands on the nurse's shoulders; the nurse backs up in desired direction while holding the client around the waist.
- • Keep call light button within client's reach, and check location of call light button before leaving the room.
- ▲ For a blind client, consider referring to a clinic for use of a blind mobility aid device that uses ultrasound.
- • Ensure access to eyeglasses or magnifying devices as needed.
- • Pay attention to the client's emotional needs. Encourage expression of feelings and expect grieving behavior.
- ▲ Refer to optometrist, ophthalmologist, or specialist in vision loss for vision care if needed.

Auditory—Hearing Loss

- • Keep background noise to a minimum. Turn off television and radio when communicating with the client. If the environment is noisy, take the client to a private room and shut the door.
- • Stand or sit directly in front of the client when communicating. Make sure adequate light is on your face, avoid chewing gum or covering the mouth or face with your hands while speaking, establish eye contact, and use nonverbal gestures.
- • Speak distinctly in lower voice tones if possible. Do not overenunciate or shout at the client.
- • State the topic of conversation before beginning the conversation; make it clear when you change conversation topics.
- • Verify that the client understands critical information by asking the client to repeat the information back.
- • If necessary, provide a communication board or personnel who know sign language.
- • Prepare pictures or diagrams depicting rests or procedures; have books with relevant pictures available for more detailed discussions.

S

- ▲ Refer to appropriate resources, such as a speech and hearing clinic; audiologist; or ear, nose, and throat physician. Refer children early for help.
- • Encourage the client to wear a hearing aid if available.
- • Avoid inserting an intravenous cannula in the deaf client's hands.
- ▲ Refer to hearing clinics.
- • Observe emotional needs and encourage expression of feelings.
- • For **Disturbed Sensory perception: kinesthetic, tactile,** see the care plan for **Risk for Injury** or **Risk for Falls.** For **Disturbed Sensory perception: olfactory, gustatory,** see the care plan for **Imbalanced Nutrition: less than body requirements.**

Pediatric

- ▲ Test hearing of infants and begin treatment/therapy early as needed.
- • For classroom learning, ensure that ambient noise is minimized and devices are used to decrease reverberation in the environment.
- • Recommend the child use a frequency-modulated system along with a hearing aid in school.
- ▲ Refer the child to a specialist who uses a Language Wizard/Player with Baldi, a computer-animated tutor for teaching vocabulary.

Geriatric

- • Keep environment quiet, soothing, and familiar. Use consistent caregivers.
- • If the client has a sensory deprivation, encourage family to provide appropriate sensory stimulation with music, voices, photographs, touch, and familiar smells.
- • Increase the amount of light in the environment for elderly eyes; ensure it is nonglare lighting.
- • Determine the origin of vision loss. If it is vision loss from a stroke, watch for hemianopia.
- ▲ Refer to low-vision clinics, or the Independent Living Program, which is designed for older individuals who are blind to help maintain independence.
- • For a hearing impairment in older adults, use the Hearing Handicap Inventory for the Elderly (HHIE-S) to determine

how individuals perceive the emotional and social problems associated with a hearing loss.
- If the client has a hearing or vision loss, work with the client to ensure contact with others and to strengthen the social network.

Home Care

- The previously listed interventions are applicable in the home care setting.

Client/Family Teaching

Low Vision

- Teach the client how to use a lighted magnification device to increase the ability to read text or see details.
- Teach the client to put a sheet of yellow acetate over text to make the text more visible.
- Put red, yellow, or orange identifiers on important items that need to be seen, such as a red strip at the edge of steps, red behind a light switch, or a red dot on a stove or washing machine to indicate how far to turn knob.
- Use a watch or clock that verbally tells time and a phone with large numbers and emergency numbers programmed into it.
- Teach blind clients new eating techniques, such as associating food on a plate with hours on a clock, so that the client can identify the location of foods.
- Use low-vision aids, including magnifying devices for near vision, telescopes for seeing objects at a distance, a closed-circuit television that magnifies print, and guides for writing checks and envelopes.
- Teach the client with vision loss to do the following:
  - Use a magnifying mirror to shave or apply makeup. Use an electric razor only.
  - Put personal care products in brightly colored pump containers (red, yellow, or orange) for identification.
  - Use tactile clues, such as safety pins or buttons placed in hems, to help client match clothing.
  - Use prefilled medication organizers with large lettering or three-dimensional (3D) markers.
- Increase lighting in the home to help vision in the following ways:
  - Ensure adequate illumination of the entire home, adding

light fixtures and increasing wattage of existing bulbs as needed.

- Decrease glare where light reflects on shiny surfaces by moving or covering reflective object.
- Use nonglare wax on the floor.
- Use motion-sensitive lights that come on automatically when a person enters the room for nighttime use.
- Add indoor strip or "runway" type of lighting to baseboards.

Hearing Loss

- • Suggest installation of such devices as ring signalers for the telephone and doorbell, sensors that detect an infant's cry, alarm clocks that vibrate the bed, and closed caption decoders for television sets. Other helpful devices include telephone amplifiers, speakerphones, pocket talker personal listening system, and FM and infrared amplification systems that connect directly to a TV or audio output jack. Also available is a telecommunication device—a typewriter keyboard with an alphanumeric display that allows the hearing-impaired person to send typed messages over the telephone line; software and modems are available that allow a home computer to be used in this fashion. Use of hearing ear dogs, which are specially trained to alert their owners to specific sound, may also be helpful.
- • Teach the client to avoid excessive noise at work and at home and wear hearing protection when necessary. Any noise that hurts the ears or is above 90 decibels is excessive.

Sexual dysfunction

NANDA Definition

The state in which an individual experiences a change in sexual function during the sexual response phases of desire, excitation, and/or orgasm, which is viewed as unsatisfying, unrewarding, or inadequate

Defining Characteristics

Actual limitations imposed by disease; actual limitations imposed by therapy; alterations in achieving perceived sex role; alterations in achieving sexual satisfaction; change of interest in others; change of interest in self; inability to achieve desired satisfaction; perceived alteration in sexual excitation; perceived deficiency of sexual desire; perceived limitations imposed by disease; perceived limitations imposed by therapy; seeking confirmation of desirability; verbalization of problem

Related Factors (r/t)

Absent role models; altered body function (e.g., pregnancy, recent childbirth, drugs, surgery, anomalies, disease process, trauma, radiation); altered body structure (e.g., pregnancy, recent childbirth, surgery, anomalies, disease process, trauma, radiation); biopsychosocial alteration of sexuality; ineffectual role models; lack of privacy; lack of significant other; misinformation or lack of knowledge; physical abuse; psychosocial abuse (e.g., harmful relationships); values conflict; vulnerability

Client Outcomes

Client Will (Specify Time Frame):

- Identify individual cause of sexual dysfunction
- Identify stressors that contribute to dysfunction
- Discuss alternative, satisfying, and acceptable sexual practices for self and partner
- Identify the degree of sexual interest by the patient and partner
- Adapt sexual technique as needed to cope with sexual problems
- Discuss with partner concerns about body image and sex role

S

Nursing Interventions

- Gather the client's sexual history, noting normal patterns of functioning and the client's vocabulary.
- Assess duration of sexual dysfunction and explore potential causes such as medications, medical problems, or psychosocial issues. Evaluate if sexual dysfunction may be related to either psychological or medical causes.
- Assess for history of sexual abuse.
- Determine the client's and partner's current knowledge and understanding.
- Assess and provide treatment for sexual dysfunction. Involve the person's partner in the process. Consider pharmacologic and nonpharmacologic interventions.

- • Observe for stress and anxiety as possible causes of dysfunction.
- • Assess for depression as a possible cause of sexual dysfunction. Sexual problems and depression are common in chronic disease and those with chronic pain.
- • Observe for grief related to loss (e.g., amputation, mastectomy, ostomy).
- • Explore physical causes such as diabetes, arteriosclerotic heart disease, arthritis, benign prostatic hypertrophy, drug or medication side effects, or smoking (males).
- • Provide privacy and be verbally and nonverbally nonjudgmental.
- • Provide privacy to allow sexual expression between the client and partner (e.g., private room, "Do Not Disturb" sign for a specified length of time).
- • Explain the need for the client to share concerns with partner.
- • Validate the client's feelings, let the client know that he or she is normal, and correct misinformation.
- ▲ Refer to appropriate medical providers for consideration of medication for premature ejaculation, erectile dysfunction, or orgasmic problems. Refer women for possible pharmacologic intervention when sexual dysfunction is present.

Geriatric

S

- ▲ Carefully assess the sexuality needs of the elderly client and refer for counseling if needed. Carefully assess sexual functioning needs of clients with dementia and provide privacy for them and their spouse.
- • Teach about normal changes that occur with aging: Female—reduction in vaginal lubrication, decrease in the degree and speed of vaginal expansion, reduction in duration and resolution of orgasm. Male—increase in time required for erection, increase in erection time without ejaculation, less firm erection, decrease in volume of seminal fluid, increase in time before another erection can occur (12-24 hours).
- ▲ Suggest the following to enhance sexual functioning: Female—use water-based vaginal lubricant, increase foreplay time, avoid direct stimulation of the clitoris if painful (clitoris may be exposed because of atrophy of the labia), practice Kegel exercises (alternately contracting and relaxing the muscles in the pelvic area), urinate immediately after coitus to prevent irritation of the urethra and bladder, and consult with a physician about use

of systemic estrogen therapy or topical estrogen cream. Male—have female partner try a new coital position by bending her knees and placing a pillow under her hips to elevate pelvis (will more easily accommodate a partially erect penis); massage penis down using pressure at base, which puts pressure on major blood vessel and keeps blood in the penis; ask the female partner to push the penis into the vagina herself and flex her vaginal muscles that have been strengthened by Kegel exercises. If one of the partners has a protruding abdomen, experiment to find a position that allows the penis to reach the vagina (e.g., have woman lie on her back with legs apart and knees sharply bent while the man places himself over her with his hips under the angle formed by the raised knees).

- • Explore various sexual gratification alternatives (e.g., caressing, sharing feelings) with the client and partner.
- • Discuss the difference between sexual function and sexuality.
- ▲ If prescribed, instruct clients with chronic pain to take the pain medication prior to sexual activity. Nitroglycerine can be used for anginal pain, if prescribed.
- • See care plan for **Ineffective Sexuality pattern.**

Multicultural

- • Assess for the influence of cultural beliefs, norms, and values on the client's perceptions of normal sexual functioning.
- • Discuss with the client those aspects of sexual health/lifestyle that remain unchanged by his or her health status.
- • Validate the client's feelings and emotions regarding the changes in sexual behavior.

Home Care

- • Previously discussed interventions may be adapted for home care use.
- • Identify specific sources of concern about sexual activity. Provide reassurance and instruction on appropriate expectations as indicated.
- • Help the client and significant other to identify a place and time in the home and daily living for privacy to share sexual or relationship activity. If necessary, help the client to communicate the need for privacy to other family members. Consider periodic escapes to desirable surroundings.

• Confirm that physical reasons for dysfunction have been addressed. Encourage participation in support groups or therapy if appropriate. Reinforce or teach the client about sexual functioning, alternative sexual practices, and necessary sexual precautions. Update teaching as the client status changes.

Client/Family Teaching

• Provide accurate information for clients concerning sexual activity after a myocardial infarction (MI); consider use of a videotape.
• Teach the client and partner about condom use, for those at risk.
• Teach the client that sexual activity can be resumed in 1 to 2 weeks after an uncomplicated MI (ACC/AHA, 2004). Also discuss being well rested, reporting any cardiac warning signs, using foreplay to determine tolerance for sexual activity, not using alcohol or eating heavy meals prior to sex, and having sex with a familiar partner and in the usual setting to decrease any stress the couple might feel.
• Provide written educational materials that address sexual issues for clients and families of clients with implantable cardiac defibrillators (ICDs).
▲ Refer to appropriate community resources, such as a clinical specialist, family counselor, or sexual counselor. If appropriate, include both partners in the discussion.
• Teach vaginal dilation to prevent stenosis. Inform the client to expect a bit of spotting after first session of intercourse.
• Teach how drug therapy affects sexual response (e.g., the possible side effects and the need to report them).
• Teach the importance of diabetic control and its effect on sexuality to clients with insulin-dependent diabetes.
▲ Refer for medical advice for ED that lasts longer than 2 months or is recurring.
• Teach the following interventions to decrease the likelihood of ED: limit or avoid the use of alcohol, stop smoking, exercise regularly, reduce stress, get enough sleep, deal with anxiety or depression, and see doctor for regular checkups and medical screening tests.
▲ Refer for medication to treat ED if necessary.
• Teach specifics if the client has a stoma: do not substitute the stoma for an anus.

- See Geriatric Interventions if a problem with erection is associated with stoma surgery.

Ineffective Sexuality pattern

NANDA Definition

Expressions of concern regarding own sexuality

Defining Characteristics

Alteration in relationship with significant other; alterations in achieving perceived sex role; conflicts involving values; reported changes in sexual activities; reported changes in sexual behaviors; reported difficulties in sexual activities; reported difficulties in sexual behaviors; reported limitations in sexual activities; reported limitations in sexual behaviors

Related Factors (r/t)

Absent role model; conflicts with sexual orientation or variant preferences; fear of acquiring a sexually transmitted disease; fear of pregnancy; impaired relationship with a significant other; ineffective role model; knowledge/skill deficit about alternative responses to health-related transitions, altered body function or structure, illness, or medical treatment; lack of privacy; lack of significant other

S

Client Outcomes

Client Will (Specify Time Frame):

- State knowledge of difficulties, limitations, or changes in sexual behaviors or activities
- State knowledge of sexual anatomy and functioning
- State acceptance of altered body structure or functioning
- Describe acceptable alternative sexual practices
- Identify importance of discussing sexual issues with significant other
- Describe practice of safe sex with regard to pregnancy and avoidance of STDs

Nursing Interventions

- Refer to the care plan **Sexual dysfunction** for additional interventions.

- After establishing rapport or therapeutic relationship, give the client permission to discuss issues dealing with sexuality. Ask the client specifically, "Have you been or are you concerned about functioning sexually because of your health status?"
- Encourage the client to discuss concerns with his or her partner.
- Assess psychosocial function such as anxiety, depression, and low self-esteem. Discuss alternative sexual expressions for altered body functioning or structure. Closeness and touching are other forms of expression.
- Some clients choose masturbation for sexual release.
- If mutual masturbation is a choice of expression, provide latex gloves.
- The following are *guidelines for sexual activity* for clients who have had total hip replacement (THR) surgery:
  - Do not bend the affected leg more than 90 degrees at the hip. When lying on your back, do not turn or roll your affected leg toward the other leg. Do not turn the toes of the affected leg inward. When lying on your side, keep both legs separated with pillows between them. Do not let your knees touch and do not let the toes of your affected leg turn downward.
- The following are **recommended sexual positions** for clients who have had THR surgery:
  1. **Bottom position for the male or female client:** Place one or two pillows under your affected thigh for support and comfort and to reduce friction on your skin, which may still be healing. Keep the toes of your affected leg pointed upward and slightly outward—but never inward.
  2. **Top position for male clients only:** Do not bend your affected hip more than 90 degrees while getting into position. Keep your affected leg out to the side with your toes pointed slightly outward. (Female clients: Do not assume this position because it will require that you bend more than 90 degrees at the hip.)
  3. **Side-lying position for the male client:** Lie on your unaffected side. Both you and your partner should face the same direction. You should be behind your partner in a "spooning" position. Your partner should place at least two pillows between her legs and your affected leg should rest on top of hers during intercourse. Do not bend your affected leg more

S

than 90 degrees, and do not let the toes of your affected leg dangle or turn downward.

4. **Side-lying position for the female client:** Lie on your unaffected side and place enough pillows between your legs to support the affected leg. Make sure the affected leg does not drop off the pillows during intercourse. Your partner should assume the spooning position behind you. Do not bend your affected hip more than 90 degrees, and do not let the toes of your affected leg turn downward.

Caution: If you dislocate your hip during sexual intercourse, you will experience pain, your affected leg will appear shorter, and your foot will turn inward. Lie down, do not move, and tell your partner to call an ambulance.

- The following are suggestions to be used for those who have had a myocardial infarction (MI):
  - ■ Sexual activity can be resumed in about 1 week to 10 days for those who had an uncomplicated MI. Sex should occur in familiar surroundings, in a comfortable room temperature, with the usual partner, and when well rested to minimize any cardiac stress. Heavy meals or alcohol should be avoided for 2 to 3 hours before sexual activity. Clients should choose the most comfortable position, one that minimizes any stress they may feel.
- The following are suggestions for those with an implantable cardioverter defibrillator (ICD):
  - ■ Assure the client and partner that fears about being shocked during sexual activity are normal. Sex can be resumed after the ICD is placed as long as strain on the implant site is avoided. If the ICD does discharge with sexual activity, the client should stop and rest and later notify the physician that the device fired so that it can be evaluated whether changes in the device settings are needed. The client should be instructed to report any dyspnea, chest pain, or dizziness with sexual activity.
- The following are suggestions for those with chronic lung disease:
  - ■ Sexual activity should be planned when energy level is highest and using positions that minimize shortness of breath, such as a semi-reclining position.

Pediatric

- Provide age-appropriate information for adolescents regarding human immunodeficiency virus (HIV) or the acquired immunodeficiency syndrome (AIDS) and sexual behavior.
- Provide support for the client's chosen ways to cope with HIV or AIDS.

Geriatric

- Carefully assess the sexuality needs of the elderly client and refer for counseling if needed. Explore possible changes in sexuality related to health status, menopause, and medications.
- Allow the client to verbalize feelings regarding loss of sexual partner or significant other. Acknowledge problems such as disapproval of children, lack of available partner for women, and environmental variables that make forming new relationships difficult.
- Provide a milieu that allows for discussion of sexual issues and a higher level of sexual satisfaction. Allow couples to room together and bring in double beds from home. Place signs on the door to ensure privacy.
- Provide clients with the following information:
  - Exercise, such as walking, swimming, cycling, and riding a stationary bike will help control flabby thighs and weak musculature and make people feel more sexually attractive.
  - Overindulgence in food or alcohol can affect sexual activity (see care plan for **Imbalanced Nutrition: more than body requirements**).
  - Resting and sleeping on a firm mattress may augment sexual desire.
  - Femininity and masculinity are still important.
  - Pay attention to cleanliness, skin care, and clothing.
  - Change the environment, and experiment with position changes.
- See care plan for **Sexual dysfunction.**

Multicultural

- Assess for the influence of cultural beliefs, norms, and values on client's perceptions of normal sexual behavior.

Home Care

- Previously discussed interventions may be adapted for home care use. Also see care plan for **Sexual dysfunction.**
- Help the client and significant other to identify a place and time in the home and daily living for privacy in sharing sexual or relationship activity. If necessary, help the client to communicate the need for privacy to other family members. Consider periodic escapes to desirable surroundings.
- Confirm that physical reasons for dysfunction have been addressed. Encourage participation in support groups or therapy if appropriate.
- Reinforce or teach about sexual functioning, alternative sexual practices, and necessary sexual precautions. Update teaching as client status changes.

Client/Family Teaching

▲ Refer to appropriate community agencies (e.g., certified sex counselor, Reach to Recovery, Ostomy Association).
- Provide information regarding self-care and sexuality for the woman who has cancer and her partner.

▲ Sexuality education is important to all populations, whether hearing or deaf, sighted or blind, disabled or not disabled. Discuss contraceptive choices. Refer to appropriate health professional (e.g., gynecologist, nurse practitioner [NP]).
- Teach safe sex to all clients including the elderly, which includes using latex condoms, washing with soap immediately after sexual contact, not ingesting semen, avoiding oral-genital contact, not exchanging saliva, avoiding multiple partners, abstaining from sexual activity when ill, and avoiding recreational drugs and alcohol when engaging in sexual activity. Adherence to antiretroviral therapy is important.

Impaired Skin integrity

NANDA Definition

Altered epidermis and/or dermis

Defining Characteristics

Destruction of skin layers; disruption of skin surface; invasion of body structures

Related Factors (r/t)

External

Chemical substance; extremes in age; humidity; hyperthermia; hypothermia; mechanical factors (e.g., friction, shearing forces, pressure, restraint); medications; moisture; physical immobilization; radiation

Internal

Changes in fluid status; changes in pigmentation; changes in turgor; developmental factors; imbalanced nutritional state (e.g., obesity, emaciation); immunological deficit; impaired circulation; impaired metabolic state; impaired sensation; skeletal prominence

Client Outcomes

Client Will (Specify Time Frame):

- Regain integrity of skin surface
- Report any altered sensation or pain at site of skin impairment
- Demonstrate understanding of plan to heal skin and prevent reinjury
- Describe measures to protect and heal the skin and to care for any skin lesion

Nursing Interventions

- • Assess site of skin impairment and determine cause (e.g., acute or chronic wound, burn, dermatological lesion, pressure ulcer, skin tear).
- • Determine that skin impairment involves skin damage only (e.g., partial-thickness wound, stage I or stage II pressure ulcer). The following classification system is for pressure ulcers:
  - ■ Stage I: Observable pressure-related alteration of intact skin with indicators as compared with the adjacent or opposite area on the body that may include changes in one or more of the following: skin temperature (warmth or coolness), tissue consistency (firm or boggy feel), and/or sensation (pain, itching). The ulcer appears as a defined area of persistent redness in lightly pigmented skin, whereas in darker skin tones, the ulcer may appear with persistent red, blue, or purple hues.

- ■ Stage II: Partial-thickness skin loss involving epidermis or dermis superficial ulcer that appears as an abrasion, blister, or shallow crater.

NOTE: For wounds deeper into subcutaneous tissue, muscle, or bone (stage III or stage IV pressure ulcers), see the care plan for **Impaired Tissue integrity.**

- • Monitor site of skin impairment at least once a day for color changes, redness, swelling, warmth, pain, or other signs of infection. Determine whether the client is experiencing changes in sensation or pain. Pay special attention to high-risk areas such as bony prominences, skinfolds, the sacrum, and heels.
- • Monitor the client's skin care practices, noting type of soap or other cleansing agents used, temperature of water, and frequency of skin cleansing.
- • Individualize plan according to the client's skin condition, needs, and preferences.
- • Monitor the client's continence status, and minimize exposure of skin impairment and other areas of moisture from incontinence, perspiration, or wound drainage.
- ▲ If the client is incontinent, implement an incontinence management plan to prevent exposure to chemicals in urine and stool that can strip or erode the skin. Refer to a continence care specialist, urologist, or gastroenterologist for incontinence assessment.
- • For clients with limited mobility, use a risk assessment tool to systematically assess immobility-related risk factors.
- • Do not position the client on site of skin impairment. If consistent with overall client management goals, turn and position the client at least every 2 hours. Transfer the client with care to protect against the adverse effects of external mechanical forces such as pressure, friction, and shear.
- • Evaluate for use of specialty mattresses, beds, or devices as appropriate. Maintain the head of the bed at the lowest possible degree of elevation to reduce shear and friction, and use lift devices, pillows, foam wedges, and pressure-reducing devices in the bed.
- ▲ Implement a written treatment plan for topical treatment of the site of skin impairment.
- ▲ Select a topical treatment that will maintain a moist wound-healing environment and that is balanced with the need to absorb exudate.

- Avoid massaging around the site of skin impairment and over bony prominences.
- ▲ Assess the client's nutritional status. Refer for a nutritional consult and/or institute dietary supplements as necessary.
- Identify the client's phase of wound healing (inflammation, proliferation, maturation) and stage of injury.

Home Care

- Some of the interventions described previously may be adapted for home care use.
- Instruct and assist the client and caregivers in how to change dressings and maintain a clean environment. Provide written instructions and observe them completing the dressing change.
- Educate client and caregivers on proper nutrition, signs and symptoms of infection, and when to call the agency and/or physician with concerns.
- ▲ It may be beneficial to initiate a consultation in a case assignment with a wound, ostomy, continence (WOC) nurse (or wounds specialist) to establish a comprehensive plan for complex wounds.

Client/Family Teaching

- Teach skin and wound assessment and ways to monitor for signs and symptoms of infection, complications, and healing.
- ▲ Teach the client why a topical treatment has been selected.
- ▲ If consistent with overall client management goals, teach how to turn and reposition at least every 2 hours.
- Teach the client to use pillows, foam wedges, and pressure-reducing devices to prevent pressure injury.

Risk for impaired Skin integrity

NANDA Definition

At risk for skin being adversely altered

Risk Factors

External

Chemical substance; excretions and/or secretions; extremes of age; humidity; hyperthermia; hypothermia; mechanical factors (e.g., shearing forces, pressure, restraint); moisture; physical immobilization; radiation

Internal

Alterations in skin turgor (change in elasticity); altered circulation; altered metabolic state; altered nutritional state (e.g., obesity, emaciation); altered pigmentation; altered sensation; developmental factors; immunological deficit; medication; psychogenetic, immunological factors; skeletal prominence

NOTE: Risk should be determined by the use of a risk assessment tool (e.g., Norton scale, Braden scale).

Client Outcomes

Client Will (Specify Time Frame):

- Report altered sensation or pain at risk areas
- Demonstrate understanding of personal risk factors for impaired skin integrity
- Verbalize a personal plan for preventing impaired skin integrity

Nursing Interventions

- • Monitor skin condition at least once a day for color or texture changes, dermatological conditions, or lesions. Determine whether the client is experiencing loss of sensation or pain.
- • Identify clients at risk for impaired skin integrity as a result of immobility, chronological age, malnutrition, incontinence, compromised perfusion, immunocompromised status, or chronic medical condition, such as diabetes mellitus, spinal cord injury, or renal failure.
- • Monitor the client's skin care practices, noting type of soap or other cleansing agents used, temperature of water, and frequency of skin cleansing.
- • Avoid harsh cleansing agents, hot water, extreme friction or force, or too-frequent cleansing.
- ▲ Monitor the client's continence status and minimize exposure of the site of skin impairment and other areas to moisture from incontinence, perspiration, or wound drainage. If the client is incontinent, implement an incontinence management plan to prevent exposure to chemicals in urine and stool that can strip or erode the skin; refer to a physician (e.g., continence care specialist, urologist, gastroenterologist) for an incontinence assessment.

S

- For clients with limited mobility, monitor condition of skin covering bony prominences.
- Use a risk assessment tool to systematically assess immobility-related risk factors.
- Implement a written prevention plan.
- If consistent with overall client management goals, turn and position the client at least every 2 hours. Transfer the client with care to protect against the adverse effects of external mechanical forces (e.g., pressure, friction, shear).
- Evaluate for use of specialty mattresses, beds, or devices as appropriate.
- Avoid massaging over bony prominences.

▲ Assess the client's nutritional status; refer for a nutritional consult, and/or institute dietary supplements.

Geriatric

- Limit number of complete baths to two or three per week, and alternate them with partial baths. Use a tepid water temperature (between 90° and 105° F) for bathing.
- Use lotions and moisturizers to prevent skin from drying out, especially in the winter.
- Increase fluid intake within cardiac and renal limits to a minimum of 1500 mL per day.
- Increase humidity in the environment, especially during the winter, by using a humidifier or placing a container of water on a warm object.

Home Care

- Assess caregiver vigilance and ability.
- Initiate a consultation in a case assignment with a wound care specialist or wound, ostomy, and continence (WOC) nurse to establish a comprehensive plan as soon as possible.
- See the care plan for **Impaired Skin integrity.**

Client/Family Teaching

- Teach the client skin assessment and ways to monitor for impending skin breakdown.
- If consistent with overall client management goals, teach how to turn and reposition the client at least every 2 hours.

• Teach the client to use pillows, foam wedges, and pressure-reducing devices to prevent pressure injury.

Sleep deprivation

NANDA Definition

Prolonged periods without sleep (sustained natural, periodic suspension of relative consciousness)

Defining Characteristics

Acute confusion; agitation; anxiety; apathy; combativeness; daytime drowsiness; decreased ability to function; fatigue; fleeting nystagmus; hallucinations; hand tremors; heightened sensitivity to pain; inability to concentrate; irritability; lethargy; listlessness; malaise; perceptual disorders (e.g., disturbed body sensation, delusions, feeling afloat); restlessness; slowed reaction; transient paranoia

Related Factors (r/t)

Aging-related sleep stage shifts; dementia; familial sleep paralysis; idiopathic central nervous system hypersomnolence; inadequate daytime activity; narcolepsy; nightmares; on-sleep inducing parenting practices; periodic limb movement (e.g., restless leg syndrome, nocturnal myoclonus); prolonged discomfort (e.g., physical, psychological); prolonged use of pharmacologic or dietary antisoporifics; sleep apnea; sleep-related enuresis; sleep-related painful erections; sleep terror; sleep walking; sun-downer's syndrome; sustained circadian asynchrony; sustained environmental stimulation; sustained inadequate sleep hygiene; sustained uncomfortable sleep environment

Client Outcomes

Client Will (Specify Time Frame):

- Wake up less frequently during night
- Awaken refreshed and be less fatigued during day
- Fall asleep without difficulty
- Verbalize plan that provides adequate time for sleep
- Identify actions that can be taken to improve quality of sleep

Nursing Interventions

- • Obtain a sleep-wake history, including work and other scheduled activities, history of sleep problems, changes in sleep with present illness, and use of medications and stimulants.
- • Ask the client to keep a sleep-wake diary for several weeks, which includes bedtime, rise time, number of awakenings, naps, and scheduled daytime events that may be depriving the client of adequate sleep time.
- ▲ Assess for underlying physiological illnesses causing sleep loss (e.g., cardiovascular, pulmonary, gastrointestinal, hyperthyroidism, nocturia occurring with benign hypertrophic prostatitis or pain).
- ▲ Assess level of anxiety. If the client is anxious, use relaxation techniques. See further Nursing Interventions for **Anxiety.**
- ▲ Assess for signs of depression: depressed mood state, flat affect, statements of hopelessness, poor appetite. Refer for counseling/treatment as appropriate.
- ▲ Assess the client for other symptoms of bipolar disorder (mania, hypomania). Refer for mental health services as indicated.
- ▲ Monitor for presence of nocturnal symptoms of restless leg syndrome with uncomfortable restless sensations in legs that occur before sleep onset or during the night. In addition, monitor for nocturnal panic attacks, presence of headaches, or gastroesophageal reflux disease. Refer for treatment as appropriate.
- • Assess and then evaluate the client's medication, diet, and caffeine intake. Look for hidden sources of caffeine, such as over-the-counter medications.
- ▲ Provide pain relief shortly before bedtime, and position the client comfortably for sleep.
- ▲ Monitor for presence of sleep disordered breathing as evidenced by loud snoring with periods of apnea, or other sleep disorders such as restless leg syndrome or periodic limb movement disorder. Refer to an accredited sleep disorder center.
- • Keep environment quiet for sleeping (e.g., avoid use of intercoms, lower the volume on radio and television, keep beepers on nonaudio mode, anticipate alarms on intravenous [IV] pumps, talk quietly on unit).
- • Use soothing sound generators with sounds of the ocean, rainfall, or waterfall to induce sleep, or use "white noise" such as a fan to block out other sounds. Also consider the use of earplugs.
- • Encourage the client to use soothing music to facilitate sleep.

Geriatric

- Assess if the client has a physiological problem that could result in sleep loss such as pain, cardiovascular disease, pulmonary disease, neurological problems such as dementia, or urinary problems.
- Assess urinary elimination patterns. Have the client decrease fluid intake in the evening, and instruct that diuretics are taken early in the morning.
- ▲ If the client is waking frequently during the night with periods of apnea or increased leg movement, consider the presence of sleep apnea problems or periodic leg movements disorder and refer to a sleep clinic for evaluation.
- Assist the client with taking a warm bath in the evening.
- Help the client recognize that changes in length of sleep occur with aging.
- Help client recognize that increasing age is associated with changes both in the nature and duration of sleep complaints.

Home Care

- Interventions discussed above may be adapted for home care use.
- Have the client or caregiver maintain a diary describing evening and nighttime activity, light, and noise levels in the home. Assess diary for potential areas of intervention to decrease interference with nighttime sleep.
- ▲ In the presence of a psychiatric disorder, refer for psychiatric home healthcare services for client reassurance and implementation of therapeutic regimen.

Client/Family Teaching

- Encourage the client to avoid coffee and other caffeinated foods and liquids and to avoid eating large high-protein or high-fat meals close to bedtime.
- Advise the client to avoid use of alcohol or hypnotics to induce sleep. Avoid alcohol ingestion 4 to 6 hours before bedtime.
- Encourage the client to develop a bedtime ritual that includes quiet activities such as reading, television, or crafts.
- Teach the following sleep hygiene guidelines for improving sleep habits:
  - ■ Go to bed only when sleepy.
  - ■ When awake in the middle of the night, go to another room, do quiet activities, and go back to bed only when sleepy.

- Use the bed only for sleeping.
- Avoid afternoon and evening naps.
- Get up at the same time every morning.
- Recognize that not everyone needs 8 hours of sleep.
- Do not associate lulls in performance with sleeplessness; sleeplessness should not be blamed for everything that goes wrong during the day.

Readiness for enhanced Sleep

NANDA Definition

A pattern of natural, periodic suspension of consciousness that provides adequate rest, sustains a desired lifestyle, and can be strengthened

Defining Characteristics

Amount of sleep is congruent with developmental needs; expresses a feeling of being rested after sleep; expresses willingness to enhance sleep; follows sleep routines that promote sleep habits; occasional use of medications to induce sleep

Client Outcomes

Client Will (Specify Time Frame):

- Awaken naturally, feeling refreshed, and is not fatigued during day
- Fall asleep without difficulty
- Verbalize plan to implement sleep promotion routines

Nursing Interventions

- • Obtain a sleep history including bedtime routines, sleep patterns, and use of medications and stimulants.
- • Determine level of anxiety. If the client is anxious, use relaxation techniques. See further Nursing Interventions for **Anxiety.**
- • Assess the client's medication, diet, and caffeine intake. Evaluate for hidden sources of caffeine, such as over-the-counter medications.
- • Provide interventions before bedtime to assist with sleep (e.g., quiet time to allow the mind to slow down, carbohydrates such as crackers).

- Provide a back massage before bedtime.
- Initiate nonpharmacologic interventions for improved sleep: control of disturbing environmental stimuli, sleep restriction, increasing sunlight exposure, acupuncture, and cognitive and educational interventions to address dysfunctional attitudes about sleep.

Geriatric

- Ask the client to keep a sleep diary for several weeks, which includes bedtime, rise time, number of awakenings, naps, and energy-using activities.
- Instruct the client in expectations for normal sleep. Elicit expectations for sleep, previous sleep patterns; correct misconceptions that influence emotional responses to deviation from expectations.
- Encourage the client to develop a bedtime ritual that includes quiet activities such as reading, television, or crafts.
- Encourage the client to take a warm bath in the evening.
- Encourage the client to use soothing music to facilitate sleep.
- Assess urinary elimination patterns. The client should decrease fluid intake in the evening and diuretics should be administered early in the morning unless contraindicated.
- Encourage social activities. Help elderly get outside for increased light exposure and to enjoy nature.
- Increase daytime physical and social activity. Encourage walking as the client is able.
- Recommend avoidance of hypnotics and alcohol to induce sleep. Avoid alcohol ingestion 4 to 6 hours before bedtime.
- Reduce daytime napping in the late afternoon; limit naps to short intervals as early in the day as possible.

Client/Family Teaching

- Teach somatic and cognitive relaxation techniques to induce the relaxation response and facilitate sleep.
- Teach the following guidelines for good sleep hygiene to improve sleep habits:
  - Go to bed only when sleepy.
  - When awake in the middle of the night, go to another room, do quiet activities, and go back to bed only when sleepy.
  - Use the bed only for sleeping.
  - Avoid afternoon and evening naps.

- Get out of bed at the same time every morning.
- Recognize that not everyone needs 8 hours of sleep.
- Move the alarm clock away from the bed so that it cannot be seen.
- Do not associate lulls in performance with sleeplessness; sleeplessness should not be blamed for everything that goes wrong during the day.

Home Care

• Interventions discussed above may be adapted for home care use.
▲ Assess the conduciveness of the home environment for both the caregivers and the care recipient's sleep.

Impaired Social interaction

NANDA Definition

Insufficient or excessive quantity or ineffective quality of social exchange

Defining Characteristics

S

Discomfort in social situations; dysfunctional interaction with others; family report of changes in interaction (e.g., style, pattern); inability to communicate a satisfying sense of social engagement (e.g., belonging, caring, interest, or shared history); inability to receive a satisfying sense of social engagement (e.g., belonging, caring, interest, or shared history); use of unsuccessful social interaction behaviors

Related Factors (r/t)

Absence of significant others; communication barriers; deficit about ways to enhance mutuality (e.g., knowledge, skills); disturbed thought processes; environmental barriers; limited physical mobility; self-concept disturbance; sociocultural dissonance; therapeutic isolation

Client Outcomes

Client Will (Specify Time Frame):

- Identify barriers that cause impaired social interactions
- Discuss feelings that accompany impaired and successful social interactions

- Use available opportunities to practice interactions
- Use successful social interaction behaviors
- Report increased comfort in social situations
- Communicate, state feelings of belonging, demonstrate caring and interest in others
- Report effective interactions with others

Nursing Interventions

- • Consider using a self rating scale to assess social functioning.
- • Monitor the client's use of defense mechanisms, and support healthy defenses (e.g., the client focuses on present and avoids placing blame on others for personal behavior).
- • Spend time with the client.
- • Use active listening skills, including assessment and clarification of the client's verbal and nonverbal responses and interactions.
- • Encourage social support for clients with visual impairments.
- • Identify client strengths. Have the client make a list of strengths and refer to it when experiencing negative feelings. He or she may find it helpful to put the list on a note card to carry at all times.
- • Have group members support each other in a group setting.
- • Model appropriate social interactions. Give positive verbal and nonverbal feedback for appropriate behavior (e.g., make statements such as, "I'm proud that you made it to work on time and did all the tasks assigned to you without saying that your supervisor was picking on you"; make eye contact). If not contraindicated, touch the client's arm or hand when speaking.
- • Use role playing to increase social skills.
- • Use client-centered humor as appropriate.
- ▲ Consider use of animal therapy; arrange for visitation.
- • Consider the use of the Internet to promote socialization.
- ▲ Refer client for behavioral interventions (life skills program) to increase social skills.
- • Refer to care plans for **Risk for Loneliness** and **Social isolation** for additional interventions.

Pediatric

- • Provide computers and the Internet access to children with chronic disabilities that limit socialization.
- • Consider use of RAP therapy (therapy using rap music) in groups to advance social skills of urban adolescents.

S

Geriatric

- • Avoid assuming that social isolation is normal for elderly clients.
- ▲ Assess the client's potential or actual sensory problems with hearing and vision and make appropriate referrals if a problem is identified.
- • Monitor for depression, a particular risk in the elderly.
- • Encourage group physical activity, such as aerobics or stretching and toning.
- • Have clients reminisce.
- • Refer to care plans for **Risk for Loneliness** and **Social isolation** for additional interventions.

Multicultural

- • Refer to care plan **Social isolation** for additional interventions.
- • Assess for the effect of racism on the client's perceptions of social interactions.
- • Approach individuals of color with respect, warmth, and professional courtesy.
- • Validate the client's feelings regarding social interaction.
- • Use interpreters as needed.

Home Care

- • Previously discussed interventions may be adapted for home care use.
- ▲ Assess family and living environment for social dynamics. Refer for medical social services to assist with family dynamics if appropriate.
- • Suggest that the client avoid contact with negative persons.
- ▲ Refer to or support involvement with supportive groups and counseling.

Client/Family Teaching

- ▲ Refer to appropriate social agencies for assistance (e.g., family therapy, self-help groups, crisis intervention), especially individuals who are seriously ill.

Social isolation

NANDA Definition

Aloneness experienced by the individual and perceived as imposed by others and as a negative or threatening state

Defining Characteristics

Objective

Absence of supportive significant other(s); developmentally inappropriate behaviors; dull affect; evidence of handicap (e.g. physical, mental) exists in a subculture; illness; meaningless actions; no eye contact; preoccupation with own thoughts; projects hostility; repetitive actions; sad affect; seeks to be alone; shows behavior unaccepted by dominant cultural group; uncommunicative; withdrawn

Subjective

Developmentally inappropriate interests; experiences feelings of differences from others; expresses feelings of aloneness imposed by others; expresses feelings of rejection; expresses values unacceptable to the dominant cultural group; inability to meet expectations of others; inadequate purpose in life; insecurity in public

Related Factors (r/t)

Alterations in mental status; alterations in physical appearance; altered state of wellness; factors contributing to the absence of satisfying personal relationships (e.g., delay in accomplishing developmental tasks); immature interests; inability to engage in satisfying personal relationships; inadequate personal resources; unaccepted social behavior; unaccepted social values

Client Outcomes

Client Will (Specify Time Frame):

- Identify feelings of isolation
- Practice social and communication skills needed to interact with others
- Initiate interactions with others; set and meet goals
- Participate in activities and programs at level of ability and desire
- Describe feelings of self-worth

Nursing Interventions

- • Establish a therapeutic relationship by being emotionally present and authentic.
- • Observe for barriers to social interaction (e.g., illness; incontinence; decreasing ability to form relationships; lack of transportation, money, support system, or knowledge).
- • Note risk factors (e.g., membership in ethnic/cultural minority, chronic physiological or psychological illness or deformities, advanced age).
- • Discuss causes of perceived or actual isolation.
- • Establish trust one on one and then gradually introduce the client to others. Allow the client opportunities to introduce issues and to describe his or her daily life.
- ▲ Promote social interactions. Support the expression of feelings. Consider the use of music therapy.
- • Involve clients in writing specific outcomes, such as identifying what is most important from their viewpoint and lifestyle.
- • Provide positive reinforcement when the client seeks out others.
- • Help the client identify appropriate diversional activities to encourage socialization.
- • Encourage physical closeness (e.g., use touch) if appropriate.
- • Identify available support systems and involve these individuals in the client's care.
- ▲ Refer clients to support groups.
- • Encourage liberal visitation for a client who is hospitalized or in an extended care facility.
- • Help the client identify role models and others with similar interests.
- • See the care plan for **Risk for Loneliness.**

S

Pediatric

- ▲ Refer obese adolescents for diet, exercise, and psychosocial support.
- • See the care plan for **Risk for Loneliness.**

Geriatric

- • Assess physical and mental status to establish a firm basis for planning social activities.
- ▲ Assess for hearing deficit. Provide aids and use adaptive techniques.

- • Involve client in goal setting and planning activities. Have them write down five activities in which they would like to participate.
- ▲ Involve nonprofessionals in activities, projects, and goal setting with the client. Practice interdisciplinary management for unit-based activities: engaging in arts and crafts projects, sewing, watching videos, reading large-print books, reading magazines, playing games, playing musical instruments, and using assistive listening devices.
- • Offer the client a choice of activities and persons with whom to sit and socialize. Introductions to strangers may need to be repeated several times.
- • Put clients in groups according to activity preferences, abilities, age, life situations, personal and cultural characteristics, and social networks.
- • Develop and display a seating chart for the common areas of each personal care unit and develop a process for both identifying needed changes and executing them promptly.
- • Provide physical activity, either aerobic or stretching and toning.
- • Provide music with active participation, such as drum and rhythm circles.
- • Consider the use of simulated presence therapy (see the care plan for **Hopelessness**).
- ▲ Refer to programs such as Foster Grandparents and Senior Companions.
- • Consider using computers and the Internet to alleviate or reduce loneliness and social isolation.

S

Multicultural

- • Acknowledge racial/ethnic differences at the onset of care.
- • Assess for the influence of cultural beliefs, norms, and values on the client's perception of social activity and relationships.
- • Approach individuals of color with respect, warmth, and professional courtesy.
- • Assess personal space needs, communication styles, acceptable body language, attitude toward eye contact, perception of touch, and paraverbal messages when communicating with the client.
- • Use a family-centered approach when working with Latino, Asian-American, African-American, and Native-American clients.

- • Promote a sense of ethnic attachment.
- • Validate the client's feelings regarding social isolation.
- ▲ Assist refugees who are relocated to access health care; support their connections with cultural, social, and religious groups.

Home Care

- • The interventions described previously may be adapted for home care use.
- • Confirm that the home setting has a telephone. Obtain one if necessary for medical safety. If the client lives alone, set up a Lifeline safety system that requires the client to answer the telephone.
- • Consider the use of the computer and Internet to decrease isolation.
- ▲ Assess options for living that allow the client privacy but not isolation (e.g., boarding home, congregate living, assertive community treatment programs).
- ▲ Assist clients to interact with neighbors in the community when they move to supported housing.

Client/Family Teaching

- • Teach role playing (practicing communication skills in specific situations).
- ▲ Encourage the client to initiate contacts with self-help groups, counselors, and therapists.
- • Provide information to the client about senior citizen services, house sharing, pets, day care centers, churches, and community resources.
- ▲ Refer socially isolated caregivers to appropriate support groups as well.

Chronic Sorrow

NANDA Definition

Cyclical, recurring, and potentially progressive pattern of pervasive sadness experienced (by parent, caregiver, individual with chronic illness or disability) in response to continual loss throughout the trajectory of an illness or disability

Defining Characteristics

Expresses feelings of sadness (e.g., periodic, recurrent); expresses feelings that interfere with ability to reach highest level of personal well-being; expresses feelings that interfere with ability to reach highest level of social well-being; expresses negative feelings (e.g., anger, being misunderstood, confusion, depression, disappointment, emptiness, fear, frustration, guilt, helplessness, hopelessness, loneliness, low self-esteem, being overwhelmed, recurring loss, self-blame)

Related Factors (r/t)

Death of a loved one; crises in management of the illness; crises related to developmental stages; experiences chronic disability (e.g., physical or mental); experiences chronic illness (e.g., physical or mental); missed milestones; missed opportunities; unending caregiving

Client Outcomes

Client Will (Specify Time Frame):

- Express appropriate feelings of guilt, fear, anger, or sadness
- Identify problems associated with sorrow (e.g., changes in appetite, insomnia, nightmares, loss of libido, decreased energy, alteration in activity levels)
- Seek help in dealing with grief-associated problems
- Plan for future one day at a time
- Function at normal developmental level

S

Nursing Interventions

- Assess the client's degree of sorrow. Use the Burke/NCRS Chronic Sorrow Questionnaire for the individual or caregiver as appropriate.
- Identify problems of eating and sleeping; ensure that basic human needs are being met.
- Spend time with the client and family.
- Develop a trusting relationship with the client by using empathetic therapeutic communication techniques.
- Help the client to understand that sorrow may be ongoing. No timetable exists for grieving, despite popular thought.
- Help the client recognize that, although sadness will occur at intervals for the rest of his or her life, it will become bearable.

- Encourage the use of positive coping techniques:
  - **Taking action:** Suggested strategies include keeping busy, keeping personal interests, going away, getting out of the house, doing something to gain a feeling of control over life.
  - **Cognitive coping:** Techniques include concentrating on the positive aspects of life, having a "can do" attitude, taking 1 day at a time, and taking responsibility for the quality of one's own life. Encourage the client to write about the experience.
  - **Interpersonal coping:** Techniques include talking to a close friend, a healthcare professional, or someone with the same condition or circumstance. Joining a support group can also help the sorrowful person to cope.
  - **Emotional coping:** Encourage the client to express feelings, cry as desired, give thanks, and pray if desired.
- Review past experiences, role changes, and coping skills. Use music if appropriate.
- Expect the client to meet responsibilities; give positive reinforcement.

▲ Refer the client to spiritual counseling if desired.

▲ Encourage the client to make time to talk to family members about the loss with the help of professional support as needed and without criticizing or belittling each other's feelings about the loss.

- Recognize that a stimulus for reactivation of sorrow in women is when a developmentally disabled child develops a healthcare crisis.
- Help the client determine the best way and place to find social support.

▲ Identify available community resources, including grief counselors or support groups available for specific losses (e.g., Multiple Sclerosis Society).

▲ Encourage the client to become active in interests such as volunteer work, service projects, or church activities.

▲ Identify whether the client is experiencing depression, suicidal tendencies, or other emotional disorders. Refer for counseling as appropriate.

- Identify whether the client had been notified of the health status of the deceased and was able to be present during illness and death.

S

Pediatric/Parent

- • Treat the child with respect, give him or her the opportunity to talk about their concerns, and answer questions honestly.
- • Listen to the child's expression of grief.
- • Help parents recognize that the child does not have to be "fixed" and that instead they need support going through an experience of grieving just as adults do.
- • Encourage children to listen to music that they enjoy.
- ▲ Consider the use of art for children in hospice care who are dying or dealing with the death of a parent, sibling, or other family member.
- ▲ Refer grieving children and parents to a program to help facilitate grieving if desired, especially if the death was traumatic.
- • Help the adolescent determine sources of support and how to use them effectively.
- ▲ Encourage parents to seek mental health services as needed, learn stress reduction, and take good care of their health.

Geriatric

- ▲ Use reminiscence therapy in conjunction with the expression of emotions. Refer to a reminiscence group if available.
- • Identify previous losses and assess the client for depression.
- • Evaluate the social support system of the elderly client. If the support system is minimal, help the client determine how to increase available support.

S

Multicultural

- • Assess for the influence of cultural beliefs, norms, and values on the client's expressions of sorrow.
- • Identify whether the client had been notified of the health status of the deceased and was able to be present during death and illness.

Home Care

- • The interventions described previously may be adapted for home care use.
- ▲ Assess the client for depression. Refer for mental health services as indicated.
- ▲ When sorrow is focused around loss of a pregnancy, encourage the client to follow through on a counseling referral.

- Encourage the client to participate in activities that are diversionary and uplifting as tolerated (e.g., outdoor activities, hobby groups, church-related activities, pet care).
- Encourage the client to participate in support groups appropriate to the area of loss or illness (e.g., Crohn's disease support group or Widow to Widow).
- Provide psychological support for family and caregivers.

▲ In the presence of a psychiatric disorder, refer for psychiatric home health care services for client reassurance and implementation of a therapeutic regimen.

- See the care plans for **Chronic low Self-esteem, Risk for Loneliness**, and **Hopelessness.**

Spiritual distress

NANDA Definition

Impaired ability to experience and integrate meaning and purpose in life through connectedness with self, others, art, music, literature, nature, and/or a power greater than oneself

S

Defining Characteristics

Connections to self: Anger; expresses lack of acceptance; expresses lack of courage; expresses lack of forgiveness of self; expresses lack of hope; expresses lack of love; expresses lack of meaning in life; expresses lack of purpose in life; expresses lack of serenity (e.g., peace); guilt; poor coping

Connections with others: Expresses alienation; refuses interactions with significant others; refuses interactions with spiritual leaders; verbalizes being separated from support system

Connections with art, music, literature, nature: Disinterest in nature; disinterest in reading spiritual literature; inability to express previous state of creativity (e.g., singing/listening to music/writing)

Connections with power greater than self: Expresses being abandoned; expresses having anger toward God; expresses hopelessness; expresses suffering; inability to be introspective; inability to experience the transcendent; inability to participate in religious activities; inability to pray; requests to see a religious leader; sudden changes in spiritual practices

Related Factors (r/t)

Active dying; anxiety; chronic illness; death; life change; loneliness; pain; self-alienation; social alienation; sociocultural deprivation

Client Outcomes

Client Will (Specify Time Frame):

- Express sense of connectedness with self, others, arts, music, literature, or power greater than oneself
- Express meaning and purpose in life
- Express sense of hope in the future
- Express ability to forgive
- Express acceptance of health status
- Discuss personal response to dying
- Discuss personal response to grieving

Nursing Interventions

- • Observe the client for loss of meaning, purpose, and hope in life.
- • Respect the client's beliefs; avoid imposing your own spiritual beliefs on the client. Be aware of your own belief systems and accept the client's spirituality. Allow for self-disclosure. Promote a sense of love, caring, and compassion.
- • Monitor and promote supportive social contacts.
- • Integrate family into spiritual practices as appropriate.
- ▲ Refer the client to a support group or counseling.
- • Coordinate or encourage attending spiritual retreats, courses, or programming.
- • Be physically present and actively listen to the client.
- • Support meditation, guided imagery, therapeutic touch, journaling, relaxation, and involvement in art, music, or poetry. Support outdoor activities.
- ▲ Offer or suggest visits with spiritual and/or religious advisors.
- • Help the client make a list of important and unimportant values.
- • Assist the client in identifying and creating his or her own meaningful experiences.
- • Help the client develop skills to deal with illness or lifestyle changes. Include the client in care planning.
- • If the client is comfortable with touch, hold the client's hand or place a hand gently on the client's arm.

S

- Help the client find a reason for living and be available for support. Promote hope.
- Listen to the client's feelings about suffering and/or death. Be nonjudgmental and allow time for grieving.
- Provide appropriate religious materials, artifacts, or music as requested.
- Promote forgiveness.
- Provide privacy or a "sacred space."
- Allow time and a place for prayer.
- Encourage the use of humor, as appropriate, to promote spiritual well-being.

Geriatric

- Discuss personal definitions of spiritual wellness with the client.
- Identify the client's past sources of spirituality. Help the client explore his or her life and identify those experiences that are noteworthy. Clients may want to read the Bible or other religious text or have it read to them.

Multicultural

S

- Assess for the influence of cultural beliefs, norms, and values on the client's ability to cope with spiritual distress.
- Encourage spirituality as a source of support.
- Validate the client's spiritual concerns and convey respect for his or her beliefs.

Home Care

- All of the nursing interventions described previously apply in the home setting.

Risk for Spiritual distress

NANDA Definition

At risk for an impaired ability to experience and integrate meaning and purpose in life through connectedness with self, others, art, music, literature, nature, and/or a power greater than oneself

Risk Factors

Developmental: Life changes
Environmental: Environmental changes; natural disasters
Physical: Chronic illness; physical illness; substance abuse
Psychosocial: Anxiety; blocks to experiencing love; change in religious rituals; change in spiritual practices; cultural conflict; depression; inability to forgive; loss; low self-esteem; poor relationships; racial conflict; separated support systems; stress

Client Outcomes

Client Will (Specify Time Frame):

- Express sense of connectedness with self, others, arts, music, literature, or power greater than oneself
- Express meaning and purpose in life
- Express sense of optimism and hope in the future
- Express ability to forgive
- Express desire to discuss health state and integrate care in lifestyle
- Discuss personal response to dying
- Discuss personal response to grieving
- Express satisfaction with life circumstances

Nursing Interventions

Refer to care plan for **Spiritual distress.**

Readiness for enhanced Spiritual well-being

NANDA Definition

Ability to experience and integrate meaning and purpose in life through connectedness with self, others, art, music, literature, nature, and/or a power greater than oneself that can be strengthened

Defining Characteristics

Connections to self: Expresses desire for enhanced acceptance; expresses desire for enhanced coping; expresses desire for enhanced courage; expresses desire for enhanced forgiveness of self; expresses desire for enhanced hope; expresses desire for enhanced joy; expresses desire for enhanced love; expresses desire for enhanced meaning in life; expresses desire for enhanced purpose in life; expresses desire for enhanced satisfying philosophy of life; expresses desire for enhanced surrender; expresses lack of serenity (e.g., peace); meditation

Connections with others: Provides service to others; requests forgiveness of others; requests interactions with significant others; request interactions with spiritual leaders

Connections with art, music, literature, nature: Displays creative energy (e.g., writing, poetry, singing); listens to music; reads spiritual literature; spends time outdoors

Connections with power greater than self: Expresses awe; expresses reverence; participates in religious activities; prays; reports mystical experiences

Client Outcomes

Client Will (Specify Time Frame):

- Express hope
- Express sense of meaning and purpose in life
- Express peace and serenity
- Express acceptance
- Express surrender
- Express forgiveness of self and others
- Express satisfaction with philosophy of life
- Express joy
- Express courage
- Describe being able to cope
- Describe use of spiritual practices
- Describe providing service to others
- Describe interaction with spiritual leaders, friends, and family
- Describe appreciation for art, music, literature, and nature

S

Nursing Interventions

- Perform a spiritual assessment that includes the client's relationship with God, meaning and purpose in life, religious affiliation, and any other significant beliefs.
- Be present for the client.
- Listen actively to the client.
- Encourage the client to pray, setting the example by praying with and for the client.

- • Encourage spiritual meditation exercises.
- ▲ Coordinate or encourage attending spiritual retreats or courses.
- • Promote hope.
- • Encourage clients to reflect on what is meaningful to them in life.
- • Encourage involvement in group religious practices.
- • Encourage increased quality of life through social support and family relationships.
- • Encourage volunteerism.
- • Assist the client in identifying religious or spiritual beliefs that encourage integration of meaning and purpose in the client's life.
- • Encourage the client to engage regularly in bibliotherapy.
- • Support involvement in expressive art.
- • Support the use of humor by the client.
- • Encourage the client to practice forgiveness.
- • Support the client in contemplating, viewing, and/or experiencing nature.
- • Encourage expressions of spirituality.
- • Encourage integration of spirituality in healthy lifestyle choices. Validate the client's spiritual concerns and convey respect for his or her beliefs.
- ▲ Help the client participate in religious rites or obtain spiritual guidance.
- • Assist the client in developing spirituality. List the most valuable qualities he or she can bring from within, the circumstances most helpful for unfolding these qualities, and the ways of incorporating these circumstances into the client's lifestyle.

S

Geriatrics

- • Refer to the care plan for **Spiritual distress.**

Multicultural

- • Assess for the influence of cultural beliefs, norms, and values on the client's perceptions of spirituality.
- • Encourage expressions of spirituality.
- • Validate the client's spiritual concerns and convey respect for his or her beliefs.

Home Care

- • All of the nursing interventions mentioned previously apply in the home setting. Refer the client to parish nurses.

Stress overload

NANDA Definition

Excessive amounts and types of demands that require action

Defining Characteristics

Demonstrates increased feelings of anger; demonstrates increased feelings of impatience; expresses a feeling of pressure; expresses a feeling of tension; expresses difficulty in functioning; expresses increased feelings of anger; expresses increased feelings of impatience; expresses problems with decision making; reports negative impact from stress (e.g., physical symptoms, psychological distress, feeling of "being sick" or of "going to get sick"); reports situational stress as excessive (e.g., rates stress level as 7 or above on a 10-point scale)

Related Factors (r/t)

Inadequate resources (e.g., financial, social, education/knowledge level); intense, repeated stressors (e.g., family violence, chronic illness, terminal illness); multiple coexisting stressors (e.g., environmental threats, demands); physical threats, demands; social threats, demands

Client Outcomes

Client Will (Specify Time Frame):

- Review the amounts and types of stressors in daily living
- Identify stressors that can be modified or eliminated
- Mobilize social supports to facilitate lower stress levels
- Reduce stress levels through use of relaxation techniques and other strategies

Nursing Interventions

- Assess for stress overload during vulnerable life events.
- Listen actively to descriptions of stressors and the stress response.
- In younger adult women, assess interpersonal stressors.
- Categorize stressors as modifiable or nonmodifiable.
- Help clients modify or mitigate stressors identified as modifiable.
- Help clients distinguish between short-term stressors and chronic stressors.
- Provide information as needed to reduce stress responses to acute and chronic illnesses.

- Explore possible therapeutic approaches such as cognitive behavior therapy, biofeedback, neurofeedback, pharmacologic agents, and complementary and alternative therapies.
- Help the client to reframe his or her perceptions of some of the stressors.
- Assist the client to mobilize social supports for dealing with recent stressors.

Pediatric

- With children, nurses should work with parents to help them to reduce children's stressors.
- Help children to manage their feelings related to self-concept.
- Help children to deal with bullies and other sources of violence in schools and neighborhoods.
- Help young children to identify and mitigate the experience of "feeling sick."
- Help children to manage the complexities of chronic illnesses.

Geriatric

- Assess for chronic stress with older adults and provide a variety of stress relief techniques.
- Encourage social support for older adults.

Multicultural

- Review cultural beliefs and acculturation level in relation to perceived stressors.
- Assess families for whether they experience high stress or low stress.
- Support social connectedness among cultural groups.

Home Care

- The above interventions may be adapted for home care use.
- Develop community-based programs for stress management as needed for groups with increased risk of stress overload (e.g., firefighters, policeman, military personnel, nurses). Support and encourage neighborhood stability.

Client/Family Teaching

- Diagnose the possibility of stress overload before teaching.
- Establish readiness for learning.

- Provide manageable amounts of information at the appropriate educational level.
- Evaluate the need for additional teaching and learning experiences.

Risk for Suffocation

NANDA Definition

Accentuated risk of accidental suffocation (inadequate air available for inhalation)

Risk Factors

External

Discarding refrigerators without removing doors; eating large mouthfuls of food; hanging a pacifier around infant's neck; household gas leaks; inserting small objects into airway; leaving children unattended in water; low-strung clothesline; pillow placed in infant's crib; playing with plastic bags; propped bottle placed in infant's crib; smoking in bed; use of fuel-burning heaters not vented to outside; vehicle warming in closed garage

Internal

Cognitive difficulties; disease process; emotional difficulties; injury process; lack of safety education; lack of safety precautions; reduced motor abilities; reduced olfactory sensation

Client Outcomes

Client Will (Specify Time Frame):

- Explain and undertake appropriate measures to prevent suffocation
- Demonstrate correct techniques for emergency rescue maneuvers (e.g., Heimlich maneuver, rescue breathing, cardiopulmonary resuscitation [CPR]) and describe situations that require them

Nursing Interventions

- Identify hospitalized clients at particular risk for suffocation, including the following:
  - Clients with altered levels of consciousness
  - Infants or young children

- Clients with developmental delays
- Clients with mental illness, especially schizophrenia

Pediatric

- Counsel families on the following:
  - Follow general safety practices such as not smoking in bed, not smoking during pregnancy, not smoking in the presence of an infant, properly disposing of large appliances, using properly functioning heating systems and ventilation, having functional smoke and carbon monoxide detectors, and opening garage doors when warming up a car.
  - Position infants on their back to sleep; do not position them in the prone position.
  - Avoid use of loose bedding such as blankets and sheets for sleeping. If blankets are used, they should be tucked in around the crib mattress so the infant's face is less likely to become covered by bedding. One strategy is to make up the bedding so that the infant's feet are able to reach the foot of the crib with the blankets tucked in around the crib mattress and reaching only the level of the infant's chest.
  - Teach parents not to sleep with an infant, especially if alcohol or medications/illicit drugs are used by the parents.
- Assess for signs and symptoms of abuse such as Munchausen syndrome by proxy (MSBP).
- Conduct risk factor identification, noting special circumstances in which preventive or protective measures are indicated. Note the presence of environmental hazards, including the following:
  - Plastic bags (e.g., dry cleaner's bags, bags used for mattress protection)
  - Cribs with slats wider than 2⅜ inches
  - Ill-fitting crib mattresses that can allow the infant to become wedged between the mattress and crib
  - Pillows in cribs
  - Abandoned large appliances such as refrigerators, dishwashers, or freezers
  - Clothing with cords or hoods that can become entangled
  - Bibs, pacifiers on a string, drapery cords, pull-toy strings
- Suffocation by airway obstruction is a leading cause of death in children younger than 6 years of age. Families need to be taught

S

child protection. Teach parents about available resources such as the Injury Prevention Program for Parents.

- Counsel families to not serve these foods to the child younger than 4 years of age: hot dogs, popcorn, nuts, pretzels, chips, peanut butter, chunks of meat, hard pieces of fruit or vegetables, raisins, whole grapes, hard candies, marshmallows.
- Provide information to parents about obtaining the "No-choke Test Tube" (no-choke tubes are sold at stores that sell baby items) or using a toilet paper roll: if an object fits in the tube or the roll, it is too small to give to a child.
- Stress water and pool safety precautions, including vigilant, uninterrupted parental supervision.
- Underscore the necessity of not allowing children to play with or near electric garage doors and of keeping garage door openers out of the reach of young children.
- For adolescents, watch for signs of depression that could result in suicide by suffocation.

Geriatric

- Assess the status of the swallow reflex. Offer appropriate foods and beverages accordingly.
- Observe the client for pocketing of food in the side of the mouth; remove food as needed.
- Position the client in high Fowler's position when eating and for 1 hour afterward.
- Use care in pillow placement when positioning frail elderly clients who are on bed rest.

Home Care

- Assess the home for potential safety hazards in systems that are not likely to be fixed (e.g., faulty pilot lights or gas leaks in gas stoves, carbon monoxide release from heating systems, kerosene fumes from portable heaters). Assist the family in having these areas assessed and making appropriate safety arrangements (e.g., installing detectors, making repairs).

Client/Family Teaching

▲ Recommend that families who are seeking day care or in-home care for children, geriatric family members, or at-risk family members with developmental or functional disabilities inspect the environment for hazards and examine the first aid preparation and vigilance of providers.

▲ Involve family members in learning and practicing rescue techniques, including treatment of choking and lack of breathing, as well as CPR. Initiate referral to formal training classes.

Risk for Suicide

NANDA Definition

At risk for self-inflicted, life-threatening injury

Related Factors (r/t)

Behavioral

Buying a gun; changing a will; giving away possessions; history of prior suicide attempt; impulsiveness; making a will; marked changes in attitude; marked changes in behavior; marked changes in school performance; stockpiling medicines; sudden euphoric recovery from major depression

S

Demographic

Age (e.g., elderly, young adult males, adolescents); divorced; male gender; race (e.g., Caucasian, Native American); widowed

Physical

Chronic pain; physical illness; terminal illness

Psychological

Childhood abuse; family history of suicide; gay or lesbian youth; guilt; psychiatric illness/disorder (e.g., depression, schizophrenia, bipolar disorder); substance abuse

Situational

Adolescents living in nontraditional settings (e.g., juvenile detention center, prison, half-way house, group home); economic instability; institutionalization; living alone; loss of autonomy; loss of independence; presence of gun in home; relocation; retired

Social

Cluster suicides; disciplinary problems; disrupted family life; grief; helplessness; hopelessness; legal problems; loneliness; loss of important relationship; poor support systems; social isolation

Verbal

States desire to die; threats of killing oneself

Client Outcomes

Client Will (Specify Time Frame):

- Not harm self
- Maintain connectedness in relationships
- Disclose and discuss suicidal ideas if present; seek help
- Express decreased anxiety and control of impulses
- Talk about feelings; express anger appropriately
- Refrain from using mood-altering substances
- Obtain no access to harmful objects
- Yield access to harmful objects
- Maintain self-control without supervision

Nursing Interventions

NOTE: Before implementation of interventions in the face of suicidal behavior, nurses should examine their own emotional responses to incidents of suicide to ensure that interventions will not be based on countertransference reactions.

- Assess for suicidal ideation when the history reveals the following: depression, substance abuse, and other psychiatric disorders; bipolar disorder, schizophrenia, panic disorder, dissociative disorder, eating disorder, antisocial personality disorder; attempted suicide, current or past; recent stressful life events (divorce and/or separation, relocation, problems with children); recent unemployment; recent bereavement; chronic pain or physical illness; childhood physical or sexual abuse; gay, lesbian, or bisexual gender orientation; family history of suicide.
- Assess medical clients and clients with chronic illnesses for their perception of health status.
- Use brief self-report measures to improve clinical management of at-risk cases. The client may complete screening instruments such as the Center for Epidemiological Studies Depression Scale

(CES-D), which indicates degree of depressed mood, or the Beck Suicide Intent Scale, which identifies a strong intent to die.

▲ Assess the client's ability to enter into a no-suicide contract. Contract (verbally or in writing) with the client for no self-harm; recontract at appropriate intervals.

• Be alert for warning signs of suicide: making statements such as, "I can't go on," "Nothing matters anymore," "I wish I were dead"; becoming depressed or withdrawn; behaving recklessly; getting affairs in order and giving away valued possessions; showing a marked change in behavior, attitudes, or appearance; abusing drugs or alcohol; suffering a major loss or life change.

• Take suicide notes seriously. Consider themes of notes in determining appropriate interventions.

• Question family members regarding the preparatory actions mentioned.

• Determine the presence and degree of suicidal risk. A number of questions will elicit the necessary information: Have you been thinking about hurting or killing yourself?, How often do you have these thoughts and how long do they last? Do you have a plan? What is it? Do you have access to the means to carry out that plan? How likely is it that you could carry out the plan? Are there people or things that could prevent you from hurting yourself? What do you see in your future a year from now? Five years from now? What do you expect would happen if you died? What has kept you alive up to now?

▲ Observe, record, and report any changes in mood or behavior that may signify increasing suicide risk and document results of regular surveillance checks.

• Develop a positive therapeutic relationship with the client; do not make promises that may not be kept.

▲ Refer for mental health counseling and possible hospitalization if evidence of suicidal intent exists, which may include evidence of preparatory actions (e.g., obtaining a weapon, making a plan, putting affairs in order, giving away prized possessions, preparing a suicide note).

• Assign a hospitalized client to a room located near the nursing station.

• Search the newly hospitalized client and the client's personal belongings for weapons or potential weapons and hoarded medications during the inpatient admission procedure, as appropriate. Remove dangerous items.

- Place the client in the least restrictive environment that allows for the necessary level of observation. Assess suicidal risk at least daily.
- Increase surveillance of a hospitalized client at times when staffing is predictably low (e.g., staff meetings, change of shift report, periods of unit disruption).
- Consider strategies to decrease isolation and opportunity to act on harmful thoughts (e.g., use of a sitter).
- Explain suicide precautions and relevant safety issues to the client and family (e.g., purpose, duration, behavioral expectations, and behavioral consequences).

▲ Refer for treatment and participate in the management of any psychiatric illness or symptoms that may be contributing to the client's suicidal ideation or behavior.

▲ Verify that the client has taken medications as ordered (e.g., conduct mouth checks after medication administration).

▲ Maintain increased surveillance of the client whenever use of an antidepressant has been initiated or the dose increased. Antidepressant medications take anywhere from 2 to 6 weeks to achieve full efficacy.

- Limit access to windows and exits unless locked and shatterproof, as appropriate.
- Monitor the client during the use of potential weapons (e.g., razor, scissors).
- Involve the client in treatment planning and self-care management of psychiatric disorders.
- Explore with the client all circumstances and motivations related to the suicidality. Listen to the client's own views on his or her problems.
- Explore with the client all perceived consequences that could act as a barrier to suicide (e.g., effect on family, religious beliefs).
- Avoid repeated discussion of the client's suicide history by keeping discussion oriented to the present and future.

▲ Discuss plans for dealing with suicidal ideation in the future (e.g., how to identify precipitating factors, whom to contact, where to go for help, how to respond to desire for self-harm).

▲ Assist the client in identifying a network of supportive persons and resources (e.g., clergy, family, care providers).

- ▲ Refer family members and friends to local mental health agencies and crisis intervention centers if the client has suicidal ideation or a suspicion of suicidal thoughts exists.
- ▲ Consider outpatient commitment or an overnight psychiatric observation program for an actively suicidal client.
- • Cognitive behavioral techniques help the client to modify thinking styles that promote depression, hopelessness, and a belief that suicide is a valid means of escaping the current situation.
- • Group interventions can be useful to address recurrent suicide attempts.
- ▲ If imminent suicide is suspected or an attempt has occurred, call for assistance and do not leave the client alone.
- ▲ With the client's consent, facilitate family-oriented crisis intervention.
- ▲ Involve the family in discharge planning (e.g., illness/medication teaching, recognition of increasing suicidal risk, client's plan for dealing with recurring suicidal thoughts, community resources).
- ▲ Before discharge from the hospital, ensure that the client has a supply of ordered medications, has a plan for outpatient follow-up, understands the plan or has a caregiver able and willing to follow the plan, and has the ability to access outpatient treatment.
- ▲ In the event of successful suicide, refer the family to a therapy group for survivors of suicide. Recommended clinical interventions include addressing psychological distress, normalizing denial as an effective coping strategy, working with concerns about family disintegration, and helping families deal with stigmatization.
- • See the care plans for **Risk for self-directed Violence, Hopelessness,** and **Risk for Self-mutilation.**

Pediatric

- • The above interventions may be appropriate for pediatric clients.
- • Use brief self-report measures to improve clinical management of at-risk cases.
- • Assess for both medical and psychiatric disturbances that may contribute to suicidality.

S

- Recognize that the developmental issues of childhood and adolescence may heighten suicide risks and involve different issues from those with adults.
- Assess specific stressors for the adolescent client.
- Assess for exposure to suicide of a significant other. Evaluate for the presence of self-mutilation and related risk factors. Refer to care plan for **Risk for Self-mutilation** for additional information.
- Be aware that complete overlap does not exist between suicidal behavior and self-mutilation. The motivation may be different (ending life rather than coping with difficult feelings), and the method is usually different.
- Assess for the presence of an eating disorder.
- Involve the adolescent in multimodal treatment programs. Before discharge from the hospital, ensure that the client's parent has a supply of ordered medications, has a plan for outpatient follow-up, has a caregiver who understands the plan or is able and willing to follow the plan, and has the ability to access outpatient treatment.
- Parental education groups can influence suicide risk factors.
- Support the implementation of school-based suicide prevention programs.
- Encourage family meals.

S

Geriatric

- Evaluate the older client's mental and physical health status and financial stressors.
- Explore with client any concerns or pressures (physical and financial) regarding ability to secure support of medical care, especially perceived pressures about being a burden on family.
- When assessing suicide risk factors, incorporate a higher degree of risk for older men and for some older adults who have lost a loved one in the previous year.
- Explore triggers of and barriers to suicidal behavior, with particular attention to real and perceived losses (e.g., professional role, health).
- An older adult who shows self-destructive behaviors should be evaluated for dementia.
- Anticipate overall responsiveness to treatment, but monitor for early relapse.

▲ Advocate for the older client with other professionals in securing treatment for suicidal states. Primary care physicians have been noted to underrecognize and undertreat older adult clients with depression.

- Encourage physical activity in older adults.
- Assist the older adult to identify protective factors that serve as resources to mitigate against suicidal ideation.
- Collaborative care management of older adults in primary care settings is a growing area for nursing intervention.
- Telephone contacts can serve as an effective intervention for suicidal older adults.

Multicultural

- Assess for the influence of cultural beliefs, norms, and values on the individual's perceptions of suicide.
- Identify and acknowledge the stresses unique to culturally diverse individuals.
- Identify and acknowledge unique cultural responses to stressors in determining sensitive interventions to prevent suicide.
- Encourage physical activity as intervention to decrease suicidal behavior.
- Encourage family members to demonstrate and offer caring and support to each other.
- Foster the client's use of available family and religious supports.
- Validate the individual's feelings regarding concerns about the current crisis and family functioning.

Home Care

- Communicate the degree of risk to family and caregivers; assess the family and caregiving situation for ability to protect the client and to understand the client's suicidal behavior. Provide the family and caregivers with guidelines on how to manage self-harm behaviors in the home environment.

▲ If the client's suicidal ideation intensifies, or if a suicide plan with access to means becomes evident, institute an emergency plan for mental health intervention.

- Counsel parents and homeowners to restrict unauthorized access to potentially lethal prescription drugs and firearms within the home.
- Identify the client's concerns and implement interventions to address the consequences of disability in a client with medical illness.

▲ Refer for homemaker or psychiatric home healthcare services

S

for respite, client reassurance, and implementation of a therapeutic regimen.

- ▲ If the client is on psychotropic medications, assess the client's and family's knowledge of medication administration and side effects. Teach as necessary.
- ▲ Evaluate the effectiveness and side effects of medications and adherence to the medication regimen. Review with the client and family all medications kept in the home; encourage discarding of old prescriptions. Monitor the amount of medications ordered/provided by the physician; limiting the amount of medications to which the client has access may be necessary.

Client/Family Teaching

- • Establish a supportive relationship with family members.
- • Explain all relevant symptoms, procedures, treatments, and expected outcomes for suicidal ideation that is illness based (e.g., depression, bipolar disorder).
- • Teach the family how to recognize that the client is at increased risk for suicide (changes in behavior and verbal and nonverbal communication, withdrawal, depression, or sudden lifting of depression).
- • Provide written instructions for treatments and procedures for which the client will be responsible.
- • Instruct the client in coping strategies (assertiveness training, impulse control training, deep breathing, progressive muscle relaxation).
- • Role play (e.g., say, "Tell me how you will respond if a friend asks why you were in the hospital").
- • Teach cognitive behavioral activities, such as active problem solving, reframing (reappraising the situation from a different perspective), or thought stopping (in response to a negative thought, picturing a large stop sign and replacing the image with a prearranged positive alternative). Teach the client to confront his or her own negative thought patterns (or cognitive distortions), such as catastrophizing (expecting the very worst), dichotomous thinking (perceiving events in only one of two opposite categories), or magnification (placing distorted emphasis on a single event).
- • Provide the client and family with phone numbers of appropriate community agencies for therapy and counseling.

Delayed Surgical recovery

NANDA Definition

Extension of the number of postoperative days required to initiate and perform activities that maintain life, health, and well-being

Defining Characteristics

Difficulty in moving about; evidence of interrupted healing of surgical area (e.g., red, indurated draining, immobilized); fatigue; loss of appetite with or without nausea; perception that more time is needed to recover; postpones resumption of work/employment activities; requires help to complete self-care

Related Factors (r/t)

Extensive surgical procedure; obesity; pain; postoperative surgical site infection; preoperative expectations; prolonged surgical procedure

Client Outcomes

Client Will (Specify Time Frame):

- Have surgical area that shows evidence of healing: no redness, induration, draining, or immobility
- State that appetite is regained
- State that no nausea is present
- Demonstrate ability to move about
- Demonstrate ability to complete self-care activities
- State that no fatigue is present
- State that pain is controlled or relieved after nursing interventions
- Resume employment activities/activities of daily living (ADLs)

S

Nursing Interventions

- • Perform a thorough assessment of the client, including risk factors. Allow time to be with the client.
- ▲ Assess for the presence of medical conditions and treat appropriately before surgery. If the client is diabetic, maintain normal blood glucose levels before surgery.
- ▲ Carefully assess client's use of dietary supplements such as feverfew, ginkgo biloba, garlic, ginseng, ginger, valerian, kava, St. John's wort, ephedra (Ma huang or metabo-lite), and echi-

nacea. It is recommended that all clients be advised to stop all dietary supplements at least 1 week before major surgical or diagnostic procedures.

- ▲ Assess and treat for depression and anxiety in a client complaining of continuing fatigue after surgery.
- • Play music of the client's choice preoperatively, intraoperatively, and postoperatively.
- ▲ Consider using healing touch in the perianesthesia setting and other mind-body-spirit interventions such as stress control and imagery.
- • Use warmed cotton blankets to reduce heat loss during surgery.
- • Use careful aseptic technique when caring for wounds.
- • Suggest the use of a semipermeable dressing and suction drainage for selected orthopedic clients.
- • Clients should be allowed to shower after surgery to maintain cleanliness if not contra-indicated because of the presence of pacemaker wires.
- • Promote early ambulation and deep breathing. Consider use of a transcutaneous electrical nerve stimulation (TENS) unit for pain relief.
- • The client should be provided with a complete, balanced therapeutic diet after the immediately postoperative period (24-48 hours).
- • Provide 20-minute foot and hand massage (5 minutes to each extremity), 1 to 4 hours after a dose of pain medication.
- ▲ Carefully consider the use of alternative therapy with a physician's order, such as application of aloe vera or aqueous cream to promote wound healing.
- • Consider the use of noetic therapies: stress management, imagery, and touch therapy.
- • Encourage the client to use prayer as a form of spiritual coping if this is comfortable for the client.
- • See the care plans for **Anxiety, Acute Pain, Fatigue, Risk for deficient Fluid volume, Risk for perioperative positioning Injury, Impaired physical Mobility,** and **Nausea.**

Pediatric

- • Support information the parents have gotten from the Internet regarding their child's condition.
- • Teach imagery and encourage distraction for children for post-surgical pain relief.

S

- Children who are at normal risk for aspiration/regurgitation should be allowed fluids prior to anesthesia.

Geriatric

- Perform a thorough preoperative assessment, including a cardiac and social support assessment.
- Assess for pain.
- Carefully evaluate the client's temperature. Know what is normal and abnormal for each client. Check baseline temperature and monitor trends.
- Teach guided imagery for pain relief.
- Offer spiritual support.

Home Care

- The above interventions may be adapted for the home setting.
- Provide supportive telephone calls from nurse to client as a means of decreasing anxiety and providing the psychosocial support necessary for recovery from surgery.

Client/Family Teaching

- Provide preoperative teaching by a nurse to decrease postoperative problems of anxiety, pain, nausea, and lack of independence.
- Provide preoperative information in verbal and written form.
- Teach systematic muscle relaxation for pain relief.
- Provide individualized teaching plans for the client with an ostomy. Consider basic needs: (1) maintenance of a pouching seal for a consistent, predictable wear time; (2) maintenance of peristomal skin integrity; and (3) social and professional support of the client.

S

Impaired Swallowing

NANDA Definition

Abnormal functioning of the swallowing mechanism associated with deficits in oral, pharyngeal, or esophageal structure or function

Defining Characteristics

Esophageal phase impairment: Abnormality in esophageal phase by swallow study; acidic smelling breath; bruxism; complaints of "something stuck"; epigastric pain; food refusal; heartburn or epigastric pain; hematemesis; hyperextension of head (e.g., arching during or after meals); nighttime awakening; nighttime coughing; observed evidence of difficulty in swallowing (e.g., stasis of food in oral cavity, coughing/choking); odynophagia; regurgitation of gastric contents (wet burps); repetitive swallowing; unexplained irritability surrounding mealtime; volume limiting; vomiting; vomitus on pillow

Oral phase impairment: Abnormality in oral phase of swallow study; coughing, choking, or gagging before a swallow; falling of food from mouth; inability to clear oral cavity; incomplete lip closure; lack of chewing; lack of tongue action to form bolus; long meals with little consumption; nasal reflux; piecemeal deglutition; pooling in lateral sulci; premature entry of bolus; pushing of food out of mouth; sialorrhea or drooling; slow bolus formation; weak suck resulting in inefficient nippling

Pharyngeal phase impairment: Abnormality in pharyngeal phase by swallowing study; altered head position; choking, coughing, or gagging; delayed swallow; food refusal; gurgly voice quality; inadequate laryngeal elevation; multiple swallows; nasal reflux; recurrent pulmonary infections; unexplained fever

Related Factors (r/t)

Congenital Defects

Behavioral feeding problems; conditions with significant hypotonia; congential heart disease; failure to thrive; history of tube feeding; mechanical obstruction (e.g., edema, tracheostomy tube, tumor); neuromuscular impairment (e.g., decreased or absent gag reflex, decreased strength or excursion of muscles involved in mastication, perceptual impairment, facial paralysis); protein energy malnutrition; respiratory disorders; self-injurious behavior; upper airway anomalies

Neurological Problems

Achalasia; acquired anatomic defects; cerebral palsy; cranial nerve involvement; developmental delay; esophageal defects; gastroesophageal reflux disease; laryngeal abnormalities; laryngeal defects; nasal defects; nasopharyngeal cavity defects; oropharynx abnormalities; prematurity; tracheal defects; traumas; traumatic head injury; upper airway anomalies

Client Outcomes

Client Will (Specify Time Frame):

- Demonstrate effective swallowing without choking or coughing
- Remain free from aspiration (e.g., lungs clear, temperature within normal range)

Nursing Interventions

- • Determine the client's readiness to eat. The client needs to be alert, able to follow instructions, able to hold the head erect, able to swallow, and able to move the tongue in the mouth.
- ▲ If the swallowing impairment is of new onset, ensure that the client receives a diagnostic workup.
- • Assess ability to swallow by positioning the thumb and index finger on the client's laryngeal protuberance. Ask the client to swallow; feel the larynx elevate. Ask the client to cough; test for a gag reflex on both sides of the posterior pharyngeal wall (lingual surface) with a tongue blade. Do not rely on the presence of a gag reflex to determine when to feed.
- • Consider the use of the Massey Bedside Swallowing Screen to screen for swallowing dysfunction.
- • Observe for signs associated with swallowing problems (e.g., coughing, choking, spitting of food, drooling, difficulty handling oral secretions, double swallowing or major delay in swallowing, watering eyes, nasal discharge, wet or gurgly voice, decreased ability to move the tongue and lips, decreased mastication of food, decreased ability to move food to the back of the pharynx, slow or scanning speech).
- ▲ If the client has impaired swallowing, refer to a speech pathologist for bedside evaluation as soon as possible. Ensure that the client is seen by a speech pathologist within 48 hours after admission if the client has had a CVA.
- ▲ To manage impaired swallowing, use a dysphagia team composed of a rehabilitation nurse, speech pathologist, dietitian, physician, and radiologist who work together.
- ▲ If the client has impaired swallowing, do not feed until an appropriate diagnostic workup is completed.
- • If client is not eating sufficient amount of food, recognize that

S

the immune system may be impaired with resultant increased risk of infection.

- If the client has an intact swallowing reflex, attempt to feed. Observe the following feeding guidelines:
  - Position the client upright at a 90-degree angle with the chin tucked forward at a 45-degree angle if this has been determined to be helpful.
  - Ensure that the client is awake, alert, and able to follow sequenced directions before attempting to feed.
  - Begin by feeding the client one third of a teaspoon of applesauce. Provide sufficient time to masticate and swallow.
  - Place the food on the unaffected side of the tongue.
  - During feeding, give the client specific directions (e.g., "Open your mouth, chew the food completely, and when you are ready, tuck your chin to your chest and swallow").
  - Avoid rushing or forcing feeding.
  - Ensure client is kept in an upright posture for an hour after eating.

▲ Watch for uncoordinated chewing or swallowing; coughing immediately after eating or delayed coughing, which may indicate silent aspiration; pocketing of food; wet-sounding voice; sneezing when eating; delay of more than 1 second in swallowing; or a change in respiratory patterns. If any of these signs is present, put on gloves, remove all food from the oral cavity, stop feedings, and consult with a speech and language pathologist and a dysphagia team.

- If the client tolerates single-textured foods such as pudding, hot cereal, or strained baby food, advance to a soft diet with guidance from the dysphagia team. Avoid foods such as hamburgers, corn, and pastas that are difficult to chew. Also avoid sticky foods such as peanut butter and white bread.
- Avoid providing liquids until the client is able to swallow effectively. Add a thickening agent to liquids to obtain a soft consistency that is similar to nectar, honey, or pudding, depending on the degree of swallowing problems.
- Thicken fluids as recommended from the swallowing evaluation. Preferably use prepackaged thickened liquids, or use a viscosimeter to ensure appropriate thickness.

▲ Work with the client on swallowing exercises prescribed by the dysphagia team (e.g., touching the palate with the tongue, stimulating the tonsillar arch and soft palate with a cold metal examination mirror [thermal stimulation], labial/lingual range-of-motion exercises).

▲ For many adult clients, avoid the use of straws if recommended by the speech pathologist.

• Provide meals in a quiet environment away from excessive stimuli such as a community dining room.

• Ensure that there is adequate time for the client to eat.

▲ Have suction equipment available during feeding. If choking occurs and suctioning is necessary, discontinue oral feeding until the client is safely assessed with a videofluoroscopic swallow study.

• Check the oral cavity for proper emptying after the client swallows and after the client finishes the meal. Provide oral care at the end of the meal. It may be necessary to manually remove food from the client's mouth. If this is the case, use gloves and keep the client's teeth apart with a padded tongue blade.

• Praise the client for successfully following directions and swallowing appropriately.

• Keep the client in an upright position for 45 minutes to an hour after a meal.

▲ Watch for signs of aspiration and pneumonia. Auscultate lung sounds after feeding. Note new crackles or wheezing, and note elevated temperature. Notify the physician as needed.

• Watch for signs of malnutrition and dehydration. Keep a record of food intake.

▲ Weigh the client weekly to help evaluate nutritional status. Evaluate nutritional status daily. If the client is not adequately nourished, work with the dysphagia team to determine whether the client needs to avoid oral intake with therapeutic feeding only or needs enteral feedings until the client can swallow adequately.

▲ If client has a tracheostomy, ask for referral to speech pathologist for swallowing studies before attempting to feed. After evaluation, decision should be made to have cuff either inflated or deflated when client eats.

Pediatric

▲ Refer to a physician and a dietician a child who has difficulty swallowing and symptoms such as difficulty manipulating food, delayed swallow response, and pocketing of a bolus of food.

- Provide oral motor stimulation that increases oral-sensory awareness by waking the mouth using exercises that focus on temperature, taste, and texture.
- For infants with poor sucking and swallowing, do the following:
  - Support the cheeks and jaw to increase sucking skills.
  - Pace or rhythmically move the bottle, which encourages better suck-swallow-breath synchrony.
- Watch for indicators of aspiration: coughing, a change in web vocal quality while feeding, perspiration and color changes during feeding, sneezing, and increased heart rate and breathing.
- Watch for warning signs of reflux: sour-smelling breath after eating, sneezing, lack of interest in feeding, crying and fussing extraordinarily when feeding, pained expressions when feeding, and excessive chewing and swallowing after eating.

Geriatric

- Recognize that being elderly does not result in dysphagia, but having medical problems including such things as arthritis, hypertension, and other chronic medical problems can result in dysphagia.

▲ Evaluate medications the client is presently taking, especially if elderly. Consult with the pharmacist for assistance in monitoring for incorrect doses and drug interactions that could result in dysphagia.

- Recognize that the elderly client with dementia needs a longer time to eat.
- Recognize that the loss of teeth can cause problems with chewing and swallowing.

Home Care

▲ Refer to speech therapy.

Client/Family Teaching

▲ Teach the client and family exercises prescribed by the dysphagia team.

- Teach the client a systematic method of swallowing effectively as prescribed by the dysphagia team.
- Educate the client, family, and all caregivers about rationales for food consistency and choices.

S

- Teach the family how to monitor the client to prevent and detect aspiration during eating.

Effective Therapeutic regimen management

NANDA Definition

Pattern of regulating and integrating into daily living a program for treatment of illness and its sequelae that is satisfactory for meeting specific health goals

Defining Characteristics

Appropriate choices of daily activities for meeting the goals of a prevention program; appropriate choices of daily activities for meeting the goals of a treatment program; illness symptoms within a normal range of expectation; verbalizes desire to manage the treatment of illness; verbalizes desire to manage prevention of sequelae; verbalizes intent to reduce risk factors for progression of illness and sequelae

Client Outcomes

T

Client Will (Specify Time Frame):

- Acknowledge appropriateness of choices for meeting goals of treatment or prevention programs
- Agree to continue making appropriate choices
- Verbalize intent to contact health provider(s) for additional information, support, or resources as needed

Nursing Interventions

- Review self-management strategies and related outcomes (e.g., changes in function and/or relief of symptoms such as pain).
- Explore the meaning of the person's illness experience and identify uncertainties and needs through open-ended questions.
- Acknowledge the congruence of choices in activities of daily living (ADLs) with health-related goals.

- Support decisions regarding the person's methods of integrating therapeutic regimens into ADLs.
- Provide information on possible illness trajectories to allow planning for future management. Help the person resolve ambivalent feelings about the illness and management of therapeutic regimens.
- Review methods of contacting health provider(s) for changes in therapeutic regimen and/or methods of incorporating therapeutic regimens into ADLs.
- Record the effectiveness of managing the therapeutic regimens.

Multicultural

- Assess health literacy in clients of diverse backgrounds.
- Assess cultural relevance of health information.
- Refer to care plan **Ineffective Therapeutic regimen management.**

Client/Family Teaching

- Teach about the disease trajectory and ways to manage disease symptoms as the trajectory changes.

T

Ineffective Therapeutic regimen management

NANDA Definition

Pattern of regulating and integrating into daily living a program for treatment of illness and the sequelae of illness that is unsatisfactory for meeting specific health goals

Defining Characteristics

Failure to include treatment regimens in daily routines; failure to take action to reduce risk factors; makes choices in daily living ineffective for meeting health goals; verbalizes desire to manage the illness; verbalizes difficulty with prescribed regimens

Related Factors (r/t)

Complexity of health care system; complexity of therapeutic regimen; decisional conflicts; economic difficulties; excessive demands made (e.g., individual, family); family conflict; family patterns of health care; inadequate number of cues to action; knowledge deficit; mistrust of healthcare personnel; mistrust of regimen; perceived barriers; powerlessness; perceived seriousness; perceived susceptibility; perceived benefits; social support deficit

Client Outcomes

Client Will (Specify Time Frame):

- Describe daily food and fluid intake that meets therapeutic goals
- Describe activity/exercise patterns that meet therapeutic goals
- Describe scheduling of medications that meets therapeutic goals
- Verbalize ability to manage therapeutic regimens
- Collaborate with health providers to decide on a therapeutic regimen that is congruent with health goals and lifestyle

Nursing Interventions

NOTE: This diagnosis does not have the same meaning as the diagnosis **Noncompliance.** This diagnosis is made with the client, so if the client does not agree with the diagnosis, it should not be made. The emphasis is on helping the client direct his or her own life and health, not on the client's compliance with the provider's instructions.

- Refer to the care plans for **Effective Therapeutic regimen management** and **Ineffective family Therapeutic regimen management.**
- Establish a collaborative partnership with the client for purposes of meeting health-related goals.
- Listen to the person's story about his or her illness self management. Explore the meaning of the person's illness experience and identify uncertainties and needs through open-ended questions.
- Help the client identify the "self" in self-management; show respect for the client's self-determination.
- Help the client enhance self-efficacy or confidence in his or her own ability to mange the illness. Involve family members in knowledge development, planning for self-management, and shared decision making.
- Review factors of the Health Belief Model (individual perceptions of seriousness and susceptibility, demographic and other

T

modifying factors, and perceived benefits and barriers) with the client.

- Identify the reasons for actions that are not therapeutic and discuss alternatives.
- Use various formats to provide information about the therapeutic regimen, including group education, brochures, videotapes, written instructions, computer-based programs, and telephone contact.
- Help the client identify and modify barriers to effective self-management.
- Help the client self-manage his or her own health through teaching about strategies for changing habits such as overeating, sedentary lifestyle, and smoking.
- Develop a contract with the client to maintain motivation for changes in behavior.
- Help the client maintain consistency in therapeutic regimen management for optimal results.
- Review how to contact health providers as needed to address issues and concerns regarding self-management.
- Implement organizational changes to facilitate shared decision making for self-management of chronic illnesses.
- Use focus groups to evaluate the implementation of self-management programs.

Multicultural

- Conduct a self-assessment of the relation of culture to ethnically based care.
- Provide support for self-management throughout the process of care.
- Assess the influence of cultural beliefs, norms, and values on the individual's perceptions of the therapeutic regimen. Discuss all strategies with the client in the context of the client's culture. Provide health information that is consistent with the health literacy of clients.
- Determine that health information is culturally relevant.
- Assess for barriers that may interfere with client follow-up of treatment recommendations.
- Discuss with the client his or her beliefs about medication and treatment to enhance self-management of medications and other treatments.

- Use electronic monitoring to improve management of medications.
- Validate the client's feelings regarding the ability to manage his or her own care and the impact on current lifestyle.

Home Care

- Prepare and instruct clients and family members in the use of a medication box. Set up an appropriate schedule for filling of the medication box, and post medication times and doses in an accessible area (e.g., attached by a magnet to the refrigerator).
- Monitor self-management of the medical regimen.

▲ Consult physician and/or pharmacist as questions arise.

Client/Family Teaching

- Identify what the client and/or family knows and adjust teaching accordingly.
- Teach ways to adjust ADLs for inclusion of therapeutic regimens.
- Teach safety in taking medications.
- Teach the client to act as a self-advocate with health providers who prescribe therapeutic regimens.

Ineffective community Therapeutic regimen management

NANDA Definition

Pattern of regulating and integrating into community processes programs for treatment of illness and the sequelae of illness that are unsatisfactory for meeting health-related goals

Defining Characteristics

Deficits in advocates for aggregates; deficits in community activities for prevention; illness symptoms above the norm expected for the population; insufficient healthcare resources (e.g., people, programs); unavailable healthcare resources for illness care; unexpected acceleration of illness

Community Outcomes

Community Members and Leaders Will (Specify Time Frame):

- Secure community members and/or health providers who will be accountable for illness care of specific groups.
- Remain involved in advocacy for illness care and prevention programs.
- Develop healthcare plans for effective prevention and treatment of illnesses.
- Make resources available for illness care and prevention.
- Initiate or improve strategies for prevention of the sequelae of illness.

Nursing Interventions

NOTE: Nursing interventions are conducted in collaboration with community leaders, community and public health nurses, and members of other disciplines.

- • Implement strategies to engage community members to be team members for health assessments and development of community programs.
- ▲ Request that a clinical nurse specialist in community health nursing work with coalitions of health providers and community leaders.
- ▲ Recruit additional health providers as needed.
- • Establish special action groups for specific problems and/or localities to address health policies and practices.
- • Evaluate community infrastructures for adequacy in serving community illness-related needs.
- • Advocate for and with the community in multiple arenas (e.g., newspapers, television, legislative bodies, community boards).
- • Provide information to public and private sources about community assessment, diagnosis, and plans of care.
- • Mobilize support for the community to obtain the resources necessary for illness care and prevention.
- • Establish culturally sensitive community health programs for self-management.
- • Provide coaching interventions in programs for chronic disease self-management.
- • Integrate the Internet with community health programs.
- • Determine the cultural appropriateness of all programs.

- Support the population of family caregivers through implementation of the National Family Support Program.
- Write grant proposals for the funding of new programs or the expansion of existing programs.
- Conduct research studies to convince others of the need to improve services or change policies.
- Avoid victim-blaming stances in efforts to promote community responsibility for health.

Multicultural

- Refer to care plan **Ineffective community Coping.**
- Hire culturally diverse staff members for community agencies.
- Identify the health services and information resources currently available in the community.
- Identify cultural barriers such as acculturation issues, lack of community support, and lack of experience with a health behavior.
- Develop a health promotion directory that lists health resources for clients.

Ineffective family Therapeutic regimen management

T

NANDA Definition

Pattern of regulating and integrating into family processes a program for treatment of illness and the sequelae of illness that is unsatisfactory for meeting specific health goals

Defining Characteristics

Acceleration of illness symptoms of a family member; failure to take actions to reduce risk factors; inappropriate family activities for meeting health goals; lack of attention to illness; verbalizes desire to manage the illness; verbalizes difficulty with therapeutic regimen

Related Factors (r/t)

Complexity of health care system; complexity of therapeutic regimen; decisional conflicts; economic difficulties; excessive demands; family conflict

Family Outcomes

Family Will (Specify Time Frame):

- Make adjustments in usual activities (e.g., diet, activity, stress management) to incorporate therapeutic regimens of its members
- Reduce illness symptoms of family members
- Desire to manage therapeutic regimens of its members
- Describe a decrease in the difficulties of managing therapeutic regimens
- Describe actions to reduce risk factors

Nursing Interventions

- • Base family interventions on knowledge of the family, family context, and family function.
- • Use a family approach when helping an individual with a health problem that requires therapeutic management.
- • Identify family interactions and their embedded contexts relative to specific health objectives.
- • Review with family members the congruence and incongruence of family behaviors and health-related goals.
- • Help family members make decisions regarding ways to integrate therapeutic regimens into daily living. Provide advice or suggestions as solicited and accepted by the family.
- • Demonstrate respect for and trust in family decisions.
- • Acknowledge the challenge of integrating therapeutic regimens with family behaviors.
- • Review the symptoms of specific illness(es) and work with the family toward development of greater self-efficacy in relation to these symptoms.
- • Support family decisions to adjust therapeutic regimens as indicated.
- ▲ Advocate for the family in negotiating therapeutic regimens with health providers.
- • Help the family mobilize social supports.
- • Help family members modify perceptions as indicated.
- • Use one or more theories of family dynamics to describe, explain, or predict family behaviors.
- ▲ Collaborate with expert nurses or other consultants regarding strategies for working with families.

- Promote and support public health programs to support families. Coaching methods can be used to help families improve their health.

Multicultural

- Acknowledge racial and ethnic differences at the onset of care.
- Ensure that all strategies for working with the family are congruent with the culture of the family.
- Approach families of color with respect, warmth, and professional courtesy.
- Give a rationale when assessing African-American families about sensitive issues.
- Support religious beliefs and the comfort role of religion.
- Use a family-centered approach when working with Latino, Asian, African-American, and Native-American clients.
- Facilitate modeling and role playing for the family regarding healthy ways to communicate and interact.
- Use the nursing intervention of cultural brokerage to help families deal with the healthcare system.

Client/Family Teaching

- Teach about all aspects of therapeutic regimens. Provide as much knowledge as family members will accept, adjust instruction to account for what the family already knows, and provide information in a culturally congruent manner.
- Teach ways to adjust family behaviors to include therapeutic regimens.

▲ Teach safety in taking medications.

▲ Teach family members to act as self-advocates with health providers who prescribe therapeutic regimens.

Readiness for enhanced Therapeutic regimen management

NANDA Definition

Pattern of regulating and integrating into daily living a program for treatment of illness and its sequelae that is sufficient for meeting health-related goals and can be strengthened

Defining Characteristics

Choices of daily living are appropriate for meeting goals (e.g., treatment, prevention); describes reduction of risk factors; expresses desire to manage the illness (e.g., treatment, prevention of sequelae); expresses little difficulty with prescribed regimens; no unexpected acceleration of illness symptoms

Client Outcomes

Client Will (Specify Time Frame):

- Describe integration of therapeutic regimen into daily living
- Demonstrate continued commitment to integration of therapeutic regimen into daily living routines

Nursing Interventions

- Acknowledge the expertise that the client and family bring to self-management.
- Review factors that contribute to the likelihood of health promotion and health protection. Use Pender's Health Promotion Model and Becker's Health Belief Model to identify contributing factors.
- Assess for depression.
- Facilitate the client and family to obtain health insurance and drug payment plans whenever needed and possible.
- Further develop and reinforce contributing factors that might change with ongoing management of the therapeutic regimen (e.g., knowledge, self-efficacy, self-esteem, and perceived benefits).
- Support all efforts to self-manage therapeutic regimens.
- Review the client's strengths in the management of the therapeutic regimen.
- Collaborate with the client to identify strategies to maintain strengths and develop additional strengths as indicated.
- Identify contributing factors that may need to be improved now or in the future.
- Provide knowledge as needed related to the pathophysiology of the disease or illness, prescribed activities, prescribed medications, and nutrition.
- Use coaching strategies such as educational reinforcement, psychosocial support, and motivational guidance.

- Support positive health-promotion and health-protection behaviors.
- Help the client maintain existing support and seek additional supports as needed.

Multicultural

- Manipulate community factors that may affect the management of the therapeutic regimen (e.g., barriers, supports, insurance, education about the illness, and provider-client relationships).
- Validate the client's feelings regarding the ability to manage his or her own care and the impact on current lifestyle.
- Use electronic monitoring to improve medication adherence.
- Discuss with clients their beliefs about medication and treatment to enhance medication and treatment adherence.

Community Teaching

- Review therapeutic regimens and their optimal integration with daily living routines.
- Teach disease processes and therapeutic regimens for management of these disease processes.

T

Ineffective Thermoregulation

NANDA Definition

Temperature fluctuation between hypothermia and hyperthermia

Defining Characteristics

Cool skin; cyanotic nail beds; fluctuations in body temperature above and below the normal range; flushed skin; hypertension; increased respiratory rate; mild shivering; moderate pallor; piloerection; reduction in body temperature below normal range; seizures; slow capillary refill; tachycardia; warm to touch

Related Factors (r/t)

Aging; fluctuating environmental temperature; illness; immaturity; trauma

Client Outcomes

Client Will (Specify Time Frame):

- Maintain temperature within normal range
- Explain measures needed to maintain normal temperature
- Explain symptoms of hypothermia or hyperthermia

Nursing Interventions

- Monitor temperature every 1 to 4 hours or use continuous temperature monitoring as appropriate.
- Measure the temperature orally or rectally. Avoid using the axillary or tympanic site.
- Take vital signs every 1 to 4 hours, noting changes associated with hypothermia: first, increased blood pressure, pulse, and respirations; then decreased values as hypothermia progresses.
- Monitor the client for signs of hypothermia (e.g., shivering, cool skin, piloerection, pallor, slow capillary refill, cyanotic nail beds, decreased mentation, dysrhythmias).
- Note changes in vital signs associated with hyperthermia: rapid, bounding pulse; increased respiratory rate; and decreased blood pressure, accompanied by orthostatic hypotension.
- Monitor the client for signs of hyperthermia (e.g., headache, nausea and vomiting, weakness, absence of sweating, delirium, and coma).
- Maintain a consistent room temperature (72° F [22.2° C]).
- Promote adequate nutrition and hydration.
- Adjust clothing to facilitate passive warming or cooling as appropriate.
- See the Nursing Interventions for **Hypothermia** or **Hyperthermia** as appropriate.

T

Pediatric

- Recognize that pediatric clients have a decreased ability to adapt to temperature extremes. Take the following actions to maintain body temperature in the infant or child:
  - Keep the head covered.
  - Use blankets to keep the client warm.
  - Keep the client covered during procedures, transport, and diagnostic testing.
  - Keep the room temperature at 72° F (22.2° C).
- Recognize that the infant and small child are both vulnerable to

heat stroke in hot weather and ensure they receive sufficient fluids and are protected from hot environments.

Geriatric

- • Do not allow an elderly client to become chilled or overheated. Keep the client covered when giving a bath and offer socks to wear in bed. Be aware of factors such as room temperature (heating/air conditioning), clothing (layered/loose), and fluid intake.
- • Ensure that elderly clients receive sufficient fluids during hot days and stay out of the sun.
- ▲ Assess the medication profile for the potential risk of drug-related altered body temperature.

Home Care

- • Prevent hypothermia in cold weather:
  - ■ Instruct the client to avoid prolonged exposure outdoors. When outdoors, the client should wear gloves and a cap on the head.
  - ■ Keep the room temperature at 68° to 72° F (20° to 22.2° C).
  - ▲ Ensure an adequate source of heat. Refer to social services if the client/family has a low income and the heat could be turned off.
  - ■ Help the elderly client locate a warm environment to which the client can go for safety in cold weather if the home environment is no longer warm.
- • Prevent hyperthermia in hot weather:
  - ■ Encourage the client to wear lightweight cotton clothing. Help the elderly client remove the usual sweater.
  - ■ Ensure that the client drinks adequate amounts of fluids (2000 mL/day).
  - ■ Help the client obtain a fan or air conditioner to increase evaporation as needed.
  - ■ Take the temperature of the elderly client in hot weather.
  - ■ Help the elderly client locate a cool environment to which the client can go for safety in hot weather.

Client/Family Teaching

- • Teach the client and family the signs of hypothermia and hyperthermia and appropriate actions to take if either condition develops.

- Teach the client and family an age-appropriate method for taking the temperature.
- Teach the client to avoid alcohol and medications that depress cerebral function.

Disturbed Thought processes

NANDA Definition

Disruption in cognitive operations and activities

Defining Characteristics

Cognitive dissonance; distractibility; egocentricity; hypervigilance; hypovigilance; inaccurate interpretation of environment; inappropriate thinking; memory deficit

Client Outcomes

Client Will (Specify Time Frame):

- Remains oriented to time, place, person, and circumstance; demonstrates improved cognitive function
- Remains free from actual and potential harm by self or others
- Performs activities of daily living (ADLs) adequately and independently
- Identifies community resources for help after discharge
- Understands the actions and side effects of medications

Nursing Interventions

- Observe for causes of altered thought processes.
- Monitor, record, and report changes in client's neurological status (level of consciousness, increased intracranial pressure), mental status (memory, cognition, judgment, and concentration), vital signs, laboratory results, and ability to follow commands.
- Obtain a medical history to rule out physical illness etiology for mental status changes.
- Complete a mental status examination of client, including a Mini Mental State Exam (MMSE).

- Report any new onset or sudden increase in confusion.
- Engage the client in conversation.
- ▲ Assess pain and promptly provide comfort measures.
- Identify and remove potentially dangerous items in the environment.
- Limit use of sedatives and drugs, which depress the central nervous system.
- ▲ Use soft restraints with discretion and physician order.
- Orient client, call client by name, and introduce self on each contact. Prominently display a clock and calendar that are easy to read in room and refer to them.
- Stay with clients if they are agitated and likely to be injured.
- Observe for therapeutic and side effects of psychotropic medications.
- Develop a therapeutic alliance to increase trust with the client.
- Assess client's assault potential and maintain staff safety.
- Establish predictable care routines and maintain continuity of client's nursing staff.
- Frequently check on client and have brief interactions to prevent sensory deprivation and/or overstimulation.
- Evaluate the client's ability to safely engage in self-care activities.
- Observe for signs and symptoms of significant depression concomitant to altered thoughts.
- Provide support and education to family during client's period of cognitive change.
- ▲ Initiate a social service referral to find help for client after discharge.
- Observe for evidence of auditory and/or visual hallucination experiences. Teach management techniques.
- Engage the psychotic client in simple, nonprobing conversation.
- Ask for clarification when necessary.
- Help client state needs and ask for assistance.
- Assess need for referrals to other healthcare services, such as physical or occupational therapy.
- Refer to care plans for **Risk for self-** and **other-directed Violence** for further nursing interventions.

T

Geriatric

- Monitor for dementia, as evidenced by gradual onset and a progressive deterioration, or for delirium, as evidenced by acute onset and generally reversible course.

Multicultural

- Assess the influence of cultural beliefs, norms, and values on the family's or caregiver's understanding of disturbed thought processes.
- Inform the client's family or caregiver of the meaning of and reasons for common behaviors observed in the client with disturbed thought processes.
- Validate the family members' feelings regarding the impact of the client's behavior on family lifestyle.

Home Care

- The interventions previously described may be adapted for home care use.
- ▲ Assess the client for the presence of a psychiatric disorder. Refer for mental health services as indicated.
- Assess the family's knowledge of the disease process and plan of care; teach as necessary and encourage participation.
- Identify the strengths of the caregiver and the caregiver's efforts to gain control of unpredictable situations. Help the caregiver to stay connected with a client who may be behaving differently than usual, to make life as routine as possible, to help the client set goals and sustain hope, and to allow the client space to experience progress.
- ▲ Assess the client's functional status as it relates to the ability for self-care; refer to a physician for evaluation of medication levels as indicated.
- Assess the home environment for the availability of distractions from hallucinations, such as playing music over headphones.
- ▲ If the client's condition deteriorates, seek acute medical or mental health intervention immediately, as appropriate.
- ▲ Identify an emergency plan and discuss criteria for its use with the family or caregivers.
- ▲ Assess the client's ability to manage his or her own medications and make plans for assistance as needed to maintain safety of client.

- • Assess and modify environmental stimuli that could be misinterpreted (e.g., use a nightlight, evaluate placement of mirrors).
- • Allow the client control over aspects of his or her environment, as he or she is able.
- • Provide an opportunity for the client to pursue interests and use skills without taxing the client's judgment and cognitive ability.
- ▲ Refer the client and family to community support groups (e.g., psychosocial rehabilitation programs for the client, National Alliance for the Mentally Ill for the client and family).
- ▲ In the presence of chronic thought process disorder, institute case management of frail elderly to support continued independent living.
- ▲ When the client has a psychiatric disorder, pay special attention to the presence of comorbid medical conditions and the need for medical care.
- ▲ When the client has a psychiatric disorder, refer for psychiatric home health care services for client reassurance and implementation of a therapeutic regimen.

Client/Family Teaching

- • Teach family members reorientation techniques and about the need to repeat instructions frequently.
- • Teach client distraction techniques to manage hallucinations.
- • Teach family members ways to support client without supporting delusional beliefs.
- • Help family identify coping skills, environmental supports, and community services for dealing with chronically mentally ill clients.
- • Discuss caregiver's need for respite. Offer support, encouragement, and information for meeting those needs.

T

Impaired Tissue integrity

NANDA Definition

Damage to mucous membrane, corneal, integumentary, or subcutaneous tissues

Defining Characteristics

Damaged tissue (e.g., cornea, mucous membrane, integumentary or subcutaneous tissue); destroyed tissue

Related Factors (r/t)

Altered circulation; chemical irritants; fluid deficit; fluid excess; impaired physical mobility; knowledge deficit; mechanical factors (e.g., pressure, shear, friction); nutritional factors (e.g., deficit or excess); radiation; temperature extremes

Client Outcomes

Client Will (Specify Time Frame):

- Report any altered sensation or pain at site of tissue impairment
- Demonstrate understanding of plan to heal tissue and prevent injury
- Describe measures to protect and heal the tissue, including wound care
- Experience a wound that decreases in size and has increased granulation tissue

Nursing Interventions

T

- Assess the site of impaired tissue integrity and determine the cause (e.g., acute or chronic wound, burn, dermatological lesion, pressure ulcer, leg ulcer, skin failure).
- Determine the size and depth of the wound (e.g., full-thickness wound, deep tissue injury, stage III or IV pressure ulcer). See **Impaired Skin integrity** for stage I and II pressure ulcers.
- Classify pressure ulcers in the following manner:
  - **Stage III:** Full-thickness skin loss involving damage to or necrosis of subcutaneous tissue that may extend down to but not through underlying fascia; ulcer appears as a deep crater with or without undermining of adjacent tissue.
  - **Stage IV:** Full-thickness skin loss with extensive destruction; tissue necrosis; or damage to muscle, bone, or supporting structures (e.g., tendons, joint capsules).
  - **Deep tissue injury:** A pressure-related injury to subcutaneous tissues under intact skin.
- Monitor the site of impaired tissue integrity at least once daily for color changes, redness, swelling, warmth, pain, or other signs of infection. Determine whether the client is experiencing changes

in sensation or pain. Pay special attention to all high-risk areas such as bony prominences, skin folds, sacrum, and heels.

- • Monitor the status of the skin around the wound. Monitor the client's skin care practices, noting type of soap or other cleansing agents used, temperature of water, and frequency of skin cleansing.
- • Monitor the client's continence status and minimize exposure of the skin impairment site and other areas to moisture from urine or stool, perspiration, or wound drainage.
- • Monitor for correct placement of tubes, catheters, and other devices. Assess the skin and tissue affected by the tape that secures these devices.
- • In an orthopedic client, check every 2 hours for correct placement of foot boards, restraints, traction, casts, or other devices, and assess skin and tissue integrity. Be alert for symptoms of compartment syndrome (refer to the care plan for **Risk for Peripheral neurovascular dysfunction**).
- • For a client with limited mobility, use a risk assessment tool to assess immobility-related risk factors systematically.
- • Implement a written treatment plan for the topical treatment of the skin impairment site.
- ▲ Identify a plan for debridement if necrotic tissue (eschar or slough) is present and if consistent with overall client management goals.
- • Select a topical treatment that maintains a moist wound-healing environment and also allows absorption of exudate and filling of dead space.
- • Do not position the client on the site of impaired tissue integrity.
- • Evaluate for the use of specialty mattresses, beds, or devices as appropriate.
- • If the goal of care is to keep the client comfortable (e.g., for a terminally ill client), turning and repositioning may not be appropriate.
- • Avoid massaging around the site of impaired tissue integrity and over bony prominences.
- • Assess the client's nutritional status; refer for a nutritional consultation and/or institute use of dietary supplements.
- ▲ A comprehensive plan of care includes a thorough wound assessment, treatment interventions, support surfaces, nutritional products, adjunctive therapies, and evaluation of the outcome of care.

T

Home Care

- • Some of the interventions previously described may be adapted for home care use.
- ▲ Assess the client's current phase of wound healing (inflammation, proliferation, maturation) and stage of injury; initiate appropriate wound management.
- • Instruct and assist the client and caregivers in understanding how to change dressings and the importance of maintaining a clean environment. Provide written instructions and observe them completing the dressing change.
- ▲ Initiate a consultation in a case assignment with a wound specialist or wound, ostomy, and continence nurse to establish a comprehensive plan as soon as possible. Plan case conferencing to promote optimal wound care.

Client/Family Teaching

- • Teach skin and wound assessment and ways to monitor for signs and symptoms of infection, complications, and healing.
- • Teach the client why a topical treatment has been selected. Explain wound bed changes that the caregiver can expect to see. Instruct on when the dressing needs to be changed.
- ▲ If it is consistent with overall client management goals, teach how to turn and reposition the client at least every 2 hours.

Ineffective Tissue perfusion (specify type: renal, cerebral, cardiopulmonary, gastrointestinal, peripheral)

NANDA Definition

Decrease in oxygen resulting in failure to nourish tissues at capillary level

Defining Characteristics

Cardiopulmonary

Abnormal arterial blood gasses; altered respiratory rate outside of acceptable parameters; arrhythmias; bronchospasm; capillary refill >3 seconds; chest pain; chest retraction; dyspnea; nasal flaring; sense of "impending doom"; use of accessory muscles

Cerebral
Altered mental status; behavior changes; changes in motor response; changes in papillary reactions; difficulty in swallowing; extremity weakness; paralysis; speech abnormalities

Gastrointestinal
Abdominal distention; abdominal pain or tenderness; absent bowel sounds; hypoactive bowel sounds; nausea

Peripheral Arterial
Altered sensation; altered skin characteristics (hair, moisture) or nails; cold extremities; diminished arterial pulses; intermittent claudication; pale skin upon elevation of leg, with color not returning upon lowering of leg; pallor; shiny, waxy skin; skin temperature changes; slow healing of lesions; weak or absent pulses

Peripheral Venous
Edema; brawny hemosideric skin discoloration; dependent blue or purple skin color; positive Homan's sign; slow healing of lesions

Renal
Altered blood pressure outside of acceptable parameters; anuria; elevation in blood urea nitrogen/creatinine ratio; hematuria; oliguria

Related Factors (r/t)
Altered affinity of hemoglobin for oxygen; decreased hemoglobin concentration in blood; enzyme poisoning; exchange problems; hypoventilation; hypovolemia; hypervolemia; impaired transport of oxygen; interruption of blood flow; mismatch of ventilation with blood flow

Client Outcomes
Client Will (Specify Time Frame):
- Demonstrate adequate tissue perfusion as evidenced by palpable peripheral pulses, warm and dry skin, adequate urinary output, and absence of respiratory distress
- Verbalize knowledge of treatment regimen, including appropriate exercise and medications and their actions and possible side effects
- Identify changes in lifestyle needed to increase tissue perfusion

Nursing Interventions

Cerebral Perfusion

▲ If the client has a period of syncope or other signs of a possible transient ischemic attack, assist the client to a resting position, perform a neurological assessment, and report to the physician. If the client experiences dizziness because of postural hypotension when getting up, teach methods to decrease dizziness, such as remaining seated for several minutes before standing, flexing feet upward several times while seated, rising slowly, sitting down immediately if feeling dizzy, and trying to have someone present when standing.

▲ If symptoms of a new cerebrovascular accident occur (e.g., slurred speech, change in vision, hemiparesis, hemiplegia, or dysphasia), notify a physician immediately.

• If symptoms of a stroke are present, use the National Institute of Health Stroke Scale to evaluate the condition of the client.

▲ If an ischemic stroke has occurred, determine the position of the head of the bed after consulting the physician. In some situations it is appropriate to raise the head of the bed 30 degrees to lower intracranial pressure. Other times it is appropriate to keep the client mostly flat to increase cerebral perfusion.

• See the care plans for **Decreased Intracranial adaptive capacity, Risk for Injury,** and **Acute Confusion.**

T

Renal Perfusion

• Be aware that renal blood flow and glomerular filtration rate may decrease in response to exercise and with a variety of medications.

Peripheral Perfusion

▲ Check the brachial, radial, dorsalis pedis, posterior tibial, and popliteal pulses bilaterally. If unable to find them, use a Doppler stethoscope and notify the physician immediately if new onset of pulses is not present.

• Note skin color and feel the temperature of the skin.

• Check capillary refill.

• Note skin texture and the presence of hair loss, ulcers, or gangrenous areas on the legs or feet.

• Note the presence of edema in the extremities and rate severity on a four-point scale. Measure the circumference of the ankle and calf at the same time each day in the early morning.

- Assess for pain in the extremities, noting severity, quality, timing, and exacerbating and alleviating factors. Differentiate venous from arterial disease.

Arterial Insufficiency

▲ Monitor peripheral pulses. If there is new onset of loss of pulses with bluish, purple, or black areas and extreme pain, notify the physician immediately.
• Do not elevate the legs above the level of the heart.
▲ For early arterial insufficiency, encourage exercise such as walking or riding an exercise bicycle from 30 to 60 minutes per day as ordered by the physician.
• Keep the client warm and have the client wear socks and shoes or sheepskin-lined slippers when mobile. Do not apply heat.
• Use a variety of leg positions after surgical intervention for peripheral arterial disease (either supine with legs extended, sitting with legs extended, or supine with legs elevated 20 degrees) when getting this population out of bed.
▲ Pay meticulous attention to foot care. Refer to a podiatrist if the client has a foot or nail abnormality.
• If the client has ischemic arterial ulcers, refer to the care plan for **Impaired Tissue integrity.**
▲ If client smokes, aggressively counsel the client to stop smoking and refer to the physician for medications to support nicotine withdrawal and a smoking withdrawal program.

T

Venous Insufficiency

- Elevate edematous legs as ordered and ensure no pressure under the knee.
- Apply graduated compression stockings as ordered. Ensure proper fit by measuring accurately. Remove the stocking at least twice a day, in the morning with the bath and in the evening, to assess the condition of the extremity, then reapply.
- Encourage the client to walk with compression stockings on and perform toe-up and point-flex exercises.
- If the client is overweight, encourage weight loss to decrease venous disease.
- If the client has venous leg ulcers, encourage the client to avoid prolonged sitting, standing, and elevation of the involved leg.
- Discuss lifestyle with the client to determine if the client's oc-

cupation requires prolonged standing or sitting, which can result in chronic venous disease.

- ▲ If the client is mostly immobile, consult with the physician regarding use of a calf-high pneumatic compression device for prevention of deep vein thrombosis.
- • Observe for signs of deep vein thrombosis, including pain, tenderness, swelling in the calf and thigh, and redness in the involved extremity. Take serial leg measurements of the thigh and calf circumferences. In some clients a tender venous cord can be felt in the popliteal fossa. Do not rely on Homans' sign.
- ▲ Note the results of a D-dimer test and ultrasounds.
- ▲ If deep vein thrombosis is present, observe for symptoms of a pulmonary embolism, including dyspnea, tachypnea, and tachycardia, especially with a history of trauma.
- • If client is receiving heparin subcutaneously, do not change the needle after drawing up the dose.
- • If client develops deep vein thrombosis, after treatment and hospital discharge recommend client wear below-the-knee elastic compression stockings during the day on the involved extremity.

Geriatric

T

- • Change the client's position slowly when getting the client out of bed.
- • Recognize that the elderly have an increased risk of developing pulmonary embolism; if it is present, the symptoms are nonspecific and often mimic those of heart failure or pneumonia.

Home Care

- • The interventions previously described may be adapted for home care use.
- • Differentiate between arterial and venous insufficiency.
- • If arterial disease is present and the client smokes, aggressively encourage smoking cessation. See the care plan for **Health-seeking behaviors.**
- • Examine the feet carefully at frequent intervals for changes and new ulcerations.
- ▲ Assess the client's nutritional status, paying special attention to obesity, hyperlipidemia, and malnutrition. Refer to a dietitian if appropriate.

- Monitor for development of gangrene, venous ulceration, and symptoms of cellulitis (redness, pain, and increased swelling in an extremity).

Client/Family Teaching

▲ Explain the importance of good foot care. Teach the client and family to wash and inspect the feet daily. Recommend that the diabetic client wear padded socks, special insoles, and jogging shoes.

▲ Teach the diabetic client that he or she should have a comprehensive foot examination at least annually, including assessment of sensation using the Semmes-Weinstein monofilaments. If good sensation is not present, refer to a footwear professional for fitting of therapeutic shoes and inserts, the cost of which is covered by Medicare.

- For arterial disease, stress the importance of not smoking, following a weight loss program (if the client is obese), carefully controlling a diabetic condition, controlling hyperlipidemia and hypertension, maintaining intake of antiplatelet therapy, and reducing stress.
- Teach the client to avoid exposure to cold; limit exposure to brief periods if going out in cold weather and wear warm clothing.
- For venous disease, teach the importance of wearing compression stockings as ordered, elevating the legs at intervals, and watching for skin breakdown on the legs.
- Teach the client to recognize the signs and symptoms that should be reported to a physician (e.g., change in skin temperature, color, or sensation or the presence of a new lesion on the foot).
- NOTE: If the client is receiving anticoagulant therapy, see the care plan for **Ineffective Protection.**

T

Impaired Transfer ability

NANDA Definition

Limitation of independent movement between two nearby surfaces

Defining Characteristics

Inability to transfer: between uneven levels; from bed to chair; from chair to bed; on or off a toilet; on or off a commode; in or out of tub; in or out of shower; from chair to car; from car to chair; from chair to floor; from floor to chair; from standing to floor; from floor to standing; from bed to standing; from standing to bed; from chair to standing; from standing to chair

Related Factors (r/t)

Cognitive impairment; insufficient muscle strength; musculoskeletal impairment (e.g., contractures); neuromuscular impairment; obesity; pain

Suggested functional level classifications include the following:

0—Completely independent

1—Requires use of equipment or device

2—Requires help from another person for assistance, supervision, or teaching

3—Requires help from another person and equipment or device

4—Dependent; does not participate in activity

Client Outcomes

Client Will (Specify Time Frame):

- Transfer from bed to chair and back successfully
- Transfer from chair to chair successfully
- Transfer from wheelchair to toilet and back successfully
- Transfer from wheelchair to car and back successfully

Nursing Interventions

▲ Request consult for a physical and/or occupational therapist (PT and OT) to develop exercise and strengthening program early in the client's recovery.

▲ Obtain a consult for a PT, OT, or orthotist to evaluate and fit clients with proper orthoses, braces, collars, and walking aids before helping them stand.

• Help client don/doff collars, prostheses, antiembolism stockings, and abdominal binders while in bed.

▲ Ergonomically assess clients' dependence, weight, strength, balance, tolerance to position change, cooperation, and cognition plus available equipment and staff ratio and experience to decide whether to do a manual or device-assisted transfer.

▲ Collaborate with PT and use algorithms to identify technological aids to handle and transfer dependent clients safely.

• Do not use the under-axilla method or manual handling to transfer dependent clients; rather, use mechanical handling equipment such as powered mechanical lifts and stand-assist lifts.

- Apply a gait belt to client's low back or under the axilla before transfers; keep the belt and client close to you during the transfer.
- ▲ Remind clients to comply with weight-bearing restrictions ordered by the physician.
- Adjust transfer surfaces so they are similar in height. For example, lower a hospital bed to equal commode height.
- Help clients don shoes and socks with nonskid soles, and educate diabetics to wear shoes before transfers.
- Nursing staff should wear positive-grip shoe covers or nonslip shoes when transferring clients off shower chairs on tile floors.
- Remove or swivel wheelchair armrests, leg rests, and footplates to the side, especially with squat or slide board transfers.
- Place wheelchair and commode at a slight angle toward the surface to which client will transfer onto.
- Teach client to consistently lock brakes on wheelchair/commode/shower chair before transferring.
- Position walking aids logistically so client can grasp and use them once he or she is standing.
- Reinforce that clients are to place one hand on walker and push with opposite hand against chair arm or surface from which they are rising.
- Give clear, simple cues and instructions, allow client time to process information, and let him or her do as much of the transfer as possible.
- ▲ Implement and document type of transfer (slide board, pivot, etc.), weight-bearing status (non-weight-bearing, partial, etc.), equipment (walker, sling lift, etc.), and level of assistance (standby, moderate, etc.) on care plan.
- Place client in set position before standing him or her; for example, sitting on edge of surface with bilateral weight bearing on buttocks and hips, with knees flexed, balls of feet aligned under knees, and head in midline.
- Support and stabilize clients weak knee(s) by placing one or both of your knees next to or encircling client's knee(s), rather than blocking them.
  - ■ Squat transfer: client leans well forward, slightly raises flexed hips off the surface, pivots, and sits down on new surface.

- Standing pivot transfer: client leans forward with hips flexed and pushes up with hands from seat surface (or arms of chair), then stands erect, pivots, and sits down on new surface.
- Slide board transfer: client should have on pants or have a pillowcase over the board. Remove arm and leg rest from wheelchair and slightly angle it toward new surface. Help client lean sideways, thus shifting his or her weight so transfer board can be placed well under the upper thigh of the leg next to new surface. Make sure board is safely angled across both surfaces. Help client return to neutral alignment and place one hand on board and the other hand on seat surface. Remind and help client perform a series of pushups with arms while leaning slightly forward and lifting (not sliding) hips in small increments across board with each pushup.

▲ Use extra staff to transfer debilitated bariatric (extremely obese) clients and place their beds against a corner wall. Help them into the set position, with both knees level with thighs (a footstool may be needed). Help clients lean well forward.

▲ Use bariatric moving devices, including mattress overlay, transfer sheet, sliding or roller board, 60-inch long gait belt or two regular gait belts buckled together, standing-lift device, overhead ceiling-mounted or A-frame lifts, and chairs/commodes (1000-pound limit).

• Perform initial and subsequent fall risk assessment.

▲ Collaborate with PT, OT, and pharmacy for early individualized preventative fall/recurrent fall plan, for example, scheduled toileting, balance and strength training, removal of hazards, chair alarms, call system in reach, and review of medications.

Home Care

▲ Obtain referral for occupational therapy and physical therapy to teach home exercises and balance as well as fall prevention and recovery and evaluate for modifications such as ramps, wide doorways, floor surfaces, lighting, grab bars, tub and toilet seats, and clutter elimination.

▲ Assess for optimal furniture placement for function, maneuverability, and stability for those using assistive devices at home. For example, fitted bedspreads help prevent tripping.

▲ Involve social worker or case manager to educate clients about potential assistive technology, financial cost and benefits, regulations of payers, and local resources.

- Implement ergonomic approaches for home care staff and family to safely handle and transfer clients.
- For further information, refer to care plans for **Impaired physical Mobility** and **Impaired Walking.**

Client/Family Teaching

- • Assess for readiness to learn and use teaching modalities conducive to personal learning styles.
- • Supervise practice sessions in which client and family apply gait belt, brace, or orthoses; check skin once aids are removed; and perform recommended transfer or lift ergonomically.
- • Teach and monitor client and family for consistent use of safety precautions for transfers, including nonskid shoes, correctly placed equipment and chairs, locked brakes, leg rests swiveled away, and so forth.
- ▲ Teach client and family how to check brakes on chairs to ensure they engage and how to check tires for adequate air pressure; advise routine inspection and annual tune-up of devices.
- ▲ Offer information on safe use of shower and commode chairs to prevent discomfort, pressure, and falls during transfer, transport, care, and hygiene.
- • For further information, refer to the care plans for **Impaired physical Mobility, Impaired Walking,** and **Impaired wheelchair Mobility.**

T

Risk for Trauma

NANDA Definition

Accentuated risk of accidental tissue injury (e.g., wound, burn, fracture)

Risk Factors

External

Accessibility of guns; bathing in very hot water (e.g., unsupervised bathing of young children); bathtub without antislip equipment; children playing with dangerous objects; children playing without gates at top of stairs; children riding in the front seat in car; contact with corrosives; contact with intense cold; contact with rapidly moving machinery; defective appliances; delayed lighting of gas appliances; driving a mechanically unsafe vehicle; driving at excessive speeds; driving while intoxicated; driving without necessary visual aids; entering unlighted rooms; experimenting with chemicals; exposure to dangerous machinery; faulty electrical plugs; flammable children's clothing; flammable children's toys; frayed wires; grease waste collected on stoves; high beds; high-crime neighborhood; inappropriate call-for-aid mechanisms for bed-resting client; inadequate stair rails; inadequately stored combustibles (e.g., matches, oily rags); inadequately stored corrosives (e.g., lye); knives stored uncovered; lack of protection from heat source; large icicles hanging from the roof; misuse of necessary headgear; misuse of seat restraints; nonuse of seat restraints; obstructed passageways; overexposure to radiation; overloaded electrical outlets; overloaded fuse boxes; physical proximity to vehicle pathways (e.g., driveways, lanes, railroad tracks); playing with explosives; pot handles facing toward front of stove; potential ignition of gas leaks; slippery floors (e.g., wet or highly waxed); smoking in bed; smoking near oxygen; struggling with restraints; unanchored electric wires; unanchored rugs; unsafe road; unsafe walkways; unsafe window protection in homes with children; use of cracked dishware; use of unsteady chairs; use of unsteady ladders; wearing flowing clothes around open flame

Internal

Balancing difficulties; cognitive difficulties; emotional difficulties; history of previous trauma; insufficient finances; lack of safety education; lack of safety precautions; poor vision; reduced muscle coordination; reduced sensation; weakness

Client Outcomes

Client Will (Specify Time Frame):

- Remain free from trauma
- Explain actions that can be taken to prevent trauma

Nursing Interventions

- Screen clients with a fall risk factor assessment tool to identify those at risk for falls.
- Provide vision aids for visually impaired clients.

- Help the client with ambulation. Allow the client to use assistive devices in ADLs as needed.
- Have a family member evaluate water temperature for the client.
- Assess the client for causes of impaired cognition.
- Provide assistive devices in bathrooms (e.g., hand rails, nonslip decals on the floor of the shower and bathtub).
- Ensure that call light systems are functioning and that the client is able to use them in conjunction with the nurse making hourly rounds.
- Use a nightlight after dark to assist in orientation and improve visual acuity.
- Teach the client to observe safety precautions in high-crime neighborhoods (e.g., lock doors, do not leave home at night without a companion, keep entryways well lighted).

▲ Instruct the client not to drive under the influence of alcohol or drugs. Assess for a substance abuse problem and refer to appropriate resources for drug and alcohol education.

▲ Review drug profile for potential side effects that may inhibit performance of ADLs.

- See Nursing Interventions in the care plans for **Risk for Aspiration, Impaired Home maintenance, Risk for Injury, Risk for Poisoning,** and **Risk for Suffocation.**

Pediatric

- Assess the client's socioeconomic status.
- Assess family interests in safety topics to identify priority areas for counseling.
- Never leave young children unsupervised around water or cooking areas.
- Keep flammable and potentially flammable articles out of the reach of young children.
- Lock up harmful objects such as guns.

Geriatric

- Assess the geriatric client's cognitive level of functioning both at admission and periodically.
- Assess for routine eye examinations and use of appropriate prescription glasses.
- Perform a home safety assessment and recommend the following preventive measures: keep electrical cords out of the flow of traffic;

remove small rugs or make sure they are slip resistant; increase lighting in hallways and other dark areas; place a light in the bathroom; keep towels, curtains, and other items that might catch fire away from the stove; store harmful products away from food products; provide at least one grab bar in tubs and showers; check prescribed medications for appropriate labels; store medications in original containers or in a dispenser of some type (e.g., egg carton, 7-day plastic dispenser); if the client cannot administer medications according to directions, secure someone to administer medications.

- • Mark stove knobs with bright colors (yellow or red) and outline the borders of steps.
- • Discourage driving at night.
- • Encourage the client to participate in resistance and impact exercise programs as tolerated.
- • Implement fall and injury prevention strategies in residential care facilities.
- • Attend a fall prevention screening clinic.

Client/Family Teaching

- • Educate the family regarding age-appropriate child safety precautions, environmental safety precautions, and intervention in an emergency.
- • Teach the family to assess the childcare provider's knowledge regarding child safety, environmental safety precautions, and assistance of a child in an emergency.
- • Educate the client and family regarding helmet use during recreation and sports activities.
- • Encourage the use of proper car seats and safety belts.
- • Teach parents to restrict nighttime driving after 10 PM for young drivers.
- • Teach how to plan safe prom and graduation parties.
- • Teach parents the importance of monitoring youths after school.
- • Teach firearm safety. Encourage the family to keep firearms and ammunition in locked storage.
- ▲ Educate that the use of psychotropic medications may increase the risk of falls and that withdrawal of psychotropic medications should be considered.
- • For further information, refer to care plans for **Risk for Aspiration, Impaired Home maintenance, Risk for Injury, Risk for Poisoning,** and **Risk for Suffocation.**

T

Impaired Urinary elimination

NANDA Definition

Disturbance in urine elimination

NOTE: This broad diagnosis may be used to describe many dysfunctional voiding conditions. Refer to **Functional urinary Incontinence, Reflex urinary Incontinence, Stress urinary Incontinence, Total urinary Incontinence, Urge urinary Incontinence,** and **Urinary retention** for information on these more specific diagnoses.

Defining Characteristics

The term *lower urinary tract symptoms* (LUTS) is now used to describe the variety of complaints associated with disorders of bladder filling/storage or altered patterns of urine elimination. Bothersome bladder filling/storage symptoms include diurnal frequency (voiding more than every 2 hours), infrequent urination (voiding less then every 6 hours), and nocturia (arising from sleep more than twice to urinate). Our understanding of the physiologic desire is incomplete, but the term *urgency* has been defined as a sudden and strong desire to urinate that is not easily deferred. Lower urinary tract pain may present as dysuria (pain associated with micturition), burning, pressure, or cramping discomfort during bladder filling and storage. Voiding symptoms may include reduced force of the urinary stream, intermittency, hesitancy, and the need to strain to evacuate the bladder. Other voiding symptoms are postvoid dribbling, feelings of incomplete bladder emptying, or the total inability to urinate (acute urinary retention).

Urinary incontinence is the uncontrolled loss of urine of sufficient magnitude to constitute a problem for the client, family, or caregivers. Stress urinary incontinence is the loss of urine with physical exertion. Urge urinary incontinence is the loss of urine associated with overactive detrusor contractions and a precipitous desire to urinate. It is part of a larger symptom syndrome called *overactive bladder.* The overactive bladder is characterized by bothersome urgency and typically associated with frequent daytime voiding and nocturia. Approximately 37% of patients with overactive bladder dysfunction experience urge urinary incontinence.

Reflex urinary incontinence is urine loss associated with neurogenic detrusor overactivity, diminished or absent sensations of bladder filling, and dyssynergia between the detrusor and striated urethral sphincter muscles. Functional urinary incontinence is urine loss associated with deficits of mobility, dexterity, cognition, or environmental barriers to timely toileting. Urine loss from an extraurethral source can be defined as total incontinence, and urinary retention is the condition where the client is unable to completely evacuate urine from the bladder despite micturition. Chronic urinary retention is defined as the inability to completely evacuate urine from the bladder after voiding, and acute urinary retention is the inability to urinate.

Related Factors (r/t)

Bothersome LUTS (urological disorders, neurological lesions, gynecological conditions, dysfunction of bowel elimination); incontinence (refer to specific diagnosis); urinary retention (refer to specific diagnosis); acute urinary retention (refer to **Urinary retention**)

Client Outcomes

Client Will (Specify Time Frame):

- Demonstrate diurnal frequency no more than every 2 hours
- Demonstrate nocturia two times or less per night
- Be able to postpone voiding until toileting facility is accessed and clothing is removed
- Be able to perceive and recognize cues for toileting, move to toilet or use urinal or portable toileting apparatus, and remove clothing as necessary for toileting
- Demonstrate postvoiding residual volumes less than 150 mL to 200 mL or 25% of total bladder capacity
- State absence of pain or excessive urgency during bladder storage or during urination

Nursing Interventions

- • Routinely screen all adult women and aging men for urinary incontinence or LUTS including bothersome urgency.
- ▲ Assess bladder function using the following techniques:
  - ■ Take a focused history including duration of bothersome LUTS, characteristics of symptoms, patterns of diurnal and nocturnal urination, frequency and volume of urine loss, alleviating and aggravating factors, and exploration of possible causative factors.

- In close consultation with a physician or advanced practice nurse, administer a validated questionnaire querying lower urinary symptoms, associated bowel elimination symptoms, and symptoms of pelvic organ prolapse in women.
- Perform a focused physical assessment of perineal skin integrity, evaluation of the vaginal vault, evaluation of urethral hypermobility, and neurological evaluation including bulbocavernosus reflex and perineal sensations.
- Review results of urinalysis for the presence of urinary infection, polyuria, hematuria, proteinuria, and other abnormalities, or obtain urine for analysis.

• Complete a more detailed assessment on selected clients including a bladder log and functional/cognitive assessment. (Refer to **Functional urinary Incontinence, Reflex urinary Incontinence**, **Stress urinary Incontinence**, **Total urinary Incontinence**, and **Urge urinary Incontinence**.)

• Assess the client for urinary retention. (Refer to **Urinary retention**.)

• Teach the client general guidelines for bladder health:
  - Clients should avoid dehydration and its irritative effects on the bladder; fluid consumption for the ambulatory, normally active adult should be approximately 30 mL/kg of body weight (0.5 oz per pound per day).
  - Clients with storage LUTS, overactive bladder dysfunction, or urinary incontinence should reduce or cease caffeine intake.
  - Clients with lower urinary tract pain or interstitial cystitis should be encouraged to eliminate potential bladder irritants: caffeine, alcohol, aspartame, carbonated beverages, alcohol, citrus juices, chocolate, vinegar, and highly spiced foods such as those flavored with curries or peppers. These foods should be reintroduced singly to the diet to determine their effect (if any) on bothersome LUTS.
  - All clients should be counseled about measures to alleviate or prevent constipation including adequate consumption of dietary fluids, dietary fiber, exercise, and regular bowel elimination patterns.
  - All clients should be strongly advised to stop smoking; it is associated with an increased risk of bladder cancer (Bjer-

U

regaard et al, 2006), urinary incontinence, and bothersome lower urinary tract symptoms in men.

- ▲ Consult the physician for culture and sensitivity testing and antibiotic treatment in the individual with evidence of a urinary infection.
- ▲ Refer the individual with chronic lower urinary tract pain to a urologist or specialist in the management of pelvic pain.
- ▲ Teach the client to recognize symptoms of UTI (dysuria that crescendos as the bladder nears complete evacuation; urgency to urinate followed by micturition of only a few drops; suprapubic aching discomfort; malaise; voiding frequency; sudden exacerbation of urinary incontinence with or without fever, chills, and flank pain).
- ▲ Teach colleagues that a cloudy or malodorous urine, in the absence of other lower urinary tract symptoms, does not indicate the presence of a urinary tract infection and that asymptomatic bacteriuria, in the elderly, does not justify the need for a course of antibiotics.
- • Teach the client to recognize hematuria and to seek help promptly if hematuria occurs.
- • Assist the individual with urinary leakage to select a product that adequately contains urine, avoids soiling clothing, is not apparent when worn under clothing, and protects the underlying skin. (See the care plan for **Total urinary Incontinence.**)
- • Teach perineal care including judicious use of soaps and use of vaginal douches only under special circumstances. (See the care plan for **Total urinary Incontinence.**)

U

Geriatric

- • Provide an environment that encourages toileting for the elderly client cared for in the home or in acute care, long-term care, or critical care units.
- • Perform urinalysis in all elderly persons who experience a sudden change in urine elimination patterns, lower abdominal discomfort, acute confusion, or a fever of unclear origin.
- • Encourage elderly women to drink at least 10 oz of cranberry juice daily, regularly consume one to two servings of fresh blueberries, or supplement the diet with cranberry concentrate capsules (usually taken in 500 mg doses with each meal).

Client/Family Teaching

- Provide all clients with the basic principles for optimal bladder function.
- Teach the community and healthcare providers that urinary incontinence is not a normal part of aging and that incontinence can be corrected or managed with proper evaluation and care.
- Provide information to healthcare providers and the community about the signs, symptoms, and management of UTIs and interstitial cystitis.
- Teach all persons the signs and symptoms of UTI and its management.
- Teach all persons to recognize hematuria and to promptly seek care if this symptom occurs.

Readiness for enhanced Urinary elimination

NANDA Definition

A pattern of urinary functions that is sufficient for meeting eliminatory needs and can be strengthened

Defining Characteristics

Amount of output is within normal limits; expresses willingness to enhance urinary elimination; fluid intake is adequate for daily needs; positions self for emptying of bladder; specific gravity is within normal limits; urine is odorless; urine is straw colored

Client Outcomes

Client Will (Specify Time Frame):

- Eliminate or reduce incontinent episodes
- Recognize sensory stimulus indicating readiness for urine elimination
- Respond to prompts for toileting

Nursing Interventions

- Assess the client for readiness for improving urine elimination patterns, focusing on need for physical assistance to access toilet, cognitive awareness of sensations indicating readiness for urine elimination, and current continence status (bladder management strategy, frequency of incontinent episodes).
- Using information from the Minimum Data Set (MDS), evaluate the client for potentially reversible or modifiable factors contributing to urinary incontinence.
- Complete a bladder diary of diurnal and nocturnal urine elimination patterns and patterns of urinary leakage.
- Begin a scheduled toileting program (usually every 2 to 3 hours) for the client who has mild to moderately impaired cognition and who requires some physical assistance to access the toilet.
- Remove environmental barriers to toilet access.
- Provide a urinal or bedside toilet as indicated.
- Assist client to remove clothing, transfer to the toilet, cleanse the perineal skin, and redress as indicated.
- Ensure that toileting opportunities are offered both during daytime hours and during hours of sleep.
- For the client experiencing urinary incontinence who has mild cognitive deficits, begin a prompted voiding program or patterned urge response toileting program. Begin a prompted toileting program based on the results of bladder log over a period of 2 to 3 days, using a check and change system as indicated.
  - Approach the client and briefly explain that it is time to toilet.
  - Assist the client to the toilet, provide assistance removing clothing and urine-containment devices (pads, adult urine-containment briefs), and check for urinary leakage since the last scheduled toileting.
  - Praise the client when toileting occurs with prompting.
  - If the client does not toilet or has evidence of an incontinence episode, refrain from praise, gently inform the client of the urine loss, remove and replace the soiled containment device, and assist the client to redress and rejoin activities or return to bed.
- Institute regular use of incontinence-containment devices combined with a structured perineal skin care program for the client with severe cognitive impairment, significant functional impairment, or no reduction in urinary incontinence frequency or sever-

U

ity with a scheduled or prompted toileting program. (Refer to **Total urinary Incontinence.**)

Urinary retention

NANDA Definition

Incomplete emptying of the bladder

Defining Characteristics

Measured urinary residual greater than 200 to 250 mL or 25% of total bladder capacity; voiding and postmicturition LUTS (slow stream, intermittency of stream, hesitancy of urination, postvoid dribbling, feelings of incomplete bladder emptying); often accompanied by storage LUTS (urgency, day and nighttime voiding frequency); occasionally accompanied by overflow incontinence (dribbling urine loss caused when intravesical pressure overwhelms the sphincter mechanism)

Related Factors (r/t)

Bladder outlet obstruction (benign prostatic hyperplasia [BPH], prostate cancer, prostatitis, acute prostatic congestion and inflammation after implantation of irradiated seeds, urethral stricture, bladder neck dyssynergia, bladder neck contracture, detrusor striated sphincter dyssynergia, high tone pelvic floor muscle dysfunction, obstructing cystocele, urethral tumor, urethral polyp, posterior urethral valves, postoperative complication)

Deficient detrusor contraction strength (sacral level spinal lesions, cauda equina syndrome, peripheral polyneuropathies, herpes zoster or simplex affecting sacral nerve roots, injury or extensive surgery causing denervation of pelvic plexus, medication side effect, complication of illicit drug use, impaction of stool)

Defining characteristics and related factors adapted from the work of NANDA-I.

Client Outcomes

Client Will (Specify Time Frame):

- Demonstrate consistent ability to urinate when desire to void is perceived or via timed schedule; measured urinary residual

U

volume is <200 to 250 mL or 25% of total bladder capacity (voided volume plus urinary residual volume)
- Experience correction or relief from voiding and postvoid LUTS
- Experience correction or alleviation of storage LUTS
- Be free of upper urinary tract distress (renal function remains sufficient; febrile urinary infections are absent)

Nursing Interventions

- • Obtain a focused urinary history emphasizing the character and duration of lower urinary tract symptoms. Query the client about episodes of acute urinary retention (complete inability to void) or chronic retention (documented elevated postvoid residual volumes).
- • Question the client concerning specific risk factors for urinary retention including:
  - ■ Disorders affecting the sacral spinal cord such as spinal cord injuries of vertebral levels T12-L2, disk problems, cauda equina syndrome, tabes dorsalis
  - ■ Acute neurological injury causing sudden loss of mobility such as spinal shock or ischemic stroke
  - ■ Metabolic disorders such as diabetes mellitus, chronic alcoholism, and related conditions associated with polyuria and peripheral polyneuropathies
  - ■ Herpetic infection involving the sacral skin and underlying spinal dermatomes
  - ■ Heavy-metal poisoning (lead, mercury) causing peripheral polyneuropathies
  - ■ Advanced stage human immunodeficiency virus (HIV)
  - ■ Medications including antispasmodics/parasympatholytics, alpha-adrenergic agonists, antidepressants, sedatives, narcotics, psychotropic medications, illicit drugs
  - ■ Recent surgery requiring general or spinal anesthesia
  - ■ Bowel elimination patterns, history of fecal impaction, encopresis
  - ■ Recent surgical procedures
  - ■ Recent prostatic biopsy or brachytherapy therapy
- ▲ Perform a focused physical assessment or review results of a recent physical including perineal skin integrity; inspection, percussion, and palpation of the lower abdomen for obvious bladder distention; a neurological examination including perineal skin

U

sensation and the bulbocavernosus reflex; and vaginal vault examination in women and digital rectal examination in men.

▲ Determine the urinary residual volume by catheterizing the client immediately after urination or by obtaining a bladder ultrasound after micturition.

• Complete a bladder log including patterns of urine elimination, urine loss (if present), nocturia, and volume and type of fluids consumed for a period of 3 to 7 days.

▲ Consult with the physician concerning eliminating or altering medications suspected of producing or exacerbating urinary retention.

• Teach the client with mild to moderate obstructive symptoms to double void by urinating, resting in the bathroom for 3 to 5 minutes, and then trying again to urinate.

• Teach the client with urinary retention and infrequent voiding to urinate by the clock.

• Advise the male client with urinary retention related to BPH to avoid risk factors associated with acute urinary retention as follows:
  - Avoid over-the-counter cold remedies containing a decongestant (alpha-adrenergic agonist).
  - Avoid taking over-the-counter dietary medications (frequently contain alpha-adrenergic agonists).
  - Discuss voiding problems with a healthcare provider before beginning new prescription medications.
  - After prolonged exposure to cool weather, warm the body before attempting to urinate.
  - Avoid overfilling the bladder by regular urination patterns and refrain from excessive intake of alcohol.

▲ Teach the elderly male client with BPH to self-administer a 5 alpha-reductase inhibitor, such as finasteride or dutasteride, or an alpha-adrenergic–blocking agent, such as tamsulosin, alfuzosin, doxazosin, or terazosin, as directed. Provide careful instruction concerning the dose, administration schedule, and side effects of these drugs, including possible adverse side effects (postural hypotension) when multiple doses are inadvertently missed.

▲ Teach the client who is unable to void specific strategies to manage this potential medical emergency as follows:
  - Attempt urination in complete privacy.
  - Place the feet solidly on the floor.

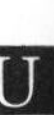

- ■ If unable to void using these strategies, take a warm sitz bath or shower and void (if possible) while still in the tub or shower.
- ■ Drink a warm cup of caffeinated coffee or tea to stimulate the bladder, which may promote voiding.
- ■ If unable to void within 6 hours or if bladder distention is producing significant pain, seek urgent or emergency care.

▲ Remove the indwelling urethral catheter at midnight in the hospitalized client to reduce the risk of acute urinary retention.

▲ Consult the physician about bladder stimulation in the client with urinary retention caused by deficient detrusor contraction strength.

▲ Perform sterile or clean intermittent catheterization as directed for clients with urinary retention.

▲ Teach the client with significant urinary retention to perform clean, self-intermittent catheterization as directed.

• Advise clients who undergo intermittent catheterization that bacteria are likely to colonize the urine but that this condition does not indicate a clinically significant urinary tract infection.

• Insert an indwelling catheter for the individual with urinary retention who is not a suitable candidate for intermittent catheterization.

• Advise clients with indwelling catheters that bacteria in the urine is an almost universal finding after the catheter has remained in place for a period of 30 days or longer and that only symptomatic infections warrant treatment.

• Use the following strategies to reduce the risk for catheter associated UTI whenever feasible:
- ■ Insert a silver impregnated catheter for short-term indwelling catheterization (<14 days).
- ■ Maintain a closed drainage system whenever feasible.
- ■ Change the catheter every 4 weeks whenever possible; more frequent catheter changes should be reserved for clients who experience catheter encrustation and blockage.
- ■ Place clients managed in an acute or long-term care facility with a catheter-associated UTI in a separate room from others managed by an indwelling catheter to reduce the risk of spreading the offending pathogen.
- ■ Educate staff about the risks of catheter-associated UTI and specific strategies to reduce this risk.

U

Geriatric

- Aggressively assess elderly clients, particularly those with dribbling urinary incontinence, UTI, and related conditions for urinary retention.
- Assess elderly clients for impaction when urinary retention is documented or suspected.
- Assess elderly male clients for retention related to prostatic enlargement (BPH or prostate cancer).

Home Care

- The interventions listed previously may be adapted for home care use.
- Encourage the client to report any inability to void.

▲ Maintain an up-to-date medication list; evaluate side effect profiles for risk of urinary retention.

▲ Refer the client for physician evaluation if urinary retention occurs.

Client/Family Teaching

- Teach techniques for intermittent catheterization including use of clean rather than sterile technique, washing using soap and water or a microwave technique, and reuse of the catheter.
- Teach the client with an indwelling catheter to assess the tube for patency, maintain the drainage system below the level of the symphysis pubis, and routinely cleanse the bedside bag.
- Teach the client with an indwelling catheter or undergoing intermittent catheterization the symptoms of a significant urinary infection including hematuria, acute-onset incontinence, dysuria, flank pain, or fever.

Impaired spontaneous Ventilation

NANDA Definition

Decreased energy reserves result in an individual's inability to maintain breathing adequate to support life

Defining Characteristics

Apprehension; decreased cooperation; decreased PO_2; decreased SaO_2; decreased tidal volume; dyspnea; increased heart rate; increased metabolic rate; increased PCO_2; increased restlessness; increased use of accessory muscles

Related Factors (r/t)

Metabolic factors; respiratory muscle fatigue

Client Outcomes

Client Will (Specify Time Frame):

- Maintain arterial blood gases within safe parameters
- Remain free of dyspnea or restlessness
- Effectively maintain airway
- Effectively mobilize secretions

Nursing Interventions

- ▲ Collaborate with the client, family, and physician regarding possible intubation and ventilation. Ask whether the client has advanced directives and, if so, integrate them into the plan of care with clinical data regarding overall health and reversibility of the medical condition.
- • Assess and respond to changes in the client's respiratory status. Monitor the client for dyspnea, increase in respiratory rate, use of accessory muscles, retraction of intercostal muscles, flaring of nostrils, decrease in O_2 saturation, and subjective complaints.
- • Have the client use a numerical scale (0-10) to rate dyspnea before and after interventions.
- • Assess for history of chronic respiratory disorders when administering oxygen.
- ▲ Collaborate with the physician and respiratory therapists in determining the appropriateness of noninvasive positive pressure ventilation (NPPV) for the decompensated client with COPD.
- ▲ Assist with implementation, client support, and monitoring if NPPV is used.
- • If the client has apnea, pH <7.25, $PaCO_2$ >50 mm Hg, PaO_2 <50 mm Hg, respiratory muscle fatigue, or somnolence, prepare the client for intubation and placement on a ventilator.

Ventilator Support

- ▲ Explain the intubation intervention to the client and family as appropriate, and during the procedure, administer sedation for client comfort according to the physician's orders.
- • Secure the endotracheal tube in place using either tape or a device, auscultate bilateral breath sounds, use a CO_2 detector, and obtain a chest radiograph to confirm endotracheal tube placement.
- • Ensure that ventilator settings are appropriate to meet the client's minute ventilation requirements.
- • Suction as needed, and hyperoxygenate and hyperventilate according to policy. Refer to the care plan **Ineffective Airway clearance** for further information on suctioning.
- • Ensure activation of all monitor alarms each shift.
- • Respond to ventilator alarms promptly. If unable to rapidly locate the source of the alarm, use a manual self-inflating resuscitation bag to ventilate the client while waiting for assistance.
- • Prevent unplanned extubation by maintaining stability of endotracheal tube and using soft wrist restraints on the client if needed and ordered.
- • Drain collected fluid from condensation out of ventilator tubing as needed.
- • Note ventilator settings of flow of inspired oxygen, peak inspiratory pressure, tidal volume, and alarm activation at intervals and when removing the client from the ventilator for any reason.
- ▲ Administer analgesics and sedatives as needed with a defined protocol to facilitate client comfort and rest. Use pain and sedation scales to provide a consistent way of monitoring sedation levels and ensuring that therapeutic outcomes are being met.

- • Assess level of sedation with such tools as the Riker Sedation-Agitation Scale, the Motor Activity Assessment Scale, or the Richmond Agitation-Sedation Scale.
- • To decrease anxiety, use music therapy with selections of the client's choice played on headphones at intervals.
- • Analyze and respond to arterial blood gas results, end-tidal CO_2 levels, and pulse oximetry values.
- • Use an effective means of verbal and nonverbal communication with the client. A variety of communication devices are available,

including electronic voice output communication aids, alphabet boards, picture boards, computers, and writing slate. Ask the client for input into care as able. Ensure client's human rights are met.

- • Move the endotracheal tube from side to side every 24 hours, and tape it or secure it with a device. Assess and document client's skin condition, and ensure correct tube placement at lip line.
- ▲ Implement steps to prevent ventilator associated pneumonia (VAP), including continuous removal of subglottic secretions, elevation of the head of bed to 30-45 degrees unless medically contraindicated, change of the ventilator circuit no more than every 48 hours, and hand washing before and after contact with each client. See details in the sections that follow.
- • Use endotracheal tubes that allow for the continuous aspiration of subglottic secretions (CASS) (if available).
- • Position the client in a semirecumbent position with the head of the bed at a 30- to 45-degree angle to decrease the aspiration of gastric secretions.
- • Perform hand washing using either soap and water (if hands are visibly soiled) or alcohol based solution before and after all client contact.
- • Provide routine oral care using toothbrushing and/or oral rinsing with an antimicrobial agent.
- • Turn the client from side to side every 2 hours or as indicated. Use rotational bed therapy in clients for whom side-to-side turning is contraindicated or difficult.
- • Assess bilateral anterior and posterior breath sounds every 2-4 hours and PRN; respond to any relevant changes.
- • Assess responsiveness to ventilator support; monitor for subjective complaints and sensation of dyspnea.
- ▲ Collaborate with the interdisciplinary team in treating clients with acute respiratory failure.

Geriatric

- • Recognize that older adults have a high rate of morbidity when mechanically ventilated.

Home Care

- ▲ Some of the interventions listed previously may be adapted for home care use. Begin discharge planning as soon as possible with the case manager or social worker to assess the need for home support systems, assistive devices, and community or home health services.

▲ With help from a medical social worker, assist the client and family to determine the fiscal affect of care in the home vs. an extended care facility.

- Assess the home setting during the discharge process to ensure the home can safely accommodate ventilator support (e.g., adequate space and electricity).
- Have the family contact the electric company and place the client residence on a high-risk list in case of a power outage.
- Assess the caregivers for commitment to supporting a ventilator-dependent client in the home.
- Be sure that the client and family or caregivers are familiar with operation of all ventilation devices, know how to suction secretions if needed, are competent in doing tracheostomy care, and know schedules for cleaning equipment. Have the designated caregiver or caregivers demonstrate care before discharge.
- Assess client and caregiver knowledge of the disease, client needs, and medications to be administered via ventilation-assistive devices. Avoid analgesics. Assess knowledge of how to use equipment. Teach as necessary.
- Establish an emergency plan and criteria for use. Identify emergency procedures to be used until medical assistance arrives. Teach and role play emergency care.

▲ Institute case management of frail elderly clients to support continued independent living.

Client/Family Teaching

- Explain to the client the potential sensations that will be experienced, including relief of dyspnea, the feeling of lung inflations, the noise of the ventilator, and the reality of alarms.
- Explain to the client and family about being unable to speak, and work out an alternative system of communication. See previously mentioned interventions.
- Demonstrate to the family how to perform simple procedures, such as suctioning secretions in the mouth with a tonsil-tip catheter, providing range-of-motion exercises, and reconnecting the ventilator immediately if it becomes disconnected.

- Offer both the client and family explanations of how the ventilator works and answer any questions.

Dysfunctional Ventilatory weaning response

NANDA Definition

Inability to adjust to lowered levels of mechanical ventilator support that interrupts and prolongs the weaning process

Defining Characteristics

Mild

Breathing discomfort; expressed feelings of increased need for oxygen; fatigue; increased concentration on breathing; queries about possible machine malfunction; restlessness; slight increase of respiratory rate from baseline; warmth

Moderate

Slight increase from baseline blood pressure (<20 mm Hg); baseline increase in respiratory rate (<5 breaths/min); slight increase from baseline heart rate (<20 beats/min); pale, slight cyanosis; slight respiratory accessory muscle use; inability to respond to coaching; inability to cooperate; apprehension; color changes; decreased air entry on auscultation; diaphoresis; eye widening, wide-eyed look; hypervigilance to activities

Severe

Deterioration in arterial blood gases from current baseline; respiratory rate increases significantly from baseline; increase from baseline blood pressure (20 mm Hg); agitation; increase from baseline heart rate (20 beats/min); paradoxical abdominal breathing; adventitious breath sounds, audible airway secretions; cyanosis; decreased level of consciousness; full respiratory accessory muscle use; shallow, gasping breaths; profuse diaphoresis; breathing uncoordinated with the ventilator

Related Factors (r/t)

Physiological

Ineffective airway clearance; sleep pattern disturbance; inadequate nutrition; uncontrolled pain or discomfort

Psychological

Knowledge deficit of the weaning process and client role; perceived inefficacy about the ability to wean; decreased motivation; decreased self-esteem; moderate or severe anxiety or fear; hopelessness; powerlessness; insufficient trust in nurse

Situational

Uncontrolled episodic energy demands or problems; inappropriate pacing of diminished ventilator support; inadequate social support; adverse environment (e.g., noise, activity, negative events in the room); low nurse-client ratio; extended nurse absence from bedside; unfamiliar nursing staff; history of ventilator dependence for >4 days to 1 week; history of multiple unsuccessful weaning attempts

Client Outcomes

Client Will (Specify Time Frame):

- Wean from ventilator with adequate arterial blood gases
- Remain free of unresolved dyspnea or restlessness
- Effectively clear secretions

Nursing Interventions

- Assess client's readiness for weaning as evidenced by the following:
  - Physiological readiness:
    - Resolution of initial medical problem that led to ventilator dependence
    - Hemodynamic stability
    - Normal hemoglobin levels
    - Absence of fever
    - Normal state of consciousness
    - Metabolic, fluid, and electrolyte balance
    - Adequate nutritional status with serum albumin levels >2.5 g/dL
    - Adequate sleep
  - Psychological readiness: There has been little research devoted to the study of psychological readiness to wean.
- For best results ensure that the client is in an optimal physiological and psychological state before introducing the stress of weaning.
- Involve family as appropriate to help the client provide a maximal effort during weaning readiness measurements.

- • Provide adequate nutrition to ventilated clients, using enteral feeding when possible.
- • Use evidence-based weaning protocols as appropriate.
- • Identify reasons for previous unsuccessful weaning attempts, and include that information in development of the weaning plan.
- ▲ Collaborate with an interdisciplinary team (physician, nurse, respiratory therapist, physical therapist, and dietician) to develop a weaning plan with a time line and goals; revise this plan throughout the weaning period. Use a communication device, such as a weaning board or flow sheet.
- • Assist client to identify personal strategies that result in relaxation and comfort (e.g., music, visualization, relaxation techniques, reading, television, family visits). Support implementation of these strategies.
- • Provide a safe and comfortable environment. Stay with the client during weaning if possible. If unable to stay, make the call light button readily available and assure the client that needs will be met responsively.
- ▲ Coordinate pain and sedation medications to minimize sedative effects.
- • Schedule weaning periods for the time of day when the client is most rested. Cluster care activities to promote successful weaning. Avoid other procedures during weaning: keep the environment quiet and promote restful activities between weaning periods.
- • Promote a normal sleep-wake cycle, allowing uninterrupted periods of nighttime sleep.
- • During weaning, monitor the client's physiological and psychological responses; acknowledge and respond to fears and subjective complaints. Validate the client's efforts during the weaning process.
- • Monitor subjective and objective data (breath sounds, respiratory pattern, respiratory effort, heart rate, blood pressure, oxygen saturation per oximetry, amount and type of secretions, anxiety, and energy level) throughout weaning to determine client tolerance and responses.
- • Involve the client and family in the weaning plan. Alert them as to possible client responses to weaning (e.g., potential feelings of dyspnea).
- • Coach the client through episodes of increased anxiety. Remain

with the client or place a supportive and calm significant other in this role. Give positive reinforcement, and with permission use touch to communicate support and concern.

- Terminate weaning when the client demonstrates predetermined criteria or when the following signs of weaning intolerance occur:
  - Tachypnea, dyspnea, or chest and abdominal asynchrony
  - Agitation or mental status changes
  - Decreased oxygen saturation: SaO_2 <90%
  - Change in pulse rate or blood pressure or onset of new dysrhythmias

▲ If the dysfunctional weaning response is severe, consider slowing weaning to brief periods (e.g., 5 minutes). Continue to collaborate with the team to determine whether an untreated physiological cause for the dysfunctional weaning pattern remains. Consider an alternative care setting (subacute, rehabilitation facility, home) for clients with prolonged ventilator dependence as a strategy that can positively affect outcomes.

Geriatric

- Recognize that older clients may require longer periods to wean.

Home Care

NOTE: Weaning from a ventilator at home should be based on client stability and comfort of the client and caregivers under an intermittent care plan. The client and/or family may be more comfortable having the client hospitalized for the process.

- Assess comfort and coping ability of the client and/or family to wean at home, fiscal implications, and home care coverage.
- Establish an emergency plan and methods of implementation. Include emergency aeration and reestablishment of the ventilation assistive device.

▲ Obtain orders for alternative routes of medication administration when medications have been administered via a ventilation device. Instruct the client and family about these changes.

Risk for other-directed Violence

NANDA Definition

At risk for behaviors in which an individual demonstrates that he or she can be physically, emotionally, and/or sexually harmful to others

Risk Factors

Body language: rigid posture, clenching of fists and jaw, hyperactivity, pacing, breathlessness, threatening stances; history of violence against others (e.g., hitting someone, kicking someone, spitting at someone, scratching someone, throwing objects at someone, biting someone, attempted rape, rape, sexual molestation, urinating/defecating on someone); history of threats of violence (e.g., verbal threats against property, verbal threats against person, social threats, cursing, threatening notes/letters, threatening gestures, sexual threats); history of violent antisocial behavior (e.g., stealing, insistent borrowing, insistent demanding of privileges, insistent interrupting of meetings, refusing to eat, refusing to take medication, ignoring instructions); history of violence, indirect (e.g., tearing off clothes, ripping objects off walls, writing on walls, urinating on floor, defecating on floor, stamping feet, displaying temper tantrum, running in corridors, yelling, throwing objects, breaking a window, slamming doors, making sexual advances); neurological impairment (e.g., positive EEG, CAT, or MRI; head trauma; positive neurological findings; seizure disorders); cognitive impairment (e.g., learning disabilities, attention deficit disorder, decreased intellectual functioning); history of childhood abuse; history of witnessing family violence; cruelty to animals; fire setting; prenatal/perinatal complications or abnormalities; history of drug or alcohol abuse; pathological intoxication; psychotic symptomatology (e.g., auditory, visual, command hallucinations; paranoid delusions; loose, rambling, or illogical thought processes); motor vehicle offenses (e.g., frequent traffic violations, use of a motor vehicle to release anger); suicidal behavior; impulsivity; availability/possession of weapon(s)

Client Outcomes

Client Will (Specify Time Frame):

- Stop all forms of abuse (physical, emotional, sexual; neglect; financial exploitation)
- Have cessation of abuse reported by victim

- Display no aggressive activity
- Refrain from verbal outbursts
- Refrain from violating others' personal space
- Refrain from antisocial behaviors
- Maintain relaxed body language and decreased motor activity
- Identify factors contributing to abusive/aggressive behavior
- Demonstrate impulse control or state feelings of control
- Identify impulsive behaviors
- Identify feelings/behaviors that lead to impulsive actions
- Identify consequences of impulsive actions to self or others
- Avoid high-risk environments and situations
- Identify and talk about feelings; express anger appropriately
- Express decreased anxiety and control of hallucinations as applicable
- Displace anger to meaningful activities
- Communicate needs appropriately
- Identify responsibility to maintain control
- Express empathy for victim
- Obtain no access or yield access to harmful objects
- Use alternative coping mechanisms for stress
- Obtain and follow through with counseling
- Demonstrate knowledge of correct role behaviors

Victim (and Children If Applicable) Will (Specify Time Frame):

- Have safe plan for leaving situation or avoiding abuse
- Resolve depression or traumatic response

Parent Will (Specify Time Frame):

- Monitor social/play contacts
- Provide supervision and nurturing environment
- Intervene to prevent high-risk social behaviors

Nursing Interventions

Client Violence

▲ Monitor the environment, evaluate situations that could become violent, and intervene early to de-escalate the situation. Consider that family members or other staff may initiate violence. Enlist support from other staff rather than attempting to handle the situation alone.

- ▲ Know and follow institution's policies and procedures concerning violence.
- • Initiate client assessment by distinguishing the broadest categories of causes of aggression: social versus biological.
- ▲ Assess the client for risk factors of violence, including those in the following categories: psychiatric disorders (particularly paranoid or bipolar disorders, substance abuse), neurological disorders (e.g., head injury, temporal lobe epilepsy), psychological precursors (e.g., low tolerance for stress, impulsivity), coping difficulties (e.g., inability to plan solutions or see long-term consequences of behavior), and personal history (e.g., past violent behavior).
- ▲ Assess for potential indicators of impending violence against others: frequent medication change, high use of sedative drugs, past violent behavior, a *Diagnostic and Statistical Manual of Mental Health IV* diagnosis of antisocial personality or borderline personality disorder, and long hospitalization. Other indicators include hypervigilance, hostility, substance use, and lack of adherence to medication regimen.
- • Assess the client with a history of previous assaults. Listen to and acknowledge feelings of anger, observe for increased motor activity, and prepare to intervene if the client becomes aggressive.
- • Assess the client for physiological signs and external signs of anger.
- • Assess for the presence of hallucinations.
- • Determine the presence and degree of homicidal or suicidal risk. A number of questions will elicit the necessary information. "Have you been thinking about harming someone? If yes, who? How often do you have these thoughts, and how long do they last? Do you have a plan? What is it? Do you have access to the means to carry out that plan? What has kept you from hurting the person until now?" Refer to the care plan for **Risk for Suicide.**
- • Take action to minimize personal risk: Use nonthreatening body language. Respect personal space and boundaries. Maintain at least an arm's length distance from the client; do not touch the client without permission (unless physical restraint is the goal). Do not allow the client to block access to an exit. If speaking with the client alone, keep the door to the room open. Be aware of where other staff is at all times. Notify other staff of where you are at all times. Take verbal threats seriously and notify

other staff. Wear clothing and accessories that are not restricting and that will not be dangerous (e.g., sandals or shoes with heels can lead to twisted ankles; necklaces or dangling earrings could be grabbed).

- • Remove potential weapons from the environment. Be prepared to remove obstructions to staff response from the environment. Search the client and his or her belongings for weapons or potential weapons on admission to the hospital as appropriate.
- • Inform the client of unit expectations for appropriate behavior and the consequences of not meeting these expectations. Emphasize that the client must comply with the rules of the unit. Give positive reinforcement for compliance.
- • Increase surveillance of the hospitalized client at smoking, meal, and medication times.
- • Assign a single room to the client with a potential for violence toward others.
- • Maintain a secluded area for the client to be placed when violent. Ensure that staff are continuously present and available to client during seclusion.
- • Maintain a calm attitude in response to the client. Provide a low level of stimulation in the client's environment; place the client in a safe, quiet place, and speak slowly and quietly.
- • Redirect possible violent behaviors into physical activities (e.g., walking, jogging) if the client is physically able.
- • Provide sufficient staff if a show of force is necessary to demonstrate control to the client.
- • Protect other clients in the environment from harm. Remove other individuals from the vicinity of a violent or potentially violent client. Follow safety protocols of the department.
- ▲ Use chemical restraints as ordered. Obtain an order for medication and administer it immediately.
- ▲ Use mechanical restraints if ordered and as necessary.
- • Follow the institution's protocol for releasing restraints. Observe the client closely, remain calm, and provide positive feedback as the client's behavior becomes controlled.
- • If restraints are necessary, provide the client with musical tapes and a headset.
- • Encourage clients to eat a balanced diet instead of junk food.
- • Form a therapeutic alliance with the client, identifying the source of anger as external to both nurse and client.

- Allow, encourage, and assist the client to verbalize feelings appropriately either one-on-one or in a group setting. Actively listen to the client; explore the source of the client's anger, and negotiate resolution when possible.
- Teach healthy ways to express feelings/anger, appropriate gender roles, and how to communicate needs appropriately.
- Have the client keep an anger diary and discuss alternative responses together. Teach cognitive-behavioral techniques.
- Identify stimuli that initiate violence and the means of dealing with the stimuli.
- Emphasize that the client is responsible for his or her choices and behavior. Introduce descriptions of possible effects of a client's aggressive/violent behavior on others.

▲ Always follow up a violent episode with a debriefing of clients and staff.

Domestic Violence

NOTE: Before implementation of interventions in the face of domestic violence, nurses should examine their own emotional responses to abuse, their knowledge base about abuse, and systemic elements within the emergency department (ED) to ensure that interventions will be compassionate and appropriate.

- Screen for possible abuse in women or children with a pattern of multiple injuries, particularly if any suspicion exists that the physical findings are inconsistent with the explanation of how the injuries were incurred.

▲ Report suspected child abuse to Child Protective Services. Refer women suspected of being in a spouse abuse situation to an area crisis center and provide phone number of area crisis hotline.

- With women who repeatedly experience injuries from domestic violence, maintain a nonjudgmental approach and continue to offer resources/referrals.

▲ In dealing with abused wives, maintain a nonjudgmental response when clients return to husbands or refuse to leave them.

- Particular attention should be paid to the potential for domestic violence during pregnancy. Women with physical or mental disabilities require extended assessment if abuse is suspected or present, to determine unique ways in which they may experience abuse. In addition to an assessment of the usual power and

V

control concerns, a comprehensive functional assessment should be conducted along with attention to cultural issues, the nature of the disability, and needed resources.

- ▲ Women with disabilities may experience abuse from multiple sources, and particular attention should be paid to the additional emotional stresses for these women.
- ▲ In cases where spouse or child abuse accompanies substance abuse, refer the abusive client to a substance abuse treatment program. Refer the spouse receiving abuse to Al-Anon and the children to Alateen.
- ▲ In cases where an adult reveals a history of unresolved/untreated sexual abuse as a child, referral to a local Adults Molested as Children (AMAC) group may be helpful.
- ▲ Intervention may include referral to a number of programs available, including parenting classes or a parental counseling support group.

Social Violence

- • Assess for acute stress disorder (ASD) and posttraumatic stress disorder (PTSD) among victims of violence.
- ▲ Assess the support network of women who become victims of violent crime and refer for appropriate levels of assistance.
- • Be aware that hate crime is increasing, particularly toward transgendered individuals, and it requires support and advocacy for victims.
- ▲ Victims of violence seen in the ED should receive an assessment for needed services and assignment to case management.

Pediatric

- • Be alert for both shaken baby syndrome and exposure of children to violence. Assess for dating violence among adolescent girls. Additional assessments may be required for sexually transmitted diseases and pregnancy.
- • Pregnant teens should be assessed for abuse, particularly if they are with an older partner.
- ▲ When physical abuse by parents is present, parent-child interaction therapy (PCIT) may be helpful.
- ▲ In the case of child abuse or neglect, refer for early childhood home visitation.

Geriatric

- Be alert to the potential for elder abuse in clients, including the possibility of psychological abuse.
- Assess for changes in physiological functions (e.g., constipation, dehydration) or impairment of the ability to meet basic needs (e.g., inadequate toileting, decreased mobility). Observe for signs of fear, anxiety, anger, and agitation, and intervene immediately.
- Observe for dementia and delirium.
- Assess sensory impairments and the influence they may have on the client's behavior.
- Be alert for the potential of sexual abuse of elders.

▲ Monitor for paradoxical drug reactions, and report any to the physician.

▲ Assess for brain insults, such as recent falls or injuries, strokes, or transient ischemic attacks.

- Decrease environmental stimuli if violence is directed at others.
- Provide hand or back rubs and calming music when an elderly client experiences agitation.

▲ If abuse or neglect of an elderly client is suspected, report the suspicion to an adult protective services agency with jurisdiction over the geographical area where the client lives.

Multicultural

- Exercise cultural competence when dealing with domestic violence.

Home Care

- Be alert to the potential for violent behavior in the home setting. Respond to verbal aggression with interventions to de-escalate negative emotional states.
- Assess family members or caregivers for their ability to protect the client and themselves.
- Include an initial and ongoing assessment and evaluation of potential abuse and neglect. Photograph evidence of abuse or neglect when possible.

▲ If neglect or abuse is suspected, identify an emergency plan that addresses the problem immediately, ensures client safety, and includes a report to the appropriate authorities. Discuss when to use hotlines and 911. Role play access to emergency resources with the client and caregivers.

- Encourage appropriate safety behaviors in abused women; call the client at intervals during a 6-month period to determine whether safety behaviors are being carried out.

- • Assess the home environment for harmful objects. Have the family remove or lock objects as able.
- ▲ Refer for homemaker or psychiatric home healthcare services for respite, client reassurance, and implementation of a therapeutic regimen.
- ▲ If the client is taking psychotropic medications, assess client and family knowledge of medication and its administration and side effects. Teach as necessary.
- ▲ Evaluate effectiveness and side effects of medications.
- • If client displays mildly intensifying aggressive behavior, attempt to diffuse anger or violence (e.g., ask for a glass of water to distract client). Later in the visit explain that aggressive behavior is not acceptable and present consequences of continued aggressive behavior (i.e., right of agency to discontinue services).
- • Document all acts or verbalizations of aggression.
- ▲ If client verbalizes or displays threatening behavior, notify your supervisor and plan to make joint visits with another staff person or a security escort.
- • If the client's behavior is not overtly threatening but makes the nurse uncomfortable, a meeting may be held outside the home in sight of others (e.g., front porch).
- • Never enter a home or remain in a home if aggression threatens your well-being.
- ▲ Never challenge a show of force, such as a gun threat. Leave and notify your supervisor and the appropriate authorities. Document the incident.
- ▲ If client behaviors intensify, refer for immediate mental health intervention.

V

Client/Family Teaching

- • Teach relaxation and exercise as ways to release anger.
- • Teach cognitive-behavioral activities, such as active problem solving, reframing (reappraising the situation from a different perspective), or thought stopping (in response to a negative thought, picture a large stop sign and replace the image with a prearranged positive alternative). Teach the client to confront his or her own negative thought patterns (or cognitive distor-

tions), such as catastrophizing (expecting the very worst), dichotomous thinking (perceiving events in only one of two opposite categories), magnification (placing distorted emphasis on a single event), or unrealistic expectations (e.g., "I should get what I want when I want it.").

- • For religious couples, encourage the use of prayer.
- ▲ Refer to individual or group therapy.
- • Teach the adolescent client violence prevention, and encourage him or her to become involved in community service activities.
- ▲ Teach the use of appropriate community resources in emergency situations (e.g., hotline, community mental health agency, ED, 911 in most places in the United States, the toll-free National Domestic Violence Hotline [1-800-799-SAFE]).
- ▲ Encourage the use of self-help groups in nonemergency situations.
- ▲ Inform the client and family about medication actions, side effects, target symptoms, and toxic reactions.

Risk for self-directed Violence

NANDA Definition

At risk for behaviors in which an individual demonstrates that he/she can be physically, emotionally and/or sexually harmful to self

V

Risk Factors

Age 15-19; age over 45; behavioral clues (e.g., writing forlorn love notes, directing angry messages at a significant other who has rejected the person, giving away personal items, taking out a large life insurance policy); conflictual interpersonal relationships; emotional problems (e.g., hopelessness, despair, increased anxiety, panic, anger, hostility); employment problems (e.g., unemployed, recent job loss/failure); engagement in autoerotic sexual acts; family background (e.g., chaotic or conflictual, history of suicide); history of multiple suicide attempts; lack of personal resources (e.g., poor achievement, poor insight, affect unavailable and poorly controlled); lack of social resources (e.g., poor rapport, socially isolated, unresponsive family); physical health problems (e.g., hypochondriasis, chronic or terminal illness); marital status (single, widowed, divorced); mental health problems (e.g., severe depression, psychosis, severe personality disorder, alcoholism, or drug abuse); occupation (executive, administrator/owner of business, professional, semiskilled worker); sexual orientation (bisexual [active], homosexual [inactive]); suicidal ideation; suicidal plan; verbal clues (e.g., talking about death, "better off without me," asking questions about lethal dosages of drugs)

Client Outcomes

Client Will (Specify Time Frame):

- Refrain from self-injury
- State appropriate ways to cope with increased psychological or physiological tension
- Talk about feelings; express anger appropriately
- Seek help when feeling self-destructive or having urges to self-mutilate
- Maintain self-control without supervision
- Use appropriate community agencies when caregivers are unable to attend to emotional needs
- Maintain connectedness in relationships
- Express decreased anxiety and control of impulses
- Refrain from using mood-altering substances
- Obtain no access to harmful objects
- Yield access to harmful objects
- Maintain self-control without supervision

Nursing Interventions

Refer to care plans for **Risk for Suicide**, **Self-mutilation**, and **Risk for Self-mutilation**.

Impaired Walking

NANDA Definition

Limitation of independent movement within the environment on foot (or artificial limb)

Defining Characteristics

Impaired ability to: climb stairs, walk on uneven surface, walk required distances, walk on even surfaces, walk on an incline or decline, navigate curbs

Related Factors (r/t)

Cognitive impairment; deconditioning; depressed mood; environmental constraints (e.g., stairs, inclines, uneven surfaces, unsafe obstacles, distances, lack of assistive devices or person, restraints); fear of falling; impaired balance; impaired vision; insufficient muscle strength; lack of knowledge; limited endurance; musculoskeletal impairment (e.g., contractures); neuromuscular impairment; obesity; pain

NOTE: These are the same as the etiologies for **Impaired physical Mobility** with the addition of lower extremity amputation.

Suggested functional level classifications follow:

0—Completely independent
1—Requires use of equipment or device
2—Requires help from another person for assistance, supervision, or teaching
3—Requires help from another person and equipment device
4—Dependent (does not participate in activity)

Client Outcomes/Goals

Client Will (Specify Time Frame):

- Demonstrate optimal independence and safety in walking
- Demonstrate the ability to direct others on how to assist with walking
- Demonstrate the ability to properly and safely use and care for assistive walking devices

Nursing Interventions

▲ Reinforce "bridging" (lifting hips up while supine); have client use it to move to side of bed and raise buttocks off bed.

▲ Progressively mobilize clients (gradual elevation of head of bed, sitting in reclined chair, standing, etc.).

• Assist clients to apply orthoses, immobilizers, splints, and braces before walking.

• Apply thromboembolic deterrent stockings (TEDs), elastic wraps, abdominal binders; raise head of bed in small increments; have clients move feet up/down, sit up/stand slowly, and avoid prolonged standing for orthostatic hypotension.

▲ Compare morning and lying/sitting/standing blood pressures. If systolic pressure falls 20 mm Hg or diastolic pressure falls 10 mm Hg from lying to standing within 3 minutes, and/or if light-headedness, dizziness, syncope, or unexplained falls occur, consult a physician.

▲ Give hydration and prescribed medications to treat orthostatic hypotension.

• Screen for and vigilantly apply compression stockings/ intermittent pneumatic compression devices; exercise feet and ankles and give prophylactic anticoagulants as ordered to persons at risk for deep vein thrombosis (DVT). Refer to the care plan for **Ineffective Tissue perfusion.**

▲ Assist persons with DVT to walk, because early ambulation may be ordered.

▲ Cue clients regarding weight-bearing restrictions and how to correctly use prescribed devices.

• As weight bearing resumes after prolonged bed rest, teach clients to ingest protein but avoid nonsteroidal antiinflammatory drugs (NSAIDs); be alert for depression.

• Encourage clients to stand and walk frequently.

• Teach clients with leg amputations to correctly don sheath, stump socks, liner, and prosthesis before walking.

▲ Use a snug gait belt and assistive devices while walking clients, as recommended by the physical therapist (PT).

• Walk clients with an appropriate number of people; have one team member state short simple motor instructions.

• Document the number of helpers, level of assistance (maximum, standby, etc.), type of assistance, and devices needed on the care plan.

• Collect baseline pulse rate/rhythm before walking clients, and reassess after 5 minutes of walking. If either are abnormal, have the client sit for 5 minutes then retake pulse rate. If it is still abnormal, walk clients more slowly and with more help, or for a shorter time.

▲ Monitor the client's tolerance for walking. Initiate a 5-minute rest period if shortness of breath, use of accessory muscles, chest pain, nausea, sweating, pale/flushed skin, dizziness, syncope, or mental confusion occurs. If signs persist, notify the physician. Refer to the care plan for **Activity intolerance.**

▲ Perform initial and subsequent screening for risk of falling.

• Individualize interventions to prevent falls and overuse of restraints. Interventions include scheduled toileting, balance/

strength training, sleep hygiene, education on risk of medication/alcohol use, and removal of hazards.

Geriatric

- • Monitor pulse, respirations, and blood pressure before and 5 minutes after the client has started a new upright activity; stop if resting heart rate >100 beats/min, exercise heart rate is 35% greater than resting rate, systolic blood pressure is 25-35 mm Hg above resting pressure, or decrease in systolic blood pressure >20 mm Hg.
- • Encourage walking and recognize that older adults often walk slowly.
- ▲ Assess risk then implement fall precautions, such as using a visual identifier to indicate clients at risk, placing a call system within reach, recommending an exercise/education program, clearing obstacles, and reviewing medication.
- • Assess for swaying, poor balance, and short first step length during standing and walking.
- ▲ Encourage participation in therapeutic exercise programs.
- • Emphasize the importance of wearing firm, low-heeled shoes with nonskid and nonfriction soles and seeking medical care for foot pain, foot problems, and diabetes.
- • Introduce and reinforce positive perceptions of old age.

Home Care

- • Establish a support system for emergency and contingency care (e.g., Lifeline).

- • Teach compensatory strategies mentioned previously for orthostatic hypotension.
- • Assess for and modify any barriers to walking in the home environment.
- • Stress the importance of adequate lighting, tacking down carpet edges, removing throw rugs, using nonskid backings with throw rugs, applying nonskid wax to floors, and removing clutter.
- ▲ Obtain referral for PT home visits for individualized strength, balance retraining, and a walking plan.
- ▲ Make referrals for home health aide services for assistance with activities of daily living (ADLs).
- ▲ Listen to and support client/caregivers; refer to case manager, social services, or support groups.

Client/Family Teaching

- Teach the client to routinely check walking devices, such as removing dirt from and replacing rubber tips of walkers and canes; checking push button locks on walkers with telescoping legs; and inspecting prostheses for cracks, rough spots inside the socket, and odd noises and movement at joints or the foot.
- ▲ Instruct men and women at risk for osteoporosis or hip fractures to bear weight, walk, take calcium and vitamin D supplements, drink milk, stop smoking, and consult a physician for estrogen replacement and antiresorptive therapy.
- For more information, please refer to the care plans for **Impaired Transfer ability** and **Impaired wheelchair Mobility.**

Wandering

NANDA Definition

Meandering; aimless or repetitive locomotion that exposes the individual to harm; frequently incongruent with boundaries, limits, or obstacles

Defining Characteristics

Frequent or continuous movement from place to place, often revisiting the same destinations; persistent locomotion in search of "missing" or unattainable people or places; haphazard locomotion; locomotion in unauthorized or private spaces; locomotion resulting in unintended leaving of a premise; long periods of locomotion without an apparent destination; fretful locomotion or pacing; inability to locate significant landmarks in a familiar setting; locomotion that cannot be easily dissuaded or redirected; following behind or shadowing a caregiver's locomotion; trespassing; hyperactivity; scanning, seeking, or searching behaviors; periods of locomotion interspersed with periods of nonlocomotion (e.g., sitting, standing, sleeping); getting lost

Related Factors (r/t)

Cognitive impairment, specifically memory and recall deficits, disorientation, poor visuoconstructive (or visuospatial) ability, and language

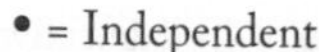

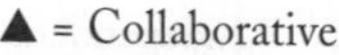

(primarily expressive) defects; cortical atrophy; premorbid behavior (e.g., outgoing, sociable personality); separation from familiar people and places; sedation; emotional state, especially fear, anxiety, boredom, or depression (agitation); overstimulating/understimulating social or physical environment; physiological state or need (e.g., hunger/thirst, pain, urination, constipation); time of day

Client Outcomes

Client Will (Specify Time Frame):

- Decrease incidence of falls (preferably free of falls)
- Decrease incidence of elopements
- Maintain appropriate body weight

Caregiver Will (Specify Time Frame):

- Be able to explain interventions he or she can use to provide a safe environment for a care receiver who displays wandering behavior

Nursing Interventions

- Assess and document the amount (frequency and duration), pattern (random, lapping, or pacing), and 24-hour distribution of wandering behavior over 3 days.
- Document particular aspects of wandering that are troubling.
- Obtain a history of personality characteristics and behavioral responses to stress.
- Evaluate for neurocognitive strengths and limitations, particularly language, attention, visuospatial skills, and perseveration.
- Assess for physical distress or needs, such as hunger, thirst, pain, discomfort, or elimination.
- Assess for emotional or psychological distress, such as anxiety, fear, or feeling lost.
- Observe wandering episodes for antecedents and consequences.
- Apply observed consequences of wandering, such as personal attention, food, and so forth, at times when the person is not wandering, and withhold them while the person is wandering.
- Assess regularly for the presence of or potential for negative outcomes of wandering, such as declining social skills, falls, elopement, and getting lost.
- Weigh the client at defined intervals to detect onset of weight loss, and watch for symptoms associated with inadequate food intake, including constipation, dehydration, muscle wasting, and starvation.

- For the client who displays wandering behavior during mealtimes, use behavioral interventions to shape behavior, including verbal statements, nonverbal social behavior, and systematic extinguishing of undesirable client behavior.
- Provide for safe ambulation with comfortable and well-fitting clothes, shoes with nonskid soles and foot support, and any necessary walking aids (e.g., a cane, walker, or Merry Walker).
- Provide safe and secure surroundings that deter accidental elopements, using perimeter control devices, camouflage, or electronic tracking systems.
- During periods of inactivity, position the wanderer so that desirable destinations (e.g., bathroom) are within the client's line of vision and undesirable destinations (e.g., exits or stairwells) are out of sight.
- If wandering takes a random or haphazard route, reduce environmental distractions and increase relevant environmental cues. Note and eliminate stimuli that distract the wanderer while in route. Provide afternoon rest periods if assessment reveals that random-pattern wandering worsens as the day progresses.
- Enhance institutional settings with areas that provide interesting views and opportunities to sit.
- Engage wanderers in social interaction and structured activity, especially when wanderers appear distressed or otherwise uncomfortable, or their wandering presents a challenge to others in the setting.
- If wandering has a pacing quality, attempt to identify and address any underlying problems or concerns. Offer stress-reducing approaches, such as music, massage, or rocking. Attempts to distract or redirect the pacing wanderer may worsen wandering.
- If wandering is a recently acquired behavior or if it increases in intensity over previous levels, evaluate for constipation, pneumonia, or acute physical problems.
- If wandering has a lapping or circuitous pattern, signs or labels may be effective. Substitute another repetitive activity, such as folding or rocking, if lapping becomes problematic or excessive.
- Provide a regularly scheduled and supervised exercise or walking program, particularly if wandering occurs excessively during the night or at times that are inconvenient in the setting.
- Use slow-stroke, hand, or foot massage before the times of day or events that induce wandering.

Multicultural

- Assess for the influence of cultural beliefs, norms, and values on the family's understanding of wandering behavior.
- ▲ Refer the family to social services or other supportive services to assist with the impact of caregiving for the wandering client.
- Encourage the family to use support groups or other service programs.
- Validate the family's feelings regarding the impact of client wandering on family lifestyle.

Home Care

- Help the caregiver set up a plan to deal with wandering behavior using the interventions mentioned in Nursing Interventions.
- Assess the home environment for modifications that will protect the client and prevent elopement.
- Assist the family to set up a plan of exercise for the client, including safe walking.
- Enroll wanderers in the Safe Return Program of the Alzheimer's Association, and help the caregiver develop a plan of action to use if the client elopes.
- Help the caregiver develop a plan of action to use if the client elopes.
- ▲ Institute case management of frail elderly clients to support continued independent living.
- ▲ Refer for homemaker or psychiatric home healthcare services for respite, client reassurance, and implementation of a therapeutic regimen. Refer to the care plan for **Caregiver role strain.**

Client/Family Teaching

- Inform the client and family of the meaning of and reasons for wandering behavior.
- Teach the caregiver/family methods to deal with wandering behavior using the interventions mentioned in Nursing Interventions.

INDEX

A

Abdomen, acute, 5
Abdominal dehiscence, 46
Abdominal distention, 2
Abdominal pain, 2
Abdominal surgery, 2, 13
Abdominal trauma, 2
Abortion, 2-3
Abruptio placentae, 3, 120
Abscess
  anorectal, 14
  formation of, 3
Abuse
  child, 33, 152
  cocaine, 37, 42
  drug, 51-52
  laxative, 86
  of spouse, parent, or significant other, 3
  substance, 78-79, 150
Accessory muscle use, 4
Accident proneness, 4
Achalasia, 4
Acidosis
  diabetic keto-, 83
  lactic, 85
  metabolic and respiratory, 4
Acne, 4
Acquired immunodeficiency syndrome, 8-9
Acromegaly, 4
Activity intolerance, 4, 168-173
Activity intolerance, risk for, 5, 173
Acute respiratory distress syndrome, 17
Addiction, nicotine, 106
Addison's disease, 5
Adenoidectomy, 5, 153
Adjustment disorder, 5-6
Adjustment impairment, 6
Adolescent
  maturational issues of, 93
  pregnant, 6
  sexuality of, 143
  substance abuse by, 150
  terminally ill, 155
Adoption, giving up child for, 6-7
Adrenal crisis, 7
Adult
  failure to thrive in, 58, 328-332
  seizure disorders in, 141
  terminally ill, 154-155
Advance directives, 7
Affect, flat, 60
Affective disorders, 7, 138
Aggressive behavior, 7
Aging, 7-8
Agitation, 8
Agoraphobia, 8
Agranulocytosis, 8
AIDS. *See* Acquired immunodeficiency syndrome.
Airway clearance, ineffective, 174-178
Airway obstruction/secretions, 9
Alcohol intoxication, acute, 5
Alcohol withdrawal, 9-10
Alcoholism, 10, 338-341
Alkalosis, metabolic, 95
Allergies, 10
Allergy response, latex, 86, 178-183
Alopecia, 10
ALS. *See* Amyotrophic lateral sclerosis.
Alzheimer's type dementia, 10-11
Amenorrhea, 11
Amnesia, 11
Amniocentesis, 11
Amputation, 11-12
Amyotrophic lateral sclerosis, 12
Analgesia, patient-controlled, 115
Anaphylactic shock, 12
Anasarca, 12
Anemia, 12
  aplastic, 16
  pernicious, 117
  sickle cell, 144
Anencephaly, 104
Aneurysm
  abdominal surgery for, 13
  dissecting, 50
Anger, 13
Angina pectoris, 13

Angioplasty, coronary, 13
Anomalies
cardiac, 39-40
fetal/newborn, 13-14
Anorectal abscess, 14
Anorexia, 14
Anorexia nervosa, 14-15
Anosmia, 15
Anterior repair, anterior colporrhaphy, 15
Anticoagulant therapy, 15
Antisocial personality disorder, 15
Anus, imperforate, 76
Anxiety, 15-16, 183-187
death, 187-189
separation, 142
Aphasia, 16
Aplastic anemia, 16
Apnea, obstructive sleep, 108
Apneustic respirations, 16
Appendectomy, 16
Appendicitis, 16
Apprehension, 16-17
ARDS. *See* Acute respiratory distress syndrome.
Arterial insufficiency, 17
Arteriolar nephrosclerosis, 91
Arthritis, 17
osteo-, 110
rheumatoid, 82-83, 137
Arthrocentesis, 17
Arthroplasty, 17
Arthroscopy, 17
Ascites, 17-18
Asphyxia, birth, 18
Aspiration
foreign body, 60
meconium, 135
risk for, 18, 189-193
Assault victim, 18
Assaultive client, 18
Asthma, 18
Ataxia, 19
Atelectasis, 19
Athlete's foot, 19
Atrophy, muscular, 100
Attachment
parent, 114
parent/child, risk for impaired, 193-196
Attention deficit disorder, 19
Autism, 19-20
Autonomic dysreflexia, 20, 196-198
Autonomic dysreflexia, risk for, 198-199

B

Back, acute, 5
Back pain, 20, 89
Bacteremia, 20
Bacteria, flesh-eating, 103
Balloon counterpulsation, intraaortic, 80
Bathing
problems in, 20
self-care deficit in, 142, 608-613
Battered child syndrome, 20
Bed mobility, impaired, 97, 488-494
Bedbug infestation, 20-21
Bedrest, prolonged, 21
Behavior
aggressive, 7
defensive, 46
destructive toward others, 47-48
health-seeking, 66, 392-296
hitting, 69
hostile, 70
infant, 78, 443-450
manipulative, 92
risk-prone health, 199-202
self-destructive, 142
smoking, 146
violent, 51, 163
wellness-seeking, 164
Bell's palsy, 21
Benign prostatic hypertrophy, 24
Bereavement, 21
Biliary atresia, 21
Biopsy, 21
bone marrow, 23
breast, 25
liver, 88
Bioterrorism, 21
Bipolar disorder, 22, 91-92
Birth
asphyxia at, 18
breech, 26
Bladder, neurogenic, 105
Bladder cancer, 22
Bladder distention, 22
Bladder training, 22
Bleeding. *See also* Hemorrhage.
gastrointestinal, 63
rectal, 132
tendency for, 22

Blepharoplasty, 22
Blindness, 22-23
Blood disorder, 23
Blood glucose, risk for unstable, 374-377
Blood sugar control, 23
Blood transfusion, 23
Body dysmorphic disorder, 23
Body image, disturbed, 23, 202-206
Body temperature
altered, 23
decreased or increased, 154
ineffective regulation of, 154, 156, 711-714
risk for imbalanced, 206-207
Bone marrow biopsy, 23
Borderline personality disorder, 23
Boredom, 23
Botulism, 23-24
Bowel incontinence, 24, 59, 77, 207-212
Bowel obstruction, 24
Bowel sounds, abnormal, 24
Bowel training, 24
BPH. *See* Benign prostatic hypertrophy.
Bradycardia, 24
Bradypnea, 24
Brain injury, traumatic, 154
Brain tumor, 25
Braxton Hicks contractions, 25
Breast biopsy, 25
Breast cancer, 25
Breast lumps, 25
Breast pumping, 25
Breastfeeding
effective, 25, 212-214
ineffective, 25, 214-216
interrupted, 25, 217-219
sore nipples in, 146
Breasts
engorgement of, 112
painful, 107, 112, 146
self-examination of, 139
Breathing pattern, ineffective, 26, 219-222
Breech birth, 26
Bronchitis, 26
Bronchopulmonary dysplasia, 26
Bronchoscopy, 26
Bruits, carotid, 26
Bulimia, 26
Bunion, 27
Bunionectomy, 27
Burns, 27
Bursitis, 27
Bypass
coronary artery, 42, 96, 109
femoral popliteal, 59

C

Cachexia, 27
Cancer, 27-28
bladder, 22
breast, 25
pancreatic, 112
skin, 145
Candidiasis, oral, 28
Capillary refill time, prolonged, 28
Carcinoma, ovarian, 111
Cardiac anomalies, 39-40
Cardiac arrest, 29
Cardiac catheterization, 29
Cardiac disorders, 29
Cardiac output, decreased, 29, 223-229
Cardiac tamponade, 30
Cardiogenic shock, 30, 144
Cardiopulmonary perfusion, ineffective, 720-725
Care plans, guide to, 167
Caregiver role strain, 30, 229-236
Caregiver role strain, risk for, 236-237
Caries, dental, 31, 47
Carotid bruits, 26
Carotid endarterectomy, 30
Carpal tunnel syndrome, 30
Casts, 30, 159
Cataract extraction, 30
Cataracts, 30
Catatonic schizophrenia, 30-31
Catheterization
cardiac, 29
urinary, 31
Cavities in teeth, 31, 47
Cellulitis, 31
Central cyanosis, 44
Central line insertion, 31
Cerebral palsy, 31
Cerebral perfusion, ineffective, 720-725
Cerebrovascular accident, 43-44
Cervicitis, 32
Cervix, incompetent, 125
Cesarean delivery, 32

Chemotherapy, 32
Chest, flail, 60
Chest pain, 32
Chest tubes, 32
Cheyne-Stokes respiration, 33
CHF. *See* Congestive heart failure.
Chickenpox, 38
Child
  AIDS in, 9
  battered, 20
  chronic condition in, 33-34
  communicable diseases in, 38
  gastroenteritis in, 62
  gastroesophageal reflux in, 62-63
  giving up for adoption of, 6-7
  grandparents raising, 64
  hospitalized, 70
  inflammatory bowel disease in, 79
  parental attachment with, 114, 193-196
  renal failure in, 134
  respiratory infections in, 135
  safety of, 138-139
  seizure disorders in, 141
  sepsis in, 142-143
  sleep pattern disturbance in, 145
  terminally ill/death of, 155-156
Child abuse, 33, 152
Chills, 35
Chloasma, 35
Choking with feeding, 35
Cholecystectomy, 35
Cholelithiasis, 35
Chorioamnionitis, 35
Chronic condition, child with, 33-34
Chronic obstructive pulmonary disease, 41
Circumcision, 35
Cirrhosis, 36
Claudication, intermittent, 80
Cleft lip/cleft palate, 36
Clotting disorder, 36-37
Cocaine abuse, 37, 42
Codependency, 37
Cognitive deficit, 37
Cold, viral, 37
Cold environment, exposure to, 58
Colectomy, 37
Colitis, 37
Colostomy, 37
Colporrhaphy, anterior, 15
Coma, 38
  diabetic, 49
  hyperosmolar hyperglycemic nonketotic, 73
Comfort
  loss of, 38
  readiness for enhanced, 237-239
Communicable diseases, childhood, 38
Communication
  impaired verbal, 38, 239-243
  readiness for enhanced, 38, 243-245
Community, ineffective therapeutic regimen management by, 39, 156, 705-707
Community coping, 38
  ineffective, 288-290
  readiness for enhanced, 292-294
Compartment syndrome, 39
Conflict
  decisional, 245-248
  parental role, 114, 248-251
  value system, 162
Confusion
  acute, 39, 251-254
  acute, risk for, 39, 260-261
  chronic, 39, 255-260
Congenital heart disease, 39-40
Congestive heart failure, 33
Conjunctivitis, 40
Consciousness, altered level of, 40
Constipation, 40, 261-266
  perceived, 40, 266-269
  risk for, 40, 269-270
Contamination, 40, 270-273
  pesticide, 117-118
  risk for, 273-275
Continent ileostomy, 40
Contraceptive method, 40
Contractions, Braxton Hicks, 25
Contrast myelogram, 101
Conversion disorder, 41
Convulsions, 41
COPD. *See* Chronic obstructive pulmonary disease.
Coping
  defensive, 279-282
  ineffective, 284-288
  readiness for enhanced, 41, 290-292
Coping, community, 38
  ineffective, 288-290
  readiness for enhanced, 292-294

Coping, family
compromised, 275-279
disabled, 282-284
readiness for enhanced, 294-296
Coping problems, 42
Corneal reflex, absent, 42
Corneal tissue damage, 157
Corneal transplant, 42
Coronary angioplasty, 13
Coronary artery bypass grafting, 42
minimally invasive direct, 96
off-pump, 109
Coronary artery stent, 148
Coughing
effective/ineffective, 42
with feeding, 35
Counterpulsation, intraaortic balloon, 80
Crack baby, 42, 78-79
Crackles in lungs, coarse or fine, 42
Craniectomy/craniotomy, 42-43
Crisis, 43
adrenal, 7
financial, 60
midlife, 96
sickle cell, 144
situational, 145
Criticism, hypersensitivity to slight, 73
Crohn's disease, 43
Croup, 135
Curettage, dilation and, 49
Cushing's syndrome, 43
CVA. *See* Cerebrovascular accident.
Cyanosis, 44
Cystic fibrosis, 44-45
Cystitis, 45, 80
Cystocele, 45
Cystoscopy, 45

D

D & C. *See* Dilation and curettage.
Deafness, 45
Death, 45
of child, 155-156
oncoming, 45
sudden infant, 144-145, 296-298
Death anxiety, 187-189
Debridement, wound, 165
Decision-making, readiness for enhanced, 299-300
Decisional conflict, 245-248
Decisions, difficulty making, 45
Deep vein thrombosis, 52
Defecation, straining with, 149
Defensive behavior, 46
Defensive coping, 279-282
Dehiscence
abdominal, 46
wound, 165
Dehydration, 46
Delirium, 46
Delivery, cesarean, 32
Delusions, 46
Dementia, 46-47
AIDS-related, 9
Alzheimer's type, 10-11
senile, 142
Denial, ineffective, 300-303
Denial of health status, 47
Dental caries, 31, 47
Dentition, impaired, 303-307
Depression
bipolar disorder with, 22
major, 47, 90
Dermatitis, 47
Despondency, 47
Destructive behavior
toward others, 47-48
toward self, 142
Development
concerns about, 48
lag in, 64-65
risk for delayed, 308-309
Diabetes insipidus, 48
Diabetes mellitus, 48
gestational, 63
infant of mother with, 78
insulin-dependent, 48-49
non-insulin-dependent, 107
Diabetic coma, 49
Diabetic ketoacidosis, 83
Diabetic retinopathy, 49
Dialysis, 67, 116
Diaphragmatic hernia, 135
Diarrhea, 49, 154, 310-314
DIC. *See* Disseminated intravascular coagulation.
Digitalis toxicity, 49
Dignity
loss of, 49
risk for compromised human, 314-316
Dilation and curettage, 49

Dilation of cervix, premature, 125
Dilemmas, ethical/moral, 98
Discharge planning, 50
Discomforts of pregnancy, 50
Dislocation, 50
Dissecting aneurysm, 50
Disseminated intravascular coagulation, 49
Dissociative identity disorder, 50, 99
Distention
  abdominal, 2
  bladder, 22
  neck vein, 102
Distress, 50
  fetal, 59
  moral, 316-317
  spiritual, 147, 674-677
Disuse syndrome, risk for, 50-51, 318-321
Diversional activity, deficient, 51, 322-325
Diverticulitis, 51
Dizziness, 51
Domestic violence, 51
Donor, renal transplantation, 134
Dressing, self-care deficit in, 51, 142, 613-616
Dribbling of urine, 51
Drooling, 51
Drowning, near-, 102
Drug abuse, 51-52
Drug withdrawal, 52, 78-79
Duodenal ulcer, 161
DVT. *See* Deep vein thrombosis.
Dyskinesia, tardive, 153
Dysmenorrhea, 52-53
Dysmorphic disorder, body, 23
Dyspareunia, 53
Dyspepsia, 53
Dysphagia, 53
Dysphasia, 53
Dyspnea, 53, 121
Dysreflexia, autonomic, 20, 196-199
Dysrhythmia, 53
Dysthymic disorder, 53
Dystocia, 53-54
Dysuria, 54

E

E. coli infection, 54
Ear surgery, 54
Earache, 54
Eating pattern, dysfunctional, 52
Eclampsia, 54
ECT. *See* Electroconvulsive therapy.
Ectopic pregnancy, 55
Eczema, 55
Edema, 55
  lymph-, 89-90
  pulmonary, 129-130
Education, patient, 115
Effusion, pleural, 120-121
Electroconvulsive therapy, 54
Emaciated person, 55
Embolectomy, 55
Embolism, pulmonary, 130
Emesis, 56
Empathy, 56
Emptiness, 56
Encephalitis, 94
Endarterectomy, carotid, 30
Endocarditis, 56
Endometriosis, 56
Endometritis, 56
Endotracheal intubation, 81
Energy field, disturbed, 325-328
Engorgement, breast, 112
Enterocolitis, necrotizing, 102-103
Enuresis, 56
Environment, exposure to hot or cold, 58. *See also* Home environment.
Environmental interpretation problems, 56-57
Environmental interpretation syndrome, impaired, 328
Epidermal necrolysis, toxic, 159
Epididymitis, 57
Epiglottitis, 135
Epilepsy, 57, 141
Episiotomy, 57
Epistaxis, 57
Erectile dysfunction, 57
Esophageal varices, 57
Esophagitis, 58
Ethical dilemmas, 98
Evisceration, wound, 165
Exposure to hot or cold environment, 58
External fixation, 58
Extremities
  pallor of, 112
  rubor of, 138
Eye surgery, 58, 86

F

Failure to thrive
adult, 58, 328-332
nonorganic, 58
Falls, risk for, 58, 332-338
Family, ineffective therapeutic regimen management by, 156, 707-709
Family coping
compromised, 275-279
disabled, 282-284
readiness for enhanced, 294-296
Family member, neglectful care of, 103
Family problems, 58-59
Family processes
dysfunctional, alcoholism, 10, 338-341
interrupted, 342-344
readiness for enhanced, 59, 344-347
Fasciitis, necrotizing, 103
Fatigue, 59, 347-351
Fear, 59, 351-354
Febrile seizures, 141
Fecal incontinence, 24, 59, 77, 207-212
Feeding
choking or coughing with, 35
formula, 61
newborn, problems with, 59
self-care deficit in, 142, 616-620
tube, 160
Feeding pattern, ineffective infant, 78, 450-453
Femoral popliteal bypass, 59
Femur fracture, open reduction with internal fixation of, 109
Fetal alcohol syndrome, 78-79
Fetal anomaly, parent dealing with, 13-14
Fetal distress, 59
Fever, 59
Filthy home environment, 60, 161
Financial crisis in home environment, 60
Fistula, tracheoesophageal, 159
Fixation, fracture
external, 58
internal, 80, 109
Flail chest, 60
Flashbacks, 60
Flat affect, 60
Flesh-eating bacteria, 103
Fluid balance, readiness for enhanced, 60, 355-356
Fluid volume
deficient, 60, 356-361
deficient, risk for, 364-366
excess, 60, 361-364
imbalanced, risk for, 60, 366-369
Foodborne illness, 60
Foreign body aspiration, 60
Formula feeding, 61
Fracture, 61
external fixation of, 58
hip, 69
internal fixation of, 80
open reduction with internal fixation of, 109
rib, 137
Frequency of urination, 61
Friction rub
pericardial, 115-116
pleural, 121
Frostbite, 61
Functional urinary incontinence, 417-421
Fusion, spinal, 61, 147

G

Gag reflex, depressed or absent, 61
Gallop rhythm, 62
Gangrene, 62
Gas exchange, impaired, 62, 370-373
Gastric surgery, 62
Gastric ulcer, 161
Gastritis, 62
Gastroenteritis, 62
in child, 62
viral, 163
Gastroesophageal reflux in child, 62-63
Gastrointestinal bleeding, 63
Gastrointestinal perfusion, ineffective, 720-725
Gastroschisis, 63
Gastrostomy, 63
Gestation
multiple, 98-99
prolonged, 128
Gestational age, small for, 106
Gestational diabetes, 63
Gingivitis, 63
Glaucoma, 63
Glomerulonephritis, 64
Glucose, blood, risk for unstable, 23, 374-377

Gonorrhea, 64
Gout, 64
Grandiosity, 64
Grandparents raising grandchildren, 64
Grieving, 64, 377-380
  complicated, 64, 380-382
  complicated, risk for, 382-383
Grooming, self-care deficit in, 64, 142, 613-616
Growth, risk for disproportionate, 386-388
Growth and development, delayed, 64-65, 383-385
Growth retardation, intrauterine, 81
Guillain-Barré syndrome, 65
Guilt, 65

H

Hair loss, 65
Halitosis, 65
Hallucinations, 65
Hands, trembling of, 160
Head injury, 65
Headache, 65, 96
Health behavior, risk-prone, 199-202
Health maintenance, ineffective, 66, 388-391
Health-seeking behaviors, 66, 392-296
Health status, denial of, 47
Hearing impairment, 66
Heart disease, congenital, 39-40
Heart failure, congestive, 33
Heart rate, nonreassuring fetal, 59
Heart surgery, open, 109
Heartburn, 66
Heat stroke, 66
Hematological disorder, 66
Hemianopia, 66
Hemiplegia, 66
Hemodialysis, 67
Hemodynamic monitoring, 67
Hemolytic uremic syndrome, 67
Hemophilia, 67
Hemoptysis, 67
Hemorrhage, 67. *See also* Bleeding.
  postpartum, 122-123
  subarachnoid, 149-150
Hemorrhoidectomy, 67-68
Hemorrhoids, 68
Hemothorax, 68
Hepatitis, 68
Hernia
  diaphragmatic, 135
  hiatal, 69
  inguinal, 79
Herpes simplex, 68
HHNC. *See* Hyperosmolar hyperglycemic nonketotic coma.
Hiatal hernia, 69
Hip fracture, 69
Hip replacement, total, 17, 158
Hirschsprung's disease, 69
Hirsutism, 69
Hitting behavior, 69
HIV. *See* Human immunodeficiency virus.
Home environment
  filthy, 60, 161
  financial crisis in, 60
  rats or rodents in, 132
  roaches in, 138
Home maintenance, impaired, 70, 396-399
Homelessness, 70
Hope, readiness for enhanced, 70, 399-400
Hopelessness, 70, 400-404
Hospitalized child, 70
Hostile behavior, 70
Hot environment, exposure to, 58
HTN. *See* Hypertension.
Human dignity, risk for compromised, 314-316
Human immunodeficiency virus, 69-70
Humiliating experience, 71
Huntington's disease, 71
Hydrocele, 71
Hydrocephalus, 71, 107
Hygiene
  problems with, 20
  self-care deficit in, 71, 142, 608-613
Hyperactive syndrome, 71-72
Hyperbilirubinemia, 72
Hypercalcemia, 72
Hypercapnia, 72
Hyperemesis gravidarum, 72
Hyperglycemia, 72
Hyperkalemia, 73
Hypernatremia, 73
Hyperosmolar hyperglycemic nonketotic coma, 73
Hyperphosphatemia, 73

Hypersensitivity to slight criticism, 73
Hypertension, 71, 73
  malignant, 91
  pregnancy-induced, 119
Hyperthermia, 73, 91, 404-408
Hyperthyroidism, 73
Hyperventilation, 73
Hypocalcemia, 73
Hypoglycemia, 73-74
Hypokalemia, 74
Hypomagnesemia, 74
Hypomania, 74
Hyponatremia, 74
Hypotension, 74
Hypothermia, 74, 408-411
Hypothyroidism, 74
Hypovolemic shock, 74, 144
Hypoxia, 74
Hysterectomy, 74-75, 162

I

IBS. *See* Irritable bowel syndrome.
ICD. *See* Implantable cardioverter/defibrillator.
IDDM. *See* Insulin-dependent diabetes mellitus.
Identity
  dissociative disorder of, 50, 99
  disturbed personal, 75, 117, 411-413
Idiopathic thrombocytopenic purpura, 81
Ileal conduit, 75
Ileostomy, 40, 75-76
Ileus, 76, 113
Immobility, 76
Immunization status, readiness for enhanced, 76, 414-416
Immunosuppression, 76
Impaction of stool, 76
Imperforate anus, 76
Impetigo, 38, 76
Implantable cardioverter/defibrillator, 75
Impotence, 76-77
Inactivity, 77
Incompetent cervix, 125
Incontinence, bowel, 24, 59, 77, 207-212
Incontinence, urinary, 77
  functional, 417-421
  overflow, 422
  reflex, 133, 423-426
  stress, 149, 427-431
Incontinence, urinary—cont'd
  total, 158, 431-434
  urge, 435-442
Indigestion, 77
Induction
  of abortion, 2
  of labor, 77
Infant. *See also* Newborn.
  of diabetic mother, 78
  premature, 125-126
  shaken syndrome in, 143
  of substance-abusing mother, 42, 78-79
  sudden death of, 144-145, 296-298
  terminally ill, 155
Infant behavior, 78
  disorganized, 443-447
  disorganized, risk for, 447-448
  organized, readiness for enhanced, 448-450
Infant feeding pattern, ineffective, 78, 450-453
Infantile spasms, 141
Infection, 79
  E. coli, 54
  maternal, 93
  opportunistic, 109
  respiratory, 135
  risk for, 79, 454-458
  urinary tract, 162
  wound, 165
Infertility, 79
Inflammatory bowel disease, 79
Influenza, 79
Inguinal hernia repair, 79
Injury, 79. *See also* Trauma.
  head, 65
  perioperative positioning, risk for, 116, 462-466
  risk for, 458-462
  spinal cord, 147
  traumatic brain, 154
Insomnia, 79, 145, 466-470
Insulin-dependent diabetes mellitus, 48-49
Interaction, impaired social, 146, 664-666
Intermittent claudication, 80
Internal fixation, 80, 109
Interstitial cystitis, 80
Intoxication, 5, 80

Intraaortic balloon counterpulsation, 80
Intracranial adaptive capacity, decreased, 471-472
Intracranial pressure, increased, 80-81
Intrauterine growth retardation, 81
Intubation
chest, 32
endotracheal or nasogastric, 81
Irritable bowel syndrome, 75
Isolation, social, 81, 146, 667-670
Itching, 81, 82
ITP. *See* Idiopathic thrombocytopenic purpura.

J

Jaundice, 81-82
Jaw surgery, 82
Jet lag prevention, 82
Jitteriness, 82
Jock itch, 82
Joint replacement, 82
total, 158
total hip, 17
Juvenile diabetes mellitus, 48-49
Juvenile rheumatoid arthritis, 82-83

K

Kaposi's sarcoma, 83
Kawasaki disease, 83
Kegel exercise, 83
Keloids, 83
Keratoconjunctivitis sicca, 83
Keratomileusis, laser-assisted in situ, 86
Ketoacidosis, diabetic, 83
Kidney stone, 83
Kidney transplant, 83, 134-135
Knee replacement, total, 158
Knowledge
deficient, 84, 472-475
readiness for enhanced, 84, 475-477
Kock pouch, 40
Korsakoff's syndrome, 84-85

L

Labor
induction of, 77
normal, 85
preterm, 127-128
Labyrinthitis, 85
Lactic acidosis, 85
Lactose intolerance, 85
Laminectomy, 85-86
Laparoscopy, 86
Laryngectomy, 86
Laser surgery, 86
LASIK eye surgery, 86
Latex allergy, 86
Latex allergy response, 178-181
Latex allergy response, risk for, 181-183
Laxative abuse, 86
Lead poisoning, 87
Legionnaire's disease, 87
Lethargy, 87
Leukemia, 87
Leukopenia, 87
Level of consciousness, altered, 40
Lice, 38, 87
Lifestyle, sedentary, 87, 141, 477-479
Ligation, tubal, 160
Limb reattachment procedures, 87-88
Lip, cleft, 36
Liposuction, 88
Listlessness, 87
Lithotripsy, 88
Liver biopsy, 88
Liver function, risk for impaired, 88, 479-482
Liver transplant, 88
Living will, 88
Loneliness, 88
Loneliness, risk for, 482-485
Loose stools, 88
Low back pain, 89
Lumbar fusion, 61
Lumbar puncture, 89
Lumpectomy, 89
Lumps, breast, 25
Lungs, crackles in, 42
Lupus erythematosus, 89
Lyme disease, 89
Lymphedema, 89-90

M

Macular degeneration, 90
Magnetic resonance imaging, 98
Major depressive disorder, 47, 90
Malabsorption syndrome, 90
Malaria, 90
Malignant hypertension, 91
Malignant hyperthermia, 91
Malnutrition, 91
Mammography, 91

Manic disorder, bipolar, 22, 91-92
Manipulation of organs, surgical incision, 92
Manipulative behavior, 92
Marfan syndrome, 92
Marshall-Marchetti-Krantz operation, 92
Mastectomy, 92-93, 97
Mastitis, 93
Maternal infection, 93
Maturational issues, adolescent, 93
Measles, 38
Meconium aspiration, 135
Melanoma, 93
Melena, 93-94
Memory, impaired, 94, 485-488
Ménière's disease, 94
Meningitis, 94
Meningocele, 104
Menopause, 94-95
Menorrhagia, 95
Mental illness, 95, 110
Mental retardation, 95
Metabolic acidosis, 4
Metabolic alkalosis, 95
MI. *See* Myocardial infarction.
Midlife crisis, 96
Migraine headache, 96
Minimally invasive direct coronary artery bypass, 96
Mitral stenosis, 96-97
Mitral valve prolapse, 97
Mobility, impaired
  bed, 97, 488-494
  physical, 76, 97, 494-499
  wheelchair, 97, 164, 499-503
Mononucleosis, 97
Mood disorders, 97-98
Moon face, 98
Moral dilemmas, 98
Moral distress, 316-317
Mottling of peripheral skin, 98
MRI. *See* Magnetic resonance imaging.
Mucocutaneous lymph node syndrome, 83
Mucous membrane, oral. *See* Oral mucous membrane.
Multiple gestation, 98-99
Multiple personality disorder, 99
Multiple sclerosis, 99
Mumps, 38
Murmurs, 100
Muscular atrophy/weakness, 100
Muscular dystrophy, 100
Mutilation, self-, 142, 632-639
Myasthenia gravis, 100-101
Myelogram, contrast, 101
Myelomeningocele, 104
Myocardial infarction, 96
Myocarditis, 101
Myringotomy, 101

N

Nail beds, cyanosis of, 44
Nails, ringworm of, 137
Narcissistic personality disorder, 101
Narcolepsy, 101-102
Narcotic use, 102
Nasogastric intubation, 81
Nasogastric suction, 102
Nausea, 102, 503-507
Near-drowning, 102
Nearsightedness, 102
Neck vein distention, 102
Necrolysis, toxic epidermal, 159
Necrotizing enterocolitis, 102-103
Necrotizing fasciitis, 103
Negative feelings about self, 103
Neglect
  of family member, 103
  suspected child, 152
  unilateral, 161, 507-510
Neonate. *See* Newborn.
Neoplasm, 103
Nephrectomy, 103
Nephrosclerosis, arteriolar, 91
Nephrostomy, percutaneous, 103
Nephrotic syndrome, 104
Neural tube defects, 104
Neuralgia, trigeminal, 160
Neuritis, 104
Neurofibromatosis, 104-105
Neurogenic bladder, 105
Neurological disorders, 105-106
Neuropathy, peripheral, 106
Neurovascular dysfunction, peripheral, 116, 559-561
Newborn. *See also* Infant.
  anomaly in, parent dealing with, 13-14
  feeding problems in, 59
  jaundice in, 82

Newborn—cont'd
 normal, 106
 postmature, 106
 respiratory conditions of, 135
 small for gestational age, 106
Nicotine addiction, 106
Nightmares, 107
Nipple soreness, 107, 112, 146
Nocturia, 107
Non-insulin-dependent diabetes mellitus, 107
Noncompliance, 107, 510-515
Normal pressure hydrocephalus, 107
Nursing diagnoses
 guide to, 1
 making accurate, 167
Nutrition
 readiness for enhanced, 107, 526-530
 total parenteral, 159
Nutrition, imbalanced, 108
 less than body requirements, 516-521
 more than body requirements, 522-526
 more than body requirements, risk for, 530-531

O

Obesity, 108
Obsessive-compulsive disorder, 108
Obstruction
 airway, 9
 bowel, 24
 peripheral vascular, 162
Obstructive sleep apnea, 108
ODD. *See* Oppositional defiant disorder.
Off-pump coronary artery bypass, 109
Oligohydramnios, 108
Oliguria, 108
Omphalocele, 63
Oophorectomy, 109
Open heart surgery, 109
Open reduction of fracture with internal fixation, 109
Opiate use, 109
Opportunistic infection, 109
Oppositional defiant disorder, 109-110
Oral candidiasis, 28
Oral mucous membrane
 cyanosis of, 44
 impaired, 98, 110, 531-535
Orchitis, 110
Organ manipulation, surgical incision, 92
Organic mental disorders, 110
Orthopedic traction, 110
Orthopnea, 110
Osteoarthritis, 110
Osteomyelitis, 110
Osteoporosis, 111
Other-directed violence, risk for, 752-760
Otitis media, 111
Ovarian carcinoma, 111
Overflow urinary incontinence, 422
Oximetry, pulse, 130

P

Pacemaker, 111
Paget's disease, 111-112
Pain
 abdominal, 2
 acute, 112, 535-542
 back, 20, 89
 breast or nipple, 107, 112, 146
 chest, 32
 chronic, 112, 542-550
 ear, 54
 head, 65, 96
 rectal, 132
 throat, 146
 tooth, 158
Palate, cleft, 36
Pallor of extremities, 112
Pancreatic cancer, 112
Pancreatitis, 112
Panic disorder, 113
Paralysis, 113
Paralytic ileus, 113
Paranoid personality disorder, 113-114
Parathyroidectomy, 114
Parent
 abuse of, 3
 dealing with fetal/newborn anomaly, 13-14
 of premature infant, 126
 sleep pattern disturbance in, 145
 suspected child abuse by, 152
 terminally ill child/death of child of, 155-156
Parent attachment, 114
Parent/child attachment, risk for impaired, 193-196
Parental role conflict, 114, 248-251

Parenteral nutrition, total, 159
Parenting, 114
  impaired, 114, 552-557
  impaired, risk for, 114, 557-559
  readiness for enhanced, 550-552
Paresthesia, 114
Parkinson's disease, 114-115
Paroxysmal nocturnal dyspnea, 121
Patient-controlled analgesia, 115
Patient education, 115
Pelvic inflammatory disease, 119
Penile prosthesis, 115
Peptic ulcer, 161
Percutaneous nephrostomy, 103
Perfusion, ineffective tissue, 158, 720-725
Pericardial friction rub, 115-116
Pericarditis, 116
Perioperative care, 151
Perioperative positioning injury, risk for, 116, 462-466
Periorbital cellulitis, 31
Peripheral cyanosis, 44
Peripheral neuropathy, 106
Peripheral neurovascular dysfunction, risk for, 116, 559-561
Peripheral perfusion, ineffective, 720-725
Peripheral vascular disease, 116
Peripheral vascular obstruction, 162
Peritoneal dialysis, 116
Peritonitis, 117
Pernicious anemia, 117
Personal identity, disturbed, 75, 117, 411-413
Personality disorder, 117
  antisocial, 15
  borderline, 23
  multiple, 99
  narcissistic, 101
  paranoid, 113-114
Pertussis, 135
Pesticide contamination, 117-118
Petit mal seizure, 118
Phenylketonuria, 120
Pheochromocytoma, 118
Phobia (specific), 118
Photosensitivity, 118
Physical mobility, impaired, 97, 494-499
Pica, 118-119
PID. *See* Pelvic inflammatory disease.
PIH. *See* Pregnancy-induced hypertension.
Piloerection, 119
Pinworms, 119-120
PKU. *See* Phenylketonuria.
Placenta abruptio, 3, 120
Placenta previa, 120
Planning care, guide to, 167
Pleural effusion, 120-121
Pleural friction rub, 121
Pleurisy, 121
PMS. *See* Premenstrual tension syndrome.
PND. *See* Paroxysmal nocturnal dyspnea.
Pneumonia, 121, 135
Pneumothorax, 122
Poisoning
  lead, 87
  risk for, 122, 561-566
Polydipsia, 122
Polyphagia, 122
Polyuria, 122
Positioning, perioperative, 116, 462-466
Post-trauma syndrome, 123, 566-569
Post-trauma syndrome, risk for, 123, 569-573
Post-traumatic stress disorder, 123-124
Postmature newborn, 106
Postoperative care, 151
Postpartum blues, 122
Postpartum hemorrhage, 122-123
Postpartum period, normal care in, 123
Power, readiness for enhanced, 124, 573-574
Powerlessness, 124, 574-580
Powerlessness, risk for, 580-581
Preeclampsia, 119
Pregnancy
  adolescent, 6
  anemia in, 12
  cardiac disorders in, 29
  diabetes in, 63
  discomforts of, 50
  ectopic, 55
  herpes in, 68
  loss of, 124-125
  normal, 125
  substance abuse in, 150
  trauma in, 160

Pregnancy-induced hypertension, 119
Premature dilation of cervix, 125
Premature infant, 125-126
Premature rupture of membranes, 126
Prematurity, retinopathy of, 136
Premenstrual tension syndrome, 121
Prenatal care, normal, 126-127
Prenatal testing, 127
Preoperative care, 152
Preoperative teaching, 127
Pressure ulcer, 127
Preterm labor, 127-128
Problem-solving ability, 128
Projection, 128
Prolapse
 mitral valve, 97
 umbilical cord, 128
Prostatic hypertrophy, 24, 128
Prostatitis, 128-129
Prosthesis, penile, 115
Protection, ineffective, 129, 581-584
Pruritus, 129, 585-587
Psoriasis, 129
Psychosis, 129
Pulmonary edema, 129-130
Pulmonary embolism, 130
Pulmonary tuberculosis, 153-154
Pulse deficit, 130
Pulse oximetry, 130
Pulses, absent or diminished peripheral, 130
Pumping, breast, 25
Purpura, idiopathic thrombocytopenic, 81
Pyelonephritis, 130
Pyloric stenosis, 130

Q

Quadriplegia, 131

R

Rabies, 131
Radial nerve dysfunction, 131
Radiation therapy, 131
Radical mastectomy, modified, 97
Rage, 131
Rape-trauma syndrome, 132, 587-591
 compound reaction in, 591-593
 silent reaction in, 593-595
Rash, 132
Rationalization, 132
Rats in home, 132
Raynaud's disease, 132
RDS. *See* Respiratory distress syndrome.
Reattachment procedures, limb, 87-88
Rectal fullness, 132
Rectal pain/bleeding, 132
Rectocele repair, 132-133
Reflex
 corneal, absent, 42
 gag, depressed or absent, 61
 sucking, 150
Reflex urinary incontinence, 133, 423-426
Regression, 133
Regret, 133
Rehabilitation, 133
Relaxation techniques, 133
Religiosity, 133
 impaired, 595-596
 impaired, risk for, 598-599
 readiness for enhanced, 596-598
Religious concerns, 133
Relocation stress syndrome, 133, 599-602
Renal failure, 133-134
Renal perfusion, ineffective, 720-725
Renal transplantation, 83
 donor in, 134
 recipient in, 134-135
Respirations
 accessory muscle use in, 4
 apneustic, 16
 Cheyne-Stokes, 33
 stertorous, 148
Respiratory acidosis, 4
Respiratory conditions of neonate, 135
Respiratory distress syndrome, 17, 135
Respiratory infections, acute childhood, 135
Respiratory syncytial virus, 135
Restless leg syndrome, 135
Retching, 136
Retinal detachment, 136
Retinopathy
 diabetic, 49
 of prematurity, 136
Reye's syndrome, 136
Rh factor incompatibility, 136
Rhabdomyolysis, 137

Rheumatoid arthritis, 82-83, 137
Rib fracture, 137
Ridicule of others, 137
Ringworm, 137, 157
Roaches in home, 138
Rodents in home, 132
Role conflict, parental, 114, 248-251
Role performance, ineffective, 138, 603-606
Role strain, caregiver, 30, 229-237
Rubella, 38
Rubor of extremities, 138
Rupture of membranes, premature, 126

S

SAD. *See* Seasonal affective disorder.
Sadness, 138
Safe sex, 138
Safety, childhood, 138-139
Salmonella, 139
Salpingectomy, 139
Sarcoidosis, 139
Sarcoma, Kaposi's, 83
SARS. *See* Severe acute respiratory syndrome.
SBE. *See* Self-examination, breast.
Scabies, 38
Scalp, ringworm of, 137
Scared feelings, 139
Schizophrenia, 30-31, 139-140
Scoliosis, 140-141
Seasonal affective disorder, 138
Secretions, airway, 9
Sedentary lifestyle, 87, 141, 477-479
Seizures
  adult or childhood, 141
  epileptic, 57
  petit mal, 118
Self-care, readiness for enhanced, 142, 606-608
Self-care deficit
  bathing/hygiene, 20, 71, 142, 608-613
  dressing/grooming, 51, 64, 142, 613-616
  feeding, 142, 616-620
  toileting, 142, 158, 621-623
Self-concept, readiness for enhanced, 142, 623-625
Self-destructive behavior, 142
Self-directed violence, risk for, 760-761
Self-esteem, low
  chronic, 142, 625-627
  situational, 142, 628-630
  situational, risk for, 630-632
Self-examination
  breast, 139
  testicular, 160
Self-mutilation, 632-634
Self-mutilation, risk for, 142, 634-639
Senile dementia, 142
Sensory perception, disturbed, 142, 640-644
Separation anxiety, 142
Sepsis in child, 142-143
Septic shock, 144
Septicemia, 143
Severe acute respiratory syndrome, 139
Sex, safe, 138
Sexual dysfunction, 143, 644-649
Sexuality, adolescent, 143
Sexuality pattern, ineffective, 143, 649-653
Sexually transmitted disease, 148
SGA. *See* Small for gestational age.
Shaken baby syndrome, 143
Shakiness, 143
Shame, 143-144
Shingles, 144
Shivering, 144
Shock, 144
  anaphylactic, 12
  cardiogenic, 30, 144
  hypovolemic, 74, 144
  septic, 144
Shoulder repair, 144
Shoulder replacement, total, 158
Sickle cell anemia/crisis, 144
SIDS. *See* Sudden infant death syndrome.
Significant other, abuse of, 3
Situational crisis, 145
Situational low self-esteem, 142, 628-632
Skin
  damage to, 157
  mottling of peripheral, 98
Skin cancer, 145
Skin disorders, 145
Skin integrity, impaired, 653-656
Skin integrity, impaired, risk for, 145, 656-659

Skin turgor, change in, 145
Sleep, readiness for enhanced, 145, 662-664
Sleep apnea, obstructive, 108
Sleep deprivation, 145, 659-662
Sleep pattern, disturbed, parent/child, 145
Sleep pattern disorders, 145
Slurring of speech, 145
Small for gestational age, 106
Smell, loss of ability to, 15, 146
Smoke inhalation, 146
Smoking behavior, 146
Social interaction, impaired, 146, 664-666
Social isolation, 81, 146, 667-670
Somatization disorder, 146
Sore nipples, 107, 112, 146
Sore throat, 146
Sorrow, 146
Sorrow, chronic, 670-674
Spasms, infantile, 141
Speech, slurring of, 145
Speech disorders, 146-147
Spina bifida, 104
Spinal cord injury, 147
Spinal fusion, 147
Spiritual distress, 147, 674-676
Spiritual distress, risk for, 676-677
Spiritual well-being, readiness for enhanced, 148, 677-679
Spontaneous abortion, 2-3
Spousal abuse, 3
Sprains, 148
Stapedectomy, 148
Stasis ulcer, 148
STD. *See* Sexually transmitted disease.
Stenosis
  mitral, 96-97
  pyloric, 130
Stent, coronary artery, 148
Sterilization surgery, 148
Stertorous respirations, 148
Stevens-Johnson syndrome, 148-149
Stomatitis, 149
Stone, kidney, 83
Stool
  hard/dry, 149
  impaction of, 76
  incontinence of, 24, 59, 77, 207-212
  loose, 88
Straining with defecation, 149
Stress, 149
Stress overload, 149, 680-682
Stress syndrome
  post-traumatic, 123-124
  relocation, 133, 599-602
Stress urinary incontinence, 149, 427-431
Stridor, 149
Stuttering, 149
Subarachnoid hemorrhage, 149-150
Subcutaneous tissue damage, 157
Substance abuse, 150
Substance-abusing mother, infant of, 42, 78-79
Sucking reflex, 150
Suction, nasogastric, 102
Sudden infant death syndrome, 144-145
Sudden infant death syndrome, risk for, 296-298
Suffocation, risk for, 150, 682-685
Suicide, risk for, 685-692
Suicide attempt, 151
Support system, 151
Surgery
  abdominal, 2, 13
  ear, 54
  eye, 58, 86
  gastric, 62
  jaw, 82
  laser, 86
  open heart, 109
  perioperative care in, 151
  postoperative care in, 151
  preoperative care in, 152
  sterilization, 148
Surgical incision, 92
Surgical recovery, delayed, 152, 693-695
Suspected child abuse and neglect, 152
Suspicion, 152-153
Swallowing, impaired, 153, 695-701
Syncope, 153

T

T & A. *See* Tonsillectomy and adenoidectomy.
Tachypnea, 153
Tamponade, cardiac, 30
Tardive dyskinesia, 153
Taste abnormality, 153